Exercise Physiology:

Energy, Nutrition, and Human Performance

Exercise
Physiology

Energy, Nutrition, and Human Performance

WILLIAM D. McARDLE
Professor, Department of Health and Physical Education
Queens College of The City University of New York
Flushing, New York

FRANK I. KATCH
Chairman, Department of Exercise Science
University of Massachusetts
Amherst, Massachusetts

VICTOR L. KATCH
Professor, Department of Physical Education
Associate Professor, Department of Pediatric Cardiology
School of Medicine
University of Michigan
Ann Arbor, Michigan

LEA & FEBIGER   PHILADELPHIA

Library of Congress Cataloging in Publication Data

McArdle, William D
    Exercise physiology.
    Bibliography: p.
    Includes index.
    1. Exercise—Physiological aspects. I. Katch,
Frank I., joint author. II. Katch, Victor L.,
joint author. III. Title.
QP301.M115   612'.044   80-20156
ISBN 0-8121-0682-2

PRINTED IN THE UNITED STATES OF AMERICA

Print No.   3

To Kathy (and Theresa, Amy, Kevin, and Jennifer); to Kerry (and David and Kevin); to Judith (and Erika and Leslie), whose lives give meaning to our own.

Preface

I N *Exercise Physiology: Energy, Nutrition, and Human Performance,* we have attempted to integrate basic concepts and relevant up-to-date scientific information to provide the foundation for understanding exercise. Our main theme is that exercise performance is largely determined by one's capacity to generate energy. This in turn is intimately related to the food nutrients consumed in the diet and the metabolic and physiologic systems of energy delivery and energy utilization. The textbook represents a holistic approach to the multidimensional study of exercise physiology, physical fitness, and health-related fitness aspects. The information is drawn from the research literature in physical education, physiology, metabolism, and health and nutrition. There are seven main sections with 29 chapters, each intimately related to the central theme.

Section I discusses food nutrients and optimal nutrition for exercise performance. Section II deals with the energy for physical activity including energy metabolism as it relates specifically to various modes of exercise. The next section is concerned with the physiologic systems involved in energy delivery and energy utilization, emphasizing pulmonary ventilation, circulation, and neuromuscular integration. In Section IV, the discussion moves to applied physiology where topics related to training, conditioning, and ergogenic aids are discussed with emphasis on the development of muscular strength and anaerobic and aerobic power. Section V deals with the environmental aspects of exercise that include diving, altitude, and thermal stress. Section VI is a particularly important section that focuses on the latest information concerning body composition, obesity, and exercise and weight control. The concluding section presents the role of exercise as it relates to cardiovascular health and aging. These topics are relevant to the emerging areas of adult fitness and cardiac prevention and rehabilitation programs.

Throughout this book, we have tried to balance our discussions between theoretical foundations and practical applications. Our aim is to provide a comprehensive teaching text that not only answers important questions but provides the underlying reasons and rationale. Because many students enter exercise physiology with only minimal science background, the material assumes no previous specialization in topic areas. However, we have tried to develop the basic introductory material into the complete picture required by the exercise specialist. This should make the text attractive to both undergraduate and graduate students as well as students in "special topics" courses dealing with exercise and weight control, environmental physiology, nutrition and sport, and physical conditioning.

We believe the field of exercise physiology is at the dawn of a new era. Recent advances in microscopic and biochemical techniques, aided by computerized technology, are opening up new frontiers in subcellular architecture, function, and adaptation to exercise and training. A cross-discipline thrust will hopefully begin to unravel the many unanswered secrets relating to the elite performer, as well as to a large segment of the population that is increasing its appreciation for involvement in sport and exercise. We have been particularly impressed by the public's keen awareness and enthusiasm, as well as thirst for knowledge about the role exercise can play in shaping one's lifestyle. We also share the commitment as scientists and educators to continually strive to challenge our students to achieve at their own level of excellence in the scientific, academic, and business communities. Not too many years ago, few were trained with a comprehensive background in exercise science. The knowledge explosion had not yet fully matured, and the leadership role for the conduct and implementation of exercise and training programs was entrusted to a handful of professionals struggling to maintain a high degree of respectability within our field.

It took a concerted effort, but now the academic domain of physical education has achieved distinction, especially within the broad spectrum of subdisciplines in the exercise sciences. Men like Clarke, Cureton, Dill, Henry, Hitchcock, Karpovitch, McCloy, Sargent, and Steinhaus were the early pioneers who provided the initial spark and lay the foundation for what is now called exercise physiology. We all must strive to spread their contagious enthusiasm for the systematic study of human exercise performance, and not let that commitment erode as we join in harmony with colleagues in medicine, physiology, psychology, and nutrition to further our understanding of the science of exercise.

Sound Beach, New York

Amherst, Massachusetts

Ann Arbor, Michigan

Many colleagues in physical education and other disciplines have had a significant impact on our lives. To J. Ball, A.R. Behnke, J.A. Faulkner, D. Fleming, G.F. Foglia, F.M. 'Doc'' Henry, H.J. Montoye, E.D. Michael, and G.Q. Rich, III, we would like to say "thank you" for the privilege of your close association as scientists, teachers, and friends. Appreciation is extended to G. Brooks, University of California at Berkeley; Robert Girandola, University of Southern California, P. Ribisl, Wake-Forest University; W. Osness, University of Kansas; J. Magel, Queens College; M. Svboda, Portland State University; and A. Weltman, University of Colorado, for their instructive comments and helpful suggestions during the preparation of the manuscript. We also wish to acknowledge our many undergraduate and graduate students who endured, notably S.S., G.B., R.G., P.F., K.C., A.W., G.L., N.W., M.T., N.G., D.G., J.C., and D.D. Finally, to J. Spahr, T. Colaiezzi, and E. Wickland at Lea & Febiger, our sincere appreciation for coping above and beyond the call of duty.

WILLIAM D. MCARDLE
FRANK I. KATCH
VICTOR L. KATCH

Contents

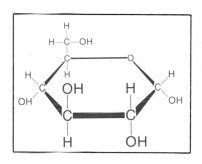
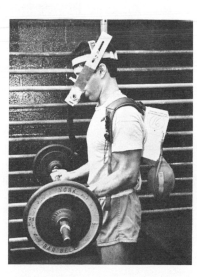

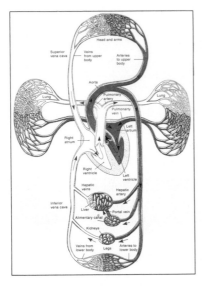
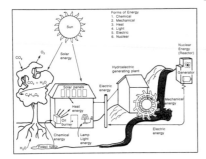
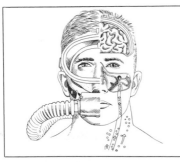

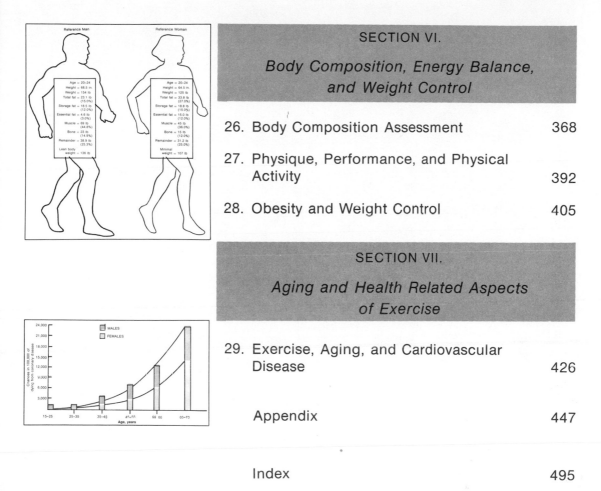

SECTION VI.

Body Composition, Energy Balance, and Weight Control

SECTION VII.

Aging and Health Related Aspects of Exercise

Exercise Physiology

SECTION I

Nutrition: The Base for Human Performance

In a textbook dealing with the physiology of human performance, it is uncommon to find a section devoted to the basics of human nutrition. We feel, however, that this topic is of such importance that it should serve as the starting point for this book.

Proper nutrition forms the foundation for physical performance; it provides both the fuel for biologic work and the chemicals for extracting and utilizing the potential energy contained within this fuel. Food also provides the essential elements for the synthesis of new tissue and the repair of existing cells.

Some may argue that adequate nutrition for exercise can easily be achieved through the intake of a well-balanced diet and that it therefore is of little consequence in the study of exercise performance. We maintain, however, that the study of exercise, especially when viewed within the framework of energy capacities, must be based on an understanding of the sources of food energy and the role of nutrients in the process of energy release. With this perspective, it becomes possible for the exercise specialist to appreciate the importance of "adequate" nutrition and to evaluate critically the validity of claims concerning nutrient supplements and special dietary modifications for enhancing physical performance. Because various food nutrients provide energy and regulate physiologic processes associated with exercise, it is tempting to link dietary modification to improvement in athletic performance. Too often individuals spend considerable time and "energy" striving for the optimum in exercise performance, only to fall short due to inadequate, counterproductive, and sometimes harmful nutritional practices.

In the chapters that follow, we will look at the six broad classifications of nutrients: carbohydrate, fat, protein, vitamins, minerals, and water. We will attempt to answer the following questions: What are they? Where are they found? What are their functions? What specific role do they play in physical activity?

Carbohydrates, Fats, and Proteins

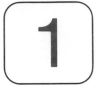

The carbohydrate, fat, and protein nutrients consumed daily provide the necessary energy to maintain body functions both at rest and during various forms of physical activity. Aside from their role as biologic fuel, these nutrients (called macronutrients by nutritionists) also play an important part in maintaining the structural and functional integrity of the organism. In this chapter, each of these nutrients is discussed in terms of general structure, function, and source in specific foods in the diet. Emphasis is placed on their importance in sustaining physiologic function during moderate and more strenuous physical activity.

BASIC STRUCTURE OF NUTRIENTS

All biologic systems are composed of cells that engage in similar activities required to maintain the integrity and life of the cell. Although different cells possess specialized functions that necessitate special structures, the basic life-sustaining processes among all cells are similar. Cells with diverse functions also have similar chemical compositions. All cells are composed of essentially the same chemicals, differing only in the proportion and arrangement of these chemicals.

Atoms: Nature's Building Blocks

Of the 103 different types of atoms or elements, hydrogen, nitrogen, oxygen, and carbon play the *major* role in the chemical composition of nutrients and comprise the structural units for most biologically active substances in the body.

Hydrogen, with its relatively low atomic weight, accounts for 10% of the body weight and 63% of all the atoms in the body; carbon, for 18% of the body weight and 9% of all the atoms; nitrogen makes up 3% of the body weight and only 1% of the total number of atoms in the body; and the relatively "heavy" oxygen atom accounts for 65% of body weight yet only 26% of the total number of atoms.

Molecules are formed from the union of two or more atoms. The specific atoms as well as the arrangement of these atoms give the molecule its properties. Glucose is glucose because of the arrangement of 24 atoms of three different kinds within its molecule. *Chemical bonding,* e.g., between atoms of hydrogen and oxygen in the water molecule, involves a common sharing of electrons between atoms. *It is this force of attraction created between the positive and negative charges of atoms that forms the basis for bonding and provides the "cement" that keeps the atoms and molecules within a substance from readily coming apart.* When these forces are altered due to the removal, transfer, or exchange of certain electrons, energy is provided to power all cellular functions. When two or more molecules are chemically bound, a larger aggregate of matter or a *substance* is formed. This substance may take the form of a gas, liquid, or a solid, depending on the force of interaction between molecules.

Carbon: The Versatile Element

All of the nutrients except water and minerals contain carbon. In fact, almost all of the biologic substances within the body are composed of compounds containing carbon. Carbon

4

atoms have an almost unlimited ability to share chemical bonds with other carbon atoms and with atoms of other elements to form large carbon chain molecules.

Fats and carbohydrates are formed from specific linkages of carbon atoms with atoms of hydrogen and oxygen. With the addition of nitrogen and certain mineral substances, a protein molecule is formed. These atoms of carbon, hydrogen, oxygen, and nitrogen are the *organic* building blocks from which the nutrients are made.

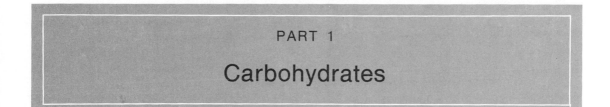

PART 1

Carbohydrates

THE NATURE OF CARBOHYDRATES

Atoms of carbon, hydrogen, and oxygen combine to form carbohydrate compounds. The basic chemical structure of a simple sugar molecule consists of a chain of from 3 to 7 carbon atoms with the hydrogen and oxygen atoms attached singly. The most typical sugar, *glucose,* is illustrated in Figure 1-1. The glucose molecule consists of 6 carbon, 12 hydrogen, and 6 oxygen atoms ($C_6H_{12}O_6$). Each of the carbon atoms has four bonding sites that can link to other atoms, including carbon atoms. Carbon atoms not linked to other carbons are "free" to hold hydrogen (which has only one bond site itself), oxygen (which has two bond sites), or an oxygen–hydrogen combination, termed a hydroxyl (OH).

Fructose and galactose are two other simple sugars that have the same chemical formula as glucose, with a slightly different carbon-to-hydrogen-to-oxygen linkage. This alteration in atomic arrangement makes fructose, galactose, and glucose different substances.

KINDS AND SOURCES OF CARBOHYDRATES

The interaction of carbon dioxide in the atmosphere with water, solar energy, and the catalyst chlorophyll provides the necessary ingredients for plants to synthesize carbohydrates. In this process, oxygen is released into the atmosphere to be used by animals in the process of energy metabolism. The total process by which the energy from sunlight is harnessed by green plants in the production of carbohydrates is known as *photosynthesis.* This process of energy transfer is discussed more fully in Chapter 5.

There are three kinds of carbohydrates: *monosaccharides, oligosaccharides,* and *polysaccharides.* Each form of carbohydrate is distinguished by the number of simple sugars in combination within the molecule.

Monosaccharides

The monosaccharides or simple sugars, glucose, fructose, and galactose, were described previously. Glucose, also called dextrose or blood sugar, is formed as a natural sugar in food or is produced in the body as a result of digestion of more complicated carbohydrates.

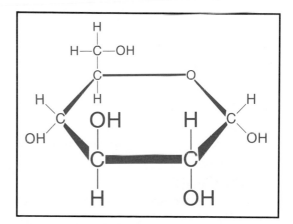

FIG. 1-1. *Three-dimensional structure of the simple sugar molecule glucose. The molecule resembles a hexagonal plate to which H and O atoms are attached.*

Fructose or fruit sugar is present in large amounts in natural form in fruits and honey and is the sweetest of the simple sugars. Galactose is not found in foods; rather, it must be produced from milk sugar in the mammary glands of lactating animals. In the body, both fructose and galactose are easily converted to glucose for energy metabolism.

Oligosaccharides

The major types of oligosaccharides are the *disaccharides* or double sugars, which are formed from the combination of two monosaccharide molecules. In the structure of each of the disaccharides, glucose is one of the simple sugars. The three principal disaccharides are:

Sucrose = glucose + fructose
Lactose = glucose + galactose
Maltose = glucose + glucose

Sucrose is the most common dietary disaccharide and contributes up to 25% of the total quantity of ingested calories in the United States. It occurs naturally in most foods containing carbohydrates, especially in beet and cane sugar, brown sugar, sorghum, maple syrup, and honey.

Lactose is found in natural form only in milk and is often called milk sugar. It is the least sweet of the disaccharides. Lactose can be artificially processed and is often found in carbohydrate-rich, high-calorie liquid meals.

Maltose occurs in malt products and in germinating cereals. It is considered a negligible carbohydrate in terms of its contribution to the carbohydrate content of the average person's diet.

Polysaccharides

Three or more simple sugar molecules form a polysaccharide. In fact, as many as 300 to 500 monosaccharide molecules can be linked to form a polysaccharide. There are generally two classifications of polysaccharides, plant and animal.

PLANT POLYSACCHARIDES. Two common forms of plant polysaccharides are *starch* and *cellulose.*

Starch is the most familiar form of plant polysaccharide. It is found in seeds, corn, and in the various grains from which bread, cereal, spaghetti, and pastries are made. Large amounts are also present in peas, beans, potatoes, and roots, where it serves as an energy store for future use by plants. Starch granules of different sizes are encased within the cellulose walls of the plant cell. Potato starch granules, for example, are relatively large, whereas the starch granules within rice are small. Plant starch is still the most important dietary source of carbohydrate in the American diet, accounting for approximately 50% of the total carbohydrate intake. It is interesting to note, however, that starch intake has decreased about 30% since the turn of the century, whereas the consumption of more simple sugars such as sucrose has correspondingly increased from 31% to about 50%.

Cellulose is another form of plant polysaccharide. It makes up the fibrous or structural part of plants and is present in leaves, stems, roots, seeds, and fruit coverings. Since cellulose is resistive to human digestive enzymes, its major function is to give "bulk" to the food residues in the small intestines. This bulk in the diet probably aids in gastrointestinal functioning and may reduce the probability of contracting colon cancer later in life.[9]

ANIMAL POLYSACCHARIDES. *Glycogen* is the polysaccharide synthesized and stored in the tissues of animals. Glycogen molecules are usually large and range in size from a few hundred to thousands of glucose molecules linked together, much like the links in a chain of sausages. In well-nourished humans, approximately 375 to 475 grams (g)* of carbohydrate are stored in the body. Of this, approximately 275 g are muscle glycogen, 100 to 120 g are liver glycogen, and only 15 to 20 g are present as blood glucose.

There are several factors that determine the rate and quantity of either glycogen synthesis or breakdown. During exercise, the carbohydrate stored as muscle glycogen is used as a source of energy for the specific muscle in which it is stored. In the liver, in contrast, glycogen is reconverted to glucose and transported in the blood for eventual use by the working

---

*(Scientific measurement is generally presented in terms of the metric system. Appendix A shows the relationship between metric units and English units that are relevant to the material presented in this book. Also presented are some common expressions of work, energy, and power.)

muscles. The term *glycogenolysis* is used to describe this reconversion process, which provides a rapid supply of glucose for muscular contraction during all forms of work. When glycogen is depleted via dietary restriction or exercise, glucose synthesis from the structural components of the other nutrients, especially proteins, tends to increase. This process is termed *gluconeogenesis*. Hormones, especially insulin, play an important part in the regulation of liver and muscle glycogen stores by controlling the level of circulating blood sugar.

Because comparatively little glycogen is stored in the body, the quantity of liver and muscle glycogen can be modified considerably through the diet. For example, a 24-hour fast results in a large reduction in liver and muscle glycogen reserves. On the other hand, maintaining a carbohydrate-rich diet for several days enhances the body's carbohydrate stores to a level almost twice that obtained with a normal, well-balanced diet.[3] The effect of enhanced carbohydrate storage on exercise performance is discussed in a later section of this chapter.

RECOMMENDED INTAKE OF CARBOHYDRATES

Almost all foods contain some carbohydrates, even if only trace amounts. Figure 1-2 illustrates the carbohydrate content of selected foods. Cereals, cookies, candies, breads, and cakes are rich carbohydrate sources. Because the values are based on carbohydrate percent-

age in relation to the total weight, including water content, fruits and vegetables appear to be less valuable sources of carbohydrates. However, the dried portion of these foods is almost pure carbohydrate.

The typical American diet consists of approximately 40% to 50% of the total calories as carbohydrate. For a sedentary 70-kilogram (kg) person, for example, this amounts to approximately 147 g of carbohydrate per day. For active people and those involved in exercise training, about 50% to 55% of the daily caloric intake should be in the form of carbohydrates.[15]

The main dietary carbohydrate source is generally fruits and vegetables. This in no way, however, represents the "state of affairs" for all individuals. A recent dietary survey of 16 moderately overweight females at the University of Michigan revealed that their daily carbohydrate intake of 375 g accounted for 53% of their total caloric intake. Fruits and vegetables represented only 20% of the carbohydrate intake, whereas cereals, bread, and especially sweets accounted for approximately 80%. Perhaps these findings should not be surprising because it has been estimated that the average American consumes more than 100 pounds (lb) of table sugar each year!

Evidence is increasing to support the contention that an excessive quantity of sucrose in the diet is a main *cause* of tooth decay. In addition, in an as yet unexplained way, excessive dietary sugar is believed to be involved in a variety of other disease processes, most notably diabetes and coronary heart disease.

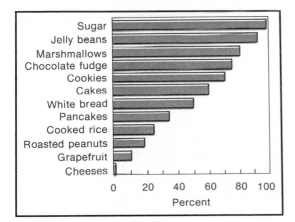

FIG. 1-2. *Percentage of carbohydrates in commonly served foods. (Adapted from Handbook No. 8: Composition of Foods. Washington, D.C., United States Department of Agriculture, 1963.)*

ROLE OF CARBOHYDRATES IN THE BODY

Carbohydrates serve several important functions related to exercise performance.

Energy Source

The main function of carbohydrate is to serve as an energy fuel for the body. The energy derived from the breakdown of carbohydrate is ultimately used to power muscular contraction as well as all other forms of biologic work.

Carbohydrates must be broken down during digestion to a simple 6-carbon sugar before they can be absorbed by the blood and used by the body. It is important that adequate amounts of carbohydrates are ingested routinely to maintain the body's relatively limited glycogen stores. If too few carbohydrates are ingested, glucose is then obtained from glycogen breakdown and the carbohydrate reserves become depleted. In contrast, following a meal, there may be excess carbohydrates that will be readily converted to muscle and liver glycogen. Once the capacity of the cell for glycogen storage is reached, the excess sugars are converted and stored as fat. This helps explain how body fat increases when excess calories in the form of carbohydrates are consumed. This process occurs even if the diet is low in fat.

Protein Sparing

Carbohydrates also provide a "protein sparing" effect. Under normal conditions, protein serves a vital role in the maintenance, repair, and growth of body tissues, and to a considerably lesser degree, as a nutrient source of energy. However, when carbohydrate reserves are reduced, metabolic pathways exist for the synthesis of glucose from protein. This process, termed gluconeogenesis, provides a metabolic option for augmenting carbohydrate availability in the face of depleted glycogen stores. We will point out shortly how this becomes increasingly important in prolonged endurance exercise. However, the price that is paid is a temporary reduction in the body's protein stores, especially muscle protein. Adequate intake and utilization of carbohydrates aid in the maintenance of tissue protein.

Metabolic Primer

Another function of carbohydrates is to serve as a "primer" for fat metabolism. Certain food fragments from the breakdown of carbohydrate must be available to facilitate the metabolism of fat. If insufficient carbohydrate metabolism exists, either through limitation in the transport of glucose into the cell, which occurs in diabetes, or depletion in glycogen through improper diet or prolonged exercise, the body begins to mobilize fat to a greater extent than it can utilize. The result is incomplete fat metabolism and the accumulation of acid by-products called *ketone bodies.* This situation can possibly lead to a harmful increase in the acidity of the body fluids, a condition called acidosis—or more specifically with regard to fat breakdown, *ketosis.* More is said of the role of carbohydrate as a primer for fat metabolism in Chapter 6.

Fuel for the Central Nervous System

Carbohydrate is essential for the proper functioning of the central nervous system. The brain uses blood glucose almost exclusively as a fuel and essentially has no stored supply of this nutrient. The symptoms of a modest reduction in blood glucose (*hypoglycemia*) include feelings of weakness, hunger, and dizziness. This condition impairs exercise performance and may partially explain the fatigue associated with prolonged exercise. Sustained and profound low blood sugar can cause irreversible brain damage. Because of the specific role played by glucose in generating energy for use by nerve tissue, blood sugar is regulated within narrow limits.

CARBOHYDRATE BALANCE IN EXERCISE

With the use of biochemical and biopsy techniques, it has been possible to study the contributions of various nutrients to the energy demands of physical activity. The biopsy technique permits the sampling of specific muscles with little interruption in exercise. Thus, through serial sampling of the same muscle in the same person, the role of intramuscular nutrients can be carefully evaluated during exercise.

Intense Exercise

Stored muscle glycogen and blood-borne glucose are the prime contributors of energy during high-intensity exercise. Blood glucose, for example, may supply 30% to 40% of the total energy of exercising muscles.[11] As illustrated in Figure 1-3, during the initial stage of exercise, the uptake of circulating blood glucose by the muscles increases sharply and continues to increase as exercise progresses. By the fortieth minute of exercise, the glucose uptake has risen to between 7 and 20 times the uptake at rest, depending on the intensity of the exercise. The increase in the percentage contribution of carbohydrate during intense exercise is explained largely by the fact that it is the *only* nutrient that provides energy when the oxygen supplied to the muscles is insufficient in relation to the oxygen needs. The specifics of this role in energy release are explained in Chapter 6.

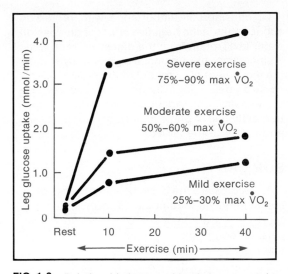

FIG. 1-3. *Relationship between blood glucose uptake by the leg muscles and exercise duration and intensity. Here intensity is expressed as a percent of one's maximum capacity to consume oxygen or max* $\dot{V}O_2$*. As exercise continues, blood-borne glucose becomes an increasingly important source of energy. If exercise continues for 10 to 40 minutes, glucose uptake by muscle rises to 7 to 20 times basal level, depending on the exercise intensity. This glucose metabolism can account for 30 to 40 percent of the total oxygen consumed by muscle. (Reprinted by permission from Felig, P., and Wahren, J.: Fuel homeostasis in exercise. Seminar in Medicine of the Beth Israel Hospital, Boston. N. Engl. J. Med., 293:1078, 1975.)*

Moderate and Prolonged Exercise

The specific nutrient fuel for muscular contraction depends not only on exercise intensity but also on the duration of the activity and, to some degree, on the diet of the individual.[6] During continuous moderate exercise, energy is derived mainly from the breakdown of the body's stores of fat and carbohydrate. In the early stages of such submaximal exercise, about 40% to 50% of the energy requirement is supplied by the glycogen stored in the liver and exercising muscles. Glucose output from the liver rises 3 to 5 times above resting values. As exercise continues and the glycogen stores become reduced, however, an increasingly greater percentage of energy is supplied through the metabolism of fat.[17]

Fatigue occurs if exercise is performed to the point where the glycogen in the liver and specific muscles becomes severely lowered, even though sufficient oxygen is available to the muscles and the potential energy from stored fat remains almost unlimited. Because enzymes are not present to allow for glycogen transfer between muscles, the relatively inactive muscles maintain their glycogen content. It is unclear why the depletion of muscle glycogen coincides with the point of fatigue in prolonged submaximal exercise. The function of carbohydrate as a "primer" in fat metabolism may provide part of the answer.

EFFECT OF DIET ON MUSCLE GLYCOGEN STORES. Figure 1-4 shows the results of one experiment in which the initial muscle glycogen stores were varied in 9 subjects through dietary manipulation.[3] In one condition, the normal caloric intake was maintained for 3 days but the major quantity of calories was supplied in the form of fat. In the second condition, the 3-day diet was normal and contained the recommended daily percentages of carbohydrate, fat, and protein. In the third diet, 82% of the calories were provided in the form of carbohydrates. The glycogen content of the *quadriceps femoris* muscle of the leg, determined by needle biopsy, averaged 0.63, 1.75, and 3.75 g of glycogen per 100 g wet muscle as a result of the high-fat, normal, and high-carbohydrate diets, respectively.

Endurance capacity on the bicycle ergometer varied considerably depending upon the diet

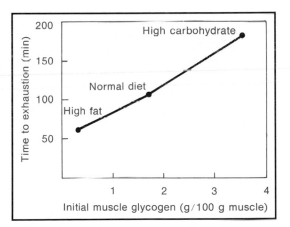

FIG. 1-4. *Effects of a mixed diet, a low-carbohydrate diet, and a high-carbohydrate diet on the glycogen content of the quadriceps femoris and the duration of exercise on a bicycle ergometer. These data clearly show that the higher the initial level of muscle glycogen, the greater is the endurance for submaximal exercise. (From Bergstrom, J. et al.: Diet, muscle glycogen and physical performance. Acta Physiol. Scand., 71:140, 1967.)*

each person consumed during the 3 days prior to the exercise test. With the normal diet, moderate exercise could be tolerated for an average of 114 minutes, whereas endurance averaged only 57 minutes with the high-fat diet. The endurance capacity of subjects fed the high-carbohydrate diet was more than three times greater than when the same subjects consumed the high-fat diet. Such results clearly demonstrate the importance of muscle glycogen for prolonged exercise lasting more than an hour, and emphasize the important role of nutrition in establishing the appropriate energy reserves.

A diet deficient in carbohydrates rapidly depletes muscle and liver glycogen and subsequently affects performance in intense short-term exercise as well as in prolonged, submaximal endurance activities. These observations are important not only for athletes but also for individuals who have modified their diet so that the normal recommended percentage of carbohydrates has become reduced. Reliance on starvation diets or on other potentially harmful diets such as high-fat, low-carbohydrate diets, "liquid-protein" diets, or water diets is counterproductive for weight control, exercise performance, optimal nutrition, and good health. Such low carbohydrate diets make it extremely difficult from the standpoint of energy supply to participate in vigorous physical activity or training.

ADMINISTRATION OF ORAL GLUCOSE. It is noteworthy that the exercise period can be extended if a solution of glucose and water is ingested at the point of fatigue from prolonged submaximal exercise.[7] This occurs even though for all practical purposes the muscles' "fuel tank" reads empty and continued energy metabolism is severely limited. In all likelihood, the additional sugar absorbed from the intestinal tract helps maintain the appropriate blood sugar level. This, in turn, supports the nutrient requirements of the central nervous system and working muscles and may forestall liver glycogen depletion during prolonged severe exertion.[8] The "sugar drink" usually recommended is an isotonic 5% glucose, fructose, or sucrose solution that can be made by adding 50 g of table sugar to one liter of water.[4] To be most effective, the fluid should be consumed at frequent intervals throughout the endurance activity.

Of considerable importance with regard to sugar drinks is the negative effect of glucose on water absorption from the digestive tract. Even a small amount of glucose significantly retards the movement of water out of the stomach. This could be deleterious during prolonged exercise in the heat, when adequate intake *and* absorption of fluid is of prime importance to the health and safety of the athlete.

SUMMARY

1. Atoms are the basic building blocks of all matter, and they combine to form molecules. Most cells are composed of the same chemicals, differing only in proportion and arrangement.

2. Carbon, hydrogen, oxygen, and nitrogen are the primary structural units of most of the biologically active substances in the body. Specific combinations of carbon with oxygen and hydrogen form carbohydrates and fats, whereas other combinations with the addition of nitrogen and minerals make proteins.

3. Simple sugars consist of a chain of from 3 to 7 carbon atoms with hydrogen and oxygen in the ratio of 2 to 1. Glucose, the most common simple sugar, contains a 6-carbon chain as $C_6H_{12}O_6$.

4. There are three kinds of carbohydrates: monosaccharides (simple sugars like glucose and fructose); oliosaccharides (disaccharides like sucrose, lactose, and maltose); and polysaccharides that contain three or more simple sugars to form starch, cellulose, and glycogen.

5. *Glycogenolysis* refers to the process of reconverting glycogen to glucose, whereas *gluconeogenesis* refers to the process of glucose synthesis, especially from protein sources.

6. Americans typically consume 40% to 50% of their total calories as carbohydrates. This is generally in the form of fruits, grains, and vegetables, although greater sugar intake in the form of sweets (simple sugars) is common and possibly harmful.

7. Carbohydrates serve (1) as a major source of energy, (2) to spare the breakdown of proteins, (3) as a metabolic primer for fat metabolism, and (4) as the fuel for the central nervous system.

8. Muscle glycogen and blood glucose are the primary fuels during intense exercise. The body's glycogen stores also serve an important

role in energy balance in sustained moderate exercise such as marathon running and distance swimming.

9. Sugar drinks may enhance exercise performance by maintaining blood sugar levels

and perhaps delaying liver and muscle glycogen depletion. These drinks, however, have been shown to retard the movement of liquid out of the stomach, which ultimately may upset the body's fluid balance.

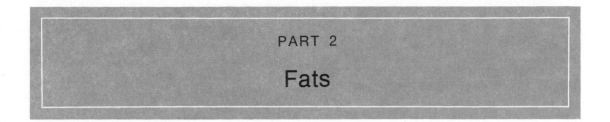

PART 2

Fats

THE NATURE OF FATS

A molecule of fat possesses the same structural elements as the carbohydrate molecule except that the linking of the specific atoms is markedly different. Specifically, the ratio of hydrogen to oxygen is considerably higher in the fat compound. For example, the common fat *stearin* has the formula $C_{57}H_{110}O_6$.

KINDS AND SOURCES OF FATS

According to common classification, fats can be placed into one of three main groups: *simple fats, compound fats,* and *derived fats.* Fats can be found in both plants and animals, are generally greasy to the touch, and are insoluble in water.

Simple Fats

The simple fats are often called *"neutral fats"* and consist primarily of *triglycerides.* Triglycerides, the most plentiful fat in the body, constitute the major storage form of fat (more than 99% of the body fat is in the form of triglycerides). A triglyceride molecule consists of two different clusters of atoms. One cluster is *glycerol,* a 3-carbon molecule. Glycerol in itself is not a fat because it is readily soluble in water. Attached to the glycerol molecule are three clusters of carbon-chained atoms termed *fatty acid.* Figure 1-5 shows the structure of glycerol and a typical 18-carbon fatty acid.

When glycerol and fatty acids are joined in the synthesis of the triglyceride molecule, three

molecules of water are formed. Conversely, during *hydrolysis,* when the fat molecule is cleaved into its constituents, three molecules of water are added at the point where the fat molecule is split. The basic structures of the two kinds of fatty acid molecules, *saturated* and *unsaturated,* are shown in Figure 1-6.

SATURATED FATTY ACIDS. A *saturated* fatty acid contains only single bonds between carbon

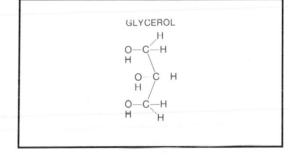

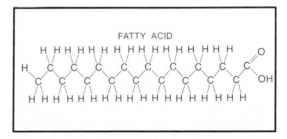

FIG. 1-5. *Chemical structure of a glycerol molecule and a fatty acid molecule. From* Nutrition, Weight Control, and Exercise *by Frank I. Katch and William D. McArdle. Copyright ⓒ 1977 by Houghton Mifflin Company. Reprinted by permission of the publisher.*

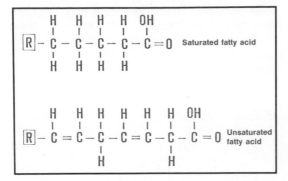

FIG. 1-6. *The major structural difference between saturated and unsaturated fatty acids is the presence or absence of double bonds between the carbon atoms. R represents the glycerol portion of the fat molecule. From* Nutrition, Weight Control, and Exercise *by Frank I. Katch and William D. McArdle. Copyright © 1977 by Houghton Mifflin Company. Reprinted by permission of the publisher.*

atoms; the remaining bonds attach to hydrogen. With this bonding arrangement, the fatty acid molecule is said to be saturated because it holds as many hydrogen atoms as is chemically possible.

Saturated fats are found primarily in animal products including beef, lamb, pork, and chicken. Saturated fats are also present in egg yolk and in the dairy fats of cream, milk, and cheese. Shellfish, such as lobster, shrimp, and crabs, also contain a large amount of saturated fatty acids.

UNSATURATED FATTY ACIDS. Fatty acids containing one or more double bonds along the main carbon chain are classified as *unsaturated*. In this case, each double bond in the carbon chain has reduced a potential hydrogen-binding site, and therefore, the molecule is said to be unsaturated with respect to hydrogen. If only one double bond is present along the main carbon chain, the fatty acid is said to be *monounsaturated*. If there are two or more double bonds along the main carbon chain, the fatty acid is said to be *polyunsaturated*.

Fats from plant sources are generally unsaturated and tend to liquify at room temperature. Unsaturated fats that are present as liquids are called oils. The more common vegetable oils are corn oil, cottonseed oil, peanut oil, and soybean oil.

The amount of saturated fat consumed in the typical American diet has steadily increased to the point that the average person now consumes over 50 lb of saturated fat per year, most of which is animal in origin. Coinciding with this increased consumption of saturated fats has been an increase in coronary heart disease. This relationship has led many nutritionists and medical personnel to suggest replacing at least a portion of the saturated fat in one's diet with fats that are unsaturated. It has become common practice to cook with and ingest fats derived primarily from vegetable sources, such as corn oil. However, this approach may be too simplistic, because increasing evidence suggests that total fat intake, both saturated and unsaturated, may be a heart disease "risk" and that all fat should be reduced. Concern has recently been expressed concerning the association of high-fat diets (both saturated and unsaturated fats) with breast and colon cancer as well as the possibility that such diets promote the growth of other cancers as well. The precise role of dietary fat in the development of heart disease is still a controversial topic and must await further research before definitive recommendations can be made. As a general recommendation, however, it is probably prudent to consume no more than 30% of the total calories in the form of fat. Of this, less than 50% should be saturated fat.

The saturated and unsaturated fatty acid contents of various sources of dietary fat of animal and plant origin are listed in Table 1-1. Of all the dietary fats, only *linoleic acid,* a polyunsaturated fatty acid present in cooking and salad oils, must be consumed in the diet, because it cannot be synthesized by the body.

Compound Fats

Compound fats are composed of a neutral fat in combination with other chemicals. One such group, the *phospholipids,* consists of a combination of one or more fatty acid molecules with phosphoric acid and a nitrogenous base. These fats are formed in all cells, though the majority are synthesized in the liver. In addition to helping maintain the structural integrity of the cell, phospholipids are important in blood clotting and in the structure of the insulating sheath around nerve fibers.

Other compound fats are the *glucolipids,* which are fatty acids bound with carbohydrate and nitrogen, and the *lipoproteins,* formed primarily in the liver from the union of either tri-

TABLE 1-1. *Common dietary sources of fat*[a]

FOOD	PERCENT FAT	PERCENT SATURATED	PERCENT UNSATURATED
Animal sources			
Beef	16–42	52	48
Chicken	10–17	30	70
Beef heart	6	50	50
Lamb	19–29	60	40
Ham, sliced	23	45	55
Pork	32	45	55
Veal cutlet	10	50	50
Butter	81	55	36
Plant sources			
Cashew nuts	48	18	82
Peanut butter	50	25	75
Carrots	0	0	0
Potato chips	35	25	75
Margarine	81	26	66
Corn oil	100	7	78
Cottonseed oil	100	21.5	71.5
Olive oil	100	14	86
Soybean oil	100	14	71.5

[a] Adapted from Handbook No. 8, Composition of Foods. Washington, D.C., U.S. Department of Agriculture, 1963.

glycerides, phospholipids, or cholesterol with protein. *The lipoproteins are important because they constitute the main form of transport for fat in the blood.* If blood lipids (Greek: lipos meaning fat) were not bound to protein or some other substance, they would float to the top like cream in milk that was not homogenized.

Derived Fats

This group of fats includes substances derived from the simple and compound fats. The most widely known of the derived fats is *cholesterol.* Cholesterol is present in all cells and is either consumed in foods (exogenous cholesterol) or is synthesized within the cell (endogenous cholesterol). Even when an individual maintains a "cholesterol-free diet," the rate of endogenous cholesterol synthesis may vary from 0.5 g to 2.0 g per day. It has been determined that this rate of synthesis is sufficient for body needs; hence, a severe reduction in dietary intake of cholesterol probably is not harmful. Cholesterol is normally required in many complex bodily functions, including the synthesis of estrogen, androgen, and progesterone, the hormones

responsible for male and female secondary sex characteristics.

The richest source of cholesterol in foods is egg yolk. Cholesterol is also plentiful in organ meats such as liver, kidney, and brains and in shellfish as well as in dairy products such as ice cream, cream cheese and whole milk. It is not present in any foods of plant origin. Because cholesterol has been implicated as a possible precursor for coronary artery disease, there has been keen interest in the relationship between the dietary intake of cholesterol and the serum levels of this fatty substance. However, the cause and effect relationship between cholesterol and heart disease has not been firmly established and awaits further study. In fact, the level of circulating triglycerides and the specific type of lipoprotein (see Chap. 29) may provide a more meaningful signal than cholesterol in predicting the probability of contracting coronary heart disease.[18]

Fats in Food

Figure 1-7 shows the approximate percentage contribution of some of the common food groups to the total fat content of the typical American diet. The "visible" fat-containing substances (butter, lard, cooking oil, and mayonnaise) contribute 30% or more to the normal dietary intake of fat, whereas "invisible" fat in meat, eggs, milk, cheese, nuts, vegetables, and cereals contributes the remaining 70%. Vegetable fat generally contributes about 34% of the daily fat intake, whereas the remaining 66% is from animal fat.

ROLE OF FAT
IN THE BODY

The most noteworthy functions of body fat include (1) providing the body's largest store of potential energy, (2) serving as a cushion for the protection of vital organs, and (3) providing insulation from the thermal stress of cold environments.

Energy Source
and Reserve

Fat constitutes the ideal cellular fuel because each molecule carries large quantities of energy per unit weight, is easily transported and stored, and is readily converted into energy. One gram of fat contains more than twice the energy storage capability of an equal quantity of carbohydrate or protein. This is largely due to the greater quantity of hydrogen in the fat molecule compared to the carbohydrate or protein molecule. As will be discussed in Chapters 6 and 7, it is the oxidation of these hydrogen atoms that provides the energy required for bodily functions at rest and during exercise. It should be recalled that three molecules of water are produced and liberated when a fat molecule is synthesized from the union of glycerol and three fatty acid molecules. In contrast, when glycogen is formed in the cell from glucose, 2.7 g of water are stored with each gram of glycogen. Thus, fat is a relatively water-free, concentrated fuel, whereas glycogen is hydrated and very heavy relative to its energy content.

Fat storage in the body constitutes approximately 15% of the body weight of males and 25% of females. Most of this fat is available for energy, especially during prolonged, moderate exercise. Excess nutrients, other than fats, are readily converted to fat for storage. In this way, fat serves as the major storehouse of excess nutrient energy. As was the case with carbohydrates, the utilization of fat as a fuel "spares" protein for its important functions of tissue synthesis and repair.

Protection
and Insulation

Fat serves as a protective shield against trauma to the vital organs such as the heart, liver, kidneys, spleen, brain, and spinal cord. Up to 4% of the total body fat serves in this capacity. Also, it does not appear that this protective fat layer can be reduced, even during long periods of semistarvation.

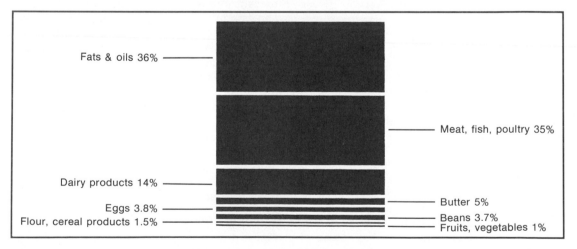

FIG. 1-7. *Percentage of fats consumed in the daily diet from various food groups. (From* Nutrition, Weight Control, and Exercise *by Frank I. Katch and William D. McArdle. Copyright © 1977 by Houghton Mifflin Company. Reprinted by permission of the publisher.)*

Body fat located in storage depots just below the skin serves an important insulating function, determining one's ability to tolerate extremes of cold exposure. An excellent indicator of an individual's adjustment to cold is the ability to maintain a fairly constant body temperature during cold stress. Swimmers who specialized in swimming the English Channel showed only a slight drop in body temperature while resting in cold water and essentially no drop in body temperature while swimming.[21] In contrast, the temperature of leaner, non-Channel swimmers dropped considerably under both conditions. The insulatory layer of fat, which in many individuals assumes a greater and greater proportion of total body weight as age increases, is probably of little value except for those engaged in cold-related activities, such as deep-sea divers, ocean or channel swimmers, or artic inhabitants. In fact, in most instances, excess body fat is a liability in terms of temperature regulation. This is especially apparent during sustained exercise in air when the body's heat production can be increased 20 times above the resting level. In this situation, heat flow from the body is greatly retarded by the shield of insulation from subcutaneous fat. For this reason, excessive body fat poses a considerable strain on the mechanisms for thermal balance.

One final point should be made concerning the insulatory and protective functions of body fat. For some athletes, such as football linemen, excess fat storage provides an additional cushion that may aid in protection from the normal hazards of the sport. However, this possible protective benefit must be evaluated against the liability imposed by the excess "dead weight" in terms of thermal regulation and its possible detrimental effects on performance.

Vitamin Carrier
and Hunger Depressor

Dietary fat serves as a carrier and transport medium for four fat-soluable vitamins—vitamins A, D, E, and K. Thus, the elimination or significant reduction of fat from the diet can lead to a reduced level of these vitamins that may ultimately lead to vitamin deficiency. Dietary fat is also believed necessary for the absorption of vitamin A precursors from nonfat sources such as carrots.

Because fat emptying from the stomach takes about $3\frac{1}{2}$ hours after ingestion, some fat in the diet helps delay the onset of "hunger pangs" and contributes to the feeling of satiety after a meal. Fat in the lower intestines stimulates the release of hormones in the stomach that in turn inhibits hunger contractions. The inclusion of a small quantity of fat increases the satiety value of low-calorie diets so that they are more easily adhered to. This is one reason why reducing diets containing moderate amounts of fat are considered more successful than *low*-fat diets.

FAT BALANCE
IN EXERCISE

Fatty acids released from triglycerides in the fat storage sites and delivered to muscle tissue by the circulation contribute considerably to the energy requirements of exercise. During brief periods of moderate exercise, energy is derived in approximately equal amounts from carbohydrate and fat. As exercise continues for an hour or more, there is a gradual increase in the quantity of fat utilized for energy, and in prolonged exercise, fat may supply nearly 80% of the total energy required.

The data in Figure 1-8 show that the uptake of fatty acids by working muscles rises about 70% during 1 to 4 hours of moderate exercise. Similar observations were made 35 years earlier for subjects on a normal diet exercising at low to moderate exercise levels.[6] In the first hour of exercise, about 50% of the energy was supplied by fat. As exercise continued into the third hour, fat contributed up to 70% of the total energy requirement.

SUMMARY

1. Fats, like carbohydrates, contain carbon, hydrogen, and oxygen atoms, but the ratio of hydrogen to oxygen is much higher. For example, the fat stearin has the formula $C_{57}H_{110}O_6$. Fat molecules are composed of one glycerol molecule and three fatty acid molecules.

2. Fats are synthesized by plants and animals. They can be classified into three groups: simple fats (glycerol + 3 fatty acids), compound fats composed of simple fats in combination with other chemicals (phospholipids, glucolipids, and lipoproteins), and derived fats like cholesterol, which is made from simple and compound fats.

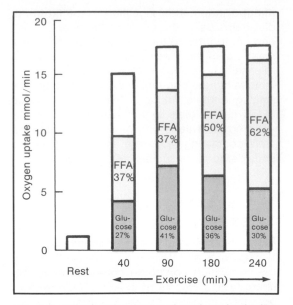

FIG. 1-8. *Uptake of oxygen and nutrients by the legs during prolonged exercise. Shaded areas represent the proportion of total oxygen uptake contributed by the oxidation of free fatty acids (FFA) and blood glucose. Open portions indicate the oxidation of non-blood-borne fuels (muscle glycogen and intramuscular fats and proteins). (From Ahlborg, G. et al.: Substrate turnover during prolonged exercise in man. J. Clin. Invest., 53:1080, 1974.)*

3. Saturated fatty acids contain as many hydrogen atoms as is chemically possible; thus, the molecule is said to be saturated with respect to hydrogen. Saturated fats are present primarily in animal meat, egg yolk, dairy fats, and cheese. High intakes of saturated fats have been linked to the development of coronary heart disease.

4. Unsaturated fatty acids contain fewer hydrogen atoms attached to the carbon chain. Instead, the carbon atoms are joined by double bonds, and they are said to be unsaturated or polyunsaturated with respect to hydrogen. Unsaturated fats liquefy easily at room temperature and are generally of vegetable origin.

5. Fats provide the largest nutrient store of potential energy to power biologic work. They protect vital organs and provide insulation from the cold. Fat also acts as the carrier of the fat-soluble vitamins, A, D, E, and K.

6. During light and moderate exercise, fat contributes about 50% of the energy requirement. As exercise continues, the role of stored fat becomes more important, and, during prolonged work, the fatty acid molecules may provide more than 80% of the energy needs of the body.

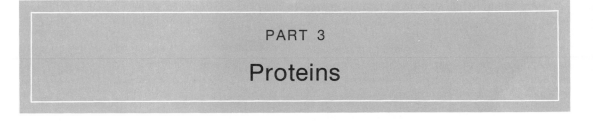

PART 3

Proteins

THE NATURE OF PROTEINS

Proteins are like carbohydrates and fats in that they contain atoms of carbon, oxygen, and hydrogen. In addition, proteins also contain nitrogen, which makes up approximately 16% of the molecule, along with sulfur, phosphorous, and iron. Just as the carbohydrate glycogen is formed by the linkage of many simpler glucose subunits, so also is the protein molecule constructed or polymerized from its "building blocks," the *amino acids*. These amino acids are linked in long chains in various forms and chemical combinations to make up the numerous protein structures.[13a]

Of the 20 different amino acids required by the body, each contains an *amino radical* and a radical called an *organic acid*. The amino radical is composed of two hydrogen atoms attached to nitrogen (NH_2), whereas the organic acid radical (technically termed a carboxyl group) is made up of one carbon atom, two oxygen atoms, and one hydrogen atom (COOH). The remainder of the amino acid molecule may take on a number of different forms and is often referred to as the *side chain* of the amino acid molecule.

Two different amino acids, *alanine* and *leucine,* are shown in Figure 1-9. Each protein contains the basic amino and organic acid group with different structural side chains. *It is the specific structure of this side chain that gives an amino acid its particular characteristics.*

Because there are so many ways the 20 amino acids can combine to form a particular protein, there is almost an infinite number of possible proteins depending on the combination of amino acids. For example, if we consider only proteins formed from the linkage of three different amino acids, there could be 20^3 or 8000 different proteins! With few exceptions, the proteins in the body are composed of numerous linkages of amino acids. Hemoglobin, for example, contains 574 amino acids whereas the muscle protein myosin is formed from the linkage of over 4500 amino acids. Insulin, a small protein, has 51 amino acids formed from 783 atoms.

KINDS AND SOURCES OF PROTEIN

Nine amino acids cannot be synthesized in the body and therefore must be provided preformed in foods. These are called *essential* amino acids. One may see them listed on food supplement labels; they are histidine, isoleucine, leucine, lysine, methionine, phenylalanine, threonine, tryptophan, and valine; in addition, cysteine and tyrosine are synthesized in the body from methionine and phenylalanine, respectively. The remaining nine amino acids that can be manufactured within the body are termed *nonessential.* This does not mean that they are unimportant, but simply that they can be synthesized in the body from compounds ordinarily available and at a rate that meets the demands for normal growth.

Proteins that contain the essential amino acids can be found in the cells of both animals and plants. There is nothing "better" about a specific amino acid from an animal compared to the same amino acid of vegetable origin. Plants make their protein by incorporating nitrogen contained in the soil to synthesize amino acids. Carbon, oxygen, and hydrogen are available from the air and water. In contrast, animals do not have a broad capability for protein synthesis and thus must derive their protein from injested sources.

Protein nutrients that contain all of the essential amino acids in terms of quantity and in the correct ratio to maintain nitrogen balance and allow for tissue growth and repair are known as *complete proteins* (higher quality). An *incomplete protein* (lower quality) lacks one or more of the essential amino acids. Diets containing predominantly incomplete protein may eventually result in protein malnutrition, even though they are adequate in caloric value and protein quantity.

Sources of complete protein are eggs, milk, meat, fish, and poultry. The mixture of essential amino acids present in eggs has been judged to be the best among food sources; hence, eggs are given the highest quality rating of 100 for comparison with other foods. Some common sources of dietary protein in the diet are rated in Table 1-2.

The "biologic value" of food refers to the completeness with which the food supplies essential amino acids. Foods of high-quality protein are largely of animal origin whereas most vegetable proteins (lentils, dried beans and peas, nuts, and cereals) are incomplete in

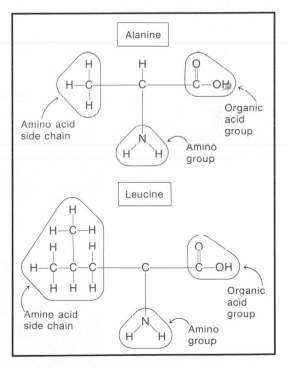

FIG. 1-9. *Two different amino acids, alanine and leucine. Each protein contains the basic amino and organic acid group with different structural side chains. It is the specific structure of the side chain that gives each amino acid its particular characteristics.*

TABLE 1-2. *Rating of common sources of dietary protein*

FOOD	PROTEIN RATING
Eggs	100
Fish	70
Cow's milk	60
Lean beef	69
Soybeans	47
Dry beans	34
Peanuts	43
Brewer's hash	45
Whole-grain wheat	44
Brown rice	57
White rice	56
White potato	34

an's nutritional problem is one of getting ample complete proteins. This is easily resolved with a *lactovegetarian* diet that allows the addition of milk and related products such as ice cream, cheese, and yogurt. The lactovegetarian approach minimizes the problem of getting sufficient protein and increases the intake of calcium and phosphorus. By adding an egg to the diet (lacto-ovovegetarian diet), an intake of high-quality protein is assured.

The contribution of various food groups to the protein content of the American diet is shown in Figure 1-10. By far, the greatest intake of protein comes from animal sources, whereas only about 30% comes from vegetable sources.

terms of protein content and thus have a relatively lower biologic value. It should be understood, however, that *all* of the essential amino acids can be obtained by consuming a *variety* of vegetable foods, each with a different quality and quantity of amino acids. Plant sources of protein meet nutritional needs for protein provided that a sufficient variety of foods such as grains, fruits, and vegetables are incorporated in the diet. There are champion athletes whose diet consists predominantly of nutrients from varied vegetable sources as well as some dairy products. In fact, two-thirds of the people in the world are adequately nourished on essentially vegetarian diets using only small amounts of animal protein. With few exceptions (calcium, phosphorus, and vitamin B_{12}), a strict vegetari-

RECOMMENDED INTAKE OF PROTEINS

There is no benefit from eating excessive amounts of proteins. For athletes, muscle mass is *not* increased simply by eating high-protein foods. Additional calories in the form of protein are converted to fat, which is stored in the subcutaneous depots. In fact, excessive protein may be harmful because the metabolism of large quantities of this nutrient may place an inordinate strain on liver and renal function.[2]

The average American consumes more than twice the protein requirement. For athletes, many of whom consume considerable quantities of food, the diet may contain more than three times the protein requirement. Table 1-3 shows the recommended daily intake of protein

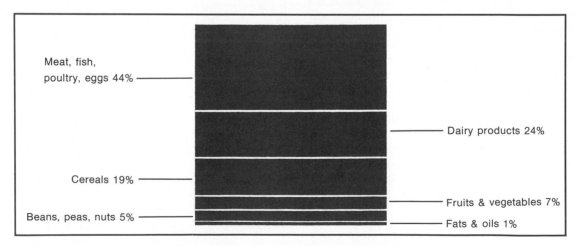

FIG. 1-10. *Protein content of major food sources in the American diet. (From* Nutrition, Weight Control, and Exercise *by Frank I. Katch and William D. McArdle. Copyright © 1977 by Houghton Mifflin Company. Reprinted by permission of the publisher.)*

TABLE 1-3. *Recommended daily allowances of protein for adolescent and adult men and women*

RECOMMENDED AMOUNT	MEN ADOLESCENT	MEN ADULT	WOMEN ADOLESCENT	WOMEN ADULT
Grams of protein per kg body weight	0.9	0.9	0.9	0.9
Grams per day based on average weight[a]	60	65	50	55

[a] Average weight is based on a ''reference'' man and woman[16]. For adolescents (age 14–18), average weight is approximately 65.8 kg (145 lb) for males and 55.7 kg (123 lb) for females. For adult men, average weight is 70 kg (154 lb). For adult women, average weight is 58 kg (128 lb).

for adolescent and adult men and women. On the average, a daily intake of about 0.9 g of protein per kg body weight is recommended. (To determine your protein requirement, multiply your body weight in pounds by 0.424.) This recommendation holds even for people who are overweight. For infants and growing children, the daily recommended intake of protein amounts to 2.0 to 4.0 g per kg body weight, whereas pregnant women and nursing mothers should increase their protein intake by 10 and 20 grams, respectively.[12]

Although little experimental evidence supports the practice of protein supplementation, it is possible that growing athletes, athletes involved in strength development programs that enhance muscle tissue growth, and those subjected to recurring trauma may need a slightly larger protein intake.[5,20] However, this requirement is more than likely met by the generally increased food intake of these athletes.

ROLE OF PROTEIN IN THE BODY

There is considerable variability in the protein content of different cells. A brain cell is only about 10% protein. Red blood cells and muscle cells, on the other hand, may contain as much as 20% of their total weight as protein. The protein content of skeletal muscle can be increased dramatically with the systematic application of strength training exercises.[13]

Amino acids provide the major substance for the synthesis of cellular components as well as of new tissue. The process of building tissue is termed *anabolism,* and the amino acid requirement for anabolic processes can vary considerably. During periods of rapid growth, as occurs in infancy and childhood, over one-third of the protein intake is retained for tissue anabolism. As the growth rate declines, so does the percentage of protein retained for growth-related processes. Once an optimal body size is attained and growth stabilizes, there is still a continuous turnover of tissue protein.

Proteins are present in all cells and are the primary constituents that make up cell membranes as well as internal cellular material. The proteins found in the nuclei of the cell (nucleoproteins) transmit hereditary characteristics and are responsible for continued protein synthesis within the cell. The hair, skin, nails, tendons, and ligaments are special forms of *structural* proteins. The *globular* proteins make up the nearly 2000 different enzymes that catalyze chemical reactions. These compounds are critical in regulating the organized breakdown of fats, carbohydrates, and proteins to release energy. Blood plasma also contains specialized proteins. For example, the plasma proteins thrombin, fibrin, and fibrinogen are intimately involved in blood clotting. Within the red blood cell, the oxygen-carrying compound hemoglobin contains the large protein molecule globin.

Proteins also play an important role in regulating the acid–base quality of the body fluids. This buffering function is important during vigorous exercise when large quantities of acid metabolites are formed. Proteins are essential for muscle contraction; actin and myosin are the structural proteins that ''slide'' past each other as the muscle shortens during movement. Amino acids are essential building blocks of certain hormones and are needed for the activation of selected vitamins that play a key role in metabolic and physiologic regulation.

DYNAMICS OF
PROTEIN METABOLISM

Although the main function of dietary protein resides in its contribution of amino acids to various anabolic processes, protein can also be broken down or catabolized for energy. During this *catabolism,* nitrogen is stripped from the amino acid molecule in the process of deamination in the liver and excreted from the body as *urea* (NH_2CONH_2). The non-nitrogenous amino acid residue is then further degraded during energy metabolism. When the intake of nitrogen (protein) equals nitrogen excretion, a *nitrogen balance* exists. If the body is in *positive nitrogen balance,* where nitrogen intake is greater than nitrogen excretion, then new tissue is being synthesized and protein is retained. This circumstance is often observed in children, during pregnancy, in recovery from illness, and as a result of intensive strength training when protein components of the muscle cell are being synthesized.

Whether the body can develop a protein reserve, as is the case with fat in adipose tissue and to some extent carbohydrate, has yet to be demonstrated and is unlikely. Nevertheless, individuals fed a diet with adequate protein have a higher content of muscle and liver protein than individuals fed a low-protein diet. Also, by use of radioactive protein (injecting protein that has one or several of its carbon atoms "tagged"), it has been shown that certain proteins are more easily recruited for energy metabolism, whereas others are relatively "fixed" as cellular constituents and cannot be used without tissue damage.[10]

The protein in nervous and connective tissue is essentially fixed whereas muscle and liver protein can be altered and used for energy. This fact helps explain the rapid muscle shrinkage or *atrophy* during periods of inactivity, and the loss in lean tissue by persons on reducing diets, especially if the diet is extremely low in carbohydrate or protein.

A greater output of nitrogen relative to its intake indicates the utilization of protein for energy and a possible encroachment on the body's available amino acids. Such a *negative nitrogen balance* can exist at levels of protein intake above the standards established as the minimum requirement. This could occur if the body catabolizes protein because of a lack of other energy nutrients. For example, an individual may consume adequate protein but too little carbohydrate and fat. Consequently, protein is used as a primary energy fuel, the result being a negative protein or nitrogen balance. The protein sparing role of dietary fat and carbohydrate discussed previously is especially important during periods of growth and high-energy output, such as occurs in intensive training. Also, in starvation, the greatest negative nitrogen balance is observed. *As a result, starvation diets or diets with reduced carbohydrate result not only in the depletion of glycogen reserves, but also in a possible protein deficiency and accompanying loss of muscle tissue.*

PROTEIN BALANCE
IN EXERCISE:
GLUCOSE–ALANINE CYCLE

For well-nourished individuals, there is some question as to whether proteins supply an appreciable portion of the energy for exercise. Physiologists have long maintained that the contribution of protein as a fuel for muscular work is minimal, even in activities as grueling as marathon running.[14,19] More recent research however, indicates that in certain situations amino acids, specifically alanine and glutamic acid, play a key role as fuels for exercise.[10,11] Figure 1-11 shows the influence of exercise on the release of alanine from the leg muscles. Clearly, there is increased alanine output related to the severity of the exercise; as exercise increases in intensity, a corresponding increase in alanine output is observed.

It has been proposed that alanine *indirectly* serves the energy requirements of exercise.[10] The alanine released from the exercising muscle is transported in the blood to the liver, where it is deaminated and converted to glucose (gluconeogenesis), which is then released to the blood and delivered to the working muscles. The sequence of this *glucose–alanine cycle* is summarized in Figure 1-12. After 4 hours of continuous exercise, the output of alanine-derived glucose can account for as much as 45% of the total glucose output from the liver. *In fact, energy derived from the glucose–alanine cycle may supply as much as 10% to 15% of the total exercise requirement.*

More data are needed before quantitative statements can be made concerning protein metabolism in exercise. Until these data are available, it appears best to acknowledge the heretofore unrecognized role of protein as an energy fuel.

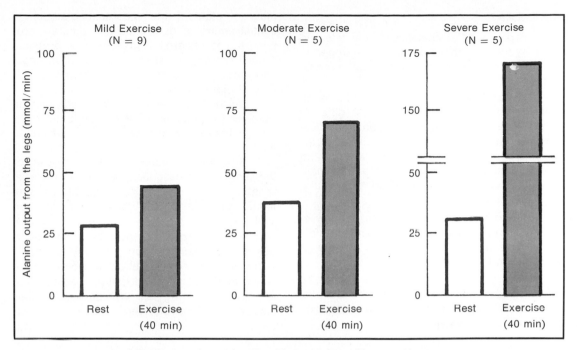

FIG. 1-11. *Influence of 40 minutes of exercise at various work intensities on estimated alanine release from the leg muscles. As the severity of exercise increases, there is a corresponding increase in alanine release. (From Felig, P., and Wahren, J.: Amino acid metabolism in exercising man. J. Clin. Invest. 50:2703, 1971.)*

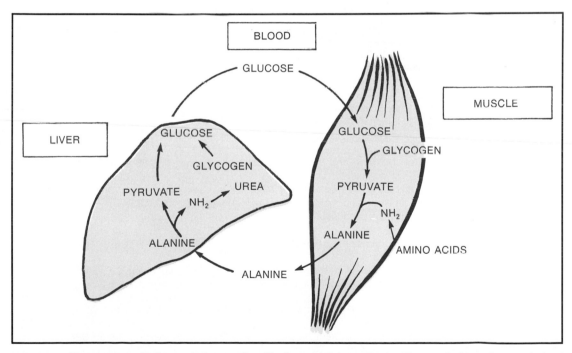

FIG. 1-12. *The glucose–alanine cycle in exercise. Alanine, which is synthesized in muscle from glucose-derived pyruvic acid, is released to the blood and converted to glucose and urea in the liver. This glucose is then released into the blood and delivered to the muscle to serve the energy needs of the cell. During exercise, the increased production and output of alanine from muscle helps supply glucose fuel molecules. (From Felig, P., and Wahren, J.: Amino acid metabolism in exercising man. J. Clin. Invest., 50:2703, 1971.)*

SUMMARY

1. Proteins differ chemically from fats and carbohydrates in that they contain nitrogen in addition to other elements such as sulfur, phosphorous, and iron.

2. Proteins are made up of subunits called amino acids. The body requires 20 different amino acids, each containing an amino radical (NH_2) and an organic acid radical called a carboxyl group (COOH). In addition to NH_2 and COOH, amino acids also contain a side-chain molecule that gives the amino acid its particular chemical characteristics.

3. There are almost an infinite number of combinations for the 20 different amino acids; thus, there are almost an infinite number of possible protein structures.

4. Nine of the 20 amino acids cannot be synthesized in the body. These are the essential amino acids and must be supplied in the diet.

5. Proteins are found in the cells of all animals and plants. Proteins containing all the essential amino acids are called complete proteins; the others are called incomplete proteins. Animal proteins such as those found in eggs, milk, cheese, meat, fish, and poultry are examples of high-quality, complete proteins.

6. All of the essential amino acids can be obtained by consuming a variety of foods, each with a different quality and quantity of amino acids.

7. Proteins provide the building blocks for the synthesis of essentially all cellular material (anabolism). Under certain conditions, the amino acids also contribute their "carbon skeletons" for energy metabolism (catabolism).

8. Certain proteins, especially those in nervous and connective tissue, are not generally sacrificed in energy metabolism. However, the amino acids alanine and glutamic acid play a key role in providing carbohydrate fuel for exercise, especially prolonged, submaximal exercise.

References

1. Ahlborg, G. et al.: Substrate turnover during prolonged exercise in man. J. Clin. Invest., *53:*1080, 1974.
2. Anderson, C.F. et al.: Nutritional therapy for adults with renal disease. *J.A.M.A., 223:*68, 1973.
3. Bergstrom, J. et al.: Diet, muscle glygogen and physical performance. Acta Physiol. Scand., *71:*140, 1967.
4. Bergstrom, J., and Hultman, E.: Nutrition for maximal sports performance. *J.A.M.A., 221:*999, 1972.
5. Bogart, J. et al.: Nutrition and Physical Fitness. Philadelphia, W.B. Saunders Co., 1979.
6. Christensen, E.H., and Hansen, O.: Zur Methodik der respiratorischen Quotient-Bestimmungen in Ruhe and Arbeit. *Skand. Arch. Physiol., 81:*152, 1939.
7. Costill, D.L.: Muscular exhaustion during distance running. Physician Sportsmed., *2:*36, 1974.
8. Costill, D.L. et al.: Glucose ingestion at rest and during prolonged exercise. J. Appl. Physiol., *34:*764, 1973.
9. Deutsch, R.M.: Realities of Nutrition. Palo Alto, Calif.: Bull Publishing Co., 1976.
10. Felig, P., and Wahren, J.: Amino acid metabolism in exercising man. J. Clin. Invest., *50:*2703, 1971.
11. Felig, P., and Wahren, J.: Fuel homeostasis in exercise. N. Engl. J. Med., *293:*1078, 1975.
12. FAO/WHO Expert Group: Protein requirements. FAO Nutrition Meeting Report Series No. 37, Rome, 1965.

13. Goldberg, A.L. et al.: Mechanism of work-induced hypertrophy of skeletal muscle. Med. Sci. Sports, *7:*185, 1975.

13a. Goodhart, R.S., and Shils, M.E.: Modern Nutrition in Health and Disease, 6th edition. Philadelphia, Lea & Febiger, 1980.

14. Hedman, R.: The available glycogen in man and the connection between rate of oxygen intake and carbohydrate usage. Acta Physiol. Scand., *40:*305, 1957.

15. Huse, D.M., and Nelson, R.A.: Basic balanced diet meets requirements of athletes. Physician Sportsmed., *5:*53, 1977.

16. Katch, F.I., and McArdle, W.D.: Nutrition, Weight Control, and Exercise. Boston, Houghton Mifflin Co., 1977.

17. Keys, A.: Physical performance in relation to diet. Fed. Proceed., *2:*164, 1943.

18. Keys, A.: Coronary heart disease—The global picture. Atherosclerosis, *22:*149, 1975.

19. Krogh, A., and Lindhard, J.: Relative value of fat and carbohydrate as sources of muscular energy. Biochem. J., *14:*290, 1920.

20. Molé, P., and Johnson, R.: Disclosure of dietary modification of an exercise-induced protein catabolism in man. J. Appl. Physiol., *31:*185, 1971.

21. Pugh, L.G.C.E., and Edholm, O.G.: The physiology of channel swimmers. Lancet, *2:*761, 1955.

Vitamins, Minerals, and Water

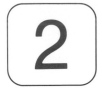

2

The effective regulation of all metabolic processes requires a delicate blending of food nutrients in the watery medium of the cell. Of special significance in the metabolic mixture are the *micronutrients*—the small quantities of vitamins and minerals that play highly specific roles in facilitating energy transfer. As we shall see, these substances are readily obtained in the foods consumed in well-balanced meals. With proper nutrition from a variety of food sources, the need to consume vitamin and mineral supplements, which is both physiologically and economically wasteful, is obviated.

PART 1

Vitamins

THE NATURE OF VITAMINS

The importance of vitamins was known long before scientists isolated and classified them. For example, Hippocrates advocated the ingestion of liver to cure night blindness, and the consumption of various citrus fruits and fresh vegetables. Cod liver oil has been used for centuries to prevent and cure specific diseases.

The formal discovery of vitamins revealed that they are organic substances needed by the body in minute amounts. The vitamins have no particular chemical structure in common and are often considered accessory foods because they neither supply energy nor contribute substantially to the body's mass. With few exceptions, the body cannot manufacture vitamins; hence, they must be supplied in the diet or via artificial supplementation.

Much of the food we consume contains an abundant quantity of vitamins. For example, green leaves and roots of plants manufacture vitamins during the process of photosynthesis. Animals obtain their vitamins from the plants, seeds, grains, and fruits they eat, or from the meat of other animals that have previously consumed these foods.

Many animals are able to manufacture certain vitamins. For example, with the exception of man, monkeys, guinea pigs, and several species of birds, vitamin C can be made by animals from blood glucose. Also, several vitamins, most notably A, D, niacin, and folacin, are activated in the presence of *provitamins.* The best known of the provitamins are the *carotenes,* the yellow and yellow-orange pigments that give color to vegetables and fruits such as carrots, squash, corn, pumpkins, apricots, and peaches.

KINDS OF VITAMINS

Fourteen different vitamins have been isolated, analyzed, classified, and synthesized, and recommended dietary intakes established. These vitamins are classified as *water-soluble* and *fat-soluble.* The water-soluble vitamins are vitamin B_6 (pyridoxine), thiamin (B_1), riboflavin (B_2), niacin (nicotinic acid), pantothenic acid, biotin, choline, folacin (folic acid), cobalamin (B_{12}), and vitamin C (ascorbic acid). The fat-soluble vitamins are vitamins A, D, E, and K.

Fat-Soluble Vitamins

The daily ingestion of fat-soluble vitamins is not absolutely necessary because these substances are dissolved and stored in the fatty tissues of the body. In fact, it may take years for symptoms of a fat-soluble vitamin insufficiency to become evident.

At the other extreme, excessive intake of fat-soluble vitamins can be harmful. For example, consuming large doses of vitamins A and D can eventually have serious toxic effects on infants and adults. These vitamins should *not* be consumed in excess without proper medical supervision. Although an "overdose" from vitamins E and K is rare, it is generally believed that intakes above the recommended level are of no benefit.

Water-Soluble Vitamins

The other group of vitamins (grouped together as vitamin B-complex and vitamin C) is classified as water-soluble. They are similar to their fat-soluble counterparts because they are composed of atoms of carbon, hydrogen, and oxygen. They also contain nitrogen and other elements such as sulfur and cobalt. Because of their water solubility, however, they are transported in the body fluids and not stored to an appreciable extent. Consequently, these vitamins should generally be consumed on a daily basis, and an excessive intake is eventually voided in the urine.

Vitamins in Food

The vitamins, bodily functions, and their major food sources are listed in Table 2-1. It is important to emphasize that an adequate quantity of all vitamins is available for those individuals who consume normal well-balanced meals.[6] This is true regardless of the level of physical activity. Indeed, there appears to be no need for individuals who expend considerable energy in vigorous exercise to consume extra vitamins in the form of special foods or supplements.[16a] Also, at high levels of physical activity, food intake is generally increased to sustain the added energy requirements of exercise. If this added food is obtained through well-balanced meals, a proportionate increase in vitamin intake is assured.[16a,21,21a]

Several possible exceptions to this general rule should be noted. Vitamin C and the B-vitamin folacin (folic acid) are found in foods that usually make only a minimal contribution to the caloric content of the American diet and whose availability varies in specific seasons. Adequate intake of these vitamins can be assured if the daily diet contains fresh fruit and uncooked or steamed vegetables. For those individuals on meatless diets, a small amount of milk, milk products, or eggs should be included, because vitamin B_{12} is only available in foods of animal origin. In fact, if milk and eggs are included in a vegetarian diet ("lacto-ovovegetarian" diet), nutritional quality will be every bit as good as the typical recommended diet that contains meat, fish, and poultry.

ROLE OF VITAMINS IN THE BODY

As shown in Table 2-1, each vitamin has several important functions. Vitamins generally serve as essential links to help regulate the chain of metabolic reactions that facilitate the release of energy bound in the food molecule and control the process of tissue synthesis. *Because vitamins can be used repeatedly in metabolic reactions, the vitamin needs of athletes are generally no greater than the requirements of sedentary people.*

VITAMIN SUPPLEMENTS: THE COMPETITIVE EDGE?

It is well established that vitamin supplements can reverse the symptoms of vitamin deficiency. However, careful research has not supported the wisdom of using such supplements to improve exercise performance in healthy

TABLE 2-1. Water- and fat-soluble vitamins, their recommended daily intake, dietary sources, major bodily functions, and effects of deficiencies and excesses[a]

VITAMIN	RDA FOR HEALTHY ADULT MALE (mg)	DIETARY SOURCES	MAJOR BODY FUNCTIONS	DEFICIENCY	EXCESS
WATER-SOLUBLE					
VITAMIN B-1 (THIAMINE)	1.5	Pork, organ meats, whole grains, legumes	Coenzyme (thiamine pyrophosphate) in reactions involving the removal of carbon dioxide	Beriberi (peripheral nerve changes, edema, heart failure)	None reported
VITAMIN B-2 (RIBOFLAVIN)	1.8	Widely distributed in foods	Constituent of two flavin nucleotide coenzymes involved in energy metabolism (FAD and FMN)	Reddened lips, cracks at corner of mouth (cheilosis), lesions of eye	None reported
NIACIN	20	Liver, lean meats, grains, legumes (can be formed from tryptophan)	Constituent of two coenzymes involved in oxidation–reduction reactions (NAD and NADP)	Pellagra (skin and gastrointestinal lesions, nervous, mental disorders)	Flushing, burning and tingling around neck, face, and hands
VITAMIN B-6 (PYRIDOXINE)	2	Meats, vegetables, whole-grain cereals	Coenzyme (pyridoxal phosphate) involved in amino acid metabolism	Irritability, convulsions, muscular twitching, dermatitis near eyes, kidney stones	None reported
PANTOTHENIC ACID	5–10	Widely distributed in foods	Constituent of coenzyme A, which plays a central role in energy metabolism	Fatigue, sleep disturbances, impaired coordination, nausea (rare in man)	None reported
FOLACIN	.4	Legumes, green vegetables, whole-wheat products	Coenzyme (reduced form) involved in transfer of single-carbon units in nucleic acid and amino acid metabolism	Anemia, gastrointestinal disturbances, diarrhea, red tongue	None reported
VITAMIN B-12	.003	Muscle meats, eggs, dairy products, (not present in plant foods)	Coenzyme involved in transfer of single-carbon units in nucleic acid metabolism	Pernicious anemia, neurologic disorders	None reported

BIOTIN	Not established. Usual diet provides .15–.3	Legumes, vegetables, meats	Coenzyme required for fat synthesis, amino acid metabolism, and glycogen (animal-starch) formation	Fatigue, depression, nausea, dermatitis, muscular pains	None reported
CHOLINE	Not established. Usual diet provides 500–900	All foods containing phospholipids (egg yolk, liver, grains, legumes)	Constituent of phospholipids. Precursor of putative neurotransmitter acetylcholine	Not reported in man	None reported
VITAMIN C (ASCORBIC ACID)	45	Citrus fruits, tomatoes, green peppers, salad greens	Maintains intercellular matrix of cartilage, bone, and dentine. Important in collagen synthesis.	Scurvy (degeneration of skin, teeth, blood vessels, epithelial hemorrhages)	Relatively nontoxic. Possibility of kidney stones
FAT SOLUBLE					
VITAMIN A (RETINOL)	1	Provitamin A (beta-carotene) widely distributed in green vegetables. Retinol present in milk, butter, cheese, fortified margarine	Constituent of rhodopsin (visual pigment). Maintenance of epithelial tissues. Role in mucopolysaccharide synthesis	Xerophthalmia (keratinization of ocular tissue), night blindness, permanent blindness	Headache, vomiting, peeling of skin, anorexia, swelling of long bones
VITAMIN D	.01	Cod-liver oil, eggs, dairy products, fortified milk, and margarine.	Promotes growth and mineralization of bones. Increases absorption of calcium	Rickets (bone deformities) in children. Osteomalacia in adults.	Vomiting, diarrhea, loss of weight, kidney damage
VITAMIN E (TOCOPHEROL)	15	Seeds, green leafy vegetables margarines, shortenings	Functions as an antioxidant to prevent cell-membrane damage.	Possibly anemia	Relatively nontoxic
VITAMIN K (PHYLLOQUINONE)	.03	Green leafy vegetables. Small amount in cereals, fruits, and meats	Important in blood clotting (involved in formation of active prothrombin)	Conditioned deficiencies associated with severe bleeding; internal hemorrhages	Relatively nontoxic. Synthetic forms at high doses may cause jaundice

aFrom Scrimshaw, N. S., and Young, V. R.: The requirements of human nutrition. Sci. Am., 235:50, 1976.

people.[15,20,22] The facts have become clouded by the "testimonials" of coaches and elite athletes to the effect that their success was due to a particular dietary modification that usually included specific vitamin supplements. This has partly contributed to the widespread use of vitamin supplements by athletes.

Vitamins and Exercise Performance

Because of the key role of the B-complex vitamins in metabolism, it has been tempting to speculate that an increase in the intake of these vitamins would enhance energy release and lead to improved physical performance.[23] The belief that "if a little is good, more must be better," has led many coaches, athletes, fitness enthusiasts, and even some scientists to advocate the use of vitamin supplements. This view is simply not supported by research findings or by the overwhelming majority of professional nutritionists.

This is also the case for vitamins other than the B-complex group such as vitamins C and E. Studies have shown that supplements of vitamin C had negligible effects on endurance performance and on the rate, severity, and duration of injuries compared to treatment with a placebo.[8] It has never been firmly established with careful research that a deficiency state for vitamin E exists, let alone that vitamin E supplements are beneficial to stamina, circulatory function, energy metabolism, aging, or sexual potency.[13,22]

Megavitamins

Although there is no need for normal people eating a well-balanced diet to take additional vitamins, most nutritionists feel that taking a multivitamin capsule of the recommended quantity of each vitamin will do no harm. For some people, the psychologic effects may even be beneficial. It is of great concern, however, that some athletes resort to taking *megavitamins,* or doses of at least *tenfold* the Recommended Dietary Allowance, in the hope of improving performance.

Except in cases of specific serious medical illness, this practice can be harmful. Once the enzyme systems that are catalyzed by specific vitamins are saturated, the excess vitamins in the megadose function as chemicals in the body.[10] For example, a megadose of the water-soluble vitamin C can raise serum uric levels and precipitate gout in people predisposed to this disease. Also, some American blacks, Asians, and Sephardic Jews have a genetic metabolic deficiency that can be activated to hemolytic anemia by excesses of vitamin C.[4] In individuals who are iron-deficient, megadoses of vitamin C destroy significant amounts of vitamin B_{12} in the diet.[11,16] In healthy people, vitamin C supplements frequently irritate the bowel and cause diarrhea.

It is now believed that an excessive intake of vitamin B_6 may produce liver disease whereas a megadose of nicotinic acid inhibits the uptake of fatty acids by cardiac muscle during exercise.[10] Possible side effects of vitamin E megadose include headache, fatigue, blurred vision, gastrointestinal disturbances, muscular weakness, and low blood sugar.[9] This is ironic because it is not known whether a lack of vitamin E per se is seriously harmful to humans.[9,22] Because vitamin E is usually found associated with unsaturated fats, it is difficult even to "construct" a vitamin E-deficient diet. The toxicity to the nervous system of megadoses of vitamin A and the damaging effects to the kidneys of excess vitamin D have been well demonstrated.[7,19]

Perhaps the misuse and abuse of vitamins by individuals hoping to improve athletic performance can be put in proper perspective by the following quotation:[16a] "The sale of vitamins is probably the biggest rip-off in our society today. Their only effect would appear to be a highly enriched sewage around athletic training or competition sites."

SUMMARY

1. Vitamins are organic substances that neither supply energy nor contribute to the body's mass but that serve crucial functions in almost all body processes. Vitamins must be obtained from food or from dietary supplementation.

2. Vitamins are synthesized by plants and are also found in animals that produce them from precursor substances known as provitamins.

3. There are 14 known vitamins classified as either water or fat soluble. The fat-soluble vitamins are vitamins A, D, E, and K; vitamin C and the B-complex vitamins are water soluble.

4. Fat-soluble vitamins taken in excess accumulate in the tissues and eventually can be

toxic. Excesses of water-soluble vitamins are eventually excreted in the urine.

5. Vitamins regulate metabolism, facilitate energy release, and are important in the process of bone and tissue synthesis.

6. Careful research generally shows that vi-tamin supplementation (above that obtained in the well-balanced diet) is not related to improved exercise performance. In fact, excessive dosage of both water- and fat-soluble vitamins can result in serious illness.

PART 2

Minerals

THE NATURE OF MINERALS

In addition to the organic elements oxygen, carbon, hydrogen, and nitrogen, approximately 4% of the body's weight, or about 6 lb for a 125-lb woman, is composed of a group of metallic elements collectively called *minerals.* Most of the minerals are found in living cells, although not all are necessarily essential for life. The minerals most important to humans are those found in enzymes, hormones, and vitamins. Minerals appear in combination with organic compounds, for example, calcium phosphate in bone, or singularly such as free calcium in intracellular fluids.

In the body, minerals are classified as *major minerals*—those present in large quantities and that have known biologic functions, and as *trace minerals*—those present in minute quantities (less than 0.05% body weight).

Most minerals, major or trace, occur freely in nature, mainly in the waters of rivers, lakes, and oceans, in topsoil, and beneath the earth's surface. Minerals can be found in the root systems of plants and trees and in the body structure of animals who consume plants and water containing the minerals.

KINDS AND SOURCES OF MINERALS

The important minerals and their functions, food sources, and daily requirements are listed in Table 2-2. As with vitamins, there generally is little need for mineral supplements because most minerals are readily available in the common foods we eat and the water we drink. Some supplementation may be necessary, however, in geographic regions where the soil or water supply of a particular mineral is poor. For example, in certain regions of the United States, particularly the basin of the Great Lakes and Pacific Northwest, sources of the mineral *iodine* are relatively poor. Iodine is taken up by the thyroid gland to become part of *thyroxine,* a hormone that exerts an accelerating influence on the cells' resting metabolic level. Severe iodine deficiency results in thyroid enlargement of up to 15 times its normal size and weight as the gland attempts to increase its hormone output. This disease, called goiter, can easily be prevented by adding iodine to the water supply or to table salt (iodized salt).

A common mineral deficiency in this country results from a lack of iron in the diet (Table 2-3). It is estimated that 30% to 50% of American women of child-bearing age suffer some form of iron insufficiency.[7] In most instances, appropriate iron supplementation can be achieved with a diet rich in iron-containing foods such as beans, peas, dried uncooked fruits, leafy green vegetables, egg yolk, and meats, especially liver, kidney, and heart.

ROLE OF MINERALS IN THE BODY

The major single function of the mineral nutrients is their role in cellular metabolism. They serve as important parts of enzymes that regulate chemical reactions within cells. Figure 2-1 shows various minerals that participate in catabolic and anabolic cellular processes.

TABLE 2-2. *The important minerals in the body, their recommended daily intake, dietary sources, major bodily functions, and the effects of deficiencies and excesses*[a]

MINERAL	AMOUNT IN ADULT BODY (g)	RDA FOR HEALTHY ADULT MALE (mg)	DIETARY SOURCES	MAJOR BODY FUNCTIONS	DEFICIENCY	EXCESS
CALCIUM	1,500	800	Milk, cheese, dark-green vegetables, dried legumes	Bone and tooth formation Blood clotting Nerve transmission	Stunted growth Rickets, osteoporosis Convulsions	Not reported in man
PHOSPHORUS	860	800	Milk, cheese, meat, poultry, grains	Bone and tooth formation Acid–base balance	Weakness, demineralization of bone Loss of calcium	Erosion of jaw (fossy jaw)
SULFUR	300	(Provided by sulfur amino acids)	Sulfur amino acids (methionine and cystine) in dietary proteins	Constituent of active tissue compounds, cartilage and tendon	Related to intake and deficiency of sulfur amino acids	Excess sulfur amino acid intake leads to poor growth
POTASSIUM	180	2,500	Meats, milk, many fruits	Acid–base balance Body water balance Nerve function	Muscular weakness Paralysis	Muscular weakness Death
CHLORINE	74	2,000	Common salt	Formation of gastric juice Acid–base balance	Muscle cramps Mental apathy Reduced appetite	Vomiting
SODIUM	64	2,500	Common salt	Acid–base balance Body water balance Nerve function	Muscle cramps Mental apathy Reduced appetite	High blood pressure
MAGNESIUM	25	350	Whole grains, green leafy vegetables	Activates enzymes. Involved in protein synthesis	Growth failure Behavioral disturbances Weakness, spasms	Diarrhea
IRON	4.5	10	Eggs, lean meats, legumes, whole grains, green leafy vegetables	Constituent of hemoglobin and enzymes involved in energy metabolism	Iron-deficiency anemia (weakness, reduced resistance to infection)	Siderosis Cirrhosis of liver
FLUORINE	2.6	2	Drinking water, tea, seafood	May be important in maintenance of bone structure	Higher frequency of tooth decay	Mottling of teeth Increased bone density Neurologic disturbances

			Sources	Functions	Deficiency	Excess/Toxicity
ZINC	2	15	Widely distributed in foods	Constituent of enzymes Involved in digestion	Growth failure Small sex glands	Fever, nausea, vomiting, diarrhea
COPPER	.1	2	Meats, drinking water	Constituent of enzymes associated with iron metabolism	Anemia, bone changes (rare in man)	Rare metabolic condition (Wilson's disease)
SILICON VANADIUM TIN NICKEL	.024 .018 .017 .010	Not established	Widely distributed in foods	Function unknown (essential for animals)	Not reported in man	Industrial exposures: Silicon—silicosis Vanadium—lung irritation Tin—vomiting Nickel—acute pneumonitis
SELENIUM	.013	Not established (Diet provides .05–.1 per day)	Seafood, meat, grains	Functions in close association with Vitamin E	Anemia (rare)	Gastrointestinal disorders, lung irritation
MANGANESE	.012	Not established (Diet provides 6–8 per day)	Widely distributed in foods	Constituent of enzymes involved in fat synthesis	In animals: poor growth, disturbances of nervous system, reproductive abnormalities	Poisoning in manganese mines: generalized disease of nervous system
IODINE	.011	.14	Marine fish and shellfish, dairy products, many vegetables	Constituent of thyroid hormones	Goiter (enlarged thyroid)	Very high intakes depress thyroid activity
MOLYBDENUM	.009	Not established (Diet provides .4 per day)	Legumes, cereals, organ meats	Constituent of some enzymes	Not reported in man	Inhibition of enzymes
CHROMIUM	.006	Not established (Diet provides .05–.12 per day)	Fats, vegetable oils, meats	Involved in glucose and energy metabolism	Impaired ability to metabolize glucose	Occupational exposures: skin and kidney damage
COBALT	.0015	(Required as vitamin B-12)	Organ and muscle meats, milk	Constituent of vitamin B-12	Not reported in man	Industrial exposure: dermatitis and diseases of red blood cells
WATER	40,000 (60% of body weight)	1.5 liters per day	Solid foods, liquids, drinking water	Transport of nutrients Temperature regulation Participates in metabolic reactions	Thirst, dehydration	Headaches, nausea Edema High blood pressure

[a]From Scrimshaw, N. S., and Young, V. R.: The requirements of human nutrition. Sci. Am. 235:50–73, 1976.

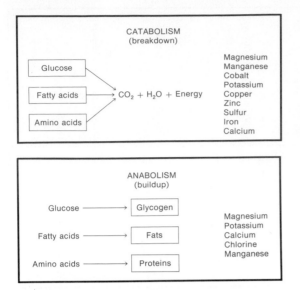

FIG. 2-1. *Minerals involved in the catabolism (breakdown) and anabolism (build-up) of nutrients. (From Nutrition, Weight Control, and Exercise by Frank I. Katch and William D. McArdle. Copyright © 1977 by Houghton Mifflin Company. Reprinted by permission of the publisher.)*

Minerals are important in activating numerous reactions that release energy during the breakdown of carbohydrates, fats, and proteins. In addition to the processes of catabolism, minerals are essential for the synthesis of biologic nutrients; glycogen from glucose, fats from fatty acids and glycerol, and proteins from amino acids. Without the essential minerals, the fine balance between catabolism and anabolism would be disrupted.

Minerals also form important constituents of hormones. An inadequate thyroxine production due to iodine deficiency could significantly slow the body's resting metabolism. In extreme cases, this reduced level of energy output could predispose a person to develop obesity. The synthesis of *insulin,* the hormone that facilitates glucose uptake by the cells, requires the mineral zinc whereas the digestive acid, hydrochloric acid, is formed from the mineral chlorine. In the subsequent sections, specific functions of several minerals are described.

Calcium

Calcium is the most abundant mineral in the body. Calcium combines with phosphorous to form the bones and teeth. In its ionized form, calcium plays an important role in the process of muscular contraction and the transmission of nerve impulses. It is also essential for blood clotting and for the transport of fluids across cell membranes.

Phosphorous

Besides its important function in combining with calcium to give rigidity to bones and teeth, phosphorous is an essential component of the high-energy compounds *adenosine triphosphate* (ATP) and creatine *phosphate* (CP). ATP and CP are crucial in supplying the energy for all forms of biologic work. Phosphorous also participates in the buffering of the acid end products of energy metabolism. For this reason, some coaches and trainers recommend the consumption of special "phosphate drinks" in the hope of improving performance by reducing the effects of acid production. To date, there is no scientific evidence to support this practice.[12]

Magnesium

Magnesium plays a vital role in glucose metabolism by facilitating the formation of muscle and liver glycogen from blood-borne glucose. Magnesium also participates in the breakdown of glucose, fatty acids, and amino acids during energy metabolism. Furthermore, magnesium is important in stabilizing the neuromuscular system in terms of nerve conduction and muscle contraction.

Iron

From 3 to 5 g or about $\frac{1}{6}$ of an ounce of iron is normally contained in the body. The largest quantity of this mineral is combined with hemoglobin in the red blood cells. This iron–protein compound increases the oxygen-carrying capacity of blood about 65 times. Iron serves other important exercise-related functions aside from its role in oxygen transport in red blood cells. Iron is a structural component of *myoglobin,* a compound similar to hemoglobin, which aids in the transport of oxygen within the muscle cell. Iron is present in small amounts in specialized substances called *cytochromes* that function as catalysts in the energy transfer systems operating within the cell.

The athlete should be sure to include iron-rich foods in the daily diet. People who do not take in enough iron or who have limited rates of iron absorption or high rates of iron loss can

TABLE 2-3. *Recommended daily allowances for iron*

	AGE	IRON (mg)
Children	1–3	15
	4–10	10
Males	11–18	18[a]
	19+	10
Females	11–50	18[a]
	51+	10
	Pregnant	18[a]
	Lactating	18[a]

[a] Generally, this increased requirement cannot be met by ordinary diets; therefore, the use of 30 to 60 mg of supplemental iron is recommended. (From Food and Nutrition Board; Recommended Dietary Allowances. Washington, D.C., National Academy of Sciences, revised, 1980.)

develop a condition in which the concentration of hemoglobin in red blood cells is reduced. This condition, commonly called *iron deficiency anemia,* is characterized by general sluggishness, loss of appetite, and a reduced capacity for sustaining even mild exercise. With "iron therapy," both the hemoglobin content of the blood and the exercise response can be brought back to normal levels.

A moderate iron deficiency anemia is common during pregnancy when there is an increased demand for iron for both mother and fetus. In addition, females usually lose between 5 and 45 milligrams (mg) of iron during the menstrual cycle. This normal iron loss increases the iron requirement of females to almost twice that of males (18 mg v. 10 mg). When this added requirement is combined with the fact that the normal American diet contains only about 6 mg of iron in each 1000 kcal of food ingested, it is not surprising that 30% to 50% of American women have significant iron insufficiencies.[7] The potential for further menstrual iron loss is increased in women who use intrauterine devices for contraception, because more than normal amounts of menstrual blood can be lost each period. For these women, the daily iron requirement is increased considerably, and some form of iron supplement may be beneficial.

It has yet to be demonstrated convincingly that the iron status of women athletes differs significantly from that of their nonathletic counterparts or that physical training increases iron requirements or aggravates existing iron deficiencies.[16a,24] Thus, one can expect about 30% of female athletes to have below normal iron stores. This may increase the risk of developing

iron deficiency anemia, which would subsequently impair exercise performance and training capacity.[3] This does not mean that *all* women athletes should take iron supplements. Rather, a proper evaluation of each woman's iron storage and hemoglobin status should be an integral part of the regular medical evaluation. For those women who are iron deficient and possibly at greater risk of developing anemia, appropriate iron supplementation should be prescribed.

Sodium, Potassium, and Chlorine

The minerals sodium, potassium, and chlorine are collectively termed *electrolytes* because they are in the body as electrically charged particles called ions. A major function of the electrolytes is to modulate body fluid exchange within the various fluid compartments of the body. This allows for a constant, well-regulated exchange of nutrients and waste products between the cell and its external fluid environment.

Perhaps the most important function of the mineral electrolytes sodium and potassium is their role in establishing the proper electrical gradients across cell membranes. This electrical difference between the interior and exterior of the cell is required for the transmission of nerve impulses, for the stimulation and contraction of muscle, and for the proper functioning of glands. The electrolytes are also important in maintaining the balance between the acid and base qualities of the body fluids, especially the blood.

MINERALS AND EXERCISE PERFORMANCE

For normal individuals receiving the Recommended Daily Allowance of minerals, there is no evidence that mineral supplementation benefits exercise performance. An important consequence of prolonged exercise, however, especially in hot weather, is the loss of water and mineral salts, primarily sodium and some potassium chloride in sweat. Excessive water and electrolyte losses impair heat tolerance and exercise performance and can lead to severe dysfunction in the form of heat cramps, heat exhaustion, or heat stroke. The yearly toll of heat-related deaths during spring and summer football practice provides a tragic illustration of the importance of fluid and electrolyte replacement. It is not uncommon for an athlete to lose anywhere from 1 to 5 kg water each practice session or during a game as a result of sweating. This fluid loss corresponds to a depletion of 1.5 to 8.0 g of salt, because each kilogram of sweat generally contains about 1.5 g of salt. *The crucial and immediate need in these situations is to replace the water lost through sweating.*

Even under extreme conditions such as marathon running in warm weather, electrolytes can usually be replenished by adding a slight amount of salt to the fluid ingested or to the normal daily food intake. In fact, research indicates that most individuals unconsciously consume more salt when the need exists. For fluid losses in excess of 4 or 5 kg and for prolonged periods of work in the heat, salt supplements may be necessary and can be achieved by adding about $\frac{1}{3}$ teaspoon of table salt per liter of water.[1] Although a potassium deficiency may occur with intense exercise,[18] the appropriate potassium level is generally assured by consuming a diet containing normal amounts of the mineral.[5]

SUMMARY

1.   About 4% of the body's weight is composed of 22 metallic elements called minerals. Minerals are a part of enzymes, hormones, and vitamins; they are found in muscles, connective tissues, and all body fluids.

2.   Minerals occur freely in nature, in the waters of rivers, lakes, and oceans, and in soil. They are absorbed into the root system of plants and eventually incorporated into the tissues of animals that consume these plants.

3.   A primary function of minerals is in metabolism where they serve as important parts of regulatory enzymes. Minerals are also important for the synthesis of the biologic nutrients, glycogen, fat, and protein.

4.   With a balanced diet, there is generally adequate mineral intake, except perhaps in geographic locations where certain minerals such as iodine are absent.

5.   There is some evidence that about 40% of the women of child-bearing age in this country suffer from iron insufficiency. This could lead to iron deficiency anemia, which would significantly affect exercise performance.

6.   As a result of excessive sweating caused by exercise, there are large losses of body water and related minerals. These should be replaced, in appropriate quantities, during and following exercise. There is no evidence that excess mineral intake benefits performance or enhances recovery.

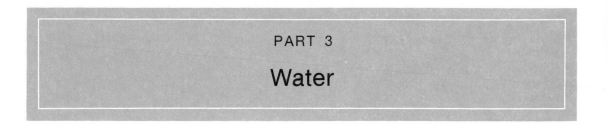

PART 3

Water

WATER IN THE BODY

Although water does not contribute to the nutrient value of food per se, it is still important in describing food composition and energy balance. The energy content of a particular food tends to be inversely related to its water content. As a general rule, foods that are high in water are low in calories. For this reason, the energy content of any food is sometimes expressed per "dry weight" of the food.

From 40% to 60% of an individual's body weight is water. Water constitutes 65% to 75% of the weight of muscle and less than 25% of the weight of fat. Consequently, differences in total body water between individuals are largely due to variations in body composition (that is, differences in lean versus fat tissue).

There are two main water "compartments" in the body; *intracellular,* referring to inside the cell and *extracellular,* referring to outside the cell. The extracellular fluid includes the blood plasma and lymph, saliva, fluids in the eyes, fluids secreted by glands and the intestines, fluids that bathe the nerves of the spinal cord, and fluids excreted from the skin and kidneys.

Of the total body water, an average of 62% is located intracellularly and 38% extracellularly.

WATER BALANCE: INTAKE VERSUS OUTPUT

The water content of the body remains relatively stable within an individual over time. Although water output may frequently exceed water intake, this imbalance is quickly adjusted with appropriate fluid intake so as to bring the body's fluid levels back into balance. The sources of water intake and output are shown in Figure 2-2.

Water Intake

Normally, about $2\frac{1}{2}$ liters of water are required each day for a fairly sedentary adult in a normal environment. This water is supplied from three sources: (1) from liquids, (2) in foods, and (3) during metabolism.

WATER FROM LIQUIDS. The average individual normally consumes 1200 milliliters (ml) (41 oz) of water each day. Of course, during exercise and thermal stress, fluid intake can increase five or six times above normal. There are reports of an individual losing 30 lb of water weight during a two-day, 17-hour 55-mile run across Death Valley, California.[17] However, with proper fluid injection, including salt supplements, the actual body weight loss was only 3 lb. In this example, fluid loss and replenishment amounted to between $3\frac{1}{2}$ and 4 gallons of liquid!

WATER IN FOODS. Most foods, especially fruits and vegetables, contain large quantities of

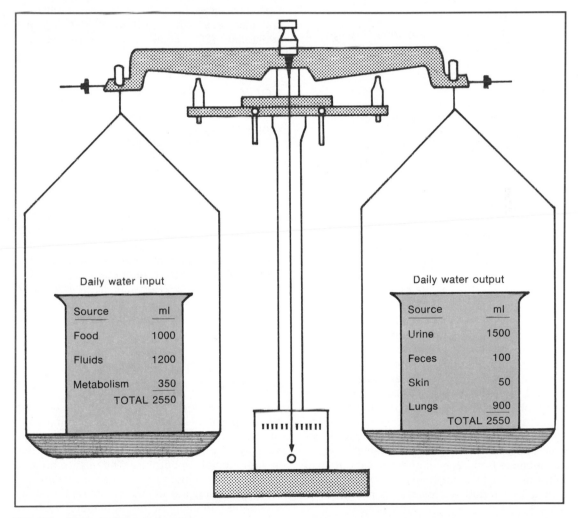

Daily water input	
Source	ml
Food	1000
Fluids	1200
Metabolism	350
TOTAL	2550

Daily water output	
Source	ml
Urine	1500
Feces	100
Skin	50
Lungs	900
TOTAL	2550

FIG. 2-2. *Water balance in humans.*

water. Such foods as lettuce, pickles, green beans, and broccoli spears are examples of foods that have a high water content, whereas the water contained in butter, oils, dried meats, and chocolate, cookies, and cakes is relatively low.

METABOLIC WATER. When food molecules are broken down for energy, carbon dioxide and water are formed. This water is termed metabolic water and accounts for about 25% of the daily water requirement of a sedentary person. The complete breakdown of 100 g of carbohydrate, protein, and fat produces 55, 100, and 107 g of metabolic water, respectively. As mentioned in Chapter 1, each gram of glycogen is hydrated with 2.7 g of water. Consequently, this water also becomes available when glycogen is used for energy.

Water Output

Water is lost from the body in urine, through the skin, as water vapor in the expired air, and in feces.

WATER LOSS IN URINE. Under normal conditions the volume of urine excreted by the kidneys ranges from 1000 to 1500 ml or about $1\frac{1}{2}$ quarts per day.

It has been estimated that 15 ml of water are required to eliminate 1 g of solute. Thus, a portion of water in urine is "obligated" in order to rid the body of metabolic solutes such as urea, an end product of protein breakdown. In this way, the use of large quantities of protein for energy (as would occur with a high-protein diet) can actually speed up the body's dehydration during exercise.

WATER LOSS THROUGH THE SKIN. A small quantity of water, perhaps 350 ml, seeps from the deeper tissues through the skin to the body's surface. This continuous loss of water has been termed *insensible perspiration.*

Water is also lost through the skin in the form of sweat produced by specialized sweat glands located beneath the skin. Evaporation of this sweat provides the refrigeration mechanism to cool the body. Under normal conditions, 500 to 700 ml of sweat are secreted each day. However, this by no means reflects sweating capacity, because 8 to 12 liters of sweat (about 25 lb at a rate of 1 liter per hour) can be produced during prolonged exercise in a hot environment.[2]

WATER LOSS AS WATER VAPOR. The amount of insensible water loss via small water droplets in exhaled air is 250 to 350 ml per day. Exercise also affects this source of water loss. For physically active persons, 2 to 5 ml of water are lost from the respiratory passages each minute during strenuous exercise.[14] This amount varies considerably with climate, being less in hot, humid weather and greatest in cold temperatures where the inspired air contains little moisture or at altitudes where ventilatory volumes are significantly elevated at rest and during exercise.

WATER LOSS IN FECES. Between 100 and 200 ml of water are lost through intestinal elimination, because approximately 70% of fecal matter is water. The remainder is composed of nondigestible material, which includes bacteria from the digestive process, and the residues of digestive juices from the intestines, stomach, and pancreas. With diarrhea or vomiting, an additional 1500 to 5000 ml of water can be lost.

FUNCTIONS OF BODY WATER

Water is truly a remarkable nutrient that is essential to life. Without water, death will occur within days. It makes up about 60% of the body weight and serves as the body's transport and reactive medium. Diffusion of gases always takes place across surfaces moistened by water. Nutrients and gases are transported in aqueous solution; waste products leave the body via the water in urine and feces. Water has tremendous heat-stabilizing qualities. It can absorb a considerable quantity of heat with only a small change in temperature. Water lubricates our joints. Because it is essentially noncompressible, it helps give structure and form to the body through the turgor it provides for body tissues.

WATER REQUIREMENT IN EXERCISE

The most serious consequence of profuse sweating is the loss of body water. The amount of water lost through sweating depends on the severity of physical activity as well as on the environmental temperature. The relative humidity of the surrounding air is also an important factor affecting the efficiency of the sweating mechanism in temperature regulation. The term *relative humidity* refers to the water content of the air. During conditions of 100% relative humidity, the air is completely saturated with water vapor. Thus, evaporation of fluid from the skin to the air is impossible, and this important avenue for body cooling is closed. Under such conditions, sweat beads on the skin and eventually rolls off. On a dry day, the air can hold a considerable amount of moisture, and the evaporation of fluid from the skin is rapid. Thus the sweat mechanism functions at optimal efficiency, and body temperature is more easily controlled. A more detailed discussion about sweating, temperature regulation, and fluid replacement with exercise is presented in Chapter 24.

SUMMARY

1. Water makes up 40 to 60% of the total body weight. Muscle is 72% water by weight whereas water represents only about 20% to 25% of the weight of fat.
2. Of the total body water, roughly 62% is located intracellularly (inside the cells) and 38% extracellularly in the plasma, lymph, and other fluids outside the cell.
3. Normal daily water intake of about 2.55 liters is supplied from (1) liquid intake (1.2 liters), (2) food (1.0 liters), and (3) metabolic water produced during energy-yielding reactions (0.35 liters).
4. Water is lost from the body each day (1) in the urine (1–1.5 liters), (2) through the skin as insensible perspiration (0.50–0.70 liters), (3) as water vapor in expired air (0.25–0.30 liters), and (4) in feces where about 70% of fecal matter is water (0.10 liters).
5. Food and oxygen are always supplied in aqueous solution and waste products always leave via a watery medium. Water also helps give structure and form to the body and plays an extremely important role in temperature regulation.
6. Exercise, especially in hot weather, greatly increases the body's water requirement. In extreme conditions the fluid needs can increase five or six times above normal.

References

1. American College of Sports Medicine. Position statement on prevention of heat injuries during distance running. Med. Sci. Sports, 7:vii, 1975.
2. Adolph, E.F.: Physiology of Man in the Desert. New York, Interscience Publishers, Inc., 1947.
3. Burskirk, E., and Haymes, E.: Nutritional requirements for women in sport. *In* Women and Sport: A National Research Conference. Edited by D. Harris. University Park, Penn State University, 1972.
4. Clinical Nutrition: Vitamin C toxicity. Nutr. Rev. 34:236, 1977.
5. Costill, D.L.: Nutritional requirements for endurance athletes. *In* Toward an Understanding of Human Performance. Edited by E.J. Burke. Ithaca, N.Y., Mouvement Publications, 1977.
6. Nutrition and athletic performance. *Dairy Council Digest, 46:*7, 1975.
7. Deutch, R.M.: Realities of Nutrition. Palo Alto, Calif., Bull Publishing Co., 1976.
8. Gey, G.O. et al.: Effect of ascorbic acid on endurance performance and athletic injury. *J.A.M.A., 211:*105, 1970.
9. Herbert, V.: Toxicity of vitamin E. Nutr. Rev., *35:*158, 1977.
10. Herbert, V.: Megavitamin therapy. *Contemp. Nutr. 2:*October, 1977.
11. Herbert, V. et al.: Destruction of vitamin B by vitamin C. Am. J. Clin. Nutr., *30:*297, 1977.
12. Johnson, W.R., and Black, D.H.: Comparison of effects of certain blood alkalizers and glucose upon competitive endurance performance. J. Appl. Physiol., *5:*577, 1953.

13. Lawrence, J.D. et al.: Effects of alpha-tocopherol acetate on the swimming endurance of trained swimmers. Am. J. Clin. Nutr., *28:*205, 1975.
14. Mitchell, J. et al: Respiratory weight losses during exercise. J. Appl. Physiol., *32:*474, 1972.
15. Nelson, R.A.: What athletes should eat? Unmixing folly and facts. The Physician and Sportsmedicine, *3:*67–72, 1975.
16. Newmark, H.L. et al.: Stability of vitamin B_{12} in the presence of ascorbic acid. Am. J. Clin. Nutr., *29:*645, 1976.
16a. Pate, R., et al.: Dietary iron supplementation in women athletes. The Physician and Sportsmedicine, *7:*16, 1979.
16b. Percy, E.C.: Ergogenic aids in athletics. Med. Sci. Sports, *10:*298, 1978.
17. Robinson, S.: Cardiovascular and respiratory reactions to heat. *In* Physiological Adaptations. Edited by M.K. Yousef et al. New York, Academic Press, 1972.
18. Rose, K. Warning for millions: Intense exercise can deplete potassium. The Physician and Sportsmedicine. *3:*67, 1975.
19. Scrimshaw, N.S., and Young, V.R.: The requirements of human nutrition. Sci. Am., *235:*50, 1976.
20. Serfass, W.C.: Nutrition for the athlete. Contemp. Nutr., 2(5): May, 1977.
21. Smith, N.J.: Food for Sport. Palo Alto, Calif., Bull Publishing Co., 1976.
21a. Strauzenberg, F., et al.: The problem of dieting in training and athletic performance. Biblthca Nuti, Dieta, *27:*133, 1979.
22. The Institute of Food Technologists' Expert Panel on Food Safety and Nutrition and the Committee on Public Information. Vitamin E. Contemp. Nutr. 2:November, 1977.
23. Van Dam, B.: Vitamins and sports. British Journal of Sports Medicine. *12:*74, 1978.
24. Wirth, J.C., et al.: The effects of physical training on the serum iron levels of college-age women. Med. Sci. Sports, *10:*223, 1978.

Optimal Nutrition
for Exercise

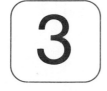

An optimal diet may be defined as one in which the supply of required nutrients is adequate for tissue maintenance, repair, and growth. Only in the last few years has it been possible to obtain a reasonable estimate of the specific nutrient needs for men and women of different ages and body sizes, with considerations for individual differences in digestion, storage capacity, nutrient metabolism, and daily levels of energy expenditure. Dietary recommendations for athletes may be further complicated by the specific energy requirements of a particular sport as well as by the athlete's dietary preferences. Truly, there is no one diet for optimal exercise performance. However, sound nutritional guidelines must be followed in planning and evaluating food intake.

NUTRIENT
REQUIREMENT

Many coaches make dietary recommendations based on their own "feelings" and past experiences rather than rely on available evidence. This problem is compounded by the fact that athletes often have either inadequate or incorrect information concerning prudent dietary practices as well as the role of specific nutrients in the diet.[10] The general consensus of researchers is that athletes do not require additional nutrients beyond those obtained in a balanced diet.[6a] In essence, sound nutrition for athletes is sound human nutrition. The extra calories required for exercise can be obtained from a variety of nutritious foods of the athlete's choice.

Recommended
Nutrient Intake

Figure 3-1 shows the recommended basic nutrient intake for protein, fat, and carbohydrate, as well as the general category of food sources for these nutrients. These guidelines provide for the necessary vitamin, mineral, and protein requirements even though the energy content of this food intake amounts to only about 1200 Calories per day. (A calorie is a unit of heat used to express the energy value of food.) In terms of average values for adult Americans, the total daily energy requirement is about 2100 and 2700 Calories for women and men, respectively. *Thus, once the basic nutrient requirements are met (as recommended in Fig. 3-1), the extra energy needs of the person can be supplied from a variety of food sources based on individual preference.*

As we discussed in Chapter 1, the standard recommendation for protein intake generally approximates 0.9 g protein per kilogram body weight. A person who weighs 170 lbs (77.1 kg) would therefore require about 69 g or 2.42 ounces of protein daily. Assuming that even during strenuous exercise there is relatively little protein loss via energy metabolism (an assumption that may not be entirely correct), the preceding protein recommendation is probably adequate for both active and sedentary persons. Also, the protein intake in the average American diet significantly exceeds the recommended protein requirement, and the athlete's diet is usually two to three times in excess of the protein intake considered optimal!

Standards for optimal fat and carbohydrate

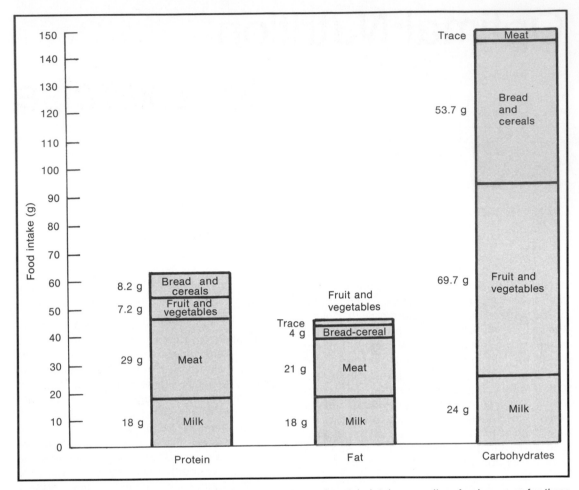

FIG. 3-1. *Recommendations for basic carbohydrate, fat, and protein intake as well as food sources for these nutrients. (From Howe, P.: Basic Nutrition in Health and Disease. Philadelphia, W.B. Saunders Co., 1971.)*

intake have not been firmly established because relatively little is known concerning the human requirement for these nutrients. The amount of dietary fat varies widely according to personal taste, money spent on food, and the availability of fat-rich foods. For example, only about 10% of the energy in the average diet of people living in Asia is furnished by fat, whereas in the United States, Canada, Scandinavia, Germany, and France, fat accounts for 40% to 45% of the caloric intake. *Many nutritionists believe that in order to promote optimal health, fat intake should not exceed more than 30% of the energy content of the diet. Of this, at least 50% should be in the form of unsaturated fats.* This recommendation is based on research that indicates that individuals with diets high in saturated fat tend to be more susceptible to coronary heart disease as well as to other diseases such as cancer (both saturated and unsatu-

rated fat) and diabetes. However, to attempt to eliminate "all" fat from the diet may be unwise and detrimental in terms of exercise performance. With low-fat diets, it is difficult to increase one's intake of carbohydrate and protein to furnish sufficient energy to maintain a stable body weight during strenuous training. Also, because the essential fatty acid, linoleic acid, and many vitamins gain entrance to the body through dietary fat, a low-fat diet could eventually result in a relative state of malnutrition.

The prominence of carbohydrates in the diet also varies widely throughout the world, depending upon factors such as the availability and relative cost of fat and protein-rich foods. Carbohydrate-rich foods such as grains, starchy roots, and dried peas and beans are usually the cheapest foods in relation to their energy value. In the Far East, carbohydrates (rice) contribute 80% of the total caloric intake, whereas in the United States only about 40% to 50% of the energy requirement comes from carbohydrates. Most evidence suggests that there is no health hazard in subsisting chiefly on carbohydrates (starches), provided that the essential amino acids, minerals, and vitamins are also present in the diet. In fact, the diet of the relatively primitive Tarahumara Indians of Mexico is very high in complex carbohydrates (75% of calories) and fiber (19 mg/day) and correspondingly low in cholesterol (71 mg/day), fat (12% of calories), and saturated fat (2% of calories).[2a] These people are noted for their remarkable physical endurance: They reportedly run distances of up to 200 miles in competitive soccer-type sports events that often last several days! This type of diet may offer health benefits to those who partake of it: Particularly notable among the Tarahumaras is the virtual absence of hypertension, obesity, and death from cardiac and circulatory complications. On the other hand, in terms of energy requirements, there is no evidence that more than a small amount of carbohydrate need be present

in the diet if daily physical activity level is low. *However, if the individual is physically active, the "prudent" diet should contain at least 50% to 60% of its calories in the form of carbohydrates, predominantly starches.* In training for specific sports and prior to competition, the carbohydrate intake may even be increased above this recommended level in order to ensure adequate glycogen stores. The specific dietary–exercise techniques for facilitating glycogen storage are presented in Chapter 22.

Carbohydrate Needs in Prolonged, Severe Training

Athletes training for endurance activities such as distance running, swimming, cross-country skiing, or cycling frequently experience a state of chronic fatigue in which successive days of hard training become exceedingly more difficult. This "staleness" may be related to a gradual depletion of the body's carbohydrate re-

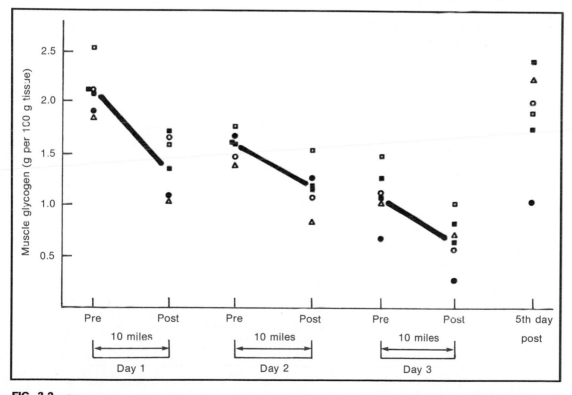

FIG. 3-2. *Changes in muscle glycogen concentration for 6 male subjects before and after each 16.1-km run performed on 3 successive days. Muscle glycogen was measured 5 days after the last run and is referred to as "fifth day post." (From Costill, D.L. et al.: Muscle glycogen utilization during prolonged exercise on successive days. J. Appl. Physiol., 31:834, 1971.)*

serves with repeated strenuous training, even though the athlete's diet contains the recommended percentage of carbohydrate.[4] As shown in Figure 3-2, after three successive days of running 16.1 km (10 miles) a day, the glycogen in the thigh muscle was nearly depleted. This occurred despite the fact that the daily food intake of the runners contained 40% to 60% carbohydrates. In addition, by the third day, the quantity of glycogen used during the run was much less than on the first day. Presumably, the energy for work was supplied predominantly by the body's fat reserves.

Even if the diet is high in carbohydrates, muscle glycogen is not rapidly restored to the preexercise level. Although liver glycogen is restored rapidly,[3] at least 48 hours are required to restore muscle glycogen levels after prolonged, exhaustive exercise.[7] From the values in Figure 3-2, some individuals may require more than 5 days to reestablish muscle glycogen levels if the diet contains only moderate amounts of carbohydrates. Unmistakably, if a person performs exercise on successive days, daily allowances must be adjusted to permit optimal glycogen resynthesis. *In addition, at least 2 days of rest and high carbohydrate intake must be provided to establish the preexercise muscle glycogen levels.*

The Four-Food-Group Plan: The Essentials of Good Nutrition

A practical approach to sound nutrition is to categorize foods that make similar nutrient contributions and then provide servings from each category in the daily diet. A key word is variety. This can be readily achieved by use of the Four-Food-Group Plan illustrated in Table 3-1. As long as the recommended number of servings from the variety provided in each group is supplied, and cooking and handling is proper, adequate nutrition is assured. More of these and other foods can be used as needed for growth, for activity, and for desirable weight.

Table 3-2 presents examples of three daily menus formulated from the guidelines of the basic diet plan shown in Table 3-1. These menus provide *all* essential nutrients, even though the energy value of each is considerably below the average adult requirement. In fact, these menus serve as excellent nutritional models for reducing diets. For active individuals whose daily energy requirement may be as large as 5000 Calories, all that need be done once the essentials are provided is to increase the quantity of food consumed; this is achieved either by increasing the size of portions, the fre-

TABLE 3-1. *The Four-Food-Group Plan—the foundation for a good diet*

FOOD CATEGORY	EXAMPLES	RECOMMENDED DAILY SERVINGS[c]
1. Milk and milk products[a]	Milk, cheese, ice cream, sour cream, yogurt	2
2. Meat and high-protein[b]	meat, fish, poultry, eggs—with dried beans, peas, nuts, or peanut butter as alternatives	2
3. Vegetables and fruits	Dark green or yellow vegetables; citrus fruits or tomatoes	4
4. Cereal and grain food	Enriched breads, cereals, flour, baked goods, or whole-grain products	4

[a] If large quantities of milk are normally consumed, *fortified* skimmed milk should be substituted to reduce the quantity of saturated fats.
[b] Fish, chicken, and high-protein vegetables contain significantly less saturated fats than other protein sources.
[c] A basic serving of meat or fish is usually 100 g or 3.5 oz of edible food; 1 cup (8 oz) milk; 1 oz cheese; ½ cup fruit, vegetables, juice; 1 slice bread; ½ cup cooked cereal or 1 cup ready-to-eat cereal.

TABLE 3-2. *Three daily menus formulated from guidelines established by the Four-Food-Group Plan*[a]

3 MEALS A DAY	5 MEALS A DAY	6 SMALL MEALS A DAY
Breakfast	**Breakfast**	**Breakfast**
½ cup unsweetened grapefruit juice	½ grapefruit	½ cup orange juice
1 poached egg 1 slice toast	⅔ cup bran flakes	¾ cup ready-to-eat cereal
1 teaspoon butter or margarine	1 cup skim or low-fat milk or	½ cup skim milk
½ cup skim milk	other beverage	tea or coffee, black
tea or coffee, black		
	Snack	**Mid-Morning Snack**
Lunch	1 small package raisins	⅓ cup low fat cottage cheese
2 ounces lean roast beef	½ bologna sandwich	
½ cup cooked summer squash		**Lunch**
1 slice rye bread	**Lunch**	2 ounces sliced turkey on
1 teaspoon butter or margarine	1 slice pizza	1 slice white toast
1 cup skim milk	carrot sticks	1 teaspoon butter or margarine
10 grapes	1 apple	2 canned drained peach halves
	1 cup skim or low-fat milk	½ cup skim milk
Dinner		
3 ounces poached haddock	**Snack**	**Mid-Afternoon Snack**
½ cup cooked spinach	1 banana	1 cup fresh spinach and lettuce salad
tomato and lettuce salad		2 teaspoons oil + vinegar or lemon
1 teaspoon oil + vinegar or lemon	**Dinner**	3 saltines
1 small biscuit	baked fish with	
1 teaspoon butter or margarine	mushrooms (3 oz.)	**Dinner**
½ cup canned drained	baked potato	1 cup clear broth
fruit cocktail	2 teaspoons margarine	3 ounces broiled chicken breast
½ cup skim milk	½ cup broccoli	⅓ cup cooked rice with
	1 cup tomato juice or skim or	1 teaspoon butter or margarine
	low-fat milk	¼ cup cooked mushrooms
		½ cup cooked broccoli
		½ cup skim milk
		Evening Snack
		1 medium apple
		½ cup skim milk
Total Calories: about 1200	Total Calories: about 1400	Total Calories: about 1200

[a]Each menu provides *all* essential nutrients; the energy or caloric value of the diet can be easily increased by increasing the size of the portions, the frequency of meals, or the variety of foods consumed at each sitting.

quency of meals or snacks, or the variety of nutritious foods consumed at each meal.

EXERCISE AND FOOD INTAKE

For individuals who engage regularly in moderate to intense physical activity, it is particularly easy to match food intake with the daily level of energy expenditure. Lumbermen, for example, who expend about 4500 Calories daily, unconsciously adjust their caloric intake to balance closely their energy output. Consequently, body weight remains stable despite an extremely large food consumption. The balancing of food intake to meet a new level of energy output takes about a day or so, during which time a new energy equilibrium is attained. Apparently, this fine balance between energy expenditure and food intake is not maintained in sedentary people.[6] Here, the caloric intake generally exceeds the daily energy expenditure. This lack of precision in the regulation of food intake at the low end of the physical activity spectrum probably accounts for the "creeping obesity" commonly observed in highly mechanized and technically advanced societies.

It was reported that the daily food intake of *athletes* in the 1936 Olympics averaged more than 7000 Calories, or roughly three times the average daily intake.[1] For these competitors, the protein intake amounted to 19% of the total caloric intake (320 g), whereas fat and carbohydrate contributed 35% (270 g) and 46% (800 g), respectively. These caloric values are often quoted and used to justify what appears to be an enormous food requirement of athletes in training. It should be noted, however, that these figures are only estimates because objective dietary data were not presented in the original report. In all likelihood, they are inflated estimates of the energy expended (and required) by the athletes. For example, distance runners who train upward of 100 miles per week (6 min per mile pace at about 15 Calories per min) probably do not expend more than 800 to 1300 Calories each day in excess of their normal energy requirement. For these endurance athletes, the daily food intake should supply about 4000 Calories.

A more objective evaluation of the nutrient intake of highly trained athletes as estimated from dietary recall is presented in Table 3-3. These relatively large athletes were in the peak of training and were in good health as judged by physiologic, medical, and performance measures. The average of 4663 Calories consumed each day exceeded the average American adult's intake by about 67%. Protein intake exceeded by 137% the recommended requirement whereas the above-average fat and carbohydrate intake supplied the energy requirements of training. The intake of all vitamins and minerals significantly exceeded recommendations of the Food and Nutrition Board. This "excess" of nutrients is due largely to the increased food intake and in no way suggests a "requirement" above the recommended guidelines.

THE PREGAME MEAL

The main purpose of the pregame meal is to provide the athlete with adequate food energy and assure optimal hydration. Within this framework, the food preferences of the athlete, the "psychologic set" of the competition, and the digestibility of the foods should be considered. As a general rule, foods that are high in fat content should be eliminated from the diet on the day of competition because these foods are digested slowly and remain in the digestive tract for a longer time than foods containing amounts of similar energy in the form of carbohydrates.

TABLE 3-3. Comparison of the nutrient intakes of United States Olympic-caliber athletes with RDA values[a,b]

	TOTAL CALORIES	PROTEIN (g)	CARBOHYDRATES (g)	FAT (g)	MINERALS (mg)		VITAMINS (mg)				
					Ca	Fe	THIAMIN	RIBOFLAVIN	NIACIN	C	A_{TU}
Athletes (N = 16) Mean	4663	237	446	203	2158	29	3.3	4.9	43	165	8850
RDA	2700 (4250)[c]	100[d]	100[e]	130[f]	800	10	1.4	1.6	18	45	5000
Absolute amount greater than RDA	+1963 (+413)[c]	+137	+346	+73	+1358	+19	+1.9	+3.3	+25	+120	+3840
Percent greater than RDA	+73 (+9.7)[c]	+137	+346	+56	+170	+190	+136	+206	+139	+267	+77

[a] From Ward, P. et al.: U.S.A. Discus Camp: Preliminary Report. Track & Field Quart. Rev. 76:29, 1976.
[b] Recommended daily allowance proposed by the Food and Nutrition Board. Recommended Dietary Allowances, 8th ed. Washington, D.C., National Academy of Sciences, 1974.
[c] Recommended daily caloric intake for persons engaged in heavy manual work or athletic training. Canadian Council on Nutrition. Dietary Standard of Canada. Can. Bull. Nutr. 6:1, 1964.
[d] Based on National Research Council standards of 0.9 g/kg body weight per day. The average weight of the athletes was 110.7 kg.
[e] Minimal requirement proposed by the Food and Nutrition Board of the National Research Council to prevent undesirable metabolic responses.

The time at which the pregame meal is eaten does not appear to be an important consideration, at least in terms of exercise performance. Table 3-4 presents data from a study of 14 high school swimmers.[2] Each athlete consumed a "typical" breakfast consisting of dry cereal, toast (2 slices), sugar, butter, and skimmed milk. The meal was eaten at either 0.5, 1.0, 1.5, 2.0, 2.5, or 3.0 hours prior to the exercise performance tests. As shown, these meal schedules had no effect on all-out swimming performance for 100 yards. In addition, none of the subjects reported adverse effects in the form of nausea or stomach cramps during or following any of the swim trials. Subsequent experiments using exercise of longer duration have essentially substantiated these observations. However, because the main function of the pregame meal is to provide food energy and water, sufficient time should be allowed for the meal to be digested and absorbed by the body.

One further consideration must be made concerning the timing of the pre-event meal. With the increased stress and tension that usually accompany competition (which may not have been the case in the research experiments), there may be a significant decrease in blood flow to the stomach and small intestines and an accompanying decrease in absorption from the digestive tract. *A 3-hour period should be sufficient to provide for adequate absorption of the pre-event meal.*

TABLE 3-4. *Effects of eating at various times upon swimming performance*[a]

FOOD CONSUMED	(g)
Protein	20.4
Carbohydrate	76.6
Fat	7.8
Calories	472 kcal

EATING TIMES BEFORE SWIM PERFORMANCE, (h)	100-YARD SWIM PERFORMANCE TIME, (s)
0.5	77.7
1.0	78.5
1.5	78.6
2.0	77.8
2.5	78.1
3.0	78.5

[a] From Ball, J.: Effects of eating at various times upon subsequent performance in swimming. Res. Quart. *33*:163–167, 1962.

Protein or Carbohydrate?

Many athletes are psychologically accustomed and even dependent on the "classic" pregame meal, which usually consists of steak and eggs. Although this meal may be satisfying to the athlete, coach, and restauranteur, its benefits in terms of exercise performance have yet to be demonstrated. In fact, such a meal, which is actually low in carbohydrates, may be detrimental to optimal performance.

There are several reasons for modifying or even abolishing the high-protein, pregame meal in favor of one high in carbohydrates. For one thing, carbohydrates are digested and absorbed more rapidly than either proteins or fats. Thus, this food is available for energy faster and may also reduce the feeling of fullness usually experienced following a meal. Furthermore, the digestion, absorption, and assimilation of a high-protein meal elevate the resting metabolic rate considerably more than similar treatment of a high-fat, high-carbohydrate meal. This metabolic heat adds additional strain to the body's heat-dissipating mechanisms that could be detrimental to exercise performance in hot weather. Concurrently, the breakdown of protein for energy facilitates dehydration during exercise. This is because the by-products of amino acid breakdown demand large amounts of water for urinary excretion.

Equally important for favoring carbohydrate intake is the fact that this is the main nutrient energy source for intense exercise and is also of crucial importance in prolonged exercise. The pregame meal must provide adequate quantities of this nutrient, to assure a normal level of blood glucose and sufficient glycogen "energy reserves" for most activities, *provided that the athlete has maintained a nutritionally sound diet throughout training.* For the endurance athlete, the pre-event meal should be high in carbohydrates to assure peak storage of liver and muscle glycogen. This is usually achieved in conjunction with other specific exercise-dietary modifications discussed more fully in Chapter 22. Although the wisdom of excessive carbohydrate intake, especially in the form of simple sugars, for prolonged periods of time has yet to be adequately established, it is certainly sound nutrition to allow athletes access to carbohydrates in a pre-event meal as well as in snacks before competition.

A moderately large glucose challenge right

before an endurance activity may actually impair subsequent performance. For example, the riding time of young men and women on a bicycle ergometer was reduced 19% when they consumed a 300-ml solution containing 75 g of glucose 30 minutes before exercise, compared to similar trials preceded by the same volume of water or a liquid meal of protein, fat, and carbohydrate.[5] The mobilization of free fatty acids for energy was depressed throughout the glucose trial. The impaired use of fats for energy in endurance exercise reduces the carbohydrate-sparing effect of fat metabolism, thereby causing the glycogen stores in the muscles to be used more rapidly. This negative effect of glucose feeding is probably mediated by an increased insulin output following the glucose challenge and the inhibitory effects of insulin on fat mobilization. Thus, if large quantities of sugars are consumed prior to competition, sufficient time must be provided to permit assimilation of this nutrient and to permit reestablishment of metabolic and hormonal balance.

Liquid Meals

Commercially prepared liquid meals such as Nutrament, Sustagen, Susta Cal, and Ensure offer an alternate and seemingly effective approach to the pre-event meal. These foods are well balanced in nutritive value. They are high in carbohydrate yet contain enough fat and protein to contribute to a feeling of satiety. Because they are in liquid form, they also contribute to the athlete's fluid needs. The liquid meal is also advantageous because it is digested rapidly and completely, leaving essentially no residue in the intestinal tract. This approach to proper nutrition on the day of competition is especially effective during day-long meets such as in swimming and track, or in some tennis and basketball tournaments. In these situations, an athlete has relatively little time (or interest) for food. Liquid meals may also provide a practical approach to the supplementation of the daily caloric intake of athletes who have difficulty maintaining body weight or who are desirous of increasing body weight.

SUMMARY

1. Many dietary options are available for obtaining the required nutrients for tissue maintenance, repair, and growth. Within rather broad limits, the nutrient requirements of athletes and other individuals engaged in training programs can be achieved with a balanced diet. With well-planned menus, the necessary vitamin, mineral, and protein requirements can be met with a food intake of about 1200 kcal a day. Additional food can then be consumed to meet the energy needs that fluctuate, depending on the daily level of physical activity.

2. The recommended protein intake is about 0.9 g of protein per kg body weight. For the average man and woman, this is a liberal requirement and represents about 15% of the daily total caloric intake.

3. Athletes generally consume two to three times the recommended protein intake. This is because the proportionately greater caloric intake of physically active people usually provides proportionately more protein.

4. Precise recommendations for fat and carbohydrate intake have not been established. A prudent recommendation is that 30% of the daily calories be obtained from fats; of this, half should be in the form of unsaturated fatty acids because excessive intake of saturated fats is related to various diseases, especially coronary heart disease. For people who are physically active, 50% to 60% of the calories should come from carbohydrates, particularly polysaccharides.

5. Successive days of prolonged, hard training may gradually deplete the body's carbohydrate reserves, even if the recommended carbohydrate intake is maintained. This could lead to a training "staleness" because muscle glycogen may take several days to return to normal levels following a single session of prolonged exercise.

6. Because sustained vigorous exercise can increase the metabolic rate 20 to 25 times, the most important factor determining the daily caloric requirement is one's level of physical activity. In all likelihood, however, the caloric requirements of athletes in the most strenuous sports do not exceed 5000 kcal per day. Such a high caloric intake usually supplies well above the RDA requirements for protein, vitamins, and minerals.

7. The pre-event meal should include foods that are readily digested and contribute to the energy and fluid requirements of exercise. For this reason, the meal should be high in carbohydrate and relatively low in fat and protein.

Clearly, the typical low-carbohydrate "steak-and-eggs diet" does not meet the requirements for optimal pre-event nutrition.

8. Commercially prepared liquid meals offer a practical approach to pregame nutrition and caloric supplementation. These "meals" are well balanced in nutritive value, contribute to fluid needs, and are absorbed rapidly, leaving practically no residue in the digestive tract.

9. Two or three hours should be sufficient time to permit digestion and absorption of the pre-event meal.

References

1. Abrahams, A.: The nutrition of athletes. Br. J. Nutr., 2:266, 1948.
2. Ball, J.R.: Effects of eating at various times upon subsequent performance in swimming. Res. Quart., 33:163, 1962.
2a. Connor, W.E. et al.: The plasma lipids, lipoproteins, and diet of the Tarahumara Indians of Mexico. Am. J. Clin. Nutr., 31:1131, 1978.
3. Costill, D.L.: Nutritional requirements for endurance athletes. In Toward an Understanding of Human Performance. Edited by E.J. Burke. Ithaca, N.Y., Mouvement Publications, 1977.
4. Costill, D.L. et al.: Muscle glycogen utilization during prolonged exercise on successive days. J. Appl. Physiol. 31:834, 1971.
5. Foster, C. et al.: Effects of pre-exercise feedings on endurance performance. Med. Sci. Sports, 11:1, 1979.
6. Mayer, J. et al.: Relation between caloric intake, body weight and physical work in an industrial male population in West Bengal. Am. J. Clin. Nutr., 4:169, 1956.
6a. Percy, E.C.: Ergogenic aids in athletics. Med. Sci. Sports, 10:298. 1978.
7. Piehl, K.: Glycogen storage and depletion in human skeletal muscle fibers. Acta Physiol. Scand., Supplement 402, 1974.
8. Smith, N.J.: Food for Sport. Palo Alto, Calif., Bull Publishing Co., 1976.
9. Ward, P. et al.: U.S.A. discus camp: Preliminary report. Track Field Quart. Rev., 76:29, 1976.
10. Werblow, J.A.: Nutritional knowledge, attitudes, and food patterns of women athletes. Journal of the American Dietetic Association, 73:242, 1978.

General References

Bogert, L.J. et al.: Nutrition and Physical Fitness. Philadelphia, W.B. Saunders Co., 1979.
Deutsch, R.M.: Realities of Nutrition. Palo Alto, Calif., Bull Publishing Co., 1976.
Goodhart, R.S., and Shils, M.E. (Eds.): Modern Nutrition in Health and Disease, 6th ed. Philadelphia, Lea & Febiger, 1980.
Higdon, H.: The Complete Diet. Mountain View, Calif., World Publications, 1978.
Pařízková, J., and Rogozkin, V.A.: Nutrition, Physical Fitness and Health. Baltimore, University Park Press, 1978.
Smith, N.J.: Food for Sport. Palo Alto, Calif., Bull Publishing Co., 1976.
Williams, M.H.: Nutritional Aspects of Human Physical and Athletic Performance. Springfield, Ill., Charles C Thomas, 1976.
Williams, R.J.: Nutrition in a Nutshell. New York, Dolphin Books, 1962.

SECTION II
Energy for Physical Activity

Considerable energy is generated rapidly for short periods of time by certain biochemical reactions that do not consume oxygen. This form of rapid anaerobic energy is crucial in maintaining a high standard of performance in sprint activities and in other all-out bursts of exercise. In comparison, in performing exercise of longer duration, energy must be extracted from food through reactions that require oxygen. To be effective, the physiologic conditioning process necessitates a basic understanding of how energy is generated to sustain exercise and of the energy requirements of a particular activity.

This section presents a broad overview of how cells extract chemical energy bound in the food nutrients and use it to power biologic work. Emphasis is placed on the importance of the food nutrients and the processes of energy transfer in sustaining physiologic function during light, moderate, and strenuous exercise.

Energy Value

of Food

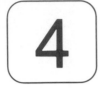

All biologic functions require energy. Because the carbohydrate, fat, and protein food nutrients contain the energy that ultimately powers biologic work, it is possible to classify both food and physical activity in terms of *energy*. This chapter deals with the quantification of food energy. In subsequent chapters, human energy expenditure during rest and physical activity is explored.

MEASUREMENT OF FOOD ENERGY

Unit of Measurement, the Calorie

A Calorie (spelled with a capital C) is a measure frequently used to express the heat or energy value of food and physical activity. It is defined as the amount of heat necessary to raise the temperature of 1 kg (1 liter) of water 1° C, from 14.5 to 15.5° C. Thus, a Calorie is more accurately termed a *kilogram Calorie,* or kilocalorie (abbreviated *kcal*). For example, if 300 kcal is the caloric value of a particular food, then the energy trapped within the chemical bonds of this food, if released, would change the temperature of 300 liters of water by 1° C. Different foods contain different amounts of energy. One-half cup of apricot nectar, for example, has a caloric value of 70 kcal and therefore contains the equivalent heat energy to increase the temperature of only 70 liters of water 1° C.

Gross Energy Value of Foods

Many laboratories throughout the world have used a *bomb calorimeter,* similar to that shown in Figure 4-1, to measure the gross or total energy value of the various food nutrients. The principle behind this method of *direct calorimetry* is simple—the food is burned and the heat liberated measured.

As depicted in the figure, a piece of food is placed inside the chamber, which is then charged with oxygen. A fuse and an electric current are used to ignite the food–oxygen mixture. As the food burns, the heat liberated is absorbed by a water jacket surrounding the bomb. Since the calorimeter is fully insulated from the outside environment, any increase in water temperature directly reflects the heat liberated during the oxidation of the specific food nutrient.

The heat liberated by the burning or *oxidation* of food is referred to as its *heat of combustion* and represents the total energy value of the food. For example, when one teaspoon of margarine is completely burned in the calorimeter, 100 kcal of heat energy is released. This is

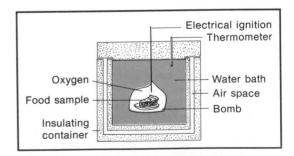

FIG. 4-1. *A bomb calorimeter is used to determine the energy value of foods. From* Nutrition, Weight Control, and Exercise *by Frank I. Katch and William D. McArdle. Copyright © 1977 by Houghton Mifflin Company. Reprinted by permission of the publisher.*

50

enough energy to raise 1.0 kg or 2.2 lb of ice water to the boiling point. It is important to point out that although the pathways for oxidation are quite different between the intact organism and the bomb calorimeter, the quantity of energy liberated in the breakdown of food is the same and is independent of the pathways by which combustion occurs.

HEAT OF COMBUSTION: FAT. The heat of combustion for fat varies somewhat depending upon the structural composition of the particular fatty acids that make up the triglycerides. For example, 1 g of either beef or pork fat yields 9.50 kcal, whereas the oxidation of 1 g of butterfat liberates 9.27 kcal. The average caloric value for one gram of fat in meat, fish, and eggs is 9.50 kcal per gram, in dairy products, 9.25 kcal per gram, and in vegetables and fruits, 9.30 kcal per gram. *The average heat of combustion per gram of fat oxidized in the calorimeter is generally considered to be 9.4 kcal.*

HEAT OF COMBUSTION: CARBOHYDRATE. The heat of combustion for a carbohydrate also varies depending upon the arrangement of atoms in the particular carbohydrate molecule. The simple carbohydrate glucose has a heat of combustion of 3.74 kcal per gram, whereas a gram of glycogen and starch liberates 4.19 and 4.20 kcal, respectively. *A value of 4.2 kcal is generally used to represent the heat of combustion for a gram of carbohydrate.*

HEAT OF COMBUSTION: PROTEIN. The heat energy released during the combustion of the protein portion of food also varies depending on two factors: (1) the kind of protein in the food, and (2) the relative proportions of the protein and nonprotein nitrogenous substances present. Many common proteins contain approximately 16% nitrogen with a corresponding heat of combustion that averages 5.75 kcal per gram. These proteins are found in foods such as eggs, meat, corn (maize), and beans (jack, lima, navy, soy). Proteins in the other food items have a somewhat higher nitrogen content such as most nuts and seeds (18.9%), whole-kernel wheat, rye, millets, and barley (17.2%), whereas other foods contain a slightly lower percentage of nitrogen such as whole milk (15.7%) or bran (15.8%). *A general value for the heat of combustion of protein is 5.65 kcal per gram.*

COMPARISON OF THE ENERGY VALUE OF NUTRIENTS. Based on the average heats of combustion for the three nutrients (carbohydrate, 4.2 kcal $\cdot$ g^{-1}; fat, 9.4 kcal $\cdot$ g^{-1}; protein, 5.65 kcal $\cdot$ g^{-1}), it is clear that the complete oxidation of fat in the bomb calorimeter liberates about 65% more energy per gram than protein, and 120% more energy than an equal weight of carbohydrate. It should be recalled from Chapter 1 that the fat molecule contains considerably more hydrogen atoms than either the carbohydrate or protein molecule. The fatty acid palmitic acid, for example, has the structural formula $C_{16}H_{32}O_2$. For this molecule as well as for other fat molecules, the ratio of hydrogen atoms to oxygen atoms is always considerably greater than 2 to 1. Thus, compared with carbohydrate and protein molecules, there are more hydrogen atoms in fat molecules that can be cleaved away and oxidized to generate energy for the body's needs.

From the previous discussion, it is evident that the energy content of food that contains a considerable amount of fat is greater than that of food that is relatively fat-free. For example, one cup of whole milk contains 160 kcal, whereas the same quantity of skimmed milk contains only 90 kcal. If someone who normally consumes one quart of whole milk each day switches to skimmed milk, the total calories ingested each year would be reduced by an amount equal to 25 pounds of fat!

Net Energy Value of Foods: Coefficient of Digestibility

The energy value of a particular food is not exactly the same when its heat of combustion (gross energy value) as determined by direct calorimetry is compared with the *net* energy actually available to the body. This is especially true for proteins because the body cannot utilize this nutrient's nitrogen component. Thus, nitrogen combines with hydrogen to form urea, which is then excreted in the urine. The elimination of hydrogen represents a loss of potential energy that reduces the heat of combustion of protein in the body to approximately 4.3 kcal per gram instead of the 5.65 kcal released during its complete oxidation in the bomb calorimeter. Because carbohydrates and fats contain no nitrogen, their physiologic fuel value is *identical* to the heat of combustion determined by bomb calorimetry.

Another consideration in determining the ultimate caloric yield from the food nutrients is the efficiency of the digestive process. The *coefficient of digestibility* refers to the proportion of ingested food that is actually digested and absorbed to serve the metabolic needs of the body. The remainder is not absorbed completely from the intestinal tract and is voided in the feces.

Table 4-1 presents the digestibility coefficients as well as the heats of combustion and net energy values of nutrients in various food groups. As can be seen, there are different coefficients of digestibility for the different food nutrients. The relative percents of each food nutrient that are completely digested and absorbed are 97%, 95%, and 92% for carbohydrate, fat, and protein, respectively. It should be kept in mind, however, that these are only averages, and some variability can be expected in efficiency percentages for any food within a particular category. This is especially true for proteins, in which the digestive efficiency ranges from a low of about 78% for legumes to a high of 97% for protein from animal sources.

From the data in Table 4-1, *the average net energy value for carbohydrates, fats, and proteins ingested in the diet can be rounded to the simple whole numbers 4, 9, and 4 kcal per gram, respectively.* These values are referred to as the *Atwater general factors* and have been traditionally used by nutritionists for nearly 50 years to represent the energy available to the body from food nutrients. Except when exact energy values are desired, as in preparing experimental or therapeutic diets, the Atwater general factors can be used to estimate the net energy value of typical foods consumed in the American diet.

Using the Atwater factors, the caloric content of any portion of food can be determined if the composition and weight of the food are known. Table 4-2 illustrates the method for calculating the kcal value of 100 grams (3.5 oz) of vanilla ice cream. Based on laboratory analysis, vanilla ice cream contains approximately 4% protein, 13% fat, and 21% carbohydrate, with the remaining 62% essentially water. Thus, each gram of ice cream contains 0.04 g protein, 0.13 g fat, and 0.21 g carbohydrate. Using these compositional values and the Atwater factors, the kcal value per gram of ice cream is determined as follows: The net kcal values indicate that 0.04 g of protein contains 0.16 kcal $(0.04 \times 4.0 \text{ kcal} \cdot \text{g}^{-1})$, 0.13 g fat equals 1.17 kcal $(0.13 \times 9 \text{ kcal} \cdot \text{g}^{-1})$, and 0.21 g carbohydrate yields 0.84 kcal $(0.21 \times 4.0 \text{ kcal} \cdot \text{g}^{-1})$. Consequently, the total energy value for each gram of vanilla ice cream equals 2.17 kcal $(0.16 + 1.17 + 0.84)$. For a 100-g serving, the caloric value is 100 times as large, or 217 kcal. This method of computation can be used to estimate the kcal value for any food serving. Of course, increasing or decreasing portion sizes, or adding extra-rich sauces or calorie-free substitutes, would affect the caloric content accordingly.

This procedure for computing the kcal of foods is time-consuming and laborious. Because of this, the United States Department of Agriculture has evaluated and compiled the nutritive value of over 2,500 food items. Appendix B presents a sample listing of some of the more common foods consumed in the American diet. One should keep in mind that caloric and nutritive values for specific food dishes such as creamed chicken are computed from standard recipes and may vary considerably, depending on taste preference and method of preparation.

If Appendix B is examined carefully, it is observed that there are large differences in the energy values of various foods. To consume an equal number of calories from different foods often requires a tremendous intake of a particular food. For example, in order to consume 100 kcal each of four common foods, carrots, green peppers, medium-sized eggs, and mayonnaise, one must eat 5 carrots, 4 cups of green peppers, $1\frac{1}{4}$ eggs, and only 1 tablespoon of mayonnaise.

To meet the daily energy requirements of an average adult, one would have to consume 120 carrots, 96 cups of green pepper, 30 eggs, but only $1\frac{1}{2}$ cup of mayonnaise. This illustrates dramatically that foods high in fat contain considerable calories compared to food low in fat and correspondingly high in water content.

Another important consideration, however, is that a calorie is a measure of food energy, regardless of its source. Thus, 100 calories from mayonnaise is no more fattening than the 100 calories contained in 5 cups of raw cabbage. The more one eats of a given food, the more calories one consumes. It is just that only a small quantity of fatty foods represents a considerable quantity of calories—thus, these foods are considered fattening. An individual's caloric intake is simply equal to the sum of *all* calories consumed, be they from a small or large quantity of food.

TABLE 4-1. *Factors for digestibility, heats of combustion, and net physiologic energy values*[a] *of protein, fat, and carbohydrate*[b]

FOOD GROUP	DIGESTIBILITY, (%)	HEAT OF COMBUSTION, (kcal·g^{-1})	NET ENERGY (kcal·g^{-1})
Protein			
Meats, fish	97	5.65	4.27
Eggs	97	5.75	4.37
Dairy products	97	5.65	4.27
Animal food	97	5.65	4.27
Cereals	85	5.80	3.87
Legumes	78	5.70	3.47
Vegetables	83	5.00	3.11
Fruits	85	5.20	3.36
Vegetable food	85	5.65	3.74
TOTAL FOOD	92	5.65	4.05
Fat			
Meat and eggs	95	9.50	9.03
Dairy products	95	9.25	8.79
Animal food	95	9.40	8.93
Vegetable food	90	9.30	8.37
TOTAL FOOD	95	9.40	8.93
Carbohydrate			
Animal food	98	3.90	3.82
Cereals	98	4.20	4.11
Legumes	97	4.20	4.07
Vegetables	95	4.20	3.99
Fruits	90	4.00	3.60
Sugars	98	3.95	3.87
Vegetable food	97	4.15	4.03
TOTAL FOOD	97	4.15	4.03

[a] Net physiologic energy values are computed as the coefficient of digestibility × heat of combustion adjusted for energy loss in urine.
[b] From Merrill, A. L., and Watt, B. K.: Energy value of foods . . . basis and derivation. Agricultural Handbook No. 74., Washington, D.C., U.S. Department of Agriculture, 1973.

TABLE 4-2. *Method of calculating the caloric value of a food when its composition of nutrients is known*

Food: ice cream (vanilla)
Weight: three-fourths cup = 100 grams

	COMPOSITION		
	PROTEIN	FAT	CARBOHYDRATE
Percentage	4%	13%	21%
Total grams	4	13	21
In one gram	.04	.13 g	.21
Calories per gram	.16	1.17	.84

$$(.04 \times 4.0 \text{ kcal}) + (.13 \times 9.0 \text{ kcal}) + (.21 \times 4.0 \text{ kcal})$$

Total calories per gram: .16 + 1.17 + .84 = 2.17 kcal
Total calories per 100 grams: 2.17 × 100 = 217 kcal

SUMMARY

1. A calorie or kilocalorie (kcal) is a measure of heat used to express the energy value of food. This food energy is directly measured in a bomb calorimeter.

2. The heat of combustion represents the heat liberated by the complete oxidation of food. For fats, carbohydrates, and proteins, these gross energy values are 9.4, 4.2 and 5.65 kcal per gram, respectively.

3. The coefficient of digestibility is the proportion of ingested food actually digested and absorbed to be used by the body. This represents about 98% for carbohydrates, 95% for fats, and 92% for proteins. Thus, the net energy values are 4, 9, and 4 kcal per gram for carbohydrates, fat, and protein, respectively. These values are referred to as the Atwater general factors and are used to estimate the net energy value of typical foods in the diet.

4. By use of these Atwater calorific values, it is possible to compute the caloric content of any food—as long as the carbohydrate, fat, and protein composition is known.

5. From an energy standpoint, a calorie is a unit of heat energy, regardless of the food source. Thus, it is incorrect to consider 100 kcal of ice cream any more fattening than 100 kcal of watermelon.

General References

Consolazio, C.F., Johnson, R., and Pecora, L.: Physiological Measurements of Metabolic Functions in Man. New York, McGraw-Hill, 1963.

Goodhart, R.S., and Shils, M.E.: Modern Nutrition in Health and Disease, 6th ed. Philadelphia, Lea & Febiger, 1980.

Guthrie, H.A.: Introductory Nutrition. St. Louis, C.V. Mosby, 1971.

Guyton, A.C.: Textbook of Medical Physiology. Philadelphia, W.B. Saunders Co., 1976.

Krause, M.V., and Hunscher, M.A.: Food, Nutrition and Diet Therapy. Philadelphia, W.B. Saunders Co., 1972.

Reed, P.B.: Nutrition: An Applied Science. St. Paul, Minn., West, 1980.

Introduction to Energy Transfer

5

The ability to swim, run, or ski long distances is framed largely by one's capacity to extract energy from the food nutrients and transfer it to the contractile elements of skeletal muscle. Likewise, specific energy-transferring capabilities determine success in weight lifting, sprinting, jumping, and football line play. Although our main frame of reference in this text is muscular activity, the direct transfer of chemical energy is required to power *all* forms of biologic work.

The sections that follow introduce general concepts dealing with bioenergetics. They provide the basis for understanding energy metabolism during various forms of physical activity.

ENERGY, THE CAPACITY FOR WORK

Unlike the physical properties of matter, it is difficult to define *energy* in concrete terms of size, shape, or mass. Rather, the term energy suggests a dynamic state related to a condition of *change*, because the presence of energy is revealed only when a change has taken place. Within this context, *energy relates to the ability to perform work*. As work increases, the transfer of energy also increases so that a change occurs.

The *first law of thermodynamics* states that energy is neither created nor destroyed, but rather is transformed from one form to another. In essence, this is the immutable principle of the *conservation of energy* that applies to both living and nonliving systems. The large amount of chemical energy in fuel oil, for example, is readily converted to heat energy in the home oil burner. In the body, however, all of the chemical energy trapped within the bonds of the food nutrients is not lost as heat; rather, a large portion is conserved as chemical energy and then changed into mechanical energy (and then ultimately heat energy) by the action of the musculoskeletal system. The underlying principle is that energy is *not* produced, consumed, or used up; it is only transformed from one form into another.

Potential and Kinetic Energy

The total energy of any system consists of two components, *potential* and *kinetic* energy. Potential energy can be energy of position, such as that possessed by a stone at the top of a hill; it can also be light energy, electric energy, or bound energy within the internal structure of a substance. *When potential energy is released, it is transformed into kinetic energy or energy of motion.* The conversion between potential and kinetic energy can take many forms. For example, the rearrangement of the chemical structure of a substance occurs when the bonds between atoms are broken. This results in the release of potential energy with a concomitant increase in kinetic energy. In some instances, the bound energy in one substance can be directly *transferred* to other substances to increase the potential energy of these molecules. Energy transfers of this type are necessary for the body's chemical work or *biosynthesis*. In this process, specific building-block molecules are activated and join other molecules in the synthesis of important biologic compounds. Some of these compounds serve structural needs, while others can then serve the energy needs of the cell.

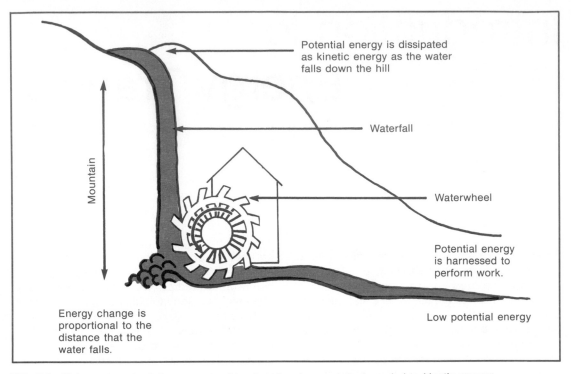

FIG. 5-1. *High-grade potential energy capable of performing work is degraded to kinetic energy.*

Figure 5-1 depicts the relationship between potential and kinetic energy as related to position. Relatively calm water at sea level has little potential energy and cannot drive the waterwheel. However, as water from a mountain stream flows downhill and over the fall, the water's potential energy is transformed into kinetic energy. Some of this energy is harnessed to turn the waterwheel. When the distance of the falling water increases, more kinetic energy is generated. Water at the top of the fall has more potential and less kinetic energy than water at the bottom, and vice versa. Thus, the potential energy stored in the water atop the fall changes into kinetic energy as it moves from a higher to a lower level.

Energy-Releasing and Energy-Conserving Processes

Any physical or chemical process that results in a release of energy to its surroundings is termed *exergonic*. Exergonic reactions can be viewed as "downhill" processes; they result in a decline in *free energy*, that is, "useful" energy that can do work. Processes that store or ab-

sorb energy are termed *endergonic;* these reactions represent "uphill" processes and proceed with an increase in free energy. In some instances, exergonic processes can be *coupled* or linked with endergonic reactions so that some of the energy is transferred to the endergonic process. *These coupled reactions are of considerable importance to the body because they serve as the means of conserving a large portion of the chemical energy in food nutrients in a usable form.* This subject is discussed more fully in the next chapter.

In exergonic chemical reactions, potential energy stored within specific atoms is released; the liberated energy is equal to the difference in the potential energy of the reactant and product substances. For example, the union of hydrogen and oxygen to form water releases 68 kcal of energy in the following reaction:

$$H_2 + O \longrightarrow H_2O \qquad -68 \text{ kcal per mole}$$

(The negative sign means that heat is lost from the system as the reaction proceeds. One mole or gram molecular weight represents the molecular weight of a substance in grams. For example, a mole of glucose weighs 180 g.)

This process is reversible. Thus, in the reverse endergonic reaction, the chemical bonds of the water molecule are broken and the original hydrogen and oxygen are set free. To achieve this, however, 68 kcal of energy must be supplied to each mole of water. This "uphill" process of energy transfer provides the hydrogen and oxygen atoms with their original energy content and thus satisfies the principle of the conservation of energy.

$$H_2 + O \longleftarrow H_2O \quad +68 \text{ kcal per mole}$$

The process of energy transfer in humans follows the same principles outlined in the waterfall–waterwheel example. The carbohydrate, fat, and protein nutrients possess considerable potential energy. Through the action of specific enzymes, there is a progressive loss of potential energy from the nutrient molecule and a corresponding increase in kinetic energy as product substances are formed. With the aid of appropriate transfer systems, a portion of this chemical energy is *conserved* in new compounds which are then utilized for biologic work.

The transfer of potential energy is unidirectional; it always proceeds so that the capacity of the total energy to perform work decreases. The tendency of potential energy to degrade to kinetic energy with a lower capacity for work represents a statement of the *second law of thermodynamics*. A good example is the car battery in which the electrochemical energy stored within the cells is slowly released, even if the battery is not used. The energy from sunlight is also continually degraded to heat energy when light strikes and is absorbed by a surface. Food and other chemicals are excellent stores of potential energy. However, this energy is eventually released as the compounds decompose through normal oxidative processes. Energy, like water, always runs downhill, whereby its potential energy is decreased. *Ultimately, all of the potential energy in a system is degraded to the nonusable form of kinetic energy or heat.*

INTERCONVERSIONS OF ENERGY

Because the total energy in an isolated system remains constant, a decrease in one form of energy is matched by an equivalent increase in another form. In the process of energy conversion, however, a loss of potential energy from one source can result in an increase in the potential energy of another source. Clearly, it has been possible to harness vast quantities of potential energy in nature for useful purposes. Even under such conditions, the tendency for *entropy* is dominant and the net flow of energy in the biologic world results in the degradation of potential energy.

Entropy is a measure of the continual process of energy change; it reflects the fact that all chemical and physical processes proceed in a direction in which total randomness or disorder increases and the energy available to do work decreases. In coupled reactions that occur during biosynthesis, part of a system may show a decrease in entropy whereas another part shows an increase. However, there is no circumventing the second law: The entire system always shows a net increase in entropy.

Forms of Energy

Energy can be categorized into six forms: chemical, mechanical, heat, light, electric, and nuclear (Fig. 5-2).

Examples of Energy Conversions

The conversion of energy from one form to another occurs readily in both the inanimate and animate worlds. The most fundamental examples of energy conversion in living cells are the processes of *photosynthesis* and *respiration.*

PHOTOSYNTHESIS. In the sun, with a temperature of several million degrees Farenheit, part of the potential energy stored in the nucleus of the hydrogen atom is released by the process of nuclear fusion. This energy in the form of gamma radiation is then converted to radiant energy.

As shown in Figure 5-3, the pigment chlorophyll in green plants absorbs solar (radiant) energy and transforms it into the chemical potential energy of carbohydrates through the reactions of photosynthesis. This endergonic process, which involves the synthesis of glucose from carbon dioxide and water and the release of oxygen, requires an input of 686 kcal of energy per mole (180 g) of glucose synthesized. Carbohydrates can be converted to fats and proteins for storage in the plant as a reserve of potential energy for future use. Animals then ingest the plant nutrients to serve

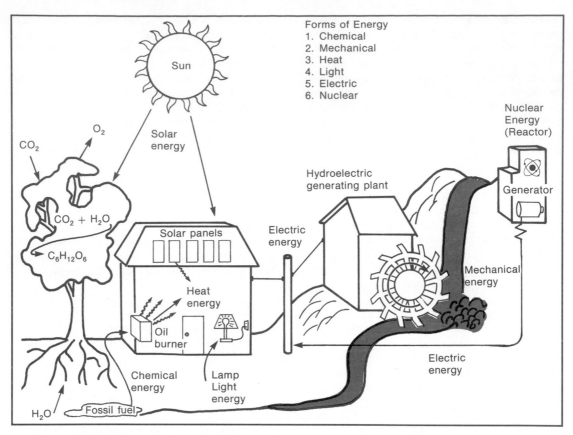

FIG. 5-2. *Interconversions of energy forms.*

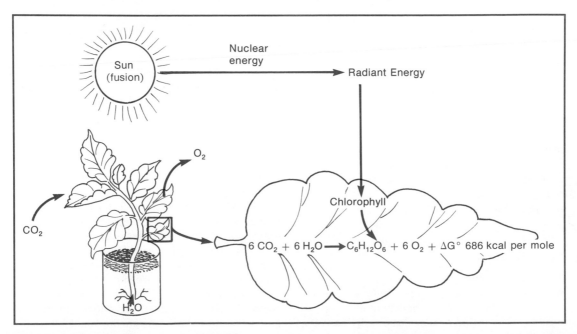

FIG. 5-3. *The endergonic process of photosynthesis. Endergonic reactions that require energy, as in the synthesis of glucose in green plants, have a positive standard free energy change (useful energy) indicated as* $+\Delta G°'$.

their own energy needs. In essence, solar energy, coupled with the process of photosynthesis, powers the animal world.

RESPIRATION. The process of respiration (Fig. 5-4) is the reverse of photosynthesis. During these exergonic reactions, the chemical energy stored in the glucose, fat, and protein molecules is extracted in the presence of oxygen. For glucose, this results in a release of 686 kcal per mole oxidized. *A portion of the energy released during respiration can be conserved in other chemical compounds and then converted to mechanical work in the body by the action of muscles; the remaining energy flows to the environment as heat.*

Biologic Work in Humans

The energy released during cellular respiration in humans is used to sustain biologic work. This work can take one of three familiar forms: (1) mechanical work of muscle contraction, (2) chemical work, which involves the synthesis of cellular molecules, or (3) transport work that concentrates various substances in the intra- and extracellular fluids.

MECHANICAL WORK. The most obvious example of energy transformation in the body is the mechanical work generated by muscle contraction. The protein filaments of the muscle fibers directly convert chemical energy into mechanical energy. However, this is not the body's only form of mechanical work. In the cell nucleus, for example, contractile elements similar to those found in muscle literally tug at the chromosomes to facilitate the process of cell division. Mechanical work is also performed by specialized structures such as cilia that are part of many cells.

CHEMICAL WORK. Chemical work is performed by all cells for growth and maintenance. Cellular components are continually synthesized as other components are destroyed. This biosynthesis opposes the tendency toward entropy and requires an input of energy for the bonding together of cellular elements.

TRANSPORT WORK. Much less conspicuous than mechanical or chemical work is the work of transporting or concentrating substances in the body. Cellular materials normally flow from an area of high concentration to one of low concentration. In this passive process, called

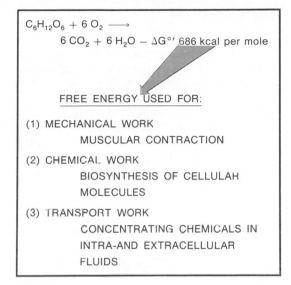

FIG. 5-4. *The exergonic process of respiration. Exergonic reactions that release potential energy, such as the burning of gasoline or the combustion of glucose, have a negative standard free energy change (i.e., reduction in total energy available to do work) indicated as* $-\Delta G°'$.

diffusion, no energy is required. However, for proper physiologic functioning, certain chemicals must also be transported "uphill" against their concentration gradients; that is, from an area of lower to one of higher concentration. The term *active transport* is usually associated with this process. Secretion and reabsorption in the kidney tubules require active transport, as does the establishment of proper electrochemical gradients about cell membranes. A continual expenditure of stored chemical energy is required to accomplish these "quiet" forms of biologic work.

FACTORS THAT AFFECT THE RATE OF BIOENERGETICS

The rate at which chemical energy in the food nutrients is extracted, conserved, and transferred to the contractile filaments of skeletal muscle determines the intensity at which exercise can progress. *The sustained pace of the marathon runner as well as the rapid speed of the sprinter is a direct expression of the body's capacity to transfer chemical energy into mechanical work.* Some factors that affect the rate of energy release during chemical reactions will now be considered.

The Mass Action Effect

The effect of the concentration of chemicals on the frequency of a particular chemical reaction reflects the *law of mass action* and is called *the mass action effect.* It is not uncommon to find certain substances in the body that are tied to several reactions; thus, the products of one reaction become reactant substances for other reactions. Thus, changing only the concentration of one substance can profoundly affect a number of reactions. Also, certain chemicals play key roles in a whole chain of chemical events. Oxygen, for example, exerts a significant mass action effect on reactions required for energy transfer. If the oxygen supply to the tissues is diminished, a number of chemical processes cease and the net energy available for biologic work is reduced dramatically.

Enzymes: The Biologic Catalysts

Enzymes are highly specific protein *catalysts* that accelerate the speed of a chemical reaction. The compound changed in an enzyme-regulated reaction is called the *substrate* for that enzyme. Enzymes do not make reactions occur that could not otherwise take place under proper conditions; rather, they facilitate the interaction of substrates that normally would occur at a much slower rate. In a way, enzymes reduce the required activation energy so that the reaction rate is changed, even though the total energy released per reaction remains unaltered.

Enzymes possess the unique property of not being readily altered by the reactions in which they participate. Consequently, the turnover of enzymes in the body is relatively slow and specific enzymes are continually reused. Because enzymes are proteins, they are adversely affected by temperature, especially heat. Another important characteristic of enzymes is their *specificity* in interacting with other substances. For example, the breakdown of glucose to carbon dioxide and water requires nineteen different chemical reactions, each catalyzed by a specific enzyme. In humans, about 900 different enzymes have been identified with each performing its specific role in a different chemical reaction. The activation of molecules is the important characteristic of enzyme-regulated processes and ensures that a reaction will occur more readily. In fact, it is only through the action of enzymes that cells function as chemical engines.

Role of Coenzymes

Some enzymes are totally inactive in the absence of additional substances termed *coenzymes.* These are complex, nonprotein, organic substances that facilitate enzyme action by helping to bind the substrate with its specific enzyme.

The action of a coenzyme is less specific than that of an enzyme because the coenzyme may act in a number of different reactions. It can act as a "co-binder," or it can serve as a temporary carrier of intermediary products of the reaction. For example, the hydrogen atoms and electrons split from the nutrient substrates during energy metabolism are temporarily carried by the coenzyme *nicotinamide adeninedinucleotide,* or NAD^+, to form NADH. The electrons are then passed to special carrier molecules that ultimately deliver them to molecular oxygen.

Vitamins serve a major role as coenzymes in the transfer of chemical energy. As coenzymes, these vitamins *do not* directly provide chemical energy, although in a sense, they "make the reactions go."

MEASURING ENERGY RELEASE IN HUMANS

The gain or loss in the heat of a system provides a simple means for determining the energy change of any process. In the breakdown of foods, for example, the energy change can be determined *directly* in a calorimeter. This heat energy is usually expressed in terms of calories or kilocalories.

Because the complete combustion of food is achieved at the expense of molecular oxygen, the heat generated in these exergonic reactions can also be conveniently and accurately estimated by measuring oxygen consumption. This forms the basis of *indirect calorimetry* and enables us to infer readily the energy metabolism of humans at rest and during almost any form of physical activity. The use of direct and indirect calorimetry for determining heat production in humans is discussed fully in Chapter 8. At this point, however, a general scheme for energy flow and subsequent measurement by these techniques is shown in Figure 5-5.

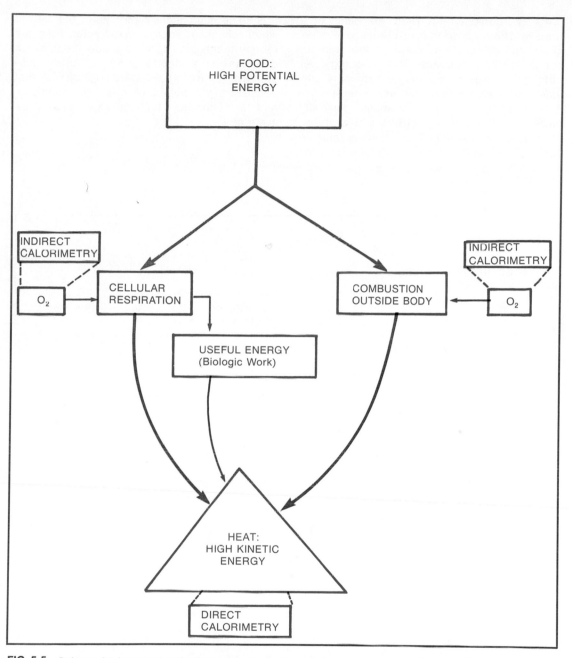

FIG. 5-5. *Scheme for heat flow and subsequent measurement of energy release by direct and indirect calorimetry. (Courtesy of Dr. G.A. Brooks, University of California, Berkeley.)*

SUMMARY

1. Energy is defined as the ability to perform work and therefore is revealed only when *change* takes place.

2. Energy exists in either a potential or kinetic form. Potential energy is the energy associated with substances because of structure or position, whereas kinetic energy is the energy of motion. Potential energy is measured when it is transformed into kinetic energy.

3. There are six forms of energy: chemical, mechanical, heat, light, electric, and nuclear. Each form of energy can be converted or transformed into another form.

4. Exergonic energy reactions result in a transfer of energy to the surroundings. Endergonic energy reactions result in the storage, conservation, or increase in free energy. All potential energy in a biologic system is ultimately degraded into kinetic heat energy.

5. Energy transfer in humans generally takes one of three forms: chemical (biosynthesis of cellular molecules), mechanical (muscle contraction), and transport (transfer of substances between cells).

6. The main factors regulating the rate at which chemical energy is extracted from the food nutrients are: (1) mass action effect, which depends on the concentration gradients of substances, (2) biologic catalysts (enzymes) that accelerate the speed of chemical reactions, and (3) coenzymes that facilitate specific enzyme action.

General References

Lehninger, A.L.: Bioenergetics. Menlo Park, Calif., W.A. Benjamin Inc., 1971.
Lehninger, A.L.: Biochemistry. New York, Worth Publishers, 1975.
Stryer, L.: Biochemistry. San Francisco, W.H. Freeman and Co., 1975.
Vander, A.J.: Human Physiology: The Mechanisms of Body Function. New York, McGraw-Hill, 1975.

Energy Transfer
in the Body

The human body must be continually supplied with chemical energy to perform its many complex functions. Energy derived from the oxidation of food is not released suddenly at some kindling temperature because the body *cannot* use heat energy. If this were the case, the body fluids would actually boil and our tissues would burst into flames. Rather, the chemical energy trapped within the bonds of carbohydrates, fats, and proteins is extracted in small amounts during complex, enzymatically controlled reactions that occur in the relatively cool, watery medium of the cell. This process reduces the loss of energy as heat and provides for much greater efficiency in energy transformations, thereby enabling the body to make direct use of chemical energy. In a sense, energy can be supplied to the cells as it is needed. The story of how the body maintains its continuous energy supply begins with the special carrier for free energy, ATP.

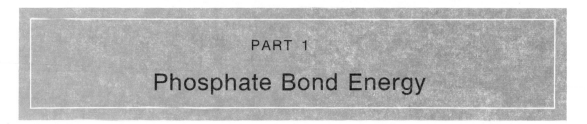

PART 1

Phosphate Bond Energy

THE ENERGY CURRENCY, ADENOSINE TRIPHOSPHATE

The energy in food is not transferred directly to the cells for biologic work. Rather, this "nutrient energy" is harvested and funneled through the energy-rich compound *adenosine triphosphate* or, simply, ATP. The potential energy within the ATP molecule is then utilized for *all* the energy-requiring processes of the cell. This cycle, in essence, represents the two major energy-transforming activities in the cell: (1) to form and conserve ATP from the potential energy in food and (2) to use the chemical energy in ATP for biologic work.

Figure 6-1 shows the ATP molecule formed from a molecule of adenine and ribose, called adenosine, linked to three phosphate molecules. The bonds linking the two outermost phosphates are termed high-energy bonds

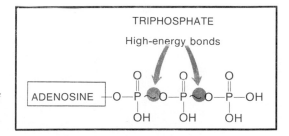

FIG. 6-1. *Simplified structure of ATP, the energy currency of the cell. The symbol ~ represents the high-energy bonds. (From* Nutrition, Weight Control, and Exercise *by Frank I. Katch and William D. McArdle. Copyright © 1977 by Houghton Mifflin Company. Reprinted by permission of the publisher.)*

63

because they represent a considerable quantity of potential energy within the ATP molecule.

When ATP joins with water in a process called *hydrolysis,* the outermost phosphate bond is broken and a new compound *adenosine diphosphate,* or *ADP,* is formed. In this reaction, approximately 7.3 kcal of free energy are liberated per mole of ATP degraded to ADP.

$$ATP + H_2O \longrightarrow ADP + P - 7.3 \text{ kcal per mole}$$

The free energy liberated in the hydrolysis of ATP is simply a measure of the energy difference between the reactants and the end products. Because considerable energy is generated in this reaction, ATP is often referred to as a *high-energy phosphate.* Infrequently, additional energy is released when another phosphate is split from ADP. In some reactions of biosynthesis, the two terminal phosphates from ATP are simultaneously donated in the construction of new cellular material. The remaining molecule with a single phosphate group is *adenosine monophosphate* or *AMP.*

The energy liberated during ATP breakdown is directly transferred to other energy-requiring molecules. In muscle, for example, this energy activates specific sites on the contractile elements causing the muscle fiber to shorten. Because energy from ATP is harnessed to power *all* forms of biologic work, ATP is considered the cell's "energy currency." The general role of ATP as energy currency is illustrated in Figure 6-2.

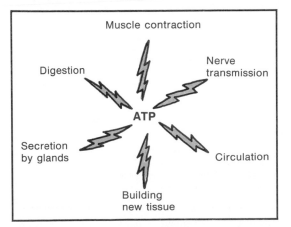

Muscle contraction

Nerve transmission

Digestion

ATP

Secretion by glands

Circulation

Building new tissue

FIG. 6-2. *ATP is the energy currency for all forms of biologic work. (From Nutrition, Weight Control, and Exercise by Frank I. Katch and William D. McArdle. Copyright © 1977 by Houghton Mifflin Company. Reprinted by permission of the publisher.)*

The splitting of the ATP molecule takes place whether oxygen is available or not. This is an immediate, *nonaerobic** energy-liberating reaction. The cell's capacity for ATP breakdown enables it to generate energy for immediate use; this would not occur if oxygen were required at all times for energy metabolism. For this reason, all types of exercise can be performed immediately without consuming oxygen, such as sprinting for a bus or lifting a heavy barbell.

THE ENERGY RESERVOIR, CREATINE PHOSPHATE

Only a small quantity of ATP is stored within the cell. This situation provides a sensitive mechanism for regulating energy metabolism in the cell. By maintaining only a small amount of ATP, its relative concentration (and corresponding concentration of ADP) is altered rapidly with any increase in a cell's energy metabolism. This change, in turn, immediately stimulates the breakdown of stored nutrients to provide energy for ATP resynthesis. In this way, energy metabolism increases rapidly in the early stages of exercise.

The total quantity of ATP within the body at any one time is about 3 oz. This amount provides only enough energy to perform maximum exercise for several seconds. Because ATP cannot be supplied via the blood or from other tissues, it must be recycled continuously within each cell. In muscle cells, some of this energy for ATP resynthesis is supplied rapidly and without oxygen by the transfer of chemical energy from another high-energy phosphate compound called creatine phosphate, or CP (Fig. 6-3). The cell's concentration of CP is about three to five times greater than that of ATP. For this reason, CP is considered the high-energy phosphate "reservoir."

The CP molecule is similar to the ATP molecule in that a large amount of free energy is released when the bond between the creatine and phosphate molecules splits. Because CP has a higher free energy of hydrolysis than ATP, its phosphate is donated directly to ADP to reform ATP. The arrows pointing in opposite directions show that the reactions are reversible.

---

*The term nonaerobic more precisely describes the breakdown of the phosphagens. The term *anaerobic* is properly used to describe reactions of glycolysis in which glucose is broken down to lactic acid.

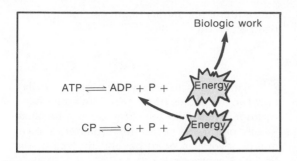

Biologic work

$$ATP \rightleftharpoons ADP + P + \text{Energy}$$

$$CP \rightleftharpoons C + P + \text{Energy}$$

FIG. 6-3. *ATP and CP are nonaerobic sources of phosphate bond energy. The energy from the breakdown of CP is used to rebond ADP and P to form ATP. (From* Nutrition, Weight Control, and Exercise *by Frank I. Katch and William D. McArdle. Copyright © 1977 by Houghton Mifflin Company. Reprinted by permission of the publisher.)*

If sufficient energy is available, creatine (C) and phosphate (P) can be joined to re-form CP. The same is true for ATP; the top reaction illustrates the union of ADP and P to re-form ATP.

It should now be apparent that human energy dynamics involves the transfer of energy by means of chemical bonds. Potential energy is released by the splitting of bonds and conserved by the formation of new bonds. Some energy lost by one molecule can be transferred to the chemical structure of another and does not appear as heat. Compounds relatively low in potential energy can be "juiced-up" by energy transfer from the high-energy phosphates to accomplish biologic work. ATP serves as the ideal energy-transfer agent; in one respect it "traps" in its phosphate bonds a large portion of potential energy in the original food molecule, yet readily transfers this energy to other compounds to raise them to a higher level of activation. This transfer of energy in the form of phosphate bonds is termed *phosphorylation.* The energy for phosphorylation is ultimately generated by the oxidation of carbohydrates, fats, and proteins consumed in the diet.

CELLULAR OXIDATION

Hydrogen atoms are continually stripped from the nutrient substrates during energy metabolism. Special carrier molecules within the cell's "energy factories," the *mitochondria,* then remove electrons from hydrogen and eventually pass them to molecular oxygen. To complete the process, oxygen also accepts hydro-

gen to form water. Much of the energy generated in cellular oxidation (that is, the transfer of electrons from hydrogen to oxygen) is trapped or conserved as chemical energy in the form of high-energy phosphates.

Electron Transport

The general scheme for the oxidation of hydrogen and the accompanying *electron transport* to oxygen is illustrated in Figure 6-4. During cellular oxidation, hydrogen atoms are not merely turned loose in the cell fluid. Rather, the release of hydrogen from the nutrient substrate is catalyzed by highly specific *dehydrogenase* enzymes. The electrons (energy) from hydrogen are picked up in pairs by the coenzyme part of the dehydrogenase, which is usually the coenzyme, *nicotinamide adeninedinucleotide* or NAD^+. While the substrate is being oxidized and losing hydrogen (electrons), NAD^+ is gaining a hydrogen and two electrons and being reduced to NADH; the other hydrogen appears in the cell fluid as H^+.

The other important electron acceptor in the oxidation of the food fragments is *flavin adenine dinucleotide,* or *FAD.* FAD is derived from the B-vitamin riboflavin. This coenzyme also catalyzes dehydrogenations and accepts pairs of electrons. Unlike NAD^+, however, FAD accepts both hydrogens to become $FADH_2$.

The NADH and $FADH_2$ formed in the breakdown of the food nutrients are energy-rich molecules because they carry electrons that have a high energy transfer potential. On the inner

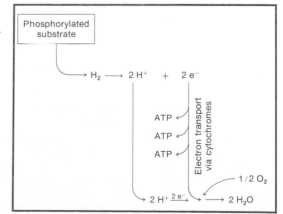

FIG. 6-4. *A general scheme for the oxidation of hydrogen and accompanying electron transport. In this process, oxygen is reduced and water is formed.*

membranes of the mitochondria, the electrons carried by NADH and $FADH_2$ are then passed in "bucket brigade" fashion by a series of iron–protein electron carriers, the *cytochromes.* The iron portion of each cytochrome can exist in either its oxidized or reduced state as ferric (Fe^{3+}) or ferrous (Fe^{2+}) ion, respectively. By accepting an electron, the ferric portion of a specific cytochrome becomes reduced to its ferrous form. In turn, this donates its electron to the next cytochrome, and so on down the line. By shuttling between these iron forms, the cytochromes transfer electrons.

The transport of electrons by specific carrier molecules constitutes the *respiratory chain.* This is the final common pathway in which the electrons extracted from hydrogen are passed to oxygen. For each pair of hydrogen atoms, two electrons flow down the chain and reduce one atom of oxygen to form water. Of the five specific cytochromes, only the last, *cytochrome oxidase* (cytochrome A_3), can discharge its electron directly to molecular oxygen. Figure 6-5A shows the route for the oxidation of hydrogen and the accompanying electron transport and energy transfer in the respiratory chain.

Free energy is released in the respiratory chain in relatively small amounts, and in several of the electron transfers, energy is conserved by the formation of high-energy phosphate bonds.

Oxidative Phosphorylation

Oxidative phosphorylation is the process by which ATP is synthesized during the transfer of electrons from NADH and $FADH_2$ to molecular oxygen. This important process represents the cell's primary means for extracting and trapping chemical energy in the form of high-energy phosphates. In fact, over 90% of ATP synthesis is accomplished in the respiratory chain by oxidative reactions coupled with phosphorylation.

In a way, the process of oxidative phosphorylation can be likened to a waterfall divided into several separate cascades by the intervention of waterwheels at different heights. As depicted in Figure 6-5B, the waterwheels harness the energy of the falling water; similarly, the energy generated in electron transport is harnessed and transferred or coupled to ADP. The energy in NADH is transferred to ADP at three distinct coupling sites during electron transport (Fig. 6-5A). This oxidation of hydrogen and subsequent phosphorylation can be summarized as follows:

$$NADH + H^+ + 3\ ADP + 3\ P + \tfrac{1}{2} O_2 \longrightarrow$$
$$NAD^+ + H_2O + 3\ ATP$$

If hydrogen is originally donated by $FADH_2$, only two molecules of ATP are formed for each hydrogen pair oxidized. This occurs because $FADH_2$ enters the respiratory chain at a lower energy level at a point beyond the site of the first ATP synthesis.

Efficiency of Electron Transport and Oxidative Phosphorylation

Approximately 7 kcal of energy are required for the synthesis of each mole of ATP. Since 3 moles of ATP are generated in the oxidation of a mole of NADH, about 21 kcal are conserved as chemical energy. In total, 52 kcal are liberated during the oxidation of a mole of NADH. Thus, the relative *efficiency* of electron transport–oxidative phosphorylation for harnessing chemical energy is approximately 40% (21 kcal ÷ 52 kcal × 100). The remaining 60% of the energy is lost to the body as heat. Considering that the steam engine transforms its fuel into useful energy with an efficiency of only about 30%, 40% represents high efficiency.

Role of Oxygen in Energy Metabolism

Three prerequisites must be met for the continual resynthesis of ATP: (1) a donor of electrons in the form of NADH (or $FADH_2$) must be available, (2) adequate oxygen, the final electron and hydrogen acceptor, must be present, and (3) enzymes must be present in sufficient concentration to make the energy transfer reactions "go." When these conditions are satisfied, hydrogen is continually shuttled down the respiratory chain to molecular oxygen during the breakdown of the food substrate.

In strenuous exercise, when the rate of oxygen delivery (prerequisite #2 above) or utilization (prerequisite #3 above) is often inadequate, a relative imbalance is created between the release of hydrogen and its final acceptance by oxygen. In a sense, electron flow down the respiratory chain begins to "back up" with an accumulation of hydrogens bound to NAD^+. As will be discussed in a subsequent section, pyruvic acid temporarily binds these excess

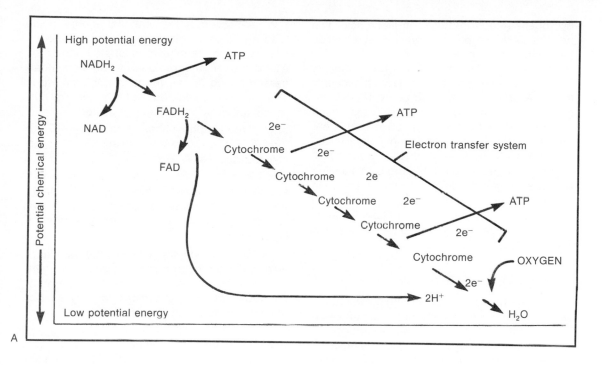

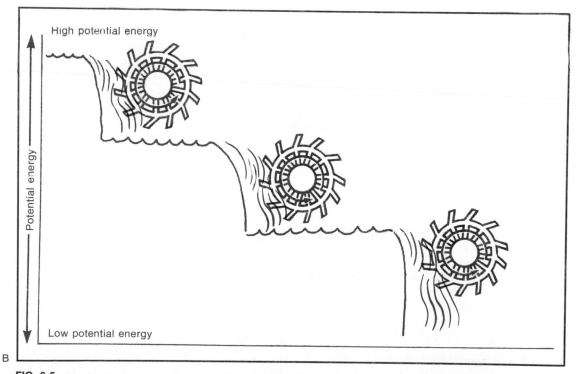

FIG. 6-5. *The harnessing of energy. A, In the respiratory chain, much of the chemical energy stored within the hydrogen atom is conserved in the formation of high-energy phosphate bonds. B, Energy from falling water is used to turn the waterwheel.*

hydrogens (electrons) to form lactic acid; this permits oxidative phosphorylation by electron transport to continue.

The function of oxygen in energy metabolism is clearly to serve as the final electron acceptor in the respiratory chain and combine with hydrogen to form water. This total process, which involves a considerable transfer of usable energy through oxidative phosphorylation in the respiratory chain, is referred to as *aerobic metabolism.* In one sense, this term is misleading because oxygen does not participate directly in the synthesis of ATP. However, the presence of oxygen at the "end of the line" largely determines one's capability for sustained aerobic energy release during exercise.

SUMMARY

1. The energy contained within the chemical structures of carbohydrates, fats, and proteins is not released in the body suddenly at some kindling temperature; rather, it is released slowly in small amounts during complex reactions. This allows for greater efficiency in energy transfer.

2. A portion of the potential energy in the food nutrients is transferred to the compound ATP. When the terminal phosphate bond of the ATP is broken, the free energy liberated is harnessed to power all forms of biologic work. Thus, ATP is considered the body's energy currency, although its quantity is limited.

3. Creatine phosphate interacts with ADP to form ATP and thus serves as an energy reservoir to replenish ATP rapidly.

4. Phosphorylation is the process by which energy is transferred in the form of phosphate bonds. It is the process by which ADP and creatine are continually recycled into ATP and CP, respectively.

5. Cellular oxidation involves the transfer of electrons from hydrogen to molecular oxygen. This process, which takes place in the mitochondria, results in the release and transfer of chemical energy in the formation of high-energy phosphates.

6. In the aerobic resynthesis of ATP, the primary role of oxygen is to serve as the final electron acceptor in the respiratory chain and to combine with hydrogen to form water.

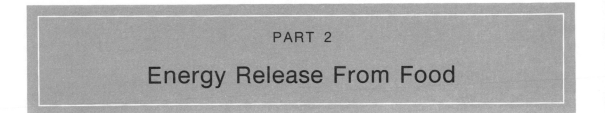

PART 2

Energy Release From Food

The energy generated in the breakdown of the food nutrients serves one purpose—to phosphorylate ADP to re-form the energy-rich compound ATP. Although the breakdown of various foods during energy metabolism is geared toward generating phosphate-bond energy, the specific pathways of degradation differ, depending on the nutrients metabolized. In the sections that follow, we will see how the potential energy in the food nutrients is extracted and utilized to synthesize ATP.

ENERGY RELEASE FROM CARBOHYDRATES

The primary function of carbohydrates is to supply energy for cellular work. Our discussion of nutrient energy metabolism begins with car-

bohydrates for several reasons: (1) Carbohydrates are the only nutrient whose stored energy can be used to generate ATP anaerobically. This is of extreme importance in vigorous exercise that requires energy above levels that can be supplied by aerobic metabolic reac-

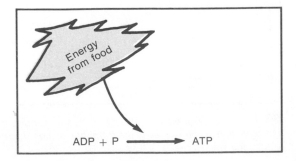

tions. In this situation, stored glycogen and blood glucose must supply the main portion of energy for ATP resynthesis. (2) In light and moderate exercise, carbohydrates supply about half of the body's energy requirements. (3) A continual breakdown of some carbohydrate seems to be required so that fat nutrients can be processed through the metabolic mill and used for energy. It is not uncommon in prolonged exercise such as marathon running for a participant to experience fatigue which is associated with a depletion of muscle and liver glycogen.

The complete breakdown of one mole (180 g) of glucose to carbon dioxide and water yields a maximum of 686 kcal of chemical energy, or energy available to do work.

$$C_6H_{12}O_6 + 6\ O_2 \longrightarrow$$
$$6\ CO_2 + 6\ H_2O,\ -\Delta G°'\ 686\ kcal\ per\ mole$$

In the cell, however, the complete breakdown of glucose to its simple, stable end products is accompanied by the conservation of energy in the form of ATP. Because 7.3 kcal are required to synthesize each mole of ATP from ADP and inorganic phosphate, it would be theoretically possible to form 94 moles of ATP per mole of glucose by coupling all of the energy in glucose to phosphorylation (686 kcal ÷ 7.3 = 94). In the muscle, however, only about 38%, or 263 kcal of energy, is actually transferred to phosphate bonds and the remainder is dissipated as heat. Consequently, 36 moles of ATP are regenerated in glucose breakdown (263 kcal ÷ 7.3 = 36) with an accompanying gain in free energy of 263 kcal.

There are two stages for glucose degradation in the body. The first stage involves the breakdown of a glucose molecule to two molecules of pyruvic acid. *These reactions involve energy transfers that do not require oxygen; they are thus anaerobic.* In the second phase of glucose catabolism, the pyruvic acid molecules are further degraded to carbon dioxide and water. *Energy transfers resulting from these reactions involve electron transport and accompanying oxidative phosphorylation; they are thus aerobic.*

Anaerobic Energy from Glucose: Glycolysis

When a glucose molecule enters a cell to be used for energy, it undergoes a series of chemical reactions collectively termed *glycolysis.*

These reactions, summarized in Figure 6-6, occur in the watery medium of the cell outside of the mitochondrion. In a sense, this process represents a more primitive form of energy transfer that is well developed in amphibia, reptiles, fish, and diving mammals.

In the first reaction, ATP acts as a phosphate donor to phosphorylate glucose to *glucose 6-phosphate*. At this point, in most tissues of the body, the glucose molecule is "trapped" in the cell. (For example, liver cells contain *phosphatase* that can split the phosphate from the glucose 6-phosphate and thus make glucose available to leave the cell and to be transported throughout the body.) The glucose molecule can now be linked together, or *polymerized*, with other glucose molecules to form glycogen, the storage form of glucose. In energy metabolism, however, glucose 6-phosphate is further phosphorylated to *fructose 1, 6-diphosphate.* At this stage, no energy has been extracted but energy has been incorporated into the original glucose molecule at the expense of two molecules of ATP. In a sense, phosphorylation has "primed the pump" so that energy metabolism can proceed. Fructose 1, 6-diphosphate then splits into *two* phosphorylated molecules with three carbon chains; these are further degraded in five successive reactions to pyruvic acid.

SUBSTRATE PHOSPHORYLATION IN GLYCOLYSIS. Most of the energy generated in the reactions of glycolysis is insufficient to resynthesize ATP and is lost to the body as heat. However, in reactions 7 and 10 the energy released from the glucose intermediates is sufficient to stimulate the direct transfer of a phosphate group to ADP. This generates a total of four molecules of ATP. *Since two molecules of ATP were lost in the initial phosphorylation of the glucose molecule, the net energy transfer from glycolysis results in a gain of two molecules of ATP.* These specific energy transfers from substrate to ADP by phosphorylation do not require oxygen. Rather, energy is directly transferred to phosphate bonds in the anaerobic process called *substrate level phosphorylation.*

Only about 5% of the total ATP generated in the complete breakdown of the glucose molecule is formed during glycolysis. Nevertheless, due to the high concentration of glycolytic enzymes and the speed of these reactions, significant energy for muscle contraction can be provided rapidly from glycolysis. The athlete

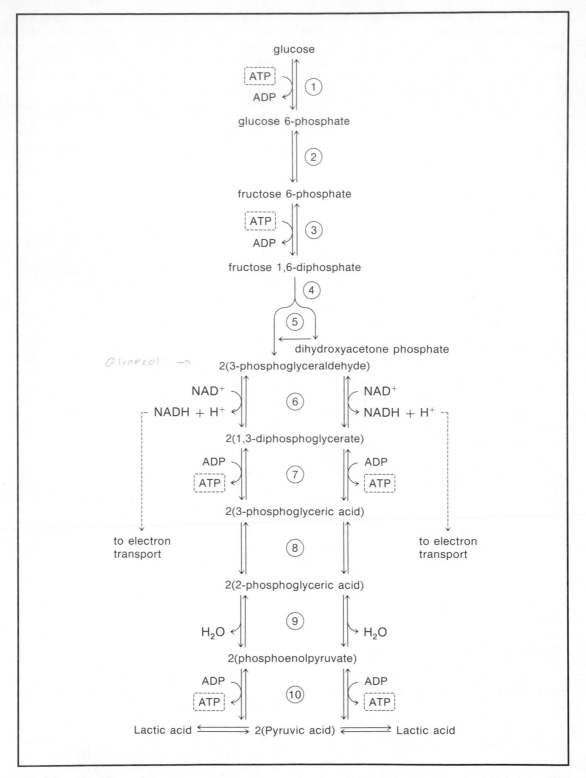

FIG. 6-6.   *Glycolysis: The breakdown of the 6-carbon glucose molecule to two, 3-carbon molecules of pyruvic acid.*

sprinting at the end of the mile run relies heavily on this form of anaerobic energy transfer—which is possible only from the breakdown of the body's carbohydrate stores by glycolytic reactions.

HYDROGEN RELEASE IN GLYCOLYSIS. During glycolysis, two pairs of hydrogen atoms are stripped from the substrate and their electrons passed to NAD^+ to form NADH (Fig. 6-6). Normally, if these electrons were processed directly through the respiratory chain, three molecules of ATP would be generated for each molecule of NADH oxidized. However, the mitochondrion is impermeable to NADH formed in the cytoplasm during glycolysis. Consequently, the electrons from extramitochondrial NADH must be *shuttled* indirectly into the mitochondria. In skeletal muscle, this route ends with electrons being passed to FAD to form $FADH_2$. This in turn transfers its electrons at a point below the first formation of ATP (see Fig. 6-5A). *Thus in skeletal muscle two, rather than three, ATP molecules are formed when cytoplasmic NADH is oxidized by the respiratory chain. Because two molecules of NADH are formed in glycolysis, four molecules of ATP are generated aerobically by subsequent electron transport–oxidative phosphorylation.*

FORMATION OF LACTIC ACID. During moderate levels of energy metabolism, sufficient oxygen is available to the cells. Consequently, most of the hydrogens (electrons) stripped from the substrate and carried by NADH are oxidized and passed to oxygen to form water. In a biochemical sense a "steady state," or more precisely a "steady rate," exists because hydrogen is oxidized at about the same rate as it is made available. Even at rest or in mild exercise, however, some lactic acid is continually formed due to limitations posed by enzyme activity and the equilibrium constants for chemical reactions. Lactic acid does not build up in this situation because its removal rate equals its rate of production.

In strenuous exercise, when the energy demands exceed either the oxygen supply or the rate of utilization, all of the hydrogen joined to NADH cannot be processed through the respiratory chain. Continued release of anaerobic energy in glycolysis depends on the availability of NAD^+ for the oxidation of *3-phosphoglyceraldehyde* (see reaction 6); otherwise, glycolysis will "grind to a halt." Under anaerobic conditions, NAD^+ is "freed" as pairs of "excess" hydrogens combine with pyruvic acid to form lactic acid in the reversible reaction:

$$CH_3-\overset{\overset{\text{O}}{\|}}{C}-COOH + NADH + H^+ \rightleftharpoons$$
(Pyruvic acid)

$$CH_3-\overset{\overset{\text{OH}}{|}}{\underset{\underset{\text{H}}{|}}{C}}-COOH + NAD^+$$
(Lactic acid)

The temporary storage of hydrogen with pyruvic acid is a unique aspect of energy metabolism because it provides a ready "sump" for the disappearance of the end products of glycolysis. Also, once lactic acid is formed in the muscle, it diffuses rapidly to the blood and away from the site of energy metabolism. In this way, glycolysis can proceed to supply additional anaerobic energy for the resynthesis of ATP. This avenue for extra energy is only temporary, however, because as the level of lactic acid in the blood and muscles increases, the regeneration of ATP cannot keep pace with its utilization, fatigue sets in, and exercise must stop. Fatigue is probably mediated by increased acidity that inactivates various enzymes involved in energy transfer.

Lactic acid should not be viewed as a metabolic "waste product." On the contrary, it is a valuable source of chemical energy that accumulates and is retained in the body during heavy physical exercise. When sufficient oxygen is once again available, as in recovery or when the pace of exercise is slowed, hydrogens attached to lactic acid are picked up by NAD^+ and eventually oxidized. Consequently, lactic acid is readily reconverted to pyruvic acid and used as an energy source or as a substrate for the resynthesis of glucose.

The Krebs Cycle

Because the anaerobic reactions of glycolysis release only about 5% of the energy within the glucose molecule, an additional means for extracting the remaining energy is available. This is provided when the pyruvic acid molecules are irreversibly converted to a form of acetic acid, *acetyl-CoA*. This intermediate compound enters the second stage of carbohydrate breakdown known as the *Krebs cycle* (or more de-

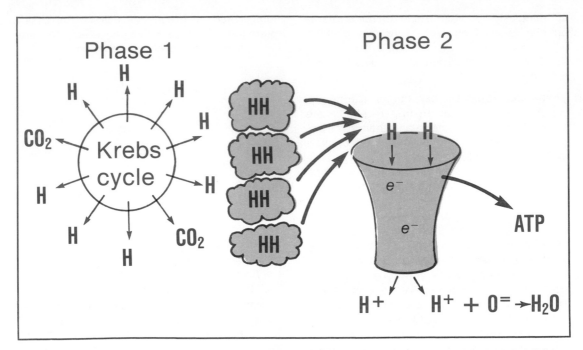

FIG. 6-7. *In the mitochondria the Krebs cycle generates hydrogen atoms in the breakdown of acetyl-CoA (Phase 1). These hydrogens are then oxidized via the aerobic process of electron transport–oxidative phosphorylation, and significant quantities of ATP are regenerated (Phase 2).*

scriptively, the citric acid or tricarboxylic acid cycle). As shown schematically in Figure 6-7, the main function of the Krebs cycle is to degrade the acetyl-CoA substrate to carbon dioxide and hydrogen atoms within the mitochondria. The hydrogen atoms are then oxidized in processes involving electron transport–oxidative phosphorylation with the subsequent regeneration of ATP.

As shown in Figure 6-8, pyruvic acid is prepared for entrance into the Krebs cycle by joining with the vitamin B-derivitive coenzyme A (A for acetic acid) to form the 2-carbon compound *acetyl-CoA.* In the process, two hydrogens are released and their electrons transferred to NAD^+, and one molecule of carbon dioxide is formed as follows:

$$\text{Pyruvic acid} + NAD^+ + CoA \longrightarrow$$
$$\text{Acetyl-CoA} + CO_2 + NADH + H^+$$

When the acetyl portion of acetyl-CoA joins with *oxaloacetic acid,* it forms *citric acid* (the same citric acid found in citrus fruits), a 6-carbon compound that then proceeds through the Krebs cycle. The cycle is continued because the original oxaloacetic molecule is retained and joins with a new 2-carbon acetyl fragment.

For each molecule of acetyl-CoA entering the Krebs cycle, two carbon dioxide molecules and four pairs of hydrogen atoms are cleaved from the substrate. One molecule of ATP is also regenerated directly by substrate level phosphorylation from Krebs cycle reactions (see reaction 6). As summarized at the bottom of Figure 6-8, for the two pyruvic acid molecules formed in glycolysis, a total of four hydrogens are released in the formation of acetyl-CoA, and 16 hydrogens are released in the Krebs cycle. *In essence, the most important function of the Krebs cycle is to generate electrons (hydrogens) for their passage to the respiratory chain by means of NAD^+ and FAD.*

Molecular oxygen does not participate directly in the reactions of the Krebs cycle. The major portion of the chemical energy in pyruvic acid is transferred to ADP through the aerobic process of electron transport–oxidative phosphorylation. As long as there is an adequate oxygen supply with enzymes and substrate available, NAD^+ and FAD will be regenerated and Krebs cycle aerobic metabolism will proceed.

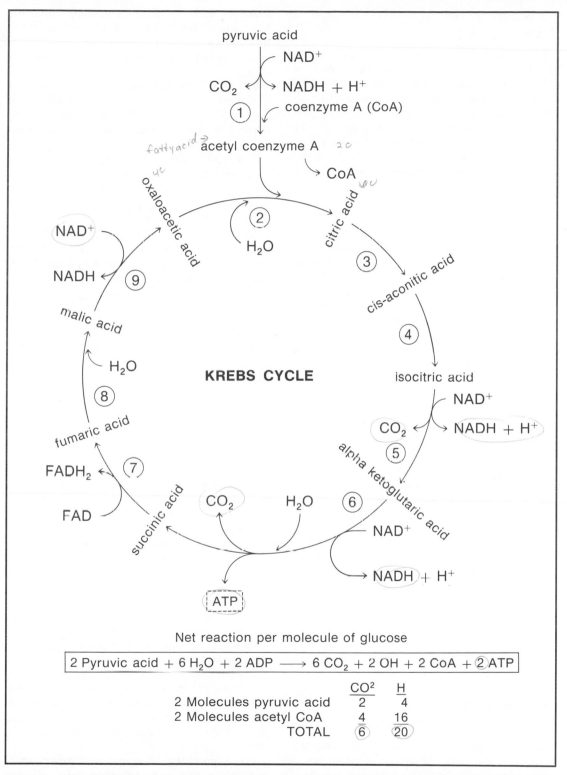

FIG. 6-8. *"Flowsheet" for release of hydrogen and carbon dioxide during the degradation of one molecule of pyruvic acid in the mitrochondrion. Since two molecules of pyruvic acid are formed from one molecule of glucose during glycolysis, all values are doubled when computing the net gain from pyruvate catabolism.*

Total Energy Transfer
from Glucose Catabolism

The pathways for energy transfer during the breakdown of a glucose molecule in skeletal muscle are summarized in Figure 6-9. A net of 2 ATP is formed from substrate phosphorylation in glycolysis and, similarly, 2 ATP are generated during acetyl-CoA degradation in the Krebs cycle. The 24 released hydrogen atoms can be accounted for as follows: (1) the 4 hydrogens (2 NADH) generated outside the mitochondria during glycolysis yield 4 ATP during oxidative phosphorylation; (2) the 4 hydrogens (2 NADH) released in the mitochondria as pyruvic acid is changed to acetyl-CoA yield 6 ATP, (3) 12 of the 16 hydrogens (6 NADH) released in the Krebs cycle yield 18 ATP, and (4) the remaining 4 hydrogens joined to FAD (2 $FADH_2$) in the Krebs cycle yield 4 ATP. *The net ATP yield from the complete breakdown of the glucose molecule in skeletal muscle is 36 molecules of ATP; 4 ATP molecules are formed directly from substrate phosphorylation (via glycolysis and the Krebs cycle) whereas 32 ATPs are generated during oxidative phosphorylation.*

ENERGY RELEASE
FROM FAT

Stored fat represents the body's greatest source of potential energy. Relative to other nutrients, the quantity of fat available for energy is almost unlimited. The actual fuel reserves from stored fat represent about 90,000 to 110,000 kcal of energy. In contrast, the carbohydrate energy reserve is less than 2000 kcal, of which 1500 kcal (375 g) are stored as muscle glycogen, 400 kcal (100 g) as liver glycogen, and about 80 kcal (20 g) of glucose are present in the extracellular fluids.

Prior to energy release from fat, the triglyceride molecule is cleaved into glycerol and three fatty acid molecules. The reaction is catalyzed by the enzyme *lipase* as follows:

$$\text{Triglyceride} + 3H_2O \xrightarrow{\textit{Lipase}}$$
$$\text{Glycerol} + 3 \text{ fatty acids}$$

Although some fat is stored in all cells, the most active supplier of fatty acid molecules is adipose tissue. *Adipocytes,* or fat cells, are specialized for the synthesis and storage of triglycerides. Triglyceride fat droplets occupy as much as 95% of the cell's volume. Once the fatty acids diffuse into the circulation, these *free fatty acids,* or *FFA,* are then delivered to active tissues where they are metabolized for energy.

Depending on a person's state of nutrition and level and duration of physical activity, 30% to 80% of the energy for biologic work is usually derived from intra- and extracellular fat molecules (see Chap. 1).

The mobilization of FFA from adipose tissue is augmented by the hormones epinephrine, norepinephrine, glucagon, and growth hormone. The injection of epinephrine into the blood, for example, results in a rapid increase in plasma FFA. Because plasma concentrations of these hormones are increased during exercise, this mechanism for lipase activation provides the muscle with a rapid supply of a potent energy substrate.

Catabolism of Glycerol and
Fatty Acids

Figure 6-10 summarizes the pathways for the degradation of the glycerol and fatty acid fragments of the triglyceride molecule.

Glycerol can be accepted into the anaerobic reactions of glycolysis as 3-phosphoglyceraldehyde and degraded to pyruvic acid. In this process, ATP is formed via substrate phosphorylation and hydrogen atoms are released to NAD^+; pyruvic acid is then oxidized in the Krebs cycle. In total, 22 ATP molecules are synthesized in the complete breakdown of the glycerol molecule.

The *fatty acid* molecule undergoes transformation to acetyl-CoA in the mitochondrion in a process called *beta oxidation*. This involves the successive release of 2-carbon acetyl fragments split from the long chain of the fatty acid. ATP is used to phosphorylate the reactions, water is added, hydrogens are passed to NAD^+ and FAD, and the acetyl fragment joins with coenzyme A to form acetyl-CoA. This process is repeated over and over until the entire fatty acid molecule is degraded to acetyl-CoA, which then enters the Krebs cycle directly to be metabolized. The hydrogens released during fatty acid catabolism are oxidized via the respiratory chain.

It is important to note that the breakdown of fatty acids is directly associated with oxygen uptake. Oxygen must be available to accept hydrogen for beta oxidation to proceed. Under

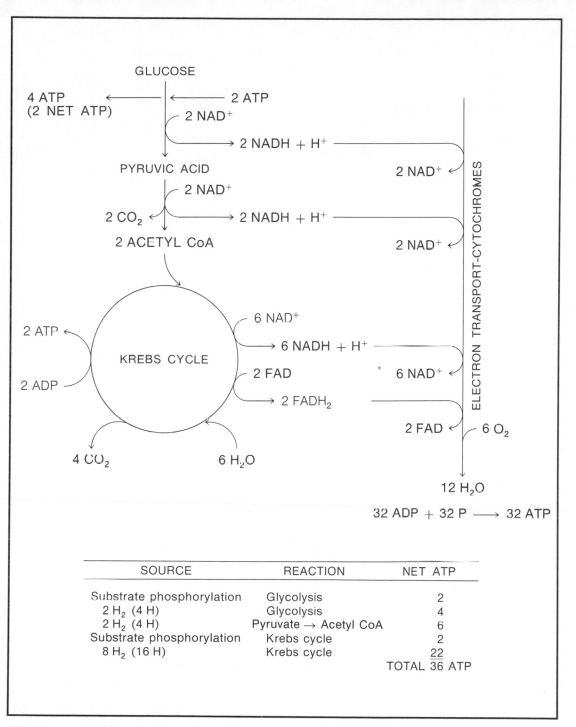

FIG. 6-9. *ATP yield from energy transfer during the complete oxidation of glucose.*

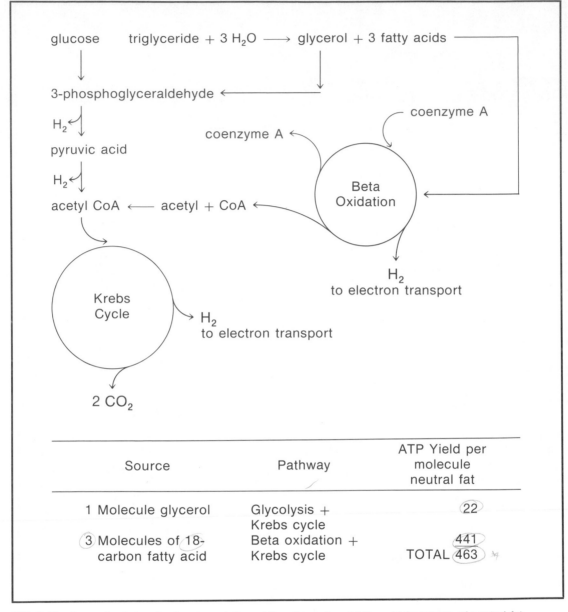

FIG. 6-10. *General scheme for the degradation of the glycerol and fatty acid fragments of neutral fat.*

anaerobic conditions, hydrogen remains with NAD+ and FAD, and fat catabolism is halted.

Total Energy Transfer
from Fat Catabolism

For each 18-carbon fatty acid molecule, 147 molecules of ADP are phosphorylated to ATP during beta oxidation and Krebs cycle metabolism. Because there are three fatty acid molecules in each triglyceride molecule, 441 ATP

molecules are formed from the fatty acid component of neutral fat (3 × 147 ATP). Since 22 molecules of ATP are also formed during glycerol catabolism, a total of 463 molecules of ATP are generated for each neutral fat molecule catabolized for energy. This is a considerable energy yield considering that only 36 ATP are formed during the catabolism of a glucose molecule in skeletal muscle. The efficiency of energy conservation for fatty acid oxidation is about 40%, a value similar to that of glucose.

ENERGY RELEASE FROM PROTEIN

As mentioned in Chapter 1, protein can serve an important role as an energy substrate during sustained exercise. To provide energy, the amino acid must first be converted to a form that can readily enter the pathways for energy release. Once the amino or nitrogen-containing group is removed from the amino acid, a process that takes place almost entirely in the liver, the remaining "carbon skeleton" is usually one of the reactive compounds that can contribute to the formation of high-energy phosphate bonds. Alanine, for example, loses its amine group and gains a double-bond oxygen to form pyruvic acid; glutamic acid forms alpha keto-glutaric acid; and aspartic acid forms oxaloacetic acid—all of these end products are Krebs cycle intermediates.

THE METABOLIC MILL—INTERRELATIONSHIPS BETWEEN CARBOHYDRATE, FAT, AND PROTEIN METABOLISM

The Krebs cycle plays a much more important role than simply the degradation of pyruvic acid produced during glucose catabolism. The Krebs cycle provides the means by which fragments of other organic compounds formed from the breakdown of fats and proteins can be effectively metabolized for energy. As illustrated in Figure 6-11, the deaminated residues of excess amino acids enter the Krebs cycle at various intermediate stages, whereas the glycerol fragment of fat catabolism gains entrance via the glycolytic pathway. Fatty acids are oxidized by beta oxidation to acetyl-CoA, which then directly enters the Krebs cycle.

This sketch of the "metabolic mill" also shows the interconversions between fragments of the various nutrients and the possible routes for substrate synthesis. Excess carbohydrates, for example, provide the glycerol and acetyl fragments for the synthesis of neutral fat. Acetyl-CoA can also function as the starting point for the synthesis of cholesterol and many hormones. However, because the conversion of pyruvic acid to acetyl-CoA is not reversible, (notice the one-way arrow), fats cannot be used to any appreciable extent to synthesize glucose. Amino acids with carbon skeletons re-sembling Krebs cycle intermediates are deaminated and synthesized to glucose. This is especially true for the amino acid alanine (see Chap. 1).

FATS BURN IN A CARBOHYDRATE FLAME

One interesting aspect of the metabolic mill is that the breakdown of fatty acids seems to depend somewhat on a continual background level of glucose catabolism. It should be recalled that acetyl-CoA enters the Krebs cycle by combining with oxaloacetic acid (generated mainly by carbohydrate catabolism) to form citric acid. The degradation of fatty acids via the Krebs cycle continues only if sufficient oxaloacetic acid is available to combine with acetyl-CoA formed during beta oxidation. The pyruvic acid formed during glucose metabolism may play an important role in furnishing this oxaloacetic intermediate: In this sense, "fats burn in a carbohydrate flame."

An appreciable reduction in carbohydrate breakdown, which could occur in prolonged exercise such as marathon running, starvation, dietary elimination of carbohydrates (as advocated with high-fat, low-carbohydrate "ketogenic diets"), or diabetes, will also seriously limit the energy transfer from fatty acids. This occurs despite the fact that large amounts of this substrate are available in the circulation. In instances of extreme carbohydrate restriction or depletion, the acetate fragments produced in beta oxidation begin to build up in the extracellular fluids, since they cannot be accommodated in the Krebs cycle. These are readily converted to ketone bodies, some of which are excreted in the urine. If this condition of *ketosis* persists, the acid quality of the body fluids can increase to potentially toxic levels.

WHAT REGULATES ENERGY METABOLISM?

By far, the most important factor controlling energy release in the cell is the concentration of cellular ADP. Under normal conditions, the transfer of electrons and subsequent release of energy are tightly coupled to ADP phosphorylation. In general, unless ADP is available and phosphorylated to ATP, electrons will not flow down the respiratory chain to oxygen. This particular mechanism for respiratory control

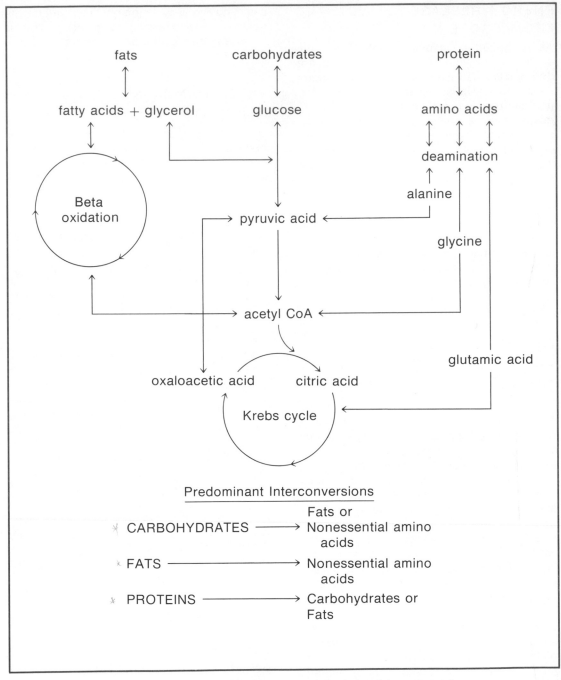

FIG. 6-11. *The metabolic mill: interconversions between carbohydrates, fats, and proteins.*

makes considerable "sense," because any increase in ADP heralds a need for energy to restore the ATP levels. Conversely, a low level of cellular ADP indicates a relatively low energy requirement.

SUMMARY

1. The food nutrients provide a source of potential energy to rejoin ADP and free phosphate to form ATP.

2. The complete breakdown of 1 mole of carbohydrate liberates 686 kcal of energy. Of this, about 263 kcal (38%) is conserved in the bonds of ATP; the remainder is dissipated as heat.

3. In the reactions of glycolysis in the cell cytoplasm, 2 ATP are formed in the anaerobic process of substrate phosphorylation.

4. In the second stage of carbohydrate breakdown, pyruvic acid is converted to acetyl-CoA, which is then processed through the Krebs cycle. The hydrogens released during glucose breakdown are oxidized via the respiratory chain and the energy generated is coupled to phosphorylation.

5. In the complete breakdown of carbohydrate in skeletal muscle a total of 36 ATP molecules are formed.

6. The complete breakdown of a fat molecule yields 463 ATP molecules. Fatty acid metabolism is directly associated with oxygen uptake; that is, the reactions are aerobic.

7. Proteins can also serve as an important energy substrate. After nitrogen is removed from the amino acid molecule, the remaining carbon skeleton can enter the Krebs cycle for the aerobic production of ATP.

8. Numerous interconversions are possible among the various food nutrients. The exception is fatty acids, which cannot be used for the synthesis of glucose.

9. In order for fats to be metabolized continually for energy in the metabolic mill, a certain level of carbohydrate breakdown is required. To this extent, "fats burn in a carbohydrate flame."

General References

Baldwin, E.: Dynamic Aspects of Biochemistry. New York, Cambridge University Press, 1963.

Giese, A.C.: Cell Physiology. Philadelphia, W.B. Saunders Co., 1979

Goodhart, R.S. and M.E. Shils. Modern Nutrition in Health and Disease, 6th ed. Philadelphia, Lea & Febiger, 1980.

Lehninger, A.L.: Bioenergetics: The Molecular Basis of Biological Energy Transfer. New York, Benjamin Press, 1965.

Lehninger, A.L.: Biochemistry. New York, Worth Publishers, 1975.

Mott-Smith, M.: The Concept of Energy Simply Explained. New York, Dover Press, 1964.

Stryer, L.: Biochemistry. San Francisco, W.H. Freeman and Co., 1975.

Vander, A.J. et al.: Human Physiology: The Mechanisms of Body Function. New York, McGraw-Hill, 1975.

Energy Transfer
in Exercise

7

Physical activity by far provides the greatest demand for energy. In sprint running and swimming, for example, the energy output from the working muscles may be as much as 120 times higher than at rest. During less intense but sustained exercise such as marathon running, the energy requirement increases some 20 to 30 times above rest. Depending on the intensity and duration of exercise, and the fitness of the participant, the relative contributions of the body's various means for energy transfer differ markedly.

IMMEDIATE ENERGY: THE ATP-CP SYSTEM

Performances of short duration and high intensity such as the 100-yard dash, 25-yard swim, or weight lifting require an immediate and rapid supply of energy. This energy is provided almost exclusively from the high-energy phosphates ATP and CP stored within the specific muscles activated during exercise.[24]

Approximately 5 millimoles (mmol) of ATP and 15 mmol of CP are stored within each kilogram of muscle.[18] For a 70-kg person with a muscle mass of 30 kg, this is between 570 and 690 mmol of high-energy phosphates. If we assume that 20 kg of muscle are activated during exercise, then there is sufficient stored phosphate energy to walk briskly for 1 minute, run a cross-country race for 20 to 30 seconds, or perform all-out exercises such as sprint running and swimming for about 6 seconds.[5] In the 100-yard dash, for example, the body cannot maintain maximum speed for longer than this time, and the runners may actually be slowing down in the last portion of the race. In this situation, the quantity of intramuscular phosphate

may significantly influence one's ability to generate intense energy for a short duration. All sports require utilization of the high-energy phosphates, but many activities rely almost exclusively on this means for energy transfer. For example, success in football, weight lifting, field events, baseball, and volleyball all require a brief maximal effort during the performance. It is difficult to imagine an end run in football or a pole vault without the capability for generating energy rapidly from the stored phosphagens. However, for sustained exercise and for recovery from an all-out effort, additional energy must be generated for ATP replenishment. To this end, the stored carbohydrates, fats, and proteins stand ready to continually recharge the phosphate pool.

SHORT-TERM ENERGY: THE LACTIC ACID SYSTEM

The high-energy phosphates must continually be resynthesized at a rapid rate in order for strenuous exercise to continue beyond a brief period of time. In such intense exercise, the energy to phosphorylate ADP comes mainly from glucose and stored glycogen during the anaerobic process of glycolysis with the resulting formation of lactic acid. In a way, this mechanism of lactic acid formation "buys time." It allows for the rapid formation of ATP by substrate phosphorylation, even though the oxygen supply is inadequate or the energy demands outstrip the capacity for ATP resynthesis aerobically. This anaerobic energy for ATP resynthesis can be thought of as reserve fuel that is brought into use by the athlete "kicking" the

80

last portion of a mile run. It is also of critical importance in supplying the rapid energy above that available from the stored phosphagens during a 440-yard run or 100-yard swim.[1] The most rapidly accumulated and highest lactic acid levels are reached during exercise that can be sustained for 60 to 180 seconds. As the intensity of "all-out" exercise decreases, thereby extending the work period, there is a corresponding decrease in both the rate of buildup and the final level of lactic acid.[21]

Lactic acid does not necessarily accumulate at all levels of exercise. Figure 7-1 illustrates the relationship between oxygen consumption, expressed as a percentage of maximum, and blood lactic acid during light, moderate, and heavy exercise in endurance athletes and untrained subjects. During light and moderate exercise, the energy demands of both groups are adequately met by reactions that use oxygen. In biochemical terms, the ATP for muscular contraction is made available predominantly through energy generated by the oxidation of hydrogen. Any lactic acid formed in light exercise is rapidly oxidized. As such, the blood lactic acid level remains fairly stable even though oxygen consumption increases.

At about 50% to 55% of the untrained subject's maximal capacity for aerobic metabolism, lactic acid begins to accumulate. This is probably due to the fact that the formation of lactic acid now exceeds its rate of removal via Krebs cycle metabolism.* This increase in lactic acid becomes greater as exercise becomes more intense and the muscle cells cannot meet the additional energy demands aerobically. This pattern is essentially similar for the trained subjects except that the threshold for lactic acid buildup, termed the *anaerobic threshold,* occurs at a higher percentage of the athlete's aerobic capacity.[10] This favorable response could be due to the endurance athlete's genetic endowment or specific adaptations with training,

*The usual explanation for a lactic acid increase is based on the assumption of a relative tissue hypoxia in heavy exercise. It is argued that under these conditions the release of hydrogen begins to exceed its oxidation down the respiratory chain. Consequently, excess hydrogens are passed to pyruvic acid and lactic acid accumulates. Studies using radioactive tracers indicate that lactic acid is formed continually at rest and in light exercise. Under aerobic conditions, however, lactic acid removal is equal to its rate of formation so that the concentration of blood lactic acid remains relatively stable.

or both. For example, it is well documented that the size and number of mitochondria increase with endurance training, as does the concentration and activity of various enzymes and transfer agents involved in aerobic metabolism.[17] Such alterations certainly enhance the cell's capability to generate ATP aerobically and may extend the percentage of one's maximum that can be sustained before the onset of lactic acid buildup. This concept of anaerobic threshold is developed more fully in Chapter 16.

The ability to generate a high lactic acid level in all-out exercise is increased with specific "anaerobic training" and subsequently reduced with detraining. Studies of well-trained athletes have shown that after they perform strenuous short-term exercise, the blood lactic acid level is 20% to 30% higher than in untrained subjects under similar circumstances.[14] The mechanism for this response is unknown, but it may be due to differences in motivation level accompanying the trained state. It is also likely that the increased intramuscular glycogen stores accompanying the trained state allow for a greater contribution of energy via anaerobic glycolysis.

LONG-TERM ENERGY: THE AEROBIC SYSTEM

Although the energy released in glycolysis is rapid and does not require oxygen, relatively little ATP is resynthesized in this manner. Consequently, aerobic reactions provide the important final stage for energy transfer, especially if vigorous exercise proceeds beyond 2 or 3 minutes.

Oxygen Consumption During Exercise

The curve in Figure 7-2 illustrates the oxygen consumption during each minute of a relatively slow jog continued at a steady pace for 10 minutes. Oxygen consumption rises rapidly during the first minutes of exercise. By the fourth minute a plateau is reached, and the oxygen consumption remains relatively stable for the rest of the exercise period. The flat portion or plateau of the oxygen consumption curve is generally considered the *steady state* or more precisely, the *steady rate.* This reflects a balance between the energy required by the working muscles and the rate of ATP production via aerobic me-

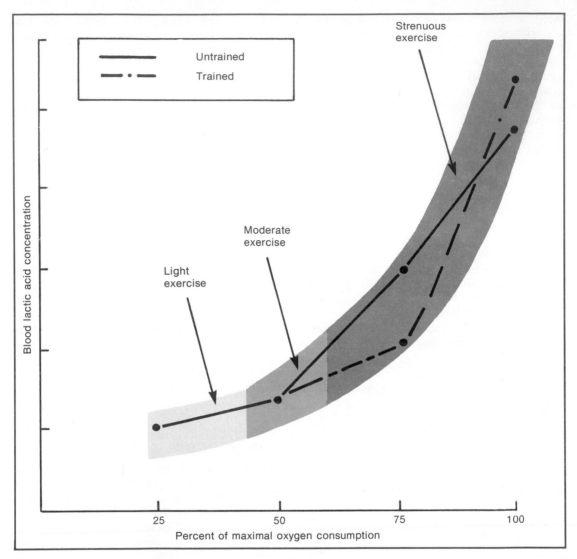

FIG. 7-1. *Increases in blood lactic acid concentration at different levels of exercise expressed as a percentage of maximal oxygen consumption for trained and untrained subjects.*

tabolism. In this region, oxygen-consuming reactions supply the energy for exercise. *Under steady-rate metabolic conditions, lactic acid accumulation is minimal.*

Many believe that once a steady rate is attained, exercise could continue indefinitely if the individual had the willpower to continue. This, of course, is based on the premise that a steady rate of aerobic metabolism is the only factor determining one's capacity for sustained submaximal exercise. Other factors, however, must be considered. Fluid loss and electrolyte depletion often become significant limiting factors, especially during work in the heat. Also of considerable importance to prolonged exercise

is maintaining adequate fuel reserves, particularly blood glucose for central nervous system function, and glycogen in the liver and in specific muscles utilized in the activity. Once a muscle's glycogen reserves are depleted, its work capabilities are dramatically reduced.

There are many steady rate levels. For some, the spectrum of steady rates might range from lying in bed to pushing a power lawn mower. On the other hand, at the upper limit the marathon runner can maintain a steady rate of aerobic metabolism throughout a 26-mile run averaging 5 minutes per mile. This magnificent accomplishment is determined largely by the athlete's ability to deliver and utilize oxygen.

OXYGEN DEFICIT. The curve of oxygen consumption shown in Figure 7-2 does not increase instantaneously to a steady rate at the start of exercise. In fact, in the beginning stages of work the oxygen uptake is considerably below the steady-rate level, even though the energy required to perform the exercise presumably remains unchanged throughout the work period. This lag in oxygen uptake should not be surprising, however, because the immediate energy for muscular work is *always* provided directly by the immediate and non-oxygen-consuming breakdown of ATP in the muscle. Oxygen becomes important only in subsequent reactions of energy transfer when it serves as an electron acceptor and combines with the hydrogens generated during glycolysis, beta oxidation of fatty acids, or the reactions of the Krebs cycle.

The oxygen deficit can be viewed quantitatively as the difference between the total oxygen actually consumed during exercise and the total that would have been consumed had a steady rate of aerobic metabolism been reached immediately at the start. The energy provided during the deficit phase of exercise represents nonaerobic energy (that is, immediate energy from the stored phosphates plus anaerobic energy from glycolysis) that is utilized until a steady rate is reached between oxygen consumption and the energy demands of exercise.

Figure 7-3 depicts the relationship between the size of the oxygen deficit and the contribution of energy from both the ATP-CP and lactic acid energy systems. As shown, the high-energy phosphates are substantially depleted by exercise that generates about a three-liter oxygen deficit. Consequently, this exercise can continue only on a "pay-as-you-go" basis with ATP being continually replenished through the breakdown of the food nutrients by oxidative phosphorylation or glycolysis. Interestingly, lactic acid begins to increase in exercising muscle well before the phosphates reach their lowest levels. This finding indicates that glycol-

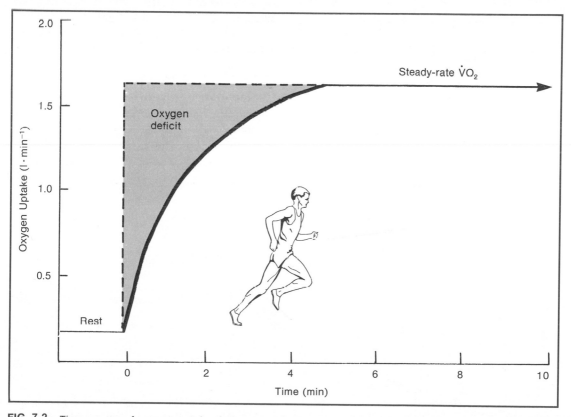

FIG. 7-2. *Time course of oxygen uptake during a continuous jog at a relatively slow pace for 10 minutes. The shaded area indicates the "oxygen deficit" or the quantity of oxygen that would have been consumed had the oxygen uptake reached a steady rate immediately.*

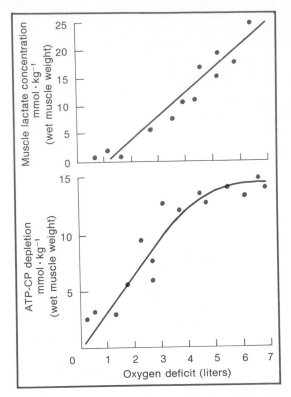

FIG. 7-3. *ATP and CP depletion and lactic acid formation in relation to the calculated oxygen deficit. (From Pernow, B., and Karlsson, J.: Muscle ATP, CP and lactate in submaximal and maximal exercise. In Muscle Metabolism During Exercise. Edited by B. Pernow, and B. Saltin. New York, Plenum Press, 1971.)*

ysis contributes anaerobic energy in the early stages of vigorous exercise, even before the full utilization of the high-energy phosphates. *These observations show that energy for exercise is not merely the result of a series of energy systems that "switch on" and "switch off," but rather, the smooth blending with considerable overlap, from one mode of energy transfer to another.*

OXYGEN DEFICIT IN TRAINED AND UNTRAINED INDIVIDUALS. It is generally observed that oxygen consumption during light and moderate exercise is similar in trained and untrained subjects once the steady rate is reached. Apparently, however, the trained person reaches the steady rate more rapidly[26] and has a *smaller* oxygen deficit for the same exercise compared to the untrained. If this is the case, the total oxygen consumed during exercise would be greater for the trained person, and, presumably, the anaerobic component of energy transfer would be proportionately smaller.[12a] It is possible that this facilitated level of aerobic metabolism in the early stages of exercise is the result of cellular adaptations with endurance training, many of which are known to increase the capacity of muscle to generate ATP aerobically.[17]

Maximal Oxygen Consumption (max $\dot{V}O_2$)

Figure 7-4 depicts the oxygen consumption response during a series of constant-speed runs up six hills, each progressively steeper than the next. (In the laboratory, these "hills"

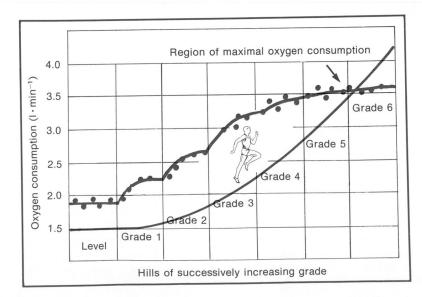

FIG. 7-4. *Oxygen consumption during exercise of increasing intensity up to the maximal oxygen consumption. This occurs in the region where a further increase in work is not accompanied by an additional increase in oxygen consumption. (From* Nutrition, Weight Control, and Exercise *by Frank I. Katch and William D. McArdle. Copyright © 1977 by Houghton Mifflin Company. Reprinted by permission of the publisher.)*

can be simulated by increasing the elevation of a treadmill or step bench or increasing the resistance to pedaling a bicycle ergometer.) Each successive hill requires a greater energy output and thus places an additional load on the runner's capacity for aerobic metabolism. During the first several hills, the increases in oxygen consumption are linear and in direct proportion to the severity of exercise. Although the runner is able to maintain running speed up the last two hills, the oxygen consumption does not increase to the same extent observed for the previous hills. In fact, no increase is noted for the run up the last hill. *The point where the oxygen consumption plateaus and shows no further increase (or increases only slightly) with an additional workload is called the maximal oxygen consumption, maximal oxygen uptake, maximal aerobic power, or, simply, max $\dot{V}O_2$.* It is generally assumed that this represents the person's capacity for the aerobic resynthesis of ATP. Additional work is accomplished only via the energy transfer reactions of glycolysis with the resulting formation of lactic acid. Under these conditions, the runner soon becomes exhausted and unable to continue.

The max $\dot{V}O_2$ provides a quantitative statement of an individual's capacity for aerobic energy transfer. As such, it is one of the more important factors determining our ability to sustain high-intensity exercise for longer than 4 or 5 minutes. In subsequent chapters, we will discuss various aspects of aerobic power, including its measurement and its role in exercise performance.

FAST- AND SLOW-TWITCH MUSCLE FIBERS

By means of surgical biopsy, biochemists and exercise physiologists have studied the functional and structural characteristics of human skeletal muscle. This has led to the identification of two distinct types of muscle fibers,[12] the proportion of which probably remains constant throughout life.[12b] One type is a *fast-twitch* (FT) fiber. This fast-contracting fiber possesses a high capability for the anaerobic production of ATP during glycolysis. These fibers are activated during change-of-pace and stop-and-go activities such as basketball and ice hockey as well as during all-out exercise that requires rapid, powerful movements that depend almost exclusively on the energy generated from anaerobic metabolism.

The second major classification is the *slow-twitch* (ST) muscle fiber. This is a predominantly aerobic fiber with a relatively slow speed of contraction compared to its fast-twitch counterpart. The capacity of these fibers to generate ATP aerobically is intimately related to their numerous mitochondria and to the high concentrations of enzymes required to sustain aerobic metabolism. The primary role of the slow-twitch fiber is to sustain continuous endurance-type activities that require a steady rate of aerobic energy transfer. In fatigue associated with distance running, glycogen depletion occurs primarily in the slow-twitch fibers. It should be kept in mind, however, that most sport activities require a blend of powerful and sustained muscular contractions and that all types of muscle fibers are utilized.

From the preceding discussion, it would seem that the predominant fiber type in specific muscles is an important factor determining success in a particular sport or activity. This idea as well as other considerations concerning each type of muscle fiber (and their various subdivisions) is discussed in Chapter 18.

THE ENERGY SPECTRUM OF EXERCISE

Figure 7-5 illustrates the relative contribution of anaerobic and aerobic energy sources during various durations of maximal exercise. In addition, the data in Table 7-1 show the approximate energy yield from these systems of energy transfer. Although these data were originally obtained from laboratory experiments involving running and bicycling, they can easily be related to other activities by drawing the appropriate relationships in terms of time. For example, a 2- to 7-second period of all-out exercise respresents the majority of plays occurring in football or a "solo dash" in soccer, ice hockey, or basketball. All-out exercise for about 1 minute incorporates the 440-yard dash in track, the 100-yard swim and, possibly, a full-court press at the end of a basketball game.

At one extreme, the total energy for exercise is supplied almost entirely by the intramuscular phosphagens. In intense exercise lasting 2 minutes, about half of the energy is supplied by the ATP-CP and lactic acid systems, whereas aerobic reactions supply the remainder. Under these conditions, it is desirable to possess a high capacity for both aerobic and anaerobic metabolism. Intense exercise of an intermedi-

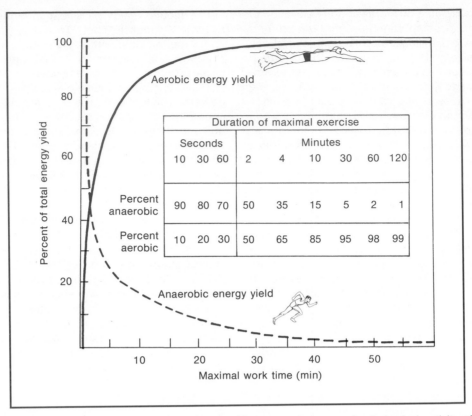

FIG. 7-5. *Relative contribution of aerobic and anaerobic energy during maximal physical activity of various durations. It should be noted that 1½ to 2 minutes of maximal effort requires 50 percent of the energy from aerobic and anaerobic processes. (Adapted from Åstrand, P.O., and Rodahl, K.: Textbook of Work Physiology. New York, McGraw-Hill Book Company, © 1977. Used with permission of McGraw-Hill Book Company).*

TABLE 7-1. *Relative contribution of anaerobic and aerobic processes to total energy output during maximal exercise of different durations*[a]

WORK TIME MAXIMAL EXERCISE	ENERGY OUTPUT (kcal)		
	ANAEROBIC PROCESSES	AEROBIC PROCESSES	TOTAL
10 s	20	4	24
1 min	30	20	50
2 min	30	45	75
5 min	30	120	150
10 min	25	245	270
30 min	20	675	695
60 min	15	1200	1215

[a] From Gollnick, P.D., and Hermansen, L.: Biochemical adaptions to exercise: Anaerobic metabolism. *In* Exercise and Sport Science Reviews. Vol. 1. Edited by J.H. Wilmore, Academic Press, New York, 1973.

ate duration performed for 5 to 10 minutes, as in middle distance running and swimming, basketball, or soccer, results in a greater demand for aerobic energy. Performances of long duration such as marathon running, distance swimming, cycling, recreational jogging, or hiking require a fairly constant supply of aerobic energy with little reliance on the mechanism of lactic acid formation.

An understanding of the energy demands of various activities provides some explanation as to why a world-record-holder in the one-mile run is not necessarily a noted distance runner. Conversely, premier marathon runners are generally unable to run a mile in less than 4 minutes yet can complete 26 miles at a 5-minute per mile pace. The appropriate approach to exercise training is to analyze an activity in terms of its specific energy components and then train those systems to assure optimal physiologic and metabolic adaptations. *An improved capacity for energy transfer directly translates into improved exercise performance.*

OXYGEN CONSUMPTION DURING RECOVERY: THE "OXYGEN DEBT"

After exercise, bodily processes do not immediately return to resting levels. In submaximal exercise, recovery is rapid and often proceeds unnoticed. If the activity is particularly stressful, such as running a half-mile race or trying to swim 200 yards as fast as possible, the body requires considerable time to return to rest. Recovery from both moderate and strenuous exercise is associated largely with the specific metabolic and physiologic processes resulting from each form of exercise.

The oxygen consumption during exercise and recovery from moderate and strenuous work is shown in Figure 7-6. During light exercise, when the oxygen deficit is small, the quantity of oxygen consumed in recovery is also small, and the preexercise metabolic rate is achieved rapidly. During the exhaustive exercise illustrated in the bottom curve, a steady rate of aerobic metabolism cannot be attained. In this situation, anaerobic energy transfer greatly exceeds aerobic reactions and lactic acid accumulates. Complete recovery from this type of exercise requires considerable time. In recovery from either light, moderate, or strenuous exercise, the oxygen consumed in excess

of the resting value has been termed the *oxygen debt*. The oxygen debt is indicated by the shaded area under the recovery curve and is calculated as the total oxygen consumed in recovery minus the total oxygen theoretically consumed at rest during the recovery period.

For example, if a total of 5.5 liters of oxygen were consumed in recovery until the resting value of .310 liters per minute was reached, and the recovery required 10 minutes, the oxygen debt would be 5.5 liters − (.310 ℓ × 10 min), or 2.4 liters. This result means that the preceding exercise caused the consumption of an additional 2.4 liters of oxygen before the preexercise state was reached. An important assumption underlying the concept of oxygen debt is that resting oxygen uptake remained essentially unchanged during exercise and recovery. As we shall see, this assumption is not entirely correct, especially in recovery from strenuous exercise.

The recovery curves in Figure 7-6 illustrate two important characteristics of oxygen debt: (1) If the previous exercise was primarily aerobic, about one-half of the total recovery oxygen consumption is repaid within 30 seconds; within several minutes, the recovery is complete. (2) Recovery from strenuous exercise, in which there has been a considerable increase in both lactic acid and body temperature, presents a somewhat different picture. In addition to the fast component of recovery oxygen consumption, there is a second, slower phase termed the "slow" component. Depending on the intensity and duration of exercise, this phase of recovery may take up to several hours, or even a day, before the preexercise oxygen consumption level is once again established.

Metabolic Dynamics of Oxygen Debt

A precise biochemical explanation of the recovery oxygen consumption, especially the role of lactic acid, is not possible because the specific chemical dynamics of oxygen debt are still unclear.

TRADITIONAL CONCEPTS. The term oxygen debt was first coined by the Nobel Prize scientist Archibald Vivian Hill in 1922. Hill, as well as others, discussed energy metabolism during exercise and recovery in financial-accounting terms.[16] Within this framework, the body's carbohydrate stores were likened to energy "cred-

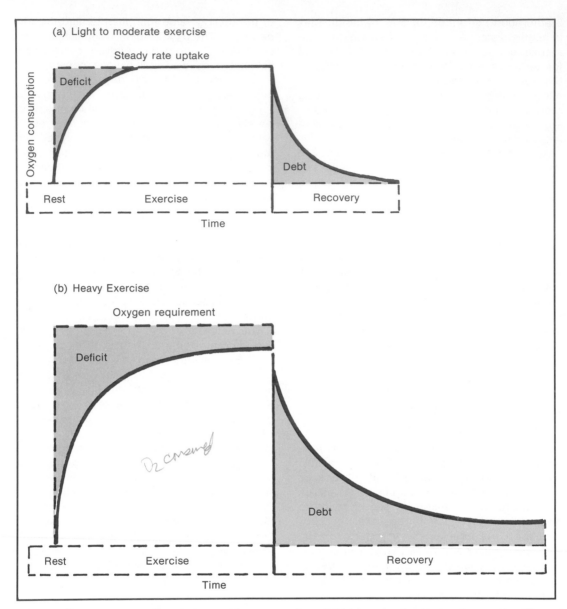

FIG. 7-6. *Oxygen consumption during and in recovery from light to moderate steady-rate exercise (A), and heavy exercise with the resulting buildup of lactic acid (B). (From Nutrition, Weight Control, and Exercise by Frank I. Katch and William D. McArdle. Copyright © 1977 by Houghton Mifflin Company. Reprinted by permission of the publisher.)*

its." If these stored credits were expended during exercise, then a "debt" was incurred. The greater the energy "deficit," or use of available stored energy credits, the larger the energy debt incurred. The recovery oxygen uptake was thought to represent the metabolic cost of repaying this debt—hence the term oxygen debt. In more concrete terms, the accumulation of lactic acid during the anaerobic component of exercise represented the utilization of the stored energy credit, glycogen. The ensuing oxygen debt was believed to serve two purposes: (1) to reestablish the original carbohydrate stores (credits) by resynthesizing approximately 80% of the lactic acid back to glycogen in the liver, and (2) to catabolize the remaining lactic acid via the pyruvic acid–Krebs cycle pathway. The ATP generated in this process presumably was used to power the resynthesis of lactic acid to glycogen. This early explanation of the dynamics of recovery oxygen consumption has often been termed the "lactic acid theory of oxygen debt."

In 1933, subsequent to the work of Hill, researchers at the Harvard Fatigue Laboratory attempted to explain their observations that the initial portion of the recovery oxygen was consumed before blood lactic acid began to decrease.[22] In fact, they showed that it was possible to incur an oxygen debt of almost three liters without any appreciable elevation in lactic acid. To resolve these findings, two phases of oxygen debt were proposed: (1) *alactic or alactacid* oxygen debt (without lactic acid buildup), and (2) *lactic acid* or *lactacid* oxygen debt. It is noteworthy that these two explanations were based on speculation, because these researchers did not measure ATP and CP replenishment or the relationship between lactic acid and glucose and glycogen levels. Essentially, the following model has served to explain the energetics of oxygen debt for nearly 40 years:

1. *Alactacid debt*—The alactacid portion of the oxygen debt depicted for steady-rate exercise in the top graph in Figure 7-6, or for the rapid phase of recovery from strenuous exercise (bottom graph), was attributed to the restoration of the high-energy phosphates ATP and CP depleted during exercise. The energy for this restoration comes from the aerobic breakdown of the food nutrients during recovery. A small portion of the recovery oxygen is also used to reload the muscle myoglobin as well as the hemoglobin in the blood returning from previously active tissues.

2. *Lactacid debt*—In keeping with the explanation by A.V. Hill, the major portion of the lactic acid oxygen debt was thought to represent the reconversion of lactic acid to glycogen in the liver.

CONTROVERSY WITH TRADITIONAL EXPLANATION OF OXYGEN DEBT. Several relationships must be established to support the contention that an aerobic energy deficit in exercise is temporarily compensated for by energy from anaerobic sources that are then resynthesized in recovery. For example, only a moderate relationship exists between the degree of anaerobiosis in exercise (oxygen deficit) and the excess oxygen uptake in recovery (oxygen debt).[4,13]

To accept the traditional explanation for the lactacid phase of the oxygen debt, it must also be clearly established that the lactic acid produced in exercise is *actually* resynthesized to glycogen in recovery, as Hill and others had speculated. This has never been shown. In fact, when radioactive lactic acid is infused into rat muscle, more than 75% of this substrate appears as radioactive carbon dioxide, whereas only 25% is synthesized to glycogen.[8] In experiments with humans, no substantial replenishment of glycogen was observed 10 minutes after strenuous exercise, even though blood lactic acid levels were significantly reduced.[26] *Apparently the major portion of lactic acid is oxidized for energy.* Indeed, it is well established that the heart, liver, kidneys, and skeletal muscle utilize lactic acid in the blood as an energy substrate.

CONTEMPORARY CONCEPTS OF OXYGEN DEBT. There is no doubt that the elevated aerobic metabolism in recovery is necessary to restore the body to its preexercise condition and is largely the result of the preceding metabolic and physiologic events during exercise.[25] In moderate exercise, this recovery oxygen consumption serves to replenish the high-energy phosphates depleted by exercise, whereas in strenuous exercise, some oxygen is utilized to resynthesize a small portion of lactic acid to glycogen. However, the main source for reestablishing preexercise glycogen levels is the carbohydrate in the diet, *not* resynthesized lactic acid.

A significant portion of the recovery oxygen consumption is also attributed to physiologic processes actually taking place *during* recovery. The considerably larger oxygen debt in relation to oxygen deficit in exhaustive exercise is probably the result of such factors. Body temperature, for example, is elevated about 3° C (5.4° F) during vigorous exercise and can remain elevated for several hours in recovery. This has a direct stimulating effect on metabolism and can cause a significant increase in recovery oxygen consumption.[2,7]

Other factors also affect recovery oxygen consumption. Perhaps as much as 10% of the recovery oxygen goes to reload the blood as it returns from the exercised muscles. An additional 2% to 5% restores the oxygen dissolved in body fluids and the oxygen bound to myoglobin in the muscle itself. In very intense exercise, the volume of air breathed increases 8 to 10 times above rest and remains elevated for some time in recovery. Thus, the respiratory muscles also require more oxygen for the work of breathing during recovery than they normally require at rest.[21a] The heart also works harder and requires a greater oxygen supply during recovery. Tissue repair and the redistribution of the ions calcium, potassium, and sodium within the muscle and other body compartments require energy, whereas the residual effects of hormones released in exercise may continue to affect metabolism for a considerable time in recovery. In essence, all of the physiologic systems that are activated to meet the demands of exercise also increase their own particular need for oxygen during recovery. *The oxygen debt, or more accurately the recovery oxygen consumption, reflects both the anaerobic metabolism of exercise and the respiratory, circulatory, hormonal, ionic, and the thermal adjustments actually occurring in recovery.*

QUANTIFYING THE OXYGEN DEBT. Table 7-2 presents theoretical estimates of the quantity of oxygen that can be ascribed to the replenishment of high-energy phosphates, reloading the body's oxygen stores, and the cost of circulation and ventilation in recovery. Based on certain reasonable assumptions in calculating

these theoretical maximums, a "true" oxygen debt in excess of 3 or 4 liters would not be anticipated. This is in direct conflict to reports of oxygen debts that frequently exceed the theoretical maximum, sometimes by as much as 18 or 19 liters of oxygen![22] More than likely, this is due to the metabolic cost of factors such as tissue repair, substrate synthesis, and ion distribution, as well as to the potentially large residual effect of an elevated body temperature caused by the previous exercise.

Implications of Oxygen Debt for Exercise and Recovery

An understanding of the dynamics of the recovery oxygen consumption provides a basis for structuring work intervals and optimizing recovery. With either steady-rate aerobic exercise or brief 5 to 10-second bouts of all-out work, no appreciable lactic acid accumulates. Consequently, recovery is rapid (fast component), and work can begin again without the hindering effects of fatigue. In contrast, longer periods of anaerobic exercise are performed at the expense of lactic acid buildup in the blood and exercising muscles. In this situation, recovery oxygen consumption consists of both fast and slow components, and considerably more time

TABLE 7-2. *Theoretical maximum recovery oxygen uptake for a 70-kg man*[a]

ASSUMPTIONS
a) Active muscle equals 20 kg
b) P/O ratio equals 3; i. e., 36 ATP are formed for 12 atoms of oxygen consumed
c) 1 mole ATP phosphorylates 1 mole creatine
d) Muscle is 80% water
e) Venous blood volume equals 4 liters
f) a-$\bar{v}$ O_2 diff after exercise is 11 ml O_2/100 ml blood
g) 10% muscle volume is blood
h) Complete desaturation of all potential sources of oxygen and hydrolysis of all ATP and CP to ADP and C, respectively

SOURCE OF RECOVERY OXYGEN CONSUMPTION	O_2 EQUIVALENT, LITERS	CUMULATIVE O_2, LITERS
ATP	0.45	0.45
CP	1.05	1.50
Resaturation of tissue H_2O	0.05	1.55
Resaturation of venous blood	0.44	1.99
Resaturation of blood in muscle	0.40	2.39
Resaturation of myoglobin	0.20	2.59
Extra cardiorespiratory work during recovery	0.40	2.99
TOTAL RECOVERY OXYGEN	2.99	

[a]From Brooks, G.A. et al.: Temperature, skeletal muscle mitochondrial functions, and oxygen debt. *Am. J. Physiol. 220*:1053, 1971.

is required for complete recovery. This can pose a problem in sports such as basketball, hockey, soccer, tennis, and badminton, because a performer pushed to a high level of anaerobic metabolism may not fully recover during brief rest periods such as times out, between points, or even half-time breaks.

Procedures for speeding recovery from exercise can generally be categorized as either *active* or *passive*. In active recovery (often called "cooling-down" or "tapering-off"), submaximal aerobic exercise is performed in the belief that this continued movement will in some way prevent muscle cramps and stiffness and facilitate the recovery process. With passive recovery, the person usually lies down with the hope that complete inactivity will reduce the resting energy requirements and thus "free" oxygen for the recovery process. Modifications of active and passive recovery have included the use of cold showers, massages, specific body positions, and the ingestion of cold liquids.

OPTIMAL RECOVERY FROM STEADY-RATE EXERCISE. Exercise performed at an oxygen consumption below 50% to 60% of max $\dot{V}O_2$ can generally be performed at a steady rate with little lactic acid buildup. Recovery from this exercise entails the resynthesis of high-energy phosphates, replenishment of oxygen in the blood, body fluids, and muscle myoglobin, and a small energy cost to sustain circulation and ventilation. In this situation, recovery is more rapid with passive procedures,[20] because exercise would only serve to elevate total metabolism and delay recovery to the resting level.

OPTIMAL RECOVERY FROM NON-STEADY-RATE EXERCISE. When exercise intensity exceeds about 50% to 60% of max $\dot{V}O_2$, a steady rate of aerobic metabolism is no longer maintained and lactic acid accumulates. As work intensity increases, the level of lactic acid rises sharply (see Fig. 7-1) and the exerciser soon becomes exhausted. Although the mechanisms of fatigue during intense anaerobic exercise are poorly understood, the level of blood lactic acid does provide a fairly objective indication of the relative strenuousness of exercise and may also reflect the adequacy of the recovery process.

Lactic acid removal is accelerated by active aerobic recovery exercise.[15,19] Apparently, the optimal level of recovery exercise is between 29% and 45% of the max $\dot{V}O_2$ for bicycle exercise[3] and 55% to 70% of max $\dot{V}O_2$ when the recovery involves treadmill running.[15] The data in Figure 7-7 illustrate the lactic acid recovery patterns for trained male and female subjects who used repeat 1-minute bouts of all-out exercise to achieve maximum lactic acid levels.

Active recovery involved 30 minutes of continuous treadmill running at different percentages of the max $\dot{V}O_2$; passive recovery consisted of 30 minutes of rest. *Clearly, all active recovery conditions facilitated lactic acid removal compared to passive recovery. The most rapid recovery (at least in terms of blood lactic acid) was achieved with continuous exercise performed at about 60% of max $\dot{V}O_2$.* In a practical sense, if left to their own choice, people voluntarily select this optimum intensity of active recovery.[6]

The reasons for the apparent benefits of active recovery compared to passive recovery are not clear. The facilitated removal of lactic acid may be the result of an increased perfusion of blood through "lactate-using" organs like the liver and heart. In addition, increased flow of blood through the muscles in active recovery would certainly enhance lactic acid removal because muscle tissue can use this substrate and oxidize it via Krebs cycle metabolism. It is important to note that if recovery exercise is too intense and above a steady rate, it will be of no benefit and may even prolong recovery by increasing lactic acid formation.

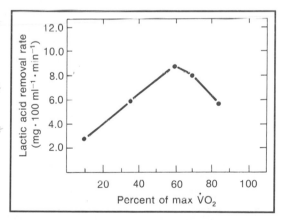

FIG. 7-7. *Lactic acid removal rate during active recovery at various percentages of max $\dot{V}O_2$. Exercise between 50 and 60 percent of max $\dot{V}O_2$ provides the optimal recovery pattern. Removal rate is expressed as mg of lactic acid per 100 ml blood per minute. (Modified from Hermansen, L., and Stensvold, I.: Production and removal of lactate during exercise in man. Acta Physiol. Scand. 86:191, 1972.)*

Intermittent Exercise

Several approaches can be taken to enable a person to perform significant amounts of normally exhaustive exercise, while at the same time reducing the contribution from anaerobic energy transfer via glycolysis and subsequent lactic acid buildup. One means is to train the aerobic systems to increase their capacity to sustain exercise at a high rate of aerobic energy transfer. A dramatic example of this high steady-rate capability is the performance of elite marathon runners, distance swimmers, and cross-country skiers. Another approach to performing work that would normally cause exhaustion within 3 to 5 minutes if performed continuously is to exercise in an intermittent manner using a preestablished spacing of work and rest intervals.[9] This technique is becoming popular in conditioning programs and is known as *interval training*. Here, various work-to-rest intervals using "supermaximal" exercise are applied to overload the various systems of energy transfer. For example, with all-out work bouts of up to 8 seconds, the intramuscular phosphates provide the major portion of energy, and reliance on the glycolytic pathway is minimal. Therefore, recovery is rapid (fast component), and another bout of heavy exercise can begin after only a brief recovery period.

The results of a series of laboratory experiments using various combinations of work and rest intervals during intermittent exercise are summarized in Table 7-3. On one day, the subject ran at a speed that would normally exhaust him within 5 minutes. About 0.8 mile was covered during this continuous run, and the runner attained a maximal oxygen consumption of 5.6 liters per minute. A relative state of exhaustion plus a high level of anaerobic metabolism were verified by the high lactic acid level shown in the last column of the table.

On another day, the same fast speed was maintained, but the exercise was performed intermittently with periods of 10 seconds of exercise and 5 seconds of recovery. With a 30-minute protocol of intermittent exercise, the actual duration of running amounted to 20 minutes and the distance covered was 4 miles compared to less than 5 minutes and 0.8 miles when the run was performed continuously! This work output capability is even more impressive if one considers that the lactic acid level remained low even though the oxygen consumption was quite high, averaging 5.1 liters per minute (91% of max $\dot{V}O_2$) throughout the 30-minute period. Thus, a relative balance had been achieved between the energy requirements of work and the level of aerobic energy transfer within the muscle during the work and rest intervals.

Clearly, by manipulating the duration of work and rest intervals, a specific energy transfer system can be emphasized and overloaded. When the rest interval was extended from 5 to 10 seconds, the oxygen consumption averaged 4.4 liters per minute; with 15-second work and 30-second recovery intervals, only a 3.6 liter oxygen consumption was noted. In each case of 30 minutes of intermittent exercise, however, the runner achieved a longer distance and much lower lactic acid levels compared to the same work performed continuously. The specific application of the principles of intermittent

TABLE 7-3. *Results of an experiment dealing with intermittent exercise*[a]

EXERCISE—REST PERIODS	TOTAL DISTANCE RUN (YARDS)	AVERAGE OXYGEN CONSUMPTION ($l \cdot min^{-1}$)	BLOOD LACTIC ACID LEVEL (mg · 100 ml blood^{-1})
4 min continuous	1422	5.6	150
10 s exercise 5 s rest	7294	5.1	44
10 s exercise 10 s rest	5468	4.4	20
15 s exercise 30 s rest	3642	3.6	16

[a]From data of Christenson, E.H. et al.: Intermittent and continuous running. Acta Physiol. Scand., *50:*269, 1960, as reported in Åstrand, P.O., and Rodahl, K.: Textbook of Work Physiology, New York, McGraw-Hill, 1970, p. 384.

exercise to both aerobic and anaerobic training and sports performance are discussed in Chapter 20.

SUMMARY

1. The major means of ATP production differ depending on the intensity and duration of exercise. In intense exercise of short duration (100-yard dash, weight lifting), the energy is derived from the already present stores of intramuscular ATP and CP (immediate energy system). For intense exercise of longer duration (1–2 min), energy is generated mainly from the anaerobic reactions of glycolysis (short-term energy system). As exercise progresses beyond several minutes, the aerobic system predominates and oxygen consumption becomes an important factor (long-term energy system).

2. Humans possess different kinds of muscle fibers, each with unique metabolic and contractile properties. The two major fiber types are (1) low oxidative–high glycolytic, *fast-twitch fibers,* and (2) low glycolytic–high oxidative, *slow-twitch fibers.* Intermediate fibers with overlapping metabolic characteristics are also present.

3. By understanding the energy spectrum of exercise, it is possible to train for specific improvement of the appropriate energy system.

4. A steady rate of oxygen uptake represents a balance between the energy requirements of the working muscles and the aerobic resynthesis of ATP. The difference between the oxygen requirement and the actual oxygen consumed is called the oxygen deficit.

5. The maximum capacity for the aerobic resynthesis of ATP is quantitatively measured as the maximum oxygen intake. This is one of the most important indicators of one's ability for sustained exercise.

6. After exercise, the oxygen uptake remains elevated above the resting level. This recovery oxygen consumption reflects the metabolic characteristics of the preceding exercise as well as the physiologic alterations caused by that exercise.

7. Moderate exercise performed during recovery (active recovery) appears to facilitate the recovery process compared to passive procedures. In most situations, this is reflected in a faster removal of lactic acid.

References

1. Alpert, N.R.: Lactate production and removal and the regulation of metabolism. Ann. N.Y. Acad. Sci., *119:*995, 1965.
2. Barclay, J.K.: The metabolism of contracting dog skeletal muscle *in situ.* Unpublished Doctoral Dissertation. The University of Michigan, 1969.
3. Belcastro, A.N., and Bonen, A.: Lactic acid removal rates during controlled and uncontrolled recovery exercise. J. Appl. Physiol., *39:*932, 1975.
4. Berg, W.E.: Individual differences in respiratory gas exchange during recovery from moderate exercise. Am. J. Physiol., *149:*597, 1947.
5. Bergstrom, J. et al.: Energy rich phosphagens in dynamic and static work. *In Muscle Metabolism During Exercise.* Edited by B. Pernow and B. Saltin. New York, Plenum Press, 1971.
6. Bonen, A., and Belcastro, A.N.: Comparison of self-selected recovery methods on lactic acid removal rates. Med. Sci. Sports, *8:*176, 1976.
7. Brooks, G.A. et al.: Temperature, skeletal muscle mitochondrial functions and oxygen debt. Am. J. Physiol., *220:*1053, 1971.
8. Brooks, G.A. et al.: Glycogen synthesis and metabolism of lactic acid after exercise. Am. J. Physiol., *224:*1162, 1973.

9. Christenson, E.H. et al.: Intermittent and continuous running. Acta Physiol. Scand., *50:*269, 1960.
10. Costill, D.L.: Metabolic responses during distance running. J. Appl. Physiol., *28:*251, 1970.
11. Costill, D. et al.: Glycogen depletion patterns in human muscle fibers during distance running. Acta Physiol. Scand., *89:*374, 1973.
12. Edgerton, V.R.: Exercise and growth and development of muscle tissue. *In* Physical Activity: Human Growth and Development. Edited by G.L. Rarick. New York: Academic Press, 1973.
12a. Girandola, R.N., and Katch, F.I.: Effects of physical conditioning on changes in exercise and recovery O_2 uptake and efficiency during constant-load ergometer exercise. Med. Sci. Sports, *5:*242, 1973.
12b. Grimby, G. Muscle morphology and function in 67–81 years old men and women. Med. Sci. Sports, (abstract) *12:*95, 1980.
13. Henry, F.M.: Aerobic oxygen consumption and alactic debt in muscular work. J. Appl. Physiol., *3:*427, 1951.
14. Hermansen, L.: Anaerobic energy release. Med. Sci. Sports, *1:*32, 1969.
15. Hermansen, L., and Stensvold, I.: Production and removal of lactate during exercise in man. Acta Physiol. Scand., *86:*191, 1972.
16. Hill, A.V. et al.: Muscular exercise, lactic acid and the supply and utilization of oxygen. Proc. R. Soc. Lond. (Biol.) *96:*438, 1924.
17. Holloszy, J.O.: Biochemical adaptation to exercise: Aerobic metabolism. *In* Exercise and Sport Science Reviews, Vol. 1. Edited by J. Wilmore. New York, Academic Press, 1973.
18. Hultman, E.: Studies on muscle metabolism of glycogen and active phosphate in man with special reference to exercise and diet. Scand. J. Clin. Lab. Invest., Suppl. 94, 1967.
19. Jervell, O.: Investigation of the concentration of lactic acid in blood and urine under physiologic and pathologic conditions. Acta Med. Scand., *24:*1, 1928.
20. Jorfeldt, L.: Metabolism of L(+)-lactate in human skeletal muscle during exercise. Acta Physiol. Scand., Suppl. 338, 1970.
21. Karlsson, J.: Lactate and phosphagen concentrations in working muscle of man. Acta Physiol. Scand., Suppl. 358, 1971.
21a. Katch, F.I., et al.: The influence of the estimated oxygen cost of ventilation on oxygen deficit and recovery oxygen intake for moderately heavy bicycle ergometer exercise. Med. Sci. Sports. *4:*71, 1972.
22. Margaria, R. et al.: The possible mechanism of contracting and paying the oxygen debt and the role of lactic acid in muscular contraction. Am. J. Physiol., *106:*687, 1933.
23. Pernow, B., and Karlsson, J.: Muscle ATP, CP and lactate in submaximal and maximal exercise. *In* Muscle Metabolism During Exercise. Edited by B. Pernow and B. Saltin. New York, Plenum Press, 1971.
24. Saltin, B.: Metabolic fundamentals in exercise. Med. Sci. Sports, *5:*137, 1973.
25. Stainsby, W.N., and Barclay, J.K.: Exercise metabolism: O_2 deficit, steady level O_2 uptake and O_2 uptake in recovery. Med. Sci. Sports, *2:*177, 1970.
26. Weltman, A., and Katch V.L.: Min-by-min respiratory exchange and oxygen uptake kinetics during steady-state exercise in subjects of high and low max $\dot{V}O_2$. Res. Quart., *47:*490, 1977.

Measurement of Human Energy Expenditure

8

METHODS OF MEASURING THE BODY'S HEAT PRODUCTION

The quantity of energy generated by the body during rest and muscular effort can be accurately determined by several different methods. These are broadly classified as *direct* and *indirect calorimetry*.

Direct Calorimetry

Human heat production can be measured directly in a calorimeter similar to the bomb calorimeter described in Chapter 4 to determine the energy content of food. The calorimeter illustrated in Figure 8-1 consists of an airtight, thermally insulated living chamber. The heat produced and radiated by the person is removed by a stream of cold water flowing at a constant rate through tubes coiled near the ceiling of the chamber. The difference in the temperature of water entering and leaving the chamber reflects the person's heat production. Humidified air is continually supplied and circulated while the expired carbon dioxide is removed by chemical absorbents. Oxygen is added to the air before it reenters the calorimeter to maintain a normal oxygen supply.

The techniques of direct calorimetry, although highly accurate and of great theoretical importance, are impractical for studies of human energy expenditure during various sport, recreational, and occupational activities. In these situations, indirect methods are almost always used.

Indirect Calorimetry

All energy metabolism in the body ultimately depends on the utilization of oxygen. Thus, by measuring a person's oxygen consumption under steady-rate conditions, it is possible to obtain an indirect estimate of energy metabolism.

Studies with the bomb calorimeter have shown that approximately 4.82 kcal of heat are liberated when a blend of carbohydrate, fat, and protein is burned in one liter of oxygen. This calorific value for oxygen varies only

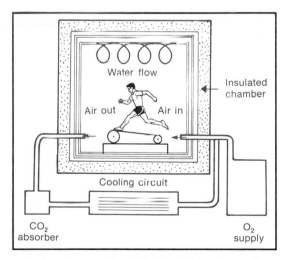

FIG. 8-1. *Human calorimeter used to measure heat production. From* Nutrition, Weight Control, and Exercise *by Frank I. Katch and William D. McArdle. Copyright © 1977 by Houghton Mifflin Company. Reprinted by permission of the publisher.*

95

slightly even with large variations in the metabolic mixture. If we assume the combustion of a mixed diet, then for convenience in calculations, a value of 5 kcal per liter of oxygen consumed can be used as an appropriate conversion factor for estimating the body's energy expenditure. This energy–oxygen equivalent, 5 kcal per liter of oxygen, is the convenient yardstick for transposing any aerobic exercise to a caloric frame of reference. In fact, indirect calorimetry via oxygen consumption measurement is the means by which the caloric stress of most activities has been evaluated.

Although the techniques for indirect calorimetry are relatively simple and inexpensive compared to direct measurement in the human calorimeter, both measures give comparable results. *Closed-circuit* and *open-circuit* spirometry represent the two applications of indirect calorimetry.

CLOSED-CIRCUIT SPIROMETRY. The method of closed-circuit spirometry illustrated in Figure 8-2 is routinely used in hospitals and other laboratory settings where resting estimates of energy expenditure are made. The subject breathes and rebreathes from a prefilled container or spirometer of oxygen. This is considered a "closed system" since the person rebreathes only the gas in the spirometer. Carbon dioxide in the exhaled air is absorbed by a cannister of soda lime (potassium hydroxide) placed in the breathing circuit. A drum that revolves at a known speed is attached to the spirometer to record changes in the volume of the system as oxygen is consumed.

During exercise, it is exceedingly difficult to measure oxygen consumption with closed-circuit spirometry. The spirometer is bulky, the subject must remain close to the equipment, resistance offered by the circuit to the large breathing volumes required by exercise is considerable, and the rate of carbon dioxide removal may be inadequate during moderate and heavy exercise. For these reasons, the method of open-circuit spirometry is the most widely used to measure exercise oxygen consumption.

OPEN-CIRCUIT SPIROMETRY. With this method the subject does not rebreathe from a container of oxygen as in the closed-circuit method but instead, inhales ambient air that has a constant composition of 20.93% oxygen, 0.03% carbon dioxide, and 79.04% nitrogen; this nitrogen fraction also includes the small quantity of inert gases. Because oxygen is utilized during energy-yielding reactions and carbon dioxide is produced, the exhaled air contains less oxygen and more carbon dioxide than the inhaled air. Thus, an analysis of the difference in composition between the exhaled air and the ambient air brought into the lungs reflects the body's constant release of energy. The open-circuit method provides a relatively simple means to measure oxygen consumption and indirectly determine energy metabolism. The two most common techniques for open-circuit spirometry in exercise make use of either (1) a lightweight, portable spirometer that is actually worn during an activity, or (2) the "Douglas bag" or balloon method, which is used routinely to collect expired air under laboratory conditions.

The box-shaped *portable spirometer* shown in Figure 8-3 was originally used to estimate the energy requirements of people working in different industrial jobs and thus provide an equitable basis for food rationing in Germany during the 1940s. The unit weighs about 8 lb and is usually worn on the back. By means of a two-way breathing valve, ambient air is inspired while the expired air passes through the gas meter that measures the volume and also collects a small gas sample. This sample is later analyzed for oxygen and carbon dioxide content, and oxygen consumption and energy expenditure are computed for the measurement period.

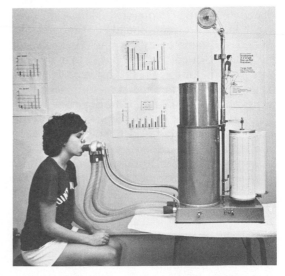

FIG. 8-2. *Spirometer used to measure oxygen consumption by the closed-circuit method.*

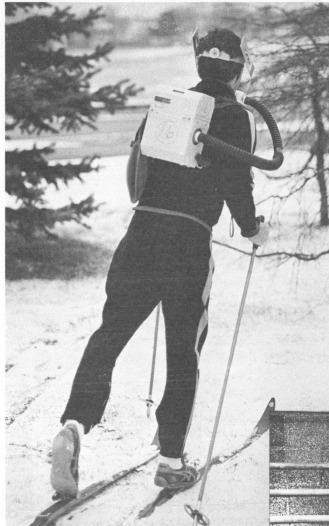

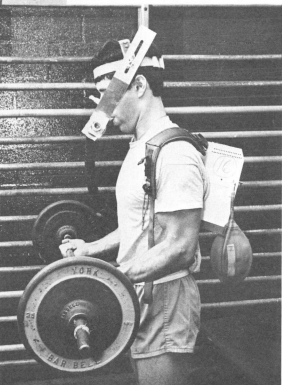

FIG. 8-3. *Portable Spirometer used to measure oxygen consumption by the open-circuit method during cross-country skiing (A) and weight lifting activities (B). (Courtesy Exercise Physiology Laboratory, Department of Exercise Science, University of Massachusetts.)*

A

B

The attractive aspect of the portable spirometer is that the subject has considerable freedom of movement in a variety of activities. Activities as diverse as mountain climbing, downhill skiing, golf, and gardening have been studied with this technique. The equipment does become cumbersome during vigorous activity, and there is some question as to the accuracy of the measurement of air flow through the meter during rapid breathing rates in heavy exercise.

The *Douglas bag method* is shown in Figure 8-4A–D. The subject shown in Figure 8-4A is running on a motor-driven treadmill. A special headgear is worn to which a two-way, high-velocity, low-resistance breathing valve is attached. Ambient air is breathed through one side of the valve while expired air moves out the other side and passes into either large canvas or plastic bags called Douglas bags or rubber meterologic balloons as illustrated, or directly through a gas meter that measures the volume of expired air. A small sample of expired air is collected and analyzed for its oxygen and carbon dioxide composition. As with all indirect calorimetric techniques, energy expenditure is computed from oxygen consumption using the appropriate calorific transformation. The photographs in Figure 8-4B, C, and D show the collection of expired air by the open-circuit method during exercise on a bicycle ergometer, in the pool prior to swimming, and during running by a world class miler on a mountain road.

Direct Versus Indirect Calorimetry

Studies of energy metabolism using both direct and indirect calorimetry provide convincing evidence for the validity of the indirect method as a means to estimate energy metabolism during rest and exercise. At the turn of the twentieth century, the two methods of calorimetry were compared in experiments conducted for 40 days on three individuals who lived in the calorimeter shown in Figure 8-1. The subjects' daily caloric output averaged 2,723 kcal when measured directly by heat exchange and 2,717 kcal when computed indirectly by closed-circuit measures of oxygen consumption, a difference of only 0.22%! Other experiments with animals and humans utilizing moderate exercise also demonstrated a close agreement between direct and indirect methods, and in most instances, the difference was less than 1%.

THE RESPIRATORY QUOTIENT

Because of inherent chemical differences in the composition of carbohydrates, fats, and proteins, different amounts of oxygen are required to oxidize completely the carbon and hydrogen atoms in the molecule to the end products, carbon dioxide and water. Thus, the quantity of carbon dioxide produced in relation to oxygen consumed varies somewhat depending on the substrate metabolized. This ratio of metabolic gas exchange is termed the *respiratory quotient* or *R.Q.*

$$R.Q. = \frac{CO_2 \text{ produced}}{O_2 \text{ consumed}}$$

The usefulness of the R.Q. during rest and submaximal aerobic exercise is that it serves as a convenient guide to the nutrient mixture being catabolized for energy. Also, because the caloric equivalent for oxygen differs somewhat depending on the nutrient oxidized, one must know the R.Q. *and* the amount of oxygen consumed to estimate *precisely* the body's heat production.

R.Q. for Carbohydrate

Because the ratio of hydrogen to oxygen atoms in all carbohydrates is always the same as that in water, that is 2 to 1, all of the oxygen consumed by the cells is used to oxidize the carbon in the carbohydrate molecule to carbon dioxide. Consequently, during the complete oxidation of a glucose molecule, *six* molecules of carbon dioxide are produced and *six* molecules of oxygen are consumed. The overall equation for this reaction is:

$$C_6H_{12}O_6 + 6\,O_2 \longrightarrow 6\,CO_2 + 6\,H_2O$$

Because the gas exchange in this reaction is equal, the R.Q. for carbohydrate is unity or 1.00:

$$R.Q. = \frac{6\,CO_2}{6\,O_2} = 1.00$$

R.Q. for Fat

The chemical composition of fats differs from that of carbohydrates in that fats contain considerably fewer oxygen atoms in proportion to atoms of carbon and hydrogen. Consequently, when fat is broken down, relatively more oxygen is required to oxidize fat to carbon dioxide and water. When palmitic acid, a typical fatty

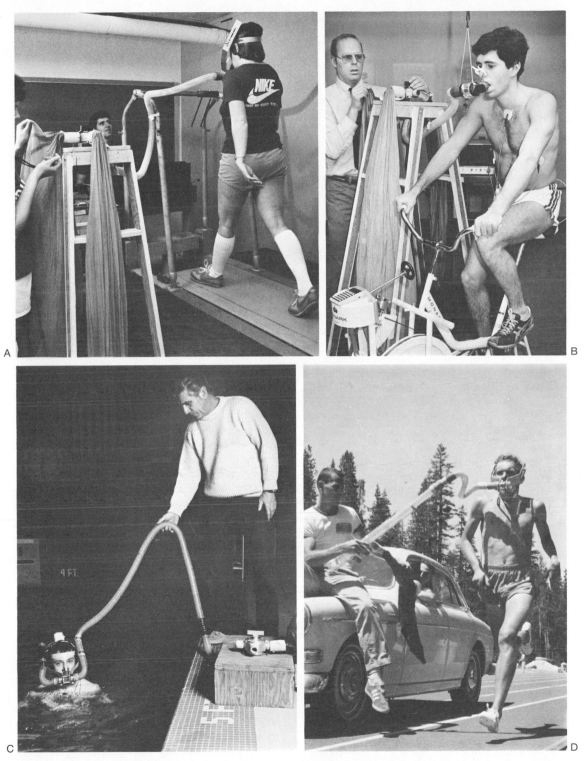

FIG. 8-4. *Measurement of oxygen consumption by open-circuit spirometry during exercise on a (A) treadmill, (B) bicycle ergometer, and while (C) swimming and (D) running. (Figures A and B are courtesy of Exercise Physiology Laboratory, University of Massachusetts, Amherst. Figures C and D are from* Nutrition, Weight Control, and Exercise *by Frank I. Katch and William D. McArdle. Copyright © 1977 by Houghton Mifflin Company. Reprinted by permission of the publisher.)*

acid, is oxidized to carbon dioxide and water, 16 carbon dioxide molecules are produced for every 23 oxygen molecules consumed. This exchange is summarized by the equation:

$$C_{16}H_{32}O_2 + 23\ O_2 \longrightarrow 16\ CO_2 + 16\ H_2O$$

Thus, the R.Q. for this fatty acid is 0.696 (16 $CO_2 \div$ 23 O_2).

$$R.Q. = \frac{16\ CO_2}{23\ O_2} = 0.696$$

Generally, the R.Q. value for fat is considered to be 0.70.

R.Q. for Protein

In the body, proteins are not simply oxidized to carbon dioxide and water during energy metabolism. Rather, the protein is first deaminated in the liver and the nitrogen and sulfur fragments are excreted in the urine and feces. The resulting "keto acid" fragments are then oxidized to carbon dioxide and water to provide energy to sustain metabolism. As was the case with fat metabolism, these short-chain keto acids require more oxygen for complete combustion in relation to carbon dioxide produced. The protein albumin oxidizes as follows:

$$C_{72}H_{112}N_2O_{22}S + 77\ O_2 \longrightarrow$$
Albumin

$$63\ CO_2 + 38\ H_2O + \underset{\text{Sulfur}}{SO_3} + 9\ \underset{\text{Urea}}{CO(NH_2)_2}$$
trioxide

The R.Q. for this particular protein is 0.818.

$$R.Q. = \frac{63\ CO_2}{77\ O_2} = 0.818$$

The general value for the R.Q. of protein is 0.82.

Nonprotein R.Q.

The R.Q. computed from the compositional analysis of expired air usually reflects some blend of carbohydrates, fats, and proteins. The precise contribution of each of these nutrients to energy metabolism can be determined. For example, approximately 1 gram of urinary nitrogen is excreted for every 6.25 grams of protein metabolized for energy. *Each gram of excreted nitrogen represents a carbon dioxide production of approximately 4.8 liters and an oxygen consumption of about 6.0 liters.* Within this framework, the following example illustrates the stepwise procedure used in calculating the *nonprotein* elements in the R.Q.: that is, that

portion of the respiratory exchange attributed to the combustion of *only* carbohydrate and fat.

The following calculation is based on data from a subject who consumes 4.0 liters of oxygen and produces 3.4 liters of carbon dioxide during a 15-minute rest period. During this time, 0.13 g of nitrogen are excreted in the urine.

Step 1. 4.8 ℓ $CO_2 \cdot g^{-1}$ protein metabolized $\times$ 0.13 g = 0.62 ℓ CO_2 produced in the catabolism of protein

Step 2. 6.0 ℓ $O_2 \cdot g^{-1}$ protein metabolized $\times$ 0.13 g = 0.78 ℓ O_2 consumed in the catabolism of protein

Step 3. Nonprotein CO_2 produced = 3.4 ℓ $CO_2 - 0.62\ \ell\ CO_2 = 2.78\ \ell\ CO_2$

Step 4. Nonprotein O_2 consumed = 4.0 ℓ $O_2 - 0.78\ \ell\ O_2 = 3.22\ \ell\ O_2$

Step 5. Nonprotein $\leftarrow$R.Q. = 2.78 $\div$ 3.22 = 0.863

Table 8-1 presents the thermal (energy) equivalents for oxygen consumption for different nonprotein R.Q. values as well as the actual percentage of fat and carbohydrate utilized for energy. For the nonprotein R.Q. of 0.863 computed in the previous example, 4.875 kcal are liberated per liter of oxygen consumed. Also, for this R.Q., 54.1% of the "nonprotein" calories are derived from carbohydrate and 45.9% from fat. The total 15-minute heat production at rest attributed to the metabolism of fat and carbohydrate is 15.70 kcal (4.875 kcal $\cdot$ ℓ^{-1} $\times$ 3.22 ℓ O_2); the energy from the breakdown of protein is equal to 3.51 kcal (4.5 kcal $\cdot$ ℓ^{-1} $\times$ 0.78 ℓO_2). Consequently, the total energy from both protein and nonprotein nutrients during the 15-minute period is 19.21 kcal (15.70 kcal nonprotein + 3.51 kcal protein).

Interestingly, had the thermal equivalent for a mixed diet with an R.Q. of 0.82 been used in the caloric transformation, or if the R.Q. had been obtained simply from the total respiratory gas exchange and applied to Table 8-1 without considering the protein component, the estimated energy expenditure during this period would have been about 19.3 kcal (4.825 kcal $\cdot$ ℓ^{-1} $\times$ 4.0 ℓ O_2; assuming a mixed diet)—a difference of only 0.5% from the value obtained with the more elaborate and time-consuming method requiring urinary nitrogen analysis. *Although the use of Table 8-1 assumes a nonprotein R.Q., in most cases the gross metabolic R.Q. calculated without measures of urinary nitro-*

TABLE 8-1. *Thermal equivalent of oxygen for nonprotein respiratory quotient, including percent kcal and grams derived from carbohydrate and fat*

NONPROTEIN RQ	KCAL PER LITER OXYGEN CONSUMED	PERCENTAGE KCAL DERIVED FROM		GRAMS PER LITER O_2 CONSUMED	
		CARBOHYDRATE	FAT	CARBOHYDRATE	FAT
0.707	4.686	0	100	0.000	.496
.71	4.690	1.10	98.9	.012	.491
.72	4.702	4.76	95.2	.051	.476
.73	4.714	8.40	91.6	.090	.460
.74	4.727	12.0	88.0	.130	.444
.75	4.739	15.6	84.4	.170	.428
.76	4.751	19.2	80.8	.211	.412
.77	4.764	22.8	77.2	.250	.396
.78	4.776	26.3	73.7	.290	.380
.79	4.788	29.9	70.1	.330	.363
.80	4.801	33.4	66.6	.371	.347
.81	4.813	36.9	63.1	.413	.330
.82	4.825	40.3	59.7	.454	.313
.83	4.838	43.8	56.2	.496	.297
.84	4.850	47.2	52.8	.537	.280
.85	4.862	50.7	49.3	.579	.263
.86	4.875	54.1	45.9	.621	.247
.87	4.887	57.5	42.5	.663	.230
.88	4.899	60.8	39.2	.705	.213
.89	4.911	64.2	35.8	.749	.195
.90	4.924	67.5	32.5	.791	.178
.91	4.936	70.8	29.2	.834	.160
.92	4.948	74.1	25.9	.877	.143
.93	4.961	77.4	22.6	.921	.125
.94	4.973	80.7	19.3	.964	.108
.95	4.985	84.0	16.0	1.008	.090
.96	4.998	87.2	12.8	1.052	.072
.97	5.010	90.4	9.58	1.097	.054
.98	5.022	93.6	6.37	1.142	.036
.99	5.035	96.8	3.18	1.186	.018
1.00	5.047	100.0	0	1.231	.000

gen introduces only minimal error because the contribution of protein to energy metabolism is usually small.

How Much Food Was Metabolized for Energy?

The last two columns of Table 8-1 present the conversions for the nonprotein R.Q. to grams of carbohydrate and fat metabolized per liter of oxygen consumed. For the subject with an R.Q. of 0.86, this represents approximately 0.62 and 0.25 g of carbohydrate and fat, respectively. For the 3.22 liters of oxygen consumed during the 15-minute period of rest, 2.00 g of carbohydrate (3.22 l O_2 × 0.62) and 0.80 g of fat (3.22 l O_2 × 0.25) were metabolized for energy.

R.Q. For a Mixed Diet

During activities ranging from complete bed rest to mild, aerobic exercise such as walking or slow jogging, the R.Q. seldom reflects the oxidation of pure carbohydrate or pure fat. Instead, a mixture of these nutrients is usually used, and the R.Q. is intermediate in value between 0.70 and 1.00. *For most purposes, an R.Q. of 0.82 from the metabolism of a mixture of 40% carbohydrate and 60% fat can be assumed, and the caloric equivalent of 4.825 kcal per liter of oxygen can be applied in energy transformations.* By use of this midpoint value, the maximum error possible in estimating energy metabolism from oxygen consumption would be only about 4%. Of course, if greater precision is required, the actual respiratory quotient can be calculated and Table 8-1 consulted to obtain the exact caloric transformation, as well as the percentage contribution of carbohydrate and fat to the metabolic mixture.

Respiratory Exchange
Ratio (R)

Because the calculation of R.Q. is based on the production of carbon dioxide and the consumption of oxygen at the cellular level, factors that disturb the normal metabolic relationship between these gases may spuriously alter this exchange ratio. Respiratory physiologists have termed the ratio of carbon dioxide produced to oxygen consumed under such conditions, when the exchange of oxygen and carbon dioxide at the lungs no longer reflects the oxidation of specific foods in the cells, the *Respiratory Exchange Ratio* or *R—even though this ratio is calculated in exactly the same manner as the R.Q.*

For example, an increase in carbon dioxide elimination occurs during hyperventilation (see Chap. 14) in which the response of breathing is disproportionate to the metabolic demands of a particular situation. As a result of this overbreathing, the normal level of carbon dioxide in the blood is reduced because the gas is "blown off" in the expired air. This increase in carbon dioxide elimination is not accompanied by a corresponding increase in oxygen consumption; thus, there is a disproportionate increase in the respiratory exchange ratio that cannot be attributed to the oxidation of foodstuffs. In such cases, the R usually increases above 1.00.

Exhaustive exercise presents another situation in which R can rise significantly above 1.00. The lactic acid generated during anaerobic exercise is buffered or "neutralized" by sodium bicarbonate in the blood in order to maintain the proper acid–base balance (see Chap. 14). During this process, carbonic acid, a weaker acid, is formed. In the pulmonary capillaries, carbonic acid breaks down to its components, carbon dioxide and water, and the carbon dioxide exits through the lungs. This buffering process adds "extra" carbon dioxide to that quantity normally released during energy metabolism, and the R moves toward and above 1.00.

In rare instances, the exchange ratio of a person gaining body fat while maintaining a high carbohydrate diet also exceeds 1.00. In this situation, oxygen is liberated when carbohydrates are converted to fat as the excess calories become stored. This extra oxygen then can be used in energy metabolism; consequently, less atmospheric oxygen is consumed even though the normal metabolic complement of carbon dioxide is released during energy metabolism. It is also possible to obtain relatively low R values. For example, carbon dioxide tends to be retained in the body fluids following very strenuous exercise to replenish the bicarbonate used to buffer lactic acid. This reduces the expired carbon dioxide and may cause the respiratory exchange ratio to dip below 0.70.

COMPUTERIZED SYSTEMS APPROACH IN METABOLIC DETERMINATIONS

The newest approach to indirect calorimetry makes use of computer technology and electronics for the collection, measurement, and computation of respiratory and metabolic data. With the system illustrated in Figure 8-5, a computer is interfaced with four measuring devices: (1) an automated system that continuously samples expired air, (2) a flow meter for measuring the volume of expired air, and (3) rapid electronic oxygen and carbon dioxide gas analyzers for measuring the fractional concentration of gases in the expired air sample. The output data from the measuring devices are either fed directly into the computer or can be "punched in" by an operator who observes and records the output from the various analyzers. The computer is "preprogrammed" to perform all of the necessary computations for oxygen consumption, carbon dioxide production, and caloric expenditure. A printed output of the subject's data can occur simultaneously during exercise and provides a record of all necessary computations by the time the data collection is completed. More advanced systems include, in addition to respiratory gas analyzers, automated blood pressure and heart rate monitors, temperature, and automatic ergometers that are preprogrammed as to workload and duration of exercise.

Although there are tremendous advantages to computerized systems in terms of ease of operation and speed of data analysis, there are also distinct disadvantages that include the high cost of equipment and delays due to sys-

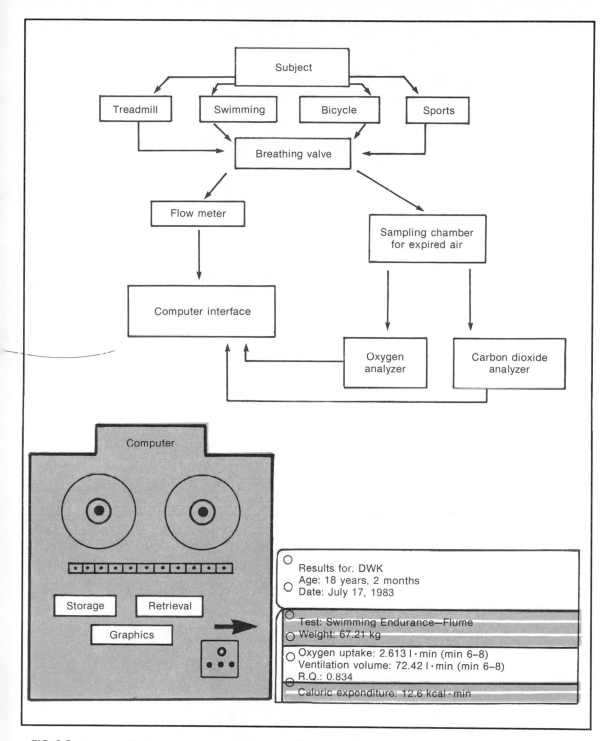

FIG. 8-5. *Computerized systems approach for the collection, analysis, and output of respiratory and metabolic data.*

tem breakdowns. *Regardless of the sophistication of a particular "automated" system, the output data are only as good as the accuracy of the measuring devices. In large part, this depends on careful and frequent calibration of the electronic equipment.*

METABOLIC CALCULATIONS

Much of the study of exercise physiology involves the measurement of *energy metabolism.* Measurement of the oxygen and carbon dioxide content of expired air and the breathing volume provide the basic data for determining the respiratory gas exchange and oxygen consumption and for inferring the body's rate of energy expenditure. Appendix C presents the step-by-step method and rationale for metabolic calculations based on experimental data utilizing methods of open-circuit spirometry.

SUMMARY

1. Direct and indirect calorimetry are the two methods for determining the body's rate of energy expenditure. With direct calorimetry, the actual heat production is measured in an appropriately insulated calorimeter. Indirect calorimetry infers energy expenditure from measurements of oxygen uptake and carbon dioxide production, using either closed or open-circuit spirometry.

2. Because of chemical composition, each nutrient requires different amounts of oxygen in relation to carbon dioxide produced during oxidation. The ratio of CO_2 produced to O_2 consumed is called the respiratory quotient and provides an important clue to the nutrient mixture catabolized for energy. The R.Q. for carbohydrate is 1.00, for fat, 0.70, and for protein 0.82.

3. For each R.Q. value, there is a corresponding calorific value for each liter of oxygen consumed. This provides for a high degree of accuracy in determining energy expenditure during exercise.

4. In strenuous exercise, the respiratory quotient may not be representative of specific substrate utilization because of nonmetabolic production of carbon dioxide, such as that which occurs during the buffering of lactic acid.

Human Energy Expenditure During Rest and Physical Activity

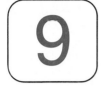

9

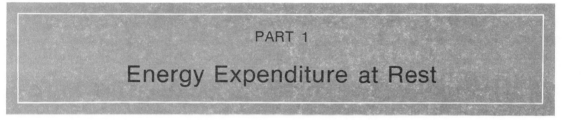

PART 1

Energy Expenditure at Rest

BASAL METABOLIC RATE

There is a minimum level of energy required to sustain the body's vital functions in the waking state. This energy requirement is called the *basal metabolic rate,* or simply *BMR*. The BMR reflects the body's heat production and is determined indirectly by measuring oxygen consumption under fairly stringent conditions. For example, the person is measured in the postabsorptive state. That is, food is not eaten for at least 12 hours prior to the measurement so that there will be no increase in metabolism due to the energy required for the digestion, absorption, and assimilation of the injested nutrients. To reduce other calorigenic influences, the person should remain relatively inactive prior to the BMR test. The actual test is conducted with the subject resting supine in a comfortable environment; after about 30 minutes, oxygen consumption is measured for a 10-minute period. Values for oxygen consumption during the BMR test usually range between 160 and 290 ml per minute (0.8 to 1.43 kcal · min^{-1}), depending upon a variety of factors, especially the size of the subject.

Use of the BMR establishes the important energy baseline for constructing a sound program of weight control by use of diet, exercise, or the effective combination of both. In most instances, so-called basal values measured under controlled conditions are only slightly lower than resting values measured 3 to 4 hours following a light meal. For our purposes, the terms basal and resting metabolic rate are used interchangeably.

Metabolism at Rest

INFLUENCE OF BODY SIZE. In the late 1800s, it was observed that the energy metabolism at rest was proportional to the surface area of the body. This "surface area law" was illustrated in a series of experiments in which the energy metabolism of a dog and a man was determined during a 24-hour period. As expected, the total amount of heat generated by the larger man was about 200% greater than that generated by the dog. However, when heat production was expressed in relation to surface area, the metabolic difference between the man and the dog was reduced to only 10%. Similar results have been obtained for other species of animals that differ considerably in size. This provided the basis for the common practice of expressing resting metabolic rate (energy expenditure) in terms of body surface area.

The results of numerous experiments have provided data with respect to average values of basal metabolism for men and women of different ages. These data are presented in Figure 9-1 and are expressed as hourly values of heat production per square meter of surface area (kcal per m² per h). Whereas they do represent averages established from measurements of large numbers of men and women, a person's BMR estimated from these curves is generally within 10% of the actual value obtained from measurements under strict laboratory conditions.

Figure 9-1 reveals that resting metabolism is about 5% to 10% lower in women than in men. This does not reflect a true sex difference in the metabolic rate of specific tissues. Rather, it is due largely to the fact that women generally possess more body fat than men of similar size, and fat is metabolically less active than muscle. In fact, the BMR differences between sexes are essentially eliminated when the metabolic rate is expressed per unit of "fat-free" or lean body weight.

Although body composition differences largely explain the BMR differences between the sexes, the curves in Figure 9-1 can be used to estimate adequately a person's resting metabolic rate. For example, between the ages of 20 to 40, the BMR of men averages about 38 kcal per m² per hour whereas for women the corresponding value is 35 kcal. For greater precision, the value for a specific age can be read directly from the appropriate curve. When this value for BMR is multiplied by the person's surface area, the estimated metabolic rate per hour is obtained. This provides important baseline information for determining daily rates of energy expenditure as well as appropriate requirements for caloric intake.

Figure 9-2 illustrates a simple method for determining surface area from height and weight. Surface area is determined by locating height on Scale I and weight on Scale II. These two points are then connected with a straight edge or piece of thread and the intersection at scale III gives the surface area expressed in square meters (m²). For example, if height is 6 feet 1 inch, and weight is 165 lb, surface area according to scale III on the nomogram would be 1.98 m².

Estimate of Daily Resting Energy Expenditure

To estimate a person's resting energy expenditure, the appropriate BMR value in Figure 9-1 should be multiplied by the surface area computed from height and weight. For a 55-year-old woman, the estimated BMR is 32 kcal per m² per hour. If her surface area was 1.40 m², the hourly energy expenditure would be 44.8 kcal per hour (32 kcal × 1.40 m²). On a daily basis, this amounts to an energy expenditure of 1075 kcal (44.8 kcal × 24).

Table 9-1 shows estimates of the relative energy needs of various body tissues under resting conditions expressed in terms of oxygen consumption. It should be noted that the brain and skeletal muscles consume about the same total quantity of oxygen during rest, even though the brain weighs only 3½ lb and the muscle mass constitutes almost 50% of the body weight. This is not the case with vigorous exercise, however, because the energy generated by muscles can increase nearly 120 times whereas the oxygen consumption of the brain remains essentially unchanged.

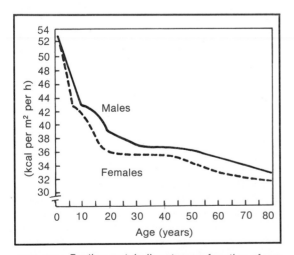

FIG. 9-1. *Resting metabolic rate as a function of age and sex. (Data from Altman, P. L., and Dittmer, D. S.: Metabolism, Bethesda, Md., Federation of American Societies for Experimental Biology, 1968.)*

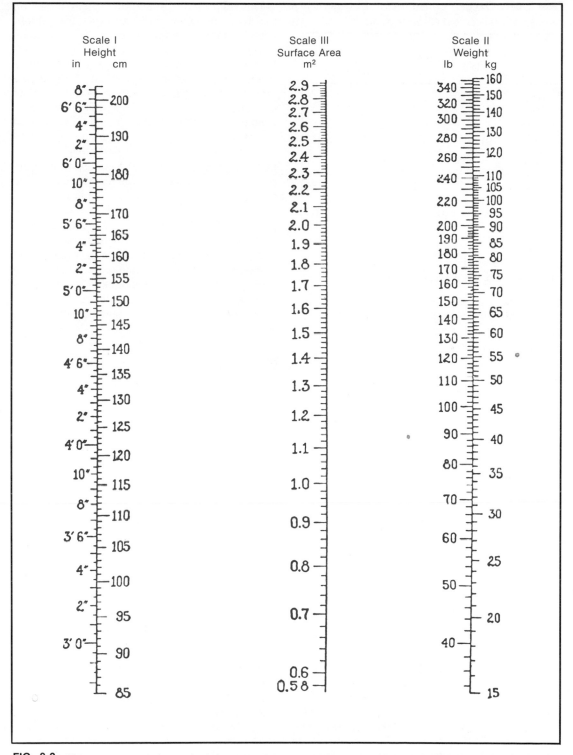

FIG. 9-2. *Nomogram to estimate body surface area from height and weight. [Reproduced from "Clinical Spirometry" (as prepared by Boothby and Sandiford of the Mayo Clinic), through the courtesy of Warren E. Collins, Inc., Braintree, Mass.]*

TABLE 9-1. *Oxygen consumption of various tissues at rest for a 143-pound man*[a]

ORGAN	OXYGEN USED (ml · min⁻¹)	PERCENT OF RESTING METABOLISM
Liver	67	27
Brain	47	19
Heart	17	7
Kidneys	26	10
Skeletal muscle	45	18
Remainder	48	19
	250	100

[a] From data of Passmore, R., and Draper, M.H.: The chemical anatomy of the human body, In Biochemical Disorders in Human Disease, 2nd ed., Edited by R.H.S. Thompson and E. J. King, London, Churchill, 1964.

FACTORS THAT AFFECT ENERGY EXPENDITURE

Many factors affect a person's rate of energy metabolism, including physical activity, dietary-induced thermogenesis, climate, and pregnancy and lactation.

Activity

Physical activity has by far the most profound effect on human energy expenditure. For example, world-class athletes nearly double their daily caloric outputs as a result of 3 or 4 hours of hard training. In fact, most of us can generate metabolic rates that are 10 times the resting value during sustained "big muscle" exercise like running and swimming.

Dietary-Induced Thermogenesis

Food has a stimulating effect on energy metabolism that is due mainly to the energy-requiring processes of digesting, absorbing, and assimilating the various nutrients. This dietary-induced thermogenesis has been termed the *specific dynamic action* effect, or SDA effect. The magnitude of the SDA effect can vary between 10% and 35% in normal individuals depending on both the quantity and type of food eaten. Protein, for example, elicits an SDA effect that is nearly 25% of the total calories in the protein itself. This large SDA, which may persist for a considerable time following a high-protein meal, is due largely to the digestive processes as well as the extra energy required by the liver to assimilate or deaminate amino acids.

The calorigenic effect of protein ingestion has been used by some to argue for a high-protein diet for weight reduction. They maintain that since protein has a relatively high SDA effect, fewer calories will ultimately be available to the body compared to a meal of similar caloric value consisting predominantly of fat or carbohydrate. Although this point has some validity, many other factors must be considered in formulating a sound program for weight loss—not to mention the potentially harmful strain on kidney and liver function that could result from excessive protein intake. For one thing, well-balanced nutrition requires a blend of carbohydrate, fat, and protein as well as appropriate quantities of vitamins and minerals. In addition, if physical activity is used in conjunction with dietary modification, it is important to maintain carbohydrate intake to power both rapid and sustained forms of exercise. Finally, if a person is physically active, the SDA effect of any food represents only a small portion of the total daily energy expenditure.

Calorigenic Effect of Food on Exercise Metabolism

A recent experiment illustrates the effects of food ingestion on energy expenditure during rest and exercise.[1] Six men performed submaximal, moderate exercise on a bicycle ergometer before breakfast on one day; then on separate days, exercise was perfomed 30 minutes after a breakfast containing either 350, 1000, or 3000 kcal. The following results were obtained: (1) Breakfast increased the resting metabolism by 10%. (2) Variations in the caloric value of the meal had no influence on the SDA effect. (3) When exercise was performed following a meal of 1000 or 3000 kcal, energy expenditure was larger compared to exercise without prior food ingestion; this calorigenic effect of food amounted to nearly two times the SDA value of the food at rest. Apparently, exercise augments the SDA effect. This is in agreement with previous findings in which the SDA response averaged 28% of the basal requirement at rest and increased to 56% of the basal requirement after exercise was performed![5]

It is tempting to speculate that the increased SDA effect with exercise could adversely affect endurance performance, since oxygen would be utilized that otherwise could serve the needs of the working muscles. Of course, one could eliminate the SDA effect by not eating before competition. In this situation, however, the possibility exists that the person would be competing with inadequate fuel reserves, especially glycogen. Certainly, more research is needed on this interesting topic.

Climate

Environmental factors also influence metabolic rate. For example, the BMR of people in a tropical climate is generally 5% to 20% higher than that of their counterparts living in a more temperate area. Exercise in the heat also imposes a small additional metabolic load, causing the oxygen consumption to be about 5% higher compared to the same work performed in a thermoneutral environment. This is probably due to the effects of an elevated core temperature per se, as well as to the additional energy required for sweat-gland activity and altered circulatory dynamics during work in the heat.

In extremely cold environments, the extent to which energy metabolism increases during exercise depends largley on a person's body fat content as well as on the amount and type of clothing that is worn. The effect of excessive fatness on the body's ability to withstand cold exposure at rest is illustrated in Figure 9-3. Two young men (lean subject, 10% body fat; fatter subject, 40% body fat) were studied on two separate occasions for 90 minutes while lying on a cot in an environmental chamber. Both men, dressed only in shorts, were first exposed to a moderate temperature of 23.3° C (74° F) for 30 minutes. The temperature was then reduced to 10° C (50° F) for an additional 45 minutes, and increased again to 23.3° C for the final 15 minutes of the experiment. The top graph shows little or no change in resting energy metabolism throughout the cold exposure for the obese subject. As shown in the bottom graph, the lean subject tripled his energy output by shivering during the 45-minute cold stress. This response is typical of lean subjects and represents the body's attempt to maintain a stable core temperature in the face of cold stress.

This temperature effect on resting metabolism also carries over to exercise in cold envi-

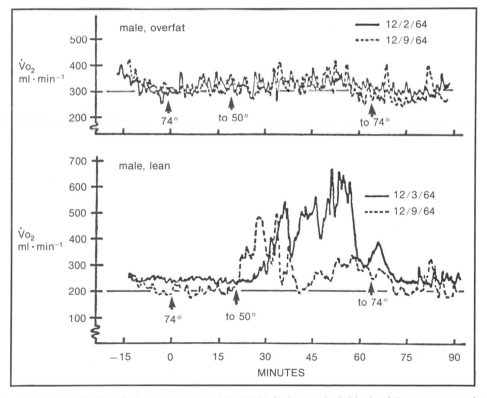

FIG. 9-3. *Energy metabolism during exposure to 50° F (10° C) for two individuals of the same age who varied widely in body fatness. (From Buskirk, E. R.: Variation in heat production during acute exposures of men and women to cold air or water. Ann. N.Y. Acad. Sci., 196:733, 1960.)*

ronments, especially in cold water where it is often difficult to maintain a stable core temperature.[4] If the water temperature is reduced to 18° C, the energy cost of exercise becomes substantially increased. This is due mainly to the energy required to sustain shivering as the body attempts to counter the heat drain to the cold water. Of course, the insulatory benefits of body fat influence the response to cold. For lean people, the thermal challenge of cold water immersion is considerable whereas for relatively fat people, immersion at the same temperature produces considerably less physiologic strain. From a recreational and sport perspective, however, a "wet" or "dry" rubber suit increases comfort in cool water and makes this an excellent medium for exercise, regardless of body composition.

Pregnancy

The response to exercise during pregnancy has been considered. In one investigation,[3a] 13 women were studied from the sixth month of pregnancy to 6 weeks after the birth of the baby. Physiologic measures taken every 4 weeks included heart rate and oxygen consumption during bicycle and treadmill exercise. As shown in Table 9-2, the increased heart rate and oxygen consumption during walking coincided with body weight changes in pregnancy, whereas no differences were noted in weight-supported bicycle exercise during the period of investigation. These findings suggest that pregnancy offers no greater physiologic stress to exercise other than that provided by the additional weight gain and possible encumbrance of fetal tissue. Certainly, when body weight is supported, the exercise response for heart rate and oxygen consumption is essentially identical prior to and following birth.

The preceding findings are complemented by a case study of a healthy 27-year-old, nonathletic woman who engaged in strenuous jogging for a 4-year period that included two pregnancies and the following lactation periods.[2] Near-maximal treadmill stress testing was conducted to within one week of delivery! The woman remained healthy throughout the study, and both pregnancies were normal and uncomplicated. Despite the high caloric cost of daily running (6 to 18 miles), milk production during lactation was normal. The only discomfort from strenuous exercise was noticed in the first trimester of pregnancy when the woman was nauseated most of the day. Although much more research in this area is needed, it does appear that healthy women can engage in aerobic exercise throughout pregnancy and after delivery and that endurance performance and physiologic capacity can be improved without harmful effects to mother or child.

SUMMARY

1.   The basal metabolic rate (BMR) is the minimum energy required to maintain vital functions in the waking state. The BMR is only slightly lower than the resting metabolism and is proportionate to the surface area of the body.

TABLE 9-2. *Heart rate and oxygen consumption in treadmill and bicycle exercise during pregnancy and following birth*[a]

		PREPARTUM	POSTPARTUM	DIFFERENCE
Body weight, kg		68.3	59.2[b]	−9.1[b]
	Treadmill			
Oxygen consumption l·min⁻¹		1.13	1.00	−0.13[b]
Heart Rate beats·min⁻¹		133	123	−10.0[b]
	Bicycle Ergometer			
Oxygen consumption l·min⁻¹		1.06	1.03	−0.03
Heart Rate beats·min⁻¹		140	137	−3.0

[a] Adapted from Knuttgen, H.G., and Emerson, K., Jr.: Physiological response to pregnancy at rest and during exercise. J. Appl. Physiol. *36*:549, 1974.
[b] Postpartum values are significantly different than prepartum values:

It is also influenced by age and is generally higher for men than for women.

2. Different organs use different amounts of oxygen during rest and exercise. At rest, muscles require about 20% of the total oxygen uptake. During exercise, however, the oxygen uptake of skeletal muscles increases 100 times above rest; this represents close to 85% of the maximal oxygen uptake.

3. Four major factors affecting a person's metabolic rate are physical activity, dietary-induced thermogenesis (SDA effect), climate, and pregnancy. Physical activity has, by far, the greatest influence.

PART 2

Energy Expenditure in Physical Activity

CLASSIFICATION OF PHYSICAL ACTIVITIES BY ENERGY EXPENDITURE

All of us at one time or another have done some type of physical work that we would classify as exceedingly "difficult." This might be walking up a flight of stairs, shoveling snow to clear the driveway, running to catch a bus, loading and unloading a truck, digging a trench to fix an underground pipe, skiing through a blizzard, or climbing a steep mountain. Intensity and duration are two important factors in rating the difficulty or strenuousness of a particular task. For example, the same number of calories may be required to complete a 26-mile marathon at various running speeds. However, one runner might exert considerable energy running at maximum pace and complete the race in a little more than 2 hours. Another runner of equal fitness might select a slower more comfortable pace and complete the run in 3 hours. In this example, the intensity of the exercise is the factor distinguishing the manner in which a specific work task is completed. In another situation, two people may run at the same speed, but one person may run twice as long as the other. In this situation, exercise duration becomes the important consideration.

Several classification systems have been proposed for rating the difficulty of sustained physical activity in terms of its strenuousness. One recommendation is that work tasks be rated by the ratio of the energy required for the work to the resting or basal energy requirement. With this system, moderate work is defined as that eliciting an oxygen consumption (or energy expenditure) up to three times the resting requirement. Hard work is categorized as that requiring three to eight times the resting metabolism, whereas maximal work is considered as any task requiring an increase in metabolism nine times or more above the resting level. As a frame of reference, most industrial jobs and household tasks require less than three times the energy expenditure at rest.

The five-level classification system presented in Table 9-3 is based on the energy required by untrained men and women performing different tasks.[3] Because 5 kcal is approximately equal to one liter of oxygen consumed, it is also possible to present this five-stage classification in terms of liters of oxygen consumed per minute, or milliliters of oxygen consumed per kilogram of body weight per minute ($ml \cdot kg^{-1} \cdot min^{-1}$), or METS, a MET being defined as a multiple of the resting metabolic rate. Thus, 1 MET is equivalent to the resting oxygen consumption that, for an average man and woman, is approximately 250 and 200 ml per minute, respectively. Work at 2 METS requires twice the resting metabolism or about 500 ml of oxygen per minute for a man, and 3 METS is three times the resting energy expenditure, and so on. For slightly more accurate classifications, the MET can be expressed in terms of oxygen consumption per unit of body weight with 1 MET equal to approximately $3.6 \ ml \cdot kg^{-1} \cdot min^{-1}$.

TABLE 9-3. *Five-level classification of physical activity in terms of exercise intensity*

LEVEL	ENERGY EXPENDITURE			
	MEN			
	kcal·min^{-1}	l·min^{-1a}	ml·kg^{-1}·min^{-1}	METS
Light	2.0–4.9	0.40–0.99	6.1–15.2	1.6–3.9
Moderate	5.0–7.4	1.00–1.49	15.3–22.9	4.0–5.9
Heavy	7.5–9.9	1.50–1.99	23.0–30.6	6.0–7.9
Very heavy	10.0–12.4	2.00–2.49	30.7–38.3	8.0–9.9
Unduly heavy	12.5–	2.50–	38.4–	10.0–
	WOMEN			
	kcal·min^{-1}	l·min^{-1}	ml·kg^{-1}·min^{-1}	METS
Light	1.5–3.4	0.30–0.69	5.4–12.5	1.2–2.7
Moderate	3.5–5.4	0.70–1.09	12.6–19.8	2.8–4.3
Heavy	5.5–7.4	1.10–1.49	19.9–27.1	4.4–5.9
Very heavy	7.5–9.4	1.50–1.89	27.2–34.4	6.0–7.5
Unduly heavy	9.5–	1.90–	34.5–	7.6–

[a]l·min^{-1} based on 5 kcal per liter of oxygen; ml·kg^{-1}·min^{-1} based on 65-kg man and 55-kg woman; one MET is equivalent to 250 ml O_2 per minute, or the average resting oxygen consumption.

DAILY RATES OF AVERAGE ENERGY EXPENDITURE

Table 9-4 shows averages for daily rates of energy expenditure for men and women living in the United States. Between the ages of 23 and 50, the "average" man expends between 2700 and 3000 kcal per day, whereas his female counterpart expends about 2000 to 2100 kcal. As can be seen in the bottom portion of this table, nearly 75% of the average person's day, regardless of sex, is spent in activities requiring only a light expenditure of energy. These observations are supported by data from the President's Council on Physical Fitness and Sports,[6] which show that walking is the most prevalent form of exercise for American men and women. For most Americans, energy expenditure rarely climbs significantly above the resting level. Our citizens have all too appropriately been termed *Homo sedentarius.*

Energy Expenditure Grouped By Occupation

Dietary surveys of nutrient intake and corresponding values of energy expenditure for various occupational groups of different ages have been reported by various teams of researchers. These surveys provide a most comprehensive evaluation of energy expenditure, as the data in Table 9-5 illustrate. Included are data based on 7-day observations of Swiss peasants and British army cadets. Daily energy expenditure was estimated by determining the time spent in each activity during the day, and the average energy expended for the activity.

Even though the average energy expenditure increases in ascending order in the job classifications presented in Table 9-5, there is considerable variability for men and women in any one classification. With university students, for example, some individuals expend less energy per day than the average for elderly retired persons, whereas other students expend energy that exceeds the average for farmers, coal miners, and forestry workers. These variations are largely explained by the intensity and duration of activities performed outside of work, especially those related to recreational pursuits.

TABLE 9-4. *Average rates of energy expenditure for men and women living in the United States*[a]

	AGE (years)	WEIGHT (kg)	WEIGHT (lbs)	HEIGHT (cm)	HEIGHT (in)	ENERGY EXPENDITURE (kcal)
Men	15–18	61	134	172	69	3000
	19–22	67	147	172	69	3000
	23–50	70	154	172	69	2700
	51+	70	154	172	69	2400
Women	15–18	54	119	162	65	2100
	19–22	58	128	162	65	2100
	23–50	58	128	162	65	2000
	51+	58	128	162	65	1800

Average time spent during the day for men and women

ACTIVITY	TIME (h)
Sleeping and lying	8
Sitting	6
Standing	6
Walking	2
Recreational: sports or exercises	2

[a]Data taken from Food and Nutrition Board, National Research Council, Recommended Dietary Allowances, 8th rev. ed., National Academy of Sciences, Washington, D.C., 1974. (Also Publ. 1146, 1964).

TABLE 9-5. *Daily rates of energy expenditure for various occupations*[a]

	OCCUPATION	AVERAGE	MINIMUM	MAXIMUM
Men	Elderly retired	2330	1750	2810
	Office workers	2520	1820	3270
	Coal mine clerks	2800	2330	3290
	Laboratory technicians	2840	2240	3820
	Older industrial workers	2840	2180	3710
	University students	2930	2270	4410
	Building workers	3000	2440	3730
	Steel workers	3280	2600	3960
	Army cadets	3490	2990	4100
	Older peasants (Swiss)	3530	2210	5000
	Farmers	3550	2450	4670
	Coal miners	3660	2970	4560
	Forestry workers	3670	2860	4600
Women	Older housewives	1990	1490	2410
	Middle-aged housewives	2090	1760	2320
	Laboratory assistants	2130	1340	2540
	Assistants in department store	2250	1820	2850
	University students	2290	2090	2500
	Factory workers	2320	1970	2980
	Bakery workers	2510	1980	3390
	Older peasants (Swiss)	2890	2200	3860

ENERGY EXPENDITURE, kcal per day

[a]From Katch, F.I., and McArdle, W.D.: Nutrition, Weight Control, and Exercise, Boston, Houghton-Mifflin, 1977. Data from Durnin, J.V.G.A., and Passmore, R.: Energy, Work and Leisure, London, Heinemann Educational Books, 1967.

Energy Expenditure

For Athletic

Competitors

Table 9-6 presents the estimated daily energy requirements of elite male competitors in training for six different groups of sport activities. The data were secured by a dietary survey of food intake, and the results were computed by multiplying the average estimated caloric expenditure per kilogram body weight by the av-
erage body weight for the group. The mean daily caloric intake of 6350 kcal for the hammer throw, shotput, and discus athletes in group 6 is probably due to their large body size and relatively intense training regime and not necessarily to the energy requirements of the actual sport competition. This value obtained from dietary recall is considerably above previous estimates of caloric intake for United States top-caliber discus athletes (see Chap. 3, Table 3-3).

TABLE 9-6. *Median energy consumption and corresponding daily food requirements (in kilocalories) of groups of elite male athletes*

Selected sports category 1	Expenditure of energy per kg of body weight per day (kcal) 2	Average body weight (kg) 3	Normative daily net needs based on computed energy requirements (column 2 × column 3) (kcal) 4	Optimal daily gross requirements, with 10% added for SDA effect (kcal) 5
Group A				
Cross-country skiing	82.14	67.5	5,550	6,105
Crew racing	69.21	80.0	5,550	6,105
Canoe racing	72.72	75.0	5,450	5,995
Swimming	69.87	76.0	5,300	5,830
Bicycle racing	80.39	68.0	5,450	5,995
Marathon racing	79.07	68.0	5,400	5,940
Average values (men)			5,450	5,995
Rounded-off norm: 6,000 kcal				
Also belonging to sports of group A are skiing, Norwegian combination; middle-distance racing; walking; ice racing; modern pentathlon; equine sports, military; and touring (alpine climbing).				
Group B				
Soccer	72.28	74.0	5,350	5,885
Handball	68.06	75.0	5,100	5,610
Basketball	67.93	75.0	5,100	5,610
Field hockey	69.18	75.0	5,200	5,720
Ice hockey	71.87	68.0	4,900	5,390
Average values (men)			5,130	5,643
Rounded-off norm: 5,600 kcal				
Also belonging to group B are rugby; water polo; volleyball; tennis; polo; and bicycle polo.				
Group C				
Canoe slalom	67.16	68.0	4,550	5,005
Shooting	62.71	72.5	4,550	5,005
Table tennis	59.96	74.0	4,450	4,895
Bowling	62.69	75.0	4,700	5,170
Sailing	63.77	74.0	4,700	5,170
Average values (men)			4,590	5,049
Rounded-off norm: 5,000 kcal				
Also belonging to group C are circuit cycle racing (1,000–4,000 meters); fencing; ice sailing; and gliding.				

TABLE 9-6. *Median energy consumption and corresponding daily food requirements (in kilocalories) of groups of elite male athletes* (continued)

Group D				
Sprinting	61.77	69.0	4,250	4,675
Running: short to middle distances	65.62	65.0	4,250	4,675
Pole vault	57.83	73.0	4,200	4,620
Diving	69.24	61.0	4,200	4,620
Boxing (middle and welter weight: to 63.5 kg)	67.25	63.0	4,250	4,675
Average values (men)			4,230	4,653

Rounded-off norm: 4,600 kcal

Also belonging to group D are hurdle races; broad- and high-jump; hop-skip-and-jump; ballet swimming; figure skating; figure roller skating; and ski, ski jump, bob sled, and tobogganing.

E				
Group I				
Judo (lightweight)	72.92	62.5	4,550	5,005
Weight lifting (light-weight)	69.15	67.5	4,650	5,115
Javelin	56.95	76.0	4,350	4,785
Gymnastics with apparatus	67.14	65.0	4,350	4,785
Steeplechase	63.96	68.0	4,350	4,785
Ski: Alpine competition	71.29	67.5	4,800	5,280
Average values (men)			4,508	4,959

Rounded-off norm: 5,000 kcal

Group II				
Hammerthrow	62.46	102.0	6,350	6,985
Shot put and discus	62.47	102.0	6,350	6,985

Rounded-off norm: 7,000 kcal

Also belonging to group E/I are wrestling; automobile rallies; motor racing; gymnastics; acrobatics; parachute jumping; equine sports, shows; decathlon; and bicycle gymnastics.

(Reprinted with permission of Macmillan Publishing Co., Inc. from *Encyclopedia of Sport Sciences and Medicine* by American College of Sports Medicine, copyright 1971.)

ENERGY COST OF HOUSEHOLD, INDUSTRIAL, AND RECREATIONAL ACTIVITIES

A list of energy expenditures, expressed in terms of body weight, for common household activities, selected industrial tasks, and popular recreational and sports activities is presented in Appendix D. These activities illustrate the large variation in energy expenditure that occurs with participation in various forms of physical activity. The caloric values represent averages that can vary considerably depending on factors such as skill, pace, and fitness level.

The value listed in the column that corresponds to a particular body weight is the caloric cost of the activity for one minute. These are gross energy values because also included is the cost of rest for the one-minute period. The total cost of participating in an activity is estimated by multiplying the value listed in the table by the number of minutes of participation. For example, if a 157-lb man spends 30 minutes vacuuming (carpet sweeping), his total caloric expenditure of 102 kcal for this household activity would be determined by multiplying the value of 3.4 kcal per minute by 30. The same individual would spend approximately 690 kcal during a 50-minute judo workout, but only 90 kcal while sitting quietly and watching television for 2 hours. Golf requires about 6.0 kcal per minute, or 360 kcal per hour, for a person who weighs 154 pounds. The same person will expend almost twice this energy, or 708 kcal per hour, while swimming the backstroke. Viewed somewhat differently, 25 minutes of swimming the backstroke requires about the same number of calories as playing golf for one hour. If the pace of either the swim or the golf game is increased, the energy expenditure also increases proportionally.

Effect of Body Weight

Body weight is an important factor that affects the energy expended in many forms of exercise. This can be seen in Appendix D, where the energy cost of a particular exercise is generally greater for heavier people, especially in weight-bearing exercise like walking and running where the person must transport his or her body weight during the activity. This is clearly illustrated in Figure 9-4, which shows that the energy cost of walking increases directly with body weight. In fact, for people of the same body weight, the variation in oxygen consumption is so small that the energy expenditure during walking can be predicted from body weight with high accuracy. With stationary cycling, however, weight is supported, and the influence of body weight on energy cost is less extreme. Certainly, for heavy people desiring to use exercise in a program for weight loss, weight-bearing forms of exercise can provide a considerable caloric expenditure.

It can be seen from Appendix D that the energy cost for cross-country running ranges between 8.2 kcal per minute for a 50 kg person to almost twice as much at 16.0 kcal for a person weighing 98 kg. However, if the energy requirement is expressed in relation to body weight as $kcal \cdot kg^{-1} \cdot min^{-1}$, this difference is essentially eliminated, and the energy cost averages about 0.164 $kcal \cdot kg^{-1} \cdot min^{-1}$. By expressing energy cost in this manner (that is, per unit of body weight), the differences between individuals are greatly reduced regardless of age, race, sex, and body weight. However, the *total* number of calories expended by the heavier person is still considerably larger than that expended by a lighter counterpart, simply because the body weight must be transported in the activity—and this requires proportionately more total energy.

Use of Heart Rate to Estimate Energy Expenditure

For each person, heart rate and oxygen consumption tend to be linearly related throughout a large portion of the aerobic work range. If this precise relationship is known, the exercise heart rate can be used to estimate oxygen consumption (and then compute energy expenditure) during other forms of *similar* activity such as exercise performed while running, walking, cycling, and swimming. This approach has been used in several research studies in which the investigators were unable to measure directly the oxygen consumption during the activity.

The data for two members of a nationally ranked women's basketball team during a laboratory treadmill test are presented in Figure 9.5. For each woman, the heart rate increased linearly, with each increase in oxygen consumption being accompanied by a proportionate increase in heart rate. Even though both heart rate–oxygen consumption lines are linear, however, the same heart rate does not correspond to the same level of oxygen consumption. This is because the slope or rate of change of the line differs considerably among people. For each increase in oxygen consumption, the heart rate of subject A increases to a much greater extent than subject B's. The significance of this difference and its relation to cardiovascular fitness are discussed in Chapters 11,

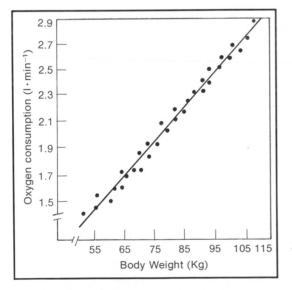

FIG. 9-4. *Relationship between body weight and oxygen consumption measured during treadmill walking. (Actual data from Laboratory of Applied Physiology, Queens College, N.Y.)*

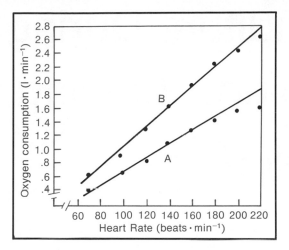

FIG. 9-5. *Linear relationship between heart rate and oxygen consumption for two subjects. Measurements were made while running on a treadmill. The elevation of the treadmill was increased by 2.5 percent every 3 minutes.*

17, and 20. The important point is that if heart rate is known, oxygen consumption can often be estimated with reasonable accuracy. For player A, an exercise heart rate of 140 beats per minute corresponds to an oxygen consumption of 1.08 liters per minute, whereas the same heart rate for player B is related to a 1.6-liter oxygen consumption.

It should be kept in mind that, although the technique for using heart rate to estimate energy expenditure is practical, it may be of limited use for research purposes because its validity has yet to be adequately established for more than a few general activities. One of the major problems is determining the degree of similarity between the laboratory test to establish the heart rate–oxygen consumption line and the specific activity to which it is applied. Factors other than oxygen consumption can influence the heart rate. These include temperature, emotions, food intake, body position, the muscle groups exercised, and whether the exercise is continuous or stop-and-go, or whether the muscles are contracting isometrically or in a more rhythmic manner.

SUMMARY

1.   Different classification systems exist for rating the strenuousness of physical activities. These include ratings based on (1) the ratio of energy cost to resting energy requirement, (2) the oxygen requirement in $ml \cdot kg^{-1} \cdot min^{-1}$, or (3) multiples of the resting metabolic rate or METS.

2.   The average daily energy expenditure is estimated to be 2700 to 3000 kcal for men and 2000 to 2100 for women between the ages of 15 and 50 years. However, great variability in daily energy expenditure exists, and this difference is directly determined by one's physical activity level.

3.   It is possible to classify different occupations, as well as athletic groups, by daily rates of energy expenditure. Within any classification, however, there is great variability. In addition, heavier individuals generally expend more energy in physical activity than their lighter counterparts.

References

1. Bray, G.: The acute effects of food intake on energy expenditure during cycle ergometry. Am. J. Clin. Nutr., 27:254, 1974.
2. Dressendorfer, R.H.: Physical training during pregnancy and lactation. *The Physician and Sportsmedicine, 6:*74, 1978.
3. Durnin, J.V.G.A., and Passmore, R.: Energy, Work and Leisure. London, Hueneman Educational Books, 1967.
3a. Knuttgen, H.G., and Emerson, K., Jr.: Physiological response to pregnancy at rest and during exercise. J. Appl. Physiol., 36:549, 1974.
4. McArdle, W.D. et al.: Metabolic and cardiovascular adjustment to work in air and water at 18, 25 and 33° C. J. Appl. Physiol., 40:85, 1976.
5. Miller, D.S., Mumford, P., and Stock, M.J.: Gluttony 2: Thermogenesis in overeating man. Am. J. Clin. Nutr., 20:1223, 1967.
6. President's Council on Physical Fitness and Sports. "National Adult Physical Fitness Survey." Washington, D.C., May 1973.

Energy Expenditure During Walking, Jogging, Running, and Swimming

10

The total amount of energy expended each day can be considerably greater than the basal requirement, depending of course on the type and duration of physical activity performed. The following sections present detailed information on the energy expenditure of the popular activities: walking, jogging and running, and swimming. Aside from being competitive sports, these forms of exercise take on special significance for they are commonly prescribed in programs of weight control, physical conditioning, and cardiac rehabilitation.

GROSS AND NET ENERGY EXPENDITURE

The following example illustrates the use of oxygen consumption measures to estimate the energy requirements of swimming. A 25-year-old man swimming at a moderate and steady pace that requires an average oxygen consumption of 2 liters per minute would, with 40 minutes of swimming, consume a total of 80 liters of oxygen. This oxygen value can easily be transposed to an energy value by using the approximate calorific transformation of 5 kcal of energy generated per liter of oxygen consumed. Thus, the swimmer would expend about 400 kcal (80 liters × 5 kcal) during the swim. This, however, is not the cost of the swim per se because this total or *gross energy expenditure* also includes energy that would have been expended if the person had rested and not swum. To obtain a clearer picture of the cost of exercise or the *net energy expenditure,* one must obtain an estimate of the resting metabolic rate and subtract this from the gross energy cost of the exercise.

$$\text{Net energy expenditure} = \text{Gross energy expenditure} - \text{Resting energy expenditure (for equivalent time period)}$$

By knowing the swimmer's size (weight, 65 kg; height, 174 cm), his surface area of 1.78 m² is computed from the nomogram in Figure 9-2. When this value is multiplied by the average basal metabolic rate for young men of 38 kcal per m² per hour (Fig. 9-1), an estimated resting energy expenditure of 67.6 kcal per hour (1.78 m² × 38 kcal) is obtained or about 45 kcal per 40-minute swimming period. The energy expended solely for the swim is then computed as gross energy expenditure (400 kcal) minus the 40-minute resting value (45 kcal). This results in a net energy expenditure for the swimming period of 355 kcal.

When a constant-load exercise is performed at light to moderate intensity, the oxygen consumption rises rapidly at the start and then levels off and remains at a relatively steady rate throughout the activity period. When exercise stops, oxygen consumption decreases rapidly with the recovery oxygen consumption being approximately equal to the quantity of oxygen not consumed in the early adjustment to exercise (oxygen deficit). Energy expenditure can therefore be estimated from only one or two measures of oxygen consumption during the steady-rate phase of relatively moderate exercise. In activities with considerable variation in pace such as tennis, soccer, or basketball, more frequent measures of oxygen consumption must be made to estimate accurately the total energy expenditure. In vigorous exercise, when the energy requirements exceed the capacity for aerobic energy transfer, considerable anaerobic energy is generated and lactic acid accumulates. In this situation, energy cost estimates require measurements of oxygen consumption in both exercise and recovery. The precision of these estimates is limited, however, because near-exhaustive exercise of long duration causes physiologic, metabolic, and thermal adjustments that can cause the oxygen consumption to remain elevated for up to 24 hours. This can increase the total energy cost by about 10% compared to the same exercise performed aerobically.

ENERGY EXPENDITURE DURING WALKING

Walking is the most common form of exercise. For most individuals, it represents the major type of physical activity that falls outside the realm of sedentary living. Figure 10-1 displays the research from five countries on the energy expenditure of men who walked at speeds ranging from 1.0 to 10 kilometers per hour (0.62 to 6.2 mph). The relationship between walking speed and oxygen consumption is approximately linear between speeds of 3.0 and 8.0 kilometers per hour (1.86 to 4.35 mph); at faster speeds, walking becomes less efficient and the relationship curves in an upward direction that indicates a greater caloric cost per unit of distance traveled.

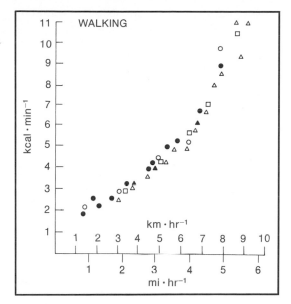

FIG. 10-1. *Energy expenditure walking on the level at different speeds. Different symbols represent the mean values from various studies reported in the literature.*

Effect of Body Weight

At horizontal walking speeds ranging from 3.2 to 6.4 km per hour (2.0 to 4.0 mph), energy expenditure for people who differ in body weight can be predicted accurately by an equation based on the combined data in Figure 10-1 and on other studies.[6,7,9,20] The predicted values for energy expenditure are listed in Table 10-1; these are accurate to within 15% of the actual energy expenditure for both men and women of different sizes. On a daily basis, therefore, estimates of the energy expended in walking could be in error by only about 50 to 100 kcal, assuming that the person walks 2 hours each day. The

TABLE 10-1. *Prediction of energy expenditure (kcal · min⁻¹) based on speed of walking and body weight*[a]

SPEED			BODY WEIGHT					
mph	km · hr⁻¹	kg lbs	36 80	45 100	54 120	64 140	73 160	82 180	91 200
2.0	3.22		1.9	2.2	2.6	2.9	3.2	3.5	3.8
2.5	4.02		2.3	2.7	3.1	3.5	3.8	4.2	4.5
3.0	4.83		2.7	3.1	3.6	4.0	4.4	4.8	5.3
3.5	5.63		3.1	3.6	4.2	4.6	5.0	5.4	6.1
4.0	6.44		3.5	4.1	4.7	5.2	5.8	6.4	7.0

[a] Data from Passmore, R., and Durnin, J.V.G.A.: Human energy expenditure. Physiolog. Rev. 35:801, 1955.

table is easy to use, is formulated on sound research, and is relatively accurate for assessing the caloric cost of walking within the speed range indicated and for body weights up to 91 kg (200 lb). For heavier individuals, extrapolations can be made but with some loss in accuracy.

Effects of Terrain and Walking Surface

The influence of terrain and surface on the energy cost of walking is summarized in Table 10-2. Efficiency is similar for level walking on a grass track or on a paved surface. Walking in the sand, however, is almost *twice* as costly as walking on a hard surface. Certainly, a brisk walk along a beach would provide an excellent exercise stress in programs designed to "burn up" calories or improve physiologic fitness.

In another series of experiments,[22] it was clearly demonstrated that the energy cost of walking on a treadmill at 5.86 km per hour (3.63 mph) and 2.93 km per hour (1.82 mph) was no different from normal walking on a hard surface at the same speeds. This indicates that people can generate essentially the same exercise stress either by walking on the level or walking at the same speed and distance on an exercise treadmill in a laboratory or exercise facility.

TABLE 10.2. *Effect of different terrain on the energy expenditure of walking between 5.2 and 5.6 km · h⁻¹*

TERRAIN	CORRECTION FACTOR[a,b]
Paved road (similar to grass track)	0.0
Ploughed field	1.5
Hard snow	1.6
Sand dune	1.8

[a] First entry from Passmore, R., and Durnin, J.V.G.A.: Human energy expenditure. Physiol. Rev., 35:801, 1955. Last three entries from Givoni, B., and Goldman, R.F.: Predicting metabolic energy cost. J. Appl. Physiol., 30:429, 1971.
[b] The correction factor is a multiple of the energy expenditure for walking on a paved road or grass track. For example, the energy cost of walking in a ploughed field is 1.5 times that of walking on the paved road.

Such results also lend further support to the use of laboratory data to quantify human energy expenditure in "real life" situations.

Competition Walkers

The energy expenditure of five Olympic-caliber walkers has been studied at various speeds while walking and running on a treadmill.[16] In actual competition, the walking speed of these athletes averaged 13.0 kilometers per hour (11.5 to 14.8 km · h⁻¹ or 7.1 to 9.2 mph) over distances ranging from 1.6 to 50 km. This was a relatively fast speed, because the winner of the 20-km walk at the 1976 Montreal Olympics averaged 14.1 km per hour (8.8 mph) during this 12.4-mile walk. As illustrated in Figure 10-2, the oxygen consumption during treadmill walking at competition speeds was only slightly lower than the highest oxygen uptake measured for these athletes during treadmill running. Also, the relationship between oxygen consumption and walking at speeds above 8 km per hour (4.97 mph) was approximately linear, but the slope of the line was twice as steep compared to running at the same speeds. Although these athletes were able to walk at velocities up to 16 kilometers per hour (9.94 mph) and attain oxygen uptakes as high as those achieved while running, *the mechanical efficiency of walking faster than 8 km per hour was one-half of that for running at similar speeds.* Competition walkers are able to achieve such high yet inefficient rates of movement by use of a special gait that involves a "rolling" of the hips.

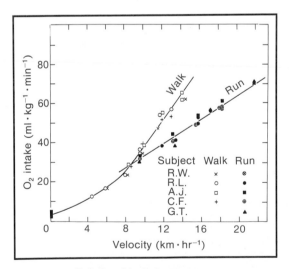

FIG. 10-2. *Relationship between oxygen consumption and velocity for walking and running on a treadmill in competition walkers. (From Menier, D.R., and Pugh, L.G.C.E.: The relation of oxygen intake and velocity of walking and running in competition walkers. J. Physiol., 197: 717, 1968.)*

ENERGY EXPENDITURE DURING JOGGING AND RUNNING

Jogging and running represent two of the most popular recreational exercise activities. They can be performed at various levels of intensity depending on terrain, weather, training goals, and the performer's fitness level. The energy expenditure for jogging and running has been quantified in two ways: (1) during performance of the actual activity, and (2) on a treadmill in the laboratory where the running speed and grade can be precisely controlled. Jogging and running are essentially qualitative terms that relate to the speed at which running is performed. This difference is determined largely by the relative aerobic energy demands required in raising and lowering the body's center of gravity and accelerating and decelerating the limbs during the run. At identical running speeds, a highly conditioned distance runner runs at a lower percentage of his or her maximal aerobic capacity than an untrained runner, even though the oxygen consumption during the run may be similar for both people. *Thus, the demarcation between what is considered jogging and running depends on the fitness level of the participant; a jog for one person could be a run for another.*

Independent of fitness, however, it is more economical from an energy standpoint to dis-continue walking and to begin to jog or run at speeds greater than about 8 km per hour (5 mph). This is illustrated in Figure 10-3, which shows the relationship between oxygen consumption and horizontal walking and running for men and women at speeds ranging from 4 to 14 km per hour (2.5 to 8.7 mph). In the data depicted by the open triangles,[11] the lines relating oxygen consumption and speed of walking and running intersect at a running speed of 8.5 km per hour (5.3 mph), whereas for the values from competition walkers shown by open circles,[16] the "break point" between the efficiency of walking and running occurs at about 9 km per hour (5.6 mph). The results of both studies confirm earlier experiments that demonstrated that at speeds below 8 km per hour, walking was more economical than running, whereas at faster speeds, running became the more economical means of locomotion.

The data for running shown in Figure 10-3 illustrate an important principle in relation to running speed and energy expenditure. *Because the relationship between oxygen consumption and speed of running is linear, the total caloric cost of running a given distance is about the same whether the pace is fast or slow.* In simple terms, if one runs a mile at a speed of 10 miles per hour, it will require about twice as much energy per minute as running at 5 miles per hour; however, the runner will finish the mile in 6 minutes whereas running at the slower speed requires twice the time, or 12 minutes. Consequently, the energy cost of the mile is about the same. This holds true not only for horizontal running at speeds between 8 and 22 km per hour (5 to 13.7 mph), but also for running at inclines that range from −45 to +15 percent.[5,11] *For horizontal running, the net energy cost (that is, excluding the resting requirement) per kilogram of body weight per kilometer traveled is approximately 1 kcal, or* $1 \ kcal \cdot kg^{-1} \cdot km^{-1}$.[11,12] Thus, for an individual who weighs 78 kg, the net energy requirement for running 1 km would be about 78 kcal, regardless of the running speed. Expressed in terms of oxygen consumption, this would amount to 15.6 liters of oxygen consumed per kilometer (1 liter O_2 = 5 kcal).

Table 10-3 presents values for the *net* energy expended during running for 1 hour at various speeds. Running speeds are expressed as kilometers per hour, miles per hour, as well as the number of minutes required to complete one mile at a particular running speed. The bold-

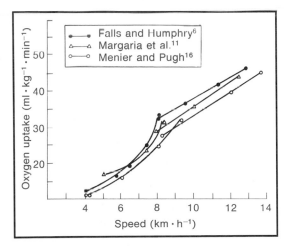

FIG. 10-3. *Relationship between oxygen uptake and speed of horizontal walking and running in men and women. (From Falls, H.B., and Humphrey, L.D.: Energy cost of running and walking in young women. Med. Sci. Sports, 8: 9, 1976.)*

TABLE 10-3. *Net energy expenditure per hour for horizontal running*[a]

BODY WEIGHT		km · hr⁻¹[b] mph min per mile **kcal per mile**	8 4.97 12:00	9 5.60 10:43	10 6.20 9:41	11 6.84 8:46	12 7.46 8:02	13 8.08 7:26	14 8.70 6:54	15 9.32 6:26	16 9.94 6:02
kg	lbs										
50	100	**80**	400	450	500	550	600	650	700	750	800
54	119	**86**	432	486	540	594	648	702	756	810	864
58	128	**93**	464	522	580	638	696	754	812	870	928
62	137	**99**	496	558	620	682	744	806	868	930	992
66	146	**106**	528	594	660	726	792	858	924	990	1056
70	154	**112**	560	630	700	770	840	910	980	1050	1120
74	163	**118**	592	666	740	814	888	962	1036	1110	1184
78	172	**125**	624	702	780	858	936	1014	1092	1170	1248
82	181	**131**	656	738	820	902	984	1066	1148	1230	1312
86	190	**138**	688	774	860	946	1032	1118	1204	1290	1376
90	199	**144**	720	810	900	990	1080	1170	1260	1350	1440
94	207	**150**	752	846	940	1034	1128	1222	1316	1410	1504
98	216	**157**	784	882	980	1078	1176	1274	1372	1470	1568
102	225	**163**	816	918	1020	1122	1224	1326	1428	1530	1632
106	234	**170**	848	954	1060	1166	1272	1378	1484	1590	1696

[a] The table is interpreted as follows: For a 50 kg person, the net energy expenditure for running for 1 hour at 8 km · hr⁻¹ or 4.97 mph is 400 kcal; this speed represents a 12-minute per mile pace. Thus, in 1 hour 5 miles would be run and 400 kcal would be expended. If the pace was increased to 12 km · hr⁻¹, 600 kcal would be expended during the hour of running.

[b] Running speeds are expressed as kilometers per hour (km · hr⁻¹), miles per hour (mph), and minutes required to complete each mile (min per mile). The values in boldface type are the net calories expended to run 1 mile for a given body weight, independent of running speed.

face values are the net calories expended to run one mile for a given body weight; as mentioned before, this energy requirement is fairly constant and independent of running speed. *Thus, for a person who weighs 62 kg, running a 26-mile marathon requires about 2600 kcal whether the run is completed in just over 2 hours or 4 hours!*

For a heavier person, the energy cost per mile increases proportionately. This certainly supports the role of exercise as a caloric stress for the relatively unfit, overfat individual who may want to increase energy expenditure for purposes of weight control. For example, if a 102-kg person jogs 5 miles each day at any comfortable pace, 163 kcal will be expended for each mile completed, or a total of 815 kcal for the 5-mile run. Increasing or decreasing the speed (within the broad range of steady-rate paces) simply alters the length of exercise period; it has little effect on the *total* energy expended.

Stride Length, Stride Frequency, and Speed

Running speed can be increased in one of three ways: (1) by increasing the number of steps taken each minute (*stride frequency*), (2) by increasing the distance between steps (*stride length*), or (3) by increasing both the length and frequency of the strides. Although the third option may seem the obvious means to increase running speed, several carefully conducted experiments have provided objective data concerning this question.

In 1944, the stride pattern of the Danish champion in the 5- and 10-km running events was evaluated.[2] At a running speed of 9.3 km per hour (5.8 mph), stride frequency for this athlete was 160 per minute with a corresponding stride length of 97 centimeters (cm) (38.2 in). When running speed was increased 91% to 17.8 km per hour (11.1 mph), stride frequency increased only 10% to 176 per minute, whereas an 83% increase was observed in stride length to 168 cm. Similarly, for another well-trained runner who performed at the same speeds, there was a 12% and 81% increase in stride frequency and stride length, respectively, as the faster speed was attained.

Figure 10-4A displays graphically the interaction betwen stride frequency and stride length as running speed increases. Doubling the running speed from 10 to 20 km per hour increases stride length by 85% whereas stride frequency only increases by about 9%. Increases in speed above 23 km per hour (14.3 mph) were achieved mainly by augmenting stride frequency. Except at rapid speeds, running speed 🏃 is increased mainly by lengthening the stride.

The competitive walker, on the other hand, does not increase speed in the same way as a runner. Figure 10-4B shows the stride length–stride frequency relationship for walking at speeds from 10 to 14.4 km per hour. The subject was an Olympic-medal-winner in the 10-km walk. When walking speed increased from 10 to 14.4 km per hour, the corresponding increase in frequency and length of stride was 27% and 13%, respectively. At faster speeds, there was an even greater increase in stride frequency because, unlike running, in which the body glides through the air, competition walking requires that the back foot remain on the ground until the front foot makes contact. Thus, lengthening the stride becomes an ineffective means to increase speed in competitive walking. Due to this standardization of style in competitive walking, additional energy must be expended to move the leg rapidly forward; this requires a corresponding involvement of the trunk and arm musculature and explains why it is more economical from an energy standpoint to run than walk at speeds greater than 8 or 9 km per hour (see Fig. 10-3).

Optimum Stride Length

For running at a constant speed, there seems to be an optimum combination of stride length and frequency that is largely dependent on the person's mechanics or "style" of running. Generally, however, it is more costly to overstride than to understride. Figure 10-5 shows values for oxygen consumption plotted in relation to different stride lengths that the runner altered during submaximal running at a relatively fast, constant speed of 14 km per hour (8.7 mph).

For this runner, a stride length of 135 cm was associated with an oxygen consumption of 3.35 liters per minute. Oxygen consumption increased 8% when stride length was *shortened* to 118 cm; a 12% increase in oxygen consumption was noted when the distance between steps *lengthened* from 135 to 153 cm. The curve in the insert graph shows a similar pattern for oxygen consumption when running speed was increased to 16 km per hour at stride lengths that varied from 135 to 169 cm. Decreasing the length of the stride from this runner's optimum of 149 cm to 135 cm increased oxygen consumption by 4.1%. Aerobic require-

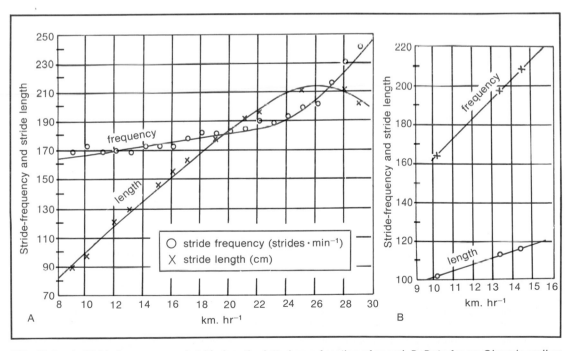

FIG. 10-4. *A, Stride frequency and stride length plotted as a function of speed. B, Data for an Olympic walker. (From Hogberg, P.: Length of stride, stride frequency, flight period and maximum distance between the feet during running with different speeds. Int. Z. Angew. Physiol., 14: 431, 1952.)*

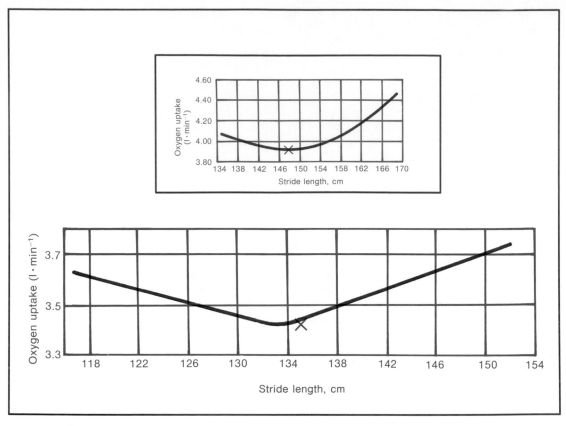

FIG. 10-5. *Oxygen consumption while running at 14 km per hour plotted as a function of different stride lengths. The insert curve is a plot of oxygen consumption at a speed of 16 km per hour at different stride lengths. (From Hogberg, P.: How do stride length and stride frequency influence the energy output during running? Int. Z. Angew. Physiol. 14: 437, 1952.)*

ments increased almost 13% by lengthening the stride to 169 cm. As might be expected, the most economical stride length for a particular running speed was the one selected by the runner (marked in the figure by an X). Lengthening the stride above that normally used by the runner produced a larger increase in oxygen consumption than when the stride was shortened below the optimum length. Thus, to urge a runner who shows signs of fatigue to, "Lengthen your stride!," in order to maintain speed is actually counterproductive in terms of mechanical efficiency and oxygen cost.

At least for well-trained runners, it would seem that the best procedure is to let them run at the stride length they have selected through years of practice; this generally produces the most efficient running performance blended to individual variations in body weight, inertia of limb segments, and anatomic development. *Consequently, there is no "best" style charac-*

teristic of elite runners! Biomechanical analysis may help the athlete correct minor irregularities in movement patterns while running;[19] this would certainly be of considerable practical importance to the competitive runner.

Air Resistance

Anyone who has run into a head wind intuitively knows that more energy is expended trying to maintain a given pace compared with running in calm weather or with the wind at one's back. The magnitude of the effect of air resistance on the energy cost of running varies with three factors: (1) air density, (2) the runner's projected surface area, and (3) the square of the wind velocity. Depending on running speed, overcoming air resistance accounts for 3% to 9% of the total energy requirement of running in *calm* weather.[8] Running into a head wind creates an

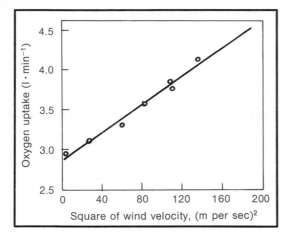

FIG. 10-6. *Oxygen consumption as a function of the square of wind velocity while running at 15.9 km per hr against various headwinds. (From Pugh, L.G.C.E.: Oxygen intake and treadmill running with observations of the effect of air resistance. J. Physiol., 207: 823, 1970.)*

additional expense. As shown in Figure 10-6, the mean oxygen consumption while running at 15.9 km per hour in calm conditions was 2.92 liters per minute.[21] This increased by 5.5% to 3.09 liters per minute against a 16-km per hour "head wind" (9.9 mph) and 4.1 liters per minute while running against the strongest wind (41 mph); this represented a 41% additional expenditure of energy in order to maintain running velocity!

At higher altitudes, wind velocity has less effect on energy expenditure than it does at sea level due to the reduced air density at higher elevations. For speed skaters, for example, the oxygen cost of skating at a particular speed is always lower at altitude compared to sea level.[1,3] Overcoming air resistance at altitude only becomes important at the faster skating speeds. In all likelihood, this altitude-effect would also be the case for running and cycling.

Treadmill Versus Track Running

Although the treadmill is used almost exclusively to evaluate the physiology of running, a question exists concerning the validity of this procedure for determining the energetics of running and for relating this to performance on a track. For example, is the energy required to run a given speed or distance on a treadmill the same as that required to run on a track in calm weather? To answer this question, eight distance runners were studied on both a treadmill and track at three submaximal speeds of 180, 210, and 260 meters per minute (6.7, 7.8, and 9.7 mph), and during a graded exercise test to determine possible differences between treadmill and track running on maximal oxygen consumption.[15] The track runs were performed under environmental conditions similar to those in the laboratory. The results for one submaximal running speed and for maximal exercise are summarized in Table 10-4.

From a practical as well as a statistical standpoint, there were no significant differences in

TABLE 10-4. *Comparison of average metabolic responses during treadmill and track running[a]*

MEASUREMENT	TREADMILL	TRACK	DIFFERENCE
Submaximal Exercise			
Oxygen consumption, $ml \cdot kg^{-1} \cdot min^{-1}$	42.2	42.7	+0.5
Respiratory exchange ratio	0.89	0.87	−0.02
Running speed, $m \cdot min^{-1}$	213.7	216.8	+3.1
Maximal Exercise			
Oxygen consumption, $l \cdot min^{-1}$	4.40	4.44	+0.04
$ml \cdot kg^{-1} \cdot min^{-1}$	66.9	66.3	−0.3
Ventilation, $l \cdot min^{-1}$, BTPS	142.5	146.5	+4.0
Respiratory exchange ratio	1.15	1.11	−0.04

[a]Adapted from McMiken, D.F., and Daniels, J.T.: Aerobic requirements and maximum aerobic power in treadmill and track running. Med. Sci. Sports. 8:14, 1976.

the aerobic requirements of submaximal running (up to 260 m per min) on the treadmill or track, or between the maximal oxygen consumption measured in both forms of exercise under similar environmental conditions. It is still possible, however, that, at the faster running speeds achieved during endurance competition, the influence of air resistance becomes considerable and the oxygen cost of track running may become greater compared to "stationary" running on a treadmill at the same speed.

Marathon Running

The average speed for the marathon during the 1980 Olympics was 5:00 minutes per mile over the 26.2-mile course. This is an incredible achievement in terms of human performance. Not only does this pace require a steady-rate aerobic metabolism that exceeds the aerobic capacity of the average male college student, but it also represents about 75% to 85% of the marathoner's aerobic power that must be maintained for just over 2 hours! These athletes have an average aerobic capacity of approximately 4.4 liters per minute or 70 to 84 ml $\cdot$ kg^{-1} $\cdot$ min^{-1}.[4]

Two long-distance runners were measured during a marathon to determine the energy expenditure per minute and the total caloric cost of the run.[13] For these racers, oxygen consumption was determined every 3 miles by use of the balloon technique of open-circuit spirometry illustrated in Figure 8-4D. Their marathon times were 2 h: 36 min: 34 s and 2 h: 39 min: 28 s; their maximal oxygen uptakes measured during treadmill running were 4.43 liters per minute (70.5 ml $\cdot$ kg^{-1} $\cdot$ min^{-1}) and 4.66 liters per minute (73.9 ml $\cdot$ kg^{-1} $\cdot$ min^{-1}), respectively. During the marathon, the first runner maintained an average speed of 270.5 meters (m) per minute (10.0 mph), which required an oxygen consumption equal to 80% of his maximal aerobic power. For the second runner, whose average speed was slower at 266.1 m per minute (9.92 mph), the aerobic energy requirement per minute averaged 78.3% of maximum. *For both men,* the energy requirement for running the marathon was 2300 to 2400 kcal.

For distance runners who train about 100 miles per week, or slightly less than the distance of four marathons at close to competitive speeds, the weekly caloric expenditure from exercise is about 10,000 kcal. For the serious marathon runner who trains year-round, the total energy expended in training for 4 years prior to an Olympic competition would be close to two million calories! It is not surprising then that these superior athletes have such a low quantity of body fat (3% to 5% of body weight). As illustrated in Table 10-3, the total expenditure of energy for a marathon run remains fairly constant for individuals of similar body size, regardless of running speed. Obviously, persons with low aerobic capacities must maintain a slower running speed; thus, they will need more time to finish the marathon.

SWIMMING

Swimming exercise differs in several important respects from walking or running.[8a] One obvious difference in swimming is that energy must be expended to maintain buoyancy and at the same time to generate horizontal movement by the use of the arms and legs, either in combination or separately. Other differences include the requirements for overcoming the *drag forces* that impede the movement of an object through a fluid. The amount of drag depends on the fluid medium and on the size, shape, and velocity of the object. All of these differences contribute to the fact that *the energy cost of swimming a given distance is about four times greater than running the same distance.*

Methods of Measurement

For short swims, such as 25 yards, swum at different velocities, subjects need not breathe during the swim, and energy expenditure has been roughly estimated from oxygen consumption during 20 to 40 minutes of recovery. For swims of longer duration, including 12- to 14-hour endurance swims, energy expenditure has been computed from oxygen consumption measured by the balloon technique (Fig. 8-4C) during portions of the swimming performance. In studies conducted in the pool, the researcher walks alongside the swimmer and carries the portable gas collection equipment.[14] In another form of swimming exercise, illustrated in Figure 10-7A, the subject remains stationary, attached or "tethered" to a cable and pulley system by means of a belt worn around the waist.[10] The amount of weight attached to the

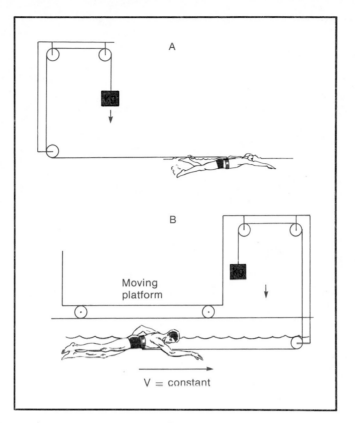

FIG. 10-7. *A, Apparatus used to measure energy expenditure during tethered swimming. B, Platform procedure to study swimming dynamics. The platform moves at a constant speed about an angular pool 60 meters in circumference. (From DiPrampero, P.E. et al.: Energetics of swimming in man. J. Physiol., 237: 1, 1974.)*

cable can be increased periodically, thereby forcing the swimmer to exert more effort to keep from being pulled back. With the ergometer illustrated in Figure 10-7B, the swimmer is paced from a moving platform. A system of pulleys is attached to the platform, which in turn connects with the subject. The platform can be positioned either in front of or behind the swimmer; the force exerted by the swimmer must be sufficient to maintain the pulley at a given height.

Figure 10-8 shows a subject swimming in a flume or "swimmill." Water is circulated and its velocity varied from the slowest swimming speeds up to 1.98 m per second, which was the record pace for the men's 100-m freestyle in the Moscow Olympics of 1980. Also, water temperature in the 38,000-liter swimmill can be varied from 10°C to 40°C, and photographic analysis of stroke mechanics is possible through windows on the side of the flume beneath the water's surface.

Energy Cost and Drag

Both the flume and platform apparatus have been particularly useful for quantifying the effects of total body drag during both tethered and "free" swimming.

The total drag force encountered by the swimmer consists of three components: (1) *Wave drag* is caused by the waves that build up in front of and form hollows behind the swimmer as he or she moves through the water. This component of drag is not a significant factor when swimming at slow velocities, but its influence becomes greater at faster swimming speeds. (2) *Skin friction drag* is produced as the water slides over the surface of the skin. Even at relatively fast swimming velocities, the quantitative contribution of skin friction drag to the total drag is minimal. *Thus, the common practice of swimmers "shaving down" to reduce skin friction drag is a questionable* procedure. (3) *Viscous pressure drag* contributes

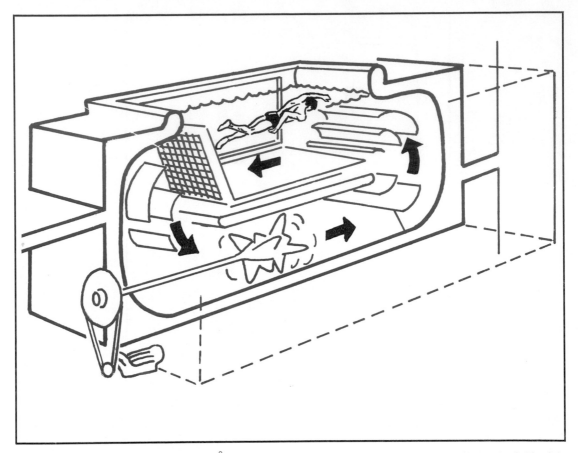

FIG. 10-8. *The swimming flume. (From Åstrand, P.O., and Englesson, S.: A swimming flume. J. Appl. Physiol., 33:514, 1972.)*

substantially to counter the propulsive efforts of the swimmer at slow velocities. It is caused by the separation of the thin sheet of water, or boundary layer, adjacent to the swimmer.[17] The pressure differential created in front of and behind the swimmer represents the viscous pressure drag. Its effect is probably reduced in highly skilled swimmers who have learned to "streamline" their stroke. Such streamlining with improved stroke mechanics reduces the separation region by moving the separation point closer to the trailing edge of the water. This is similar to what occurs when an oar slices through the water with the blade parallel rather than perpendicular to the flow of water.

As shown in Figure 10-9, a curvilinear relationship exists between body drag and the velocity at which a swimmer is towed through the water. As velocity increased above 0.8 m per second, drag was reduced when the legs and arms were supported by flotation devices that placed the entire body in a horizontal position. In general, the drag force is about 2 to 2.5 times higher in swimming than in passive towing.

Significant differences exist between men and women for body drag, mechanical efficiency, and net oxygen consumption when swimming the overarm crawl.[23] Values for drag and net oxygen consumption were all lower for the *women* at various swimming speeds. These findings indicate that women can swim a given distance at about 30% lower energy cost than men; expressed another way, women can achieve a much higher swimming velocity than men for the same energy expenditure. If women swimmers develop their maximal aerobic and anaerobic capacities to the same extent as men, they will probably swim the overarm crawl at faster speeds.

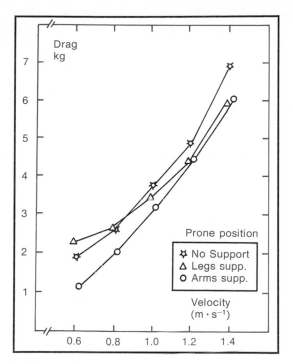

FIG. 10-9. *Water drag in three different prone positions in relation to towing velocity. (From Holmér, I.: Energy cost of arm stroke, leg kick, and the whole stroke in competitive swimming styles. Eur. J. Appl. Physiol., 33: 105, 1974.)*

Energy Cost, Swimming Velocity, and Skill

Elite swimmers are able to swim a particular stroke at a given velocity at a lower oxygen consumption than are relatively untrained or recreational swimmers. This is illustrated in Figure 10-10 for the breaststroke, front crawl, and back crawl with subjects representing three levels of ability. One subject was a recreational swimmer who did not participate in swim training; the trained subject swam on a daily basis and was a top Swedish swimmer; the elite swimmer was a European champion. Except for the breaststroke, the elite swimmer was able to swim at a given speed with a lower oxygen uptake than his trained and untrained counterpart. Figure 10-10B shows that for the two trained athletes swimming at any particular speed, the breaststroke was the most costly; this was followed by the backstroke, with the front crawl being the least "expensive" of the three strokes studied.

Effects of Water Temperature

Swimming in relatively cold water places the swimmer under thermal stress and brings about metabolic and cardiovascular adjustments that are different from those observed in warmer water.[8a] These responses are geared primarily toward maintaining a relative consistency in core temperature, because heat flow from the body is considerable, especially at water temperatures below 25° C (77° F). Heat loss is especially apparent in lean subjects who benefit less from the insulation of subcutaneous fat.[18]

Figure 10-11 shows the oxygen consumption during breaststroke swimming at water temperatures of 18, 26, and 33° C. As seen, oxygen consumption increases in an essentially linear fashion with swimming speed, with the highest values for oxygen consumption at submaximal swimming speeds occurring in cold water. This "extra" oxygen cost of swimming in cold water is due almost entirely to the energy expended in shivering as the body attempts to regulate core temperature. From the results of several experiments with swimming and other forms of exercise in water, it appears that the optimal water temperature for most competitive swimming for individuals of average body composition is 28 to 30° C (82 to 86° F). Within this temperature range, the metabolic heat generated in exercise is easily transferred to the water, yet the gradient for heat flow is not so severe as to result in a significant increases in energy cost or changes in core temperature due to cold stress.

Effects of Buoyancy: Men Versus Women

As is shown in the discussion of body composition in Chapter 26, women of all ages possess on the average significantly more total body fat than men. Because fat floats and muscle and bone sink in the water, the average woman therefore gains a hydrodynamic lift and floats more easily than her male counterpart. It is possible that this difference in body fat and thus in buoyancy is responsible for the higher swimming efficiency observed in women.

It is also possible that the distribution of body fat in women is such that their legs float high in the water, making them more horizontal or "streamlined," whereas the leaner men's legs tend to swing down and float lower in the water. This lowering of the legs to a deeper position

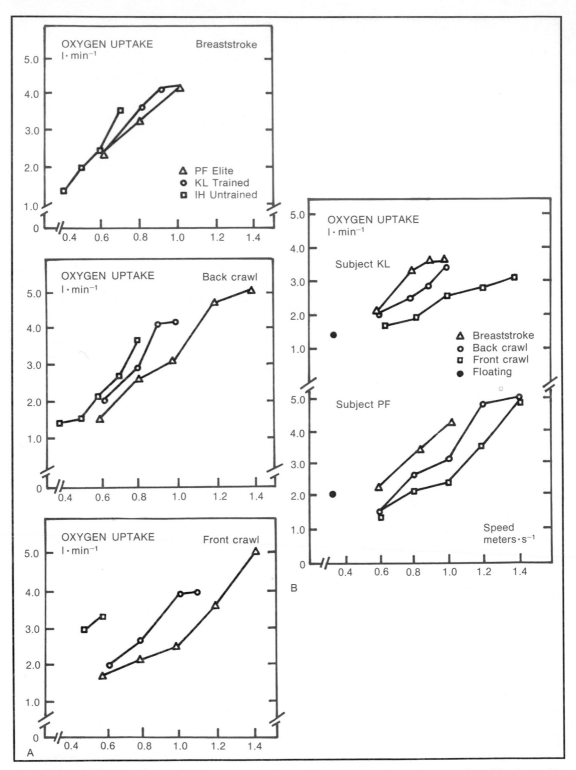

FIG. 10-10. *A, Oxygen consumption as a function of speed for the breaststroke, front crawl, and back crawl in subjects who represented three levels of skill ability. B, Oxygen consumption for two trained swimmers during three competitive strokes. (From Holmér, I.: Oxygen uptake during swimming in man. J. Appl. Physiol. 33: 502, 1972.)*

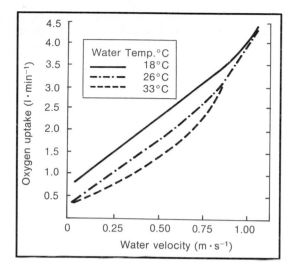

FIG. 10-11. *Energy expenditure for the breaststroke at three water temperatures in relation to velocity. (From Nadel, E.R. et al.: J. Appl. Physiol. 36: 465, 1974.)*

would increase body drag and thus reduce swimming efficiency. Such differences in flotation may help explain the "sex difference" in swimming efficiency.

Endurance Swimmers

Distance swimming in ocean water poses a severe metabolic, physiologic, and thermal challenge to the swimmer. Researchers have been intrigued by the fact that channel swimmers are able to swim up to 22 hours in water at 15.5° C (60° F), whereas the average person after a shipwreck or plane crash can survive in this water for only about 4 to 6 hours.

In one investigation, performance, metabolic, and body composition data were obtained from nine distance swimmers.[21] These data were secured both under race conditions and in a salt-water pool at swimming speeds ranging from 2.6 to 4.9 km per hour. During the race, the competitors maintained a constant stroke rate and pace until the last few hours, when fatigue set in. From detailed observations on one male subject, the average speed of 2.85 km per hour during a 12-hour swim required an average oxygen consumption of approximately 1.7 liters per minute, or an equivalent energy expenditure of 8.5 kcal per minute. Consequently,

the gross caloric requirement for the 12-hour swim was about 6120 kcal (8.5 kcal × 60 min × 12 h). The net caloric cost of swimming the Channel, assuming a resting energy expenditure of 1.2 kcal per minute (0.260 liter $O_2 \cdot min^{-1}$), was slightly in excess of 5200 kcal.

SUMMARY

1. Energy expenditure can be expressed in gross as well as net terms. Total or gross values include the resting energy requirement, whereas net energy expenditure is the energy cost of the activity per se excluding the resting value.

2. The relationship between walking speed and oxygen consumption is essentially linear. Walking surface also has an influence, because walking on sand requires twice the energy expenditure as walking on hard surfaces. The energy cost is proportionally larger for heavier people.

3. It is more economical, from an energy standpoint, to jog–run rather than to walk at speeds greater than 8 km · h⁻¹. The difference between jogging and running depends on the fitness level of the participant; a jog for one person may be a run for another.

4. The total caloric cost for running a given distance is about the same whether the pace is fast or slow. For horizontal running, the net energy expenditure is about 1 kcal · kg⁻¹ · km⁻¹.

5. It generally costs less energy to shorten running stride and to increase the number of steps in order to maintain a constant running speed rather than to lengthen the stride and reduce stride frequency.

6. Overcoming air resistance accounts for 3% to 9% of the cost of running in calm weather. This percentage increases considerably if a runner attempts to maintain pace while running into a head wind.

7. The energy required to run a given distance or speed on a treadmill is about the same as that required to run on a track under identical weather conditions.

8. The energy expended swimming a given distance is about four times greater than that expended running the same distance. This is because the swimmer must expend considerable energy to maintain buoyancy and overcome the drag forces that impede movement.

9. There are significant differences between men and women for body drag, mechani-

cal efficiency, and net oxygen consumption during swimming. Women swim a given distance at about 30% lower energy cost than men.

10. Elite swimmers expend fewer calories to swim a given stroke at any velocity. The optimal water temperatue for most competitive swimming is 28 to 30° C (82–86° F).

References

1. Åstrand, P.O., and Rodahl, K.: Textbook of Work Physiology. 2nd Edition. New York, McGraw-Hill Book Co., 1977.
2. Bøje, O.: Energy production, pulmonary ventilation, and length of steps in well-trained runners working on a treadmill. *Acta Physiol. Scand., 7:*362, 1944.
3. Cerretelli, P.: Limiting factors to oxygen transport on Mount Everest. J. Appl. Physiol., *40:*658, 1976.
4. Costill, D.L., and Fox, E.L.: Energetics of marathon running. Med. Sci. Sports, *1:*81, 1969.
5. Davies, C.T.M., Sargeant, A.J., and Smith, B.: The physiological response to running downhill. Eur. J. Appl. Physiol., *32:*187, 1974.
6. Falls, H.B., and Humphrey, L.D.: Energy cost of running and walking in young women. Med. Sci. Sports, *8:*9, 1976.
7. Godin, G., and Shephard, R.J.: Body weight and the energy cost of activity. Arch. Environ. Health, *27:*289, 1973.
8. Hill, A.V.: The air resistance to a runner. Proc. R. Soc. Lond. (Biol.) *102:*380, 1927.
8a. Holmér, I.: Physiology of swimming man. Exercise and Sport Sciences Reviews, Vol. 7. Edited by R.S. Hutton and D.I. Miller. Philadelphia, Franklin Institute Press, 1980.
9. Jankowski, L. et al.: Accuracy of methods for estimating O_2 cost of walking in coronary patients. J. Appl. Physiol., *33:*672, 1972.
10. Magel, J.R. et al: The specificity of swim training on maximum oxygen uptake. J. Appl. Physiol. *36:*753, 1974.
11. Margaria, R. et al.: Energy cost of running. J. Appl. Physiol., *18:*367, 1963.
12. Margaria, R.: Biomechanics and Energetics of Muscular Exercise. Oxford, Clarendon Press, 1976.
13. Maron, M. et al.: Oxygen uptake measurements during competitive marathon running. J. Appl. Physiol., *40:*836, 1976.
14. McArdle, W.D. et al.: Metabolic and cardiorespiratory response during free swimming and treadmill walking. J. Appl. Physiol., *30:*733, 1971.
15. McMiken, D.F., and Daniels, J.T.: Aerobic requirements and maximum aerobic power in treadmill and track running. Med. Sci. Sports, *8:*14, 1976.
16. Menier, D.R., and Pugh, L.G.C.E.: The relation of oxygen intake and velocity of walking and running in competition walkers. J. Physiol., *197:*717, 1968.
17. Miller, D.L.: Biomechanics of swimming. *In* Exercise and Sport Sciences Reviews, Vol. 3. Edited by J.H., Wilmore and J. Keogh. New York, Academic Press, 1975.
18. Nadel, E. et al.: Energy exchanges of swimming man. J. Appl. Physiol., *36:*465, 1974.
19. Nelson, R.C., and Gregor, R.J.: Biomechanics of distance running: A longitudinal study. Res. Quart., *47:*471, 1976.
20. Pandolf, K.B., Givoni, B., and Goldman, R.F.: Predicting energy expenditure with loads while standing or walking very slowly. J. Appl. Physiol., *43:*577, 1977.
21. Pugh, L.G.C.E., and Edholm, O.G.: The physiology of channel swimmers. Lancet *2:*761, 1955.
22. Ralston, H.J.: Comparison of energy expenditure during treadmill walking and floor walking. J. Appl. Physiol., *15:*1156, 1960.
23. Rennie, D.W., et al.: Energetics of swimming in man. *In* Swimming II. Edited by L. Lewille and J. Clarys. Baltimore, University Park Press, 1975.

Individual Differences and Measurement of Energy Capacities

11

We all possess the capability for anaerobic and aerobic energy metabolism, although the capacity for each form of energy transfer varies considerably among individuals.[19] This between-individual variability underlies the concept of *individual differences* in metabolic capacity for exercise. It also appears that a person's capacity for energy transfer (and for many physiologic functions, for that matter) is not simply a general factor, but is highly dependent on the form of exercise with which it is trained and evaluated.[33,34,41,43] A high maximum oxygen uptake in running, for example, does not necessarily assure a similar metabolic power when different muscle groups are activated, as in swimming and rowing. This *specificity* of metabolic capacity is observed even in activities that utilize similar muscles, such as bicycling and running. In addition, training for high aerobic power probably contributes little to one's capacity to generate anaerobic energy, and vice versa. The effects of systematic training are highly specific in terms of neurologic, physiologic, and metabolic demands. Terms such as "speed," "power," and "endurance" must therefore be defined carefully within the context of the specific metabolic and physiologic requirements of an activity.

In this chapter, the capacity of the various energy transfer systems discussed in Chapters 6 and 7 are evaluated, with special reference to *measurement, specificity,* and *individual differences.*

ANAEROBIC ENERGY: THE IMMEDIATE AND SHORT-TERM ENERGY SYSTEMS

All-out exercise for up to 2 minutes duration is powered mainly by the *immediate* and *short-term* energy systems. Both systems operate anaerobically because their transfer of chemical energy does not require molecular oxygen. Generally, there is greater reliance on anaerobic energy for fast movements or when there is resistance to movement at a given speed. This principle is shown in Figure 11-1, which illustrates the relative involvement of the anaerobic and aerobic energy transfer systems for different durations of all-out exercise. At the initiation of movement performed at high or low speed, the stored phosphates, ATP and CP, provide immediate energy for muscle contraction. After the first few seconds of movement, an increasingly greater proportion of energy is generated by the short-term energy transfer reactions of glycolysis. As exercise continues, a greater demand is then placed on the aerobic metabolic pathways for purposes of ATP resynthesis.

Evaluation of the Immediate Energy System

Performance tests that apparently cause maximal activation of the ATP–CP energy system have been developed to provide practical "field

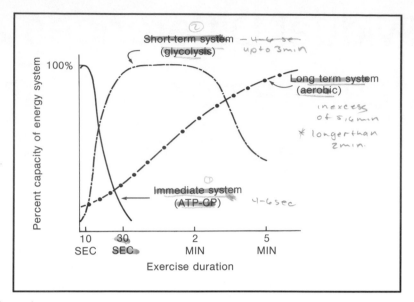

FIG. 11-1. *The various energy systems and their involvement during all-out exercise of different durations.*

tests'' to evaluate the capacity of this immediate means for energy transfer.[24,25,46] These tests are generally referred to as *power tests;* power in this context is defined as the time-rate of doing work, or work accomplished per unit time. The appropriate formula for determining power output is:

$$P = \frac{F \times D}{T}$$

where F is the force generated, D is the distance through which the force is moved or applied, and T is the duration of the work period. Depending on the units of measurement, P or power can be expressed as foot pounds, kilogram meters, or kcal per second or per minute, or even in power terms of watts and horsepower.

MARGARIA POWER TEST. Researchers have proposed that muscular power can be measured by sprinting up a flight of stairs.[23,37] As illustrated in Figure 11-2, the subject runs up a staircase as fast as possible, taking three steps at a time. The external work done in this test is the total vertical distance the body is lifted up the stairs; this distance for six stairs is usually about 1.05 m.

The power output of a 60-kg woman who traverses six steps in 0.52 seconds is computed as follows:

F = 60 kg
D = 1.05 m
T = 0.52 s

$$Power = \frac{60 \text{ kg} \times 1.05 \text{ m}}{0.52 \text{ s}}$$

Power = 121.1 kgm per s

Table 11-1 presents standards for classifying men and women of different ages in terms of immediate energy output capacity.

Because the power score in the Margaria test is influenced significantly by the person's body weight, the heavier person will necessarily have a higher power score if several individuals achieve the same speed. This implies that the heavier person has a more highly developed immediate energy system than a lighter person who may cover the same vertical distance in the same time. Because there is no direct evidence to support this contention, caution is urged in interpreting differences in scores on the Margaria power test and making inferences about individual differences in energy capacities. *The test may be better suited for evaluating individuals of similar body weight, or the same people before and after a specific training program designed to develop rapid anaerobic leg power.*

JUMPING-POWER TESTS. For years, jump tests such as the *Sargent jump-and-reach test*[47] or a *standing broad jump* have been common ele-

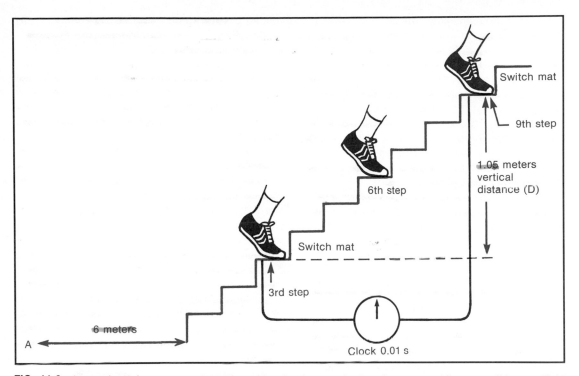

FIG. 11-2. *Margaria–Kalamen power test. The subject begins at point A and runs as rapidly as possible up a flight of stairs, taking three steps at a time. The time to cover the distance between stair 3 and stair 9 is recorded to the nearest 0.01 second by the use of switch mats placed on the steps. Power output is the product of the subject's weight (F) and vertical distance (D), divided by the time (T). From Mathews, D.K., and Fox, E.L.: The Physiological Basis of Physical Education and Athletics. Philadelphia, W.B. Saunders, 2nd Edition, 1976.*

TABLE 11-1. *Guidelines for classifying men and women in terms of power output capacity[a]*

	MEN AGE GROUPS (years)				
CLASSIFICATION	15–20	20–30	30–40	40–50	OVER 50
Poor	Under 113[b]	Under 106	Under 85	Under 65	Under 50
Fair	113–149	106–139	85–111	65–84	50–65
Average	150–187	140–175	112–140	85–105	66–82
Good	188–224	176–210	141–168	106–125	83–98
Excellent	Over 224	Over 210	Over 168	Over 125	Over 98
	WOMEN AGE GROUPS (years)				
CLASSIFICATION	15–20	20–30	30–40	40–50	OVER 50
Poor	Under 92	Under 85	Under 65	Under 50	Under 38
Fair	92–120	85–111	65–84	50–65	38–48
Average	121–151	112–140	85–105	66–82	49–61
Good	152–182	141–168	106–125	83–98	62–75
Excellent	Over 182	Over 168	Over 125	Over 98	Over 75

[a] From Mathews, D.K., and Fox, E.L.: The Physiological Basis of Physical Education and Athletics. Philadelphia, W.B. Saunders, 2nd Edition, 1976. Data from Kalamen J.: Measurement of maximum muscular power in man. Doctoral dissertation. The Ohio State University, 1968, and from Margaria, R. et al.: Measurement of muscular power (anaerobic) in man. J. Appl. Physiol. *21*:1662, 1966.
[b] Values are kilogram meters of work per second (kgm · s^{-1})

ments in many physical fitness test batteries. The Sargent jump is scored as the difference between a person's standing reach and the maximum jump-and-touch height. In the case of the broad jump, the score is the horizontal distance covered in a leap from a semicrouched position. Although both tests purport to measure leg power, they probably fail to achieve this goal. For one thing, with the jump tests, power generated in propelling the body from the crouched position occurs only in the time the feet are in contact with the surface. *It is doubtful whether this brief period is sufficient to evaluate a person's anaerobic ATP and CP capacities.* Also, no relationship has ever been established between jump-test scores and ATP–CP levels or depletion patterns.

OTHER POWER TESTS. As indicated in Figure 11-1, any performance involving all-out exercise of 4 to 6 seconds duration can probably be considered indicative of the person's immediate anaerobic power from the high-energy phosphates in the specific muscles activated.[12] Examples of such tests are sprint running or cycling, shuttle runs, or even certain more localized movements such as arm cranking.

INTERRELATIONSHIPS AMONG POWER TESTS. If the various power tests measure the same metabolic capacity, then individuals ranking high on one test should rank correspondingly high on a second or third test. Although information on this topic is incomplete, the available data indicate that those who do well on one power performance test tend to do well on another, but the correlation is moderate at best and certainly not strong. Table 11-2 shows the interrelationship (expressed statistically as a correlation coefficient) between several tests that supposedly measure immediate power output. The relationship ranges from poor to good, in-

dicating some commonality between tests and suggesting that each may be measuring a similar metabolic quality. Of practical significance is the fairly strong relationship between scores on the Margaria power test and the 40-yard dash. *Clearly, almost the same information can be obtained by sprint running on a track, compared with the more elaborate set-up in the Margaria test.*

Several factors may explain why the interrelationship between the other test scores is not higher. *For one thing, human performance is highly task-specific.* From a metabolic and performance standpoint, this means the best sprint runner is not necessarily the best sprint swimmer, sprint cyclist, or "stair sprinter." Even though the energy to power each performance is generated by the same metabolic reactions, these reactions are isolated within the specific muscles activated by the exercise. It is also important to emphasize that each specific test requires different neurologic or skill components that tend to cause the scores to be more variable.

We have suggested that power tests might be used to show changes in an athlete's performance resulting from specific training. Such tests also offer an excellent means for self-testing and motivation and often provide the actual exercise for training the immediate energy system. With many football teams, for example, the 40-yard dash is often used as a criterion to evaluate a player's *speed.* Although there are many types of "speed" that need to be evaluated, these test scores may provide some information for the evaluation of a player, even though it has yet to be established that 40-yard speed is related to overall football ability for players at similar positions! A run test of shorter duration (up to 20 yards) may turn out to be an equally or more suitable running performance.

TABLE 11-2. *Correlations among tests that are supposed to measure immediate anaerobic power output*[a]

VARIABLES (n = 31 males)	40-YARD DASH	SARGENT JUMP TEST	POWER BICYCLE TEST
1. Margaria power test	.88[b]	.56	.69
2. 40-yard dash	—	−.48[b]	−.62[b]
3. Sargent jump test	—	—	.31

[a] From Physical Performance Research Laboratory, The University of Michigan.
[b] A negative correlation coefficient means that for the group of individuals, a high score earned on one test is associated with a low score on the other test. For the correlations with the 40-yard dash, a negative correlation means a good performance on one test is associated with a low 40-yard run time, and a low score in running (time) is a good performance.

Short-Term Energy System

As depicted in Figure 11-1, when all-out exercise continues longer than a few seconds, increasingly more energy for ATP resynthesis is generated from the *short-term energy system* through the anaerobic reactions of glycolysis. This is not to say that aerobic metabolism is unimportant at this stage of exercise or that the oxygen-consuming reactions have not been "switched-on." On the contrary, Figure 11-1 shows an increase in the contribution of aerobic energy very early in exercise. However, it is in all-out exercise that the energy requirement significantly exceeds the energy generated by the oxidation of hydrogen in the respiratory chain. As a result, the anaerobic reactions of glycolysis predominate and large quantities of lactic acid are formed. It is not difficult to imagine how speed in the 100-meter swim or 1000-meter run, as well as strategies in a variety of sports contests, would suffer if humans were unable to generate power through the anaerobic reactions of glycolysis.

The level of blood lactic acid is the most common indicator of the activation of the short-term energy system. To some extent, the depletion of glycogen in specific muscles also reflects reliance on glycolytic pathways during exercise.

BLOOD LACTIC ACID LEVELS. As was shown previously in Figure 7-3, the blood lactic acid level remains relatively low during steady-rate exercise up to about 55% of the maximum oxygen uptake. As exercise becomes more intense and the max $\dot{V}O_2$ is approached, there is a precipitous increase in the amount of lactic acid in the blood. Work cannot be maintained for more than a few minutes under such conditions.

The data in Figure 11-3 were obtained from 10 college men who performed nine all-out bicycle ergometer rides of different durations on different days. The subjects were highly motivated, many were involved in conditioning programs, and some were varsity athletes. The men were unaware of the duration of each test but were instructed and urged to turn as many revolutions as possible. Venous blood lactic acid was measured before and immediately after each test and throughout recovery. The plotted points are the peak values for lactic acid obtained for each of the nine tests. Blood lactic acid levels increased in direct proportion with

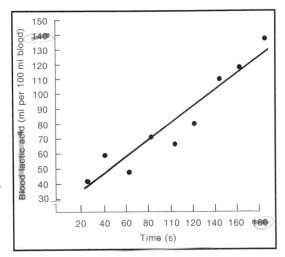

FIG. 11-3. *Blood lactic acid levels in all-out bicycle exercise of different durations. Each value represents the average of 10 subjects. (From Physical Performance Research Laboratory, The University of Michigan.)*

the duration (and total work output) of the all-out exercise. At the end of 3 minutes of cycling, the amount of lactic acid in the blood was highest and averaged about 140 mg in each 100 ml of blood.

GLYCOGEN DEPLETION. Because the short-term energy system is largely dependent on glycogen stored in the specific muscles activated by exercise, the pattern of glycogen depletion in these muscles also provides an indication of the contribution of glycolysis to exercise. Figure 11-4 illustrates that the rate of glycogen depletion in the quadriceps femoris muscle during bicycle exercise is closely related to exercise intensity. With steady-rate exercise at about 30% of max $\dot{V}O_2$, a considerable reserve of muscle glycogen remains, even after 180 minutes of exercise. Because metabolism in this relatively light exercise is essentially aerobic, large quantities of fatty acids are used for energy and the drain on stored glycogen is only moderate. At the two heaviest workloads, however, the most rapid and pronounced glycogen depletion is observed. This makes sense from a metabolic standpoint because glycogen is the only stored nutrient that provides anaerobic energy for the resynthesis of ATP; clearly, this substrate has high priority in the "metabolic mill" during strenuous exercise.

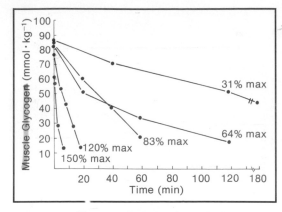

FIG. 11-4. *Glycogen depletion from the lateral portion of the quadriceps femoris muscle in bicycle exercise of different intensities and durations. The lightest workload results in some depletion of muscle glycogen. However, the most rapid and greatest glycogen depletion occurs with short-term, intense exercise. (Adapted from Gollnick, P.D.: Selective glycogen depletion pattern in human muscle fibers after exercise of varying intensity and at varying pedalling rates. J. Physiol., 241:45, 1974.)*

Changes in total muscle glycogen such as those illustrated in Figure 11-4, however, may not give a precise indication of the degree of glycogen breakdown in *specific fibers* within the muscle. It appears that glycogen depletion occurs selectively in fast- and slow-twitch fibers, depending on the intensity of exercise.[44] For example, during all-out exercise (1-min sprints on a bicycle ergometer at a very heavy load), the fast-twitch fibers are activated to provide the predominant power for the exercise. Because of the anaerobic nature of this work, glycogen in these fibers is almost totally depleted. In contrast, during moderate to heavy prolonged exercise, the slow-twitch fibers are always the first to become glycogen-depleted.[18] This *specificity* in glycogen utilization (and depletion) makes it difficult to evaluate glycolytic involvement from changes in a muscle's total glycogen content before and after exercise.

PERFORMANCE TESTS FOR GLYCOLYTIC POWER. Performances requiring substantial activation of the short-term energy system are those demanding maximal work for up to 3 minutes. All-out runs have usually been used to test this energy capacity, although weight lifting (repetitive lifting of a certain percentage of maximum), cycling, and shuttle-runs have also been used.

Because of the effects that factors such as age, skill, motivation, and body size have on performance, it is difficult to choose a suitable criterion test and to develop appropriate norms to evaluate the glycolytic energy system. Also, within the framework of exercise specificity, short-term anaerobic capacity for an arm and upper body activity like rowing or swimming cannot be adequately assessed with a test that makes maximum use of the leg muscles. The performance test must be similar to the activity for which the energy capacity is being evaluated. In most cases the actual activity can serve as the test.

Individual Differences in the Capacity for Anaerobic Energy Transfer

Several factors are often mentioned as contributing to differences among individuals in their capacity to generate short-term anaerobic energy. These include differences in previous training, motivation, and the capacity to buffer acid metabolites.

EFFECTS OF TRAINING. A comparison of the anaerobic capabilities of trained and untrained subjects is presented in Figure 11-5.[25] After short-term maximal exercise on the bicycle ergometer, the trained subjects always exhibited higher levels of muscle and blood lactic acid, as well as greater depletion of muscle glycogen and ATP and CP. These results support the belief that training for short-term, all-out exercise enhances one's capacity to generate energy anaerobically.[11] This is important, because in sprint- and middle-distance activities, individual differences in anaerobic capacity can account for large performance differences.

BUFFERING OF ACID METABOLITES. When anaerobic energy transfer predominates, lactic acid is formed, and the acidity of muscle and blood increases. This has led to the speculation that anaerobic training may enhance short-term energy capacity by the mechanism of increasing the body's alkaline reserve. This would theoretically enable greater lactic acid production because it could be buffered more effectively. Although this reasoning seems appealing, only a small increase of about 1% in alkaline reserve has been noted in athletes as compared to sedentary counterparts.[17] Furthermore, there is no appreciable change in alka-

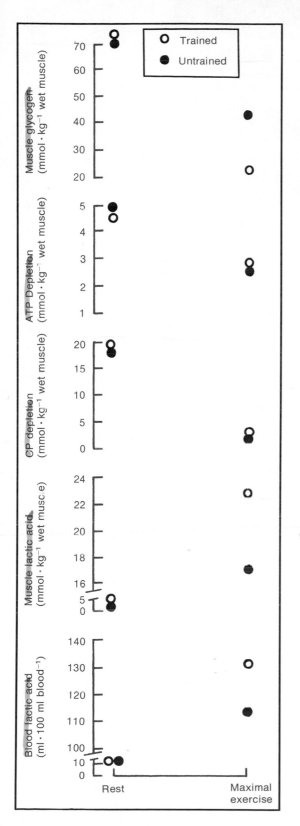

line reserve following hard physical training.[45] *The general consensus is that trained people have a buffering capability within the range expected for healthy untrained individuals.*

MOTIVATION. Individuals with greater "pain tolerance," "toughness," or ability to "push" beyond the discomforts of fatiguing exercise will definitely accomplish more anaerobic work. These people usually generate greater levels of blood lactic acid and glycogen depletion; they also score higher on tests of short-term energy capacity. Motivational factors, which are difficult to categorize or quantify, play a key role in superior performance at all levels of competition.

AEROBIC ENERGY: THE LONG-TERM ENERGY SYSTEM

As shown in Figure 11-6, persons with a large capacity for aerobic energy transfer (that is, a large max $\dot{V}O_2$) generally excell in performances requiring sustained, high-intensity exercise. The highest maximal oxygen uptakes are generally recorded for men and women competing in distance running, swimming, bicycling, and cross-country skiing. These athletes have almost double the aerobic capacity of a sedentary group! This is not to say that the max $\dot{V}O_2$ is the only determinant of aerobic work capacity. Other factors, especially those at the muscular level, such as the number of capillaries, enzymes, and fiber type, exert a strong influence on the capacity to *sustain* high levels of aerobic exercise. However, the max $\dot{V}O_2$ provides important information on the capacity of the long-term energy system. In addition, the attainment of max $\dot{V}O_2$ requires integration of the ventilatory, cardiovascular, and neuromuscular systems; this gives maximal oxygen uptake significant physiologic as well as metabolic meaning.[42] *In many ways, it has become one of the fundamental measures in exercise physiology.*

FIG. 11-5. *Depletion of various anaerobic substrates and increases in muscle and blood lactic acid during maximal exercise for trained and nontrained subjects. In each case, the trained subjects exhibited a greater increase in anaerobic metabolism or a depletion in anaerobic substrates. (From Karlsson, J. et al.: Muscle metabolites during submaximal and maximal exercise in man. Scand. J. Clin. Lab. Invest., 26:382, 1971.)*

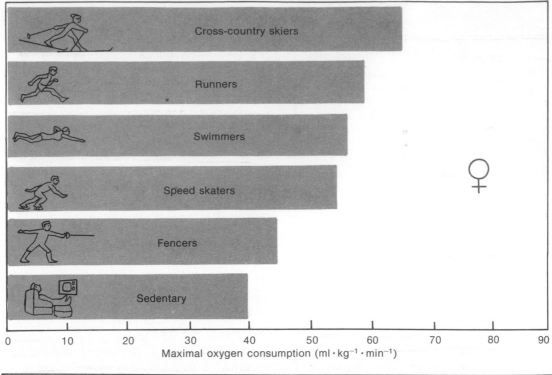

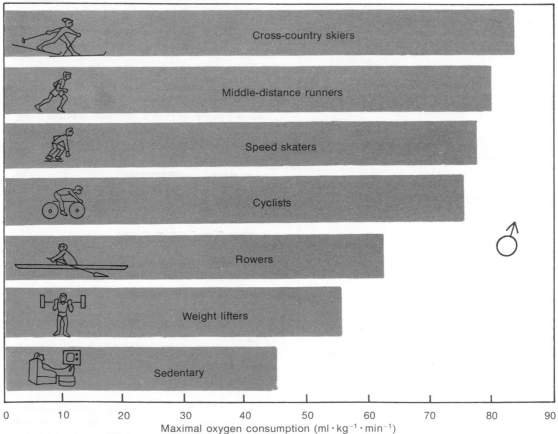

FIG. 11-6. *Maximal oxygen consumption of male and female olympic-caliber athletes and healthy sedentary subjects. (Adapted from Saltin, B., and Åstrand, P.O.: Maximal oxygen uptake in athletes. J. Appl. Physiol. 23:353, 1967.)*

Measurement of Maximal Aerobic Power

The maximal oxygen uptake can be determined by a variety of work tasks that activate large muscle groups as long as the exercise is of sufficient intensity and duration to engage maximal aerobic energy transfer. The usual forms of exercise include treadmill walking or running, bench stepping, or cycling. However, the max $\dot{V}O_2$ has also been measured during swimming,[22,32] rowing[8], and ice skating[15] as well as during arm ergometry.[7,34] Considerable research effort has been directed toward the development and standardization of tests for maximal aerobic power and toward the establishment of norms for this measure in relation to age, sex, state of training, and body composition.

To be reasonably sure that a person has reached his or her maximum capacity for aerobic metabolism during specific exercise (that is, achieved a "true" max $\dot{V}O_2$), a levelling-off or peaking-over in oxygen uptake should be achieved (Fig. 11-7).

The max $\dot{V}O_2$ test shown in Figure 11-7 involved progressive increases in treadmill exercise, and the test was terminated when the subject could not complete the full duration of a particular work block. For the average oxygen consumption values of 18 subjects plotted in Figure 11-7, the highest oxygen uptake was reached before the subjects attained their maximum work level. This peaking-over criterion

generally substantiates the fact that the max $\dot{V}O_2$ has been reached.

In many instances, however, a peaking-over or slight decrease in oxygen consumption at the highest work level is not observed. Often, the highest oxygen consumption is recorded in the last minute of exercise. Consequently, additional criteria based on changes in oxygen consumption with increasing work have been suggested. In one regard, max $\dot{V}O_2$ is considered to have been reached when oxygen consumption fails to increase by some value usually expected from previous observations with the particular test.[42,49] It is also argued that to accept an oxygen uptake value as being maximum, blood lactic acid levels should reach 70 or 80 mg per 100 ml of blood, or higher. Of course, the use of this criterion is limited because it requires blood sampling, and equipment to measure lactic acid levels must be available. Consequently, less precise but more easily measured criteria are usually applied that are reasonable indicators that the oxygen consumption is near-maximum. These include the attainment of the age-predicted maximum heart rate (Fig. 20-5), or a respiratory exchange ratio (R) in excess of 1.00.

Tests of Aerobic Power

Numerous tests have been devised and standardized for the measurement of max $\dot{V}O_2$. Performance on these tests is generally independ-

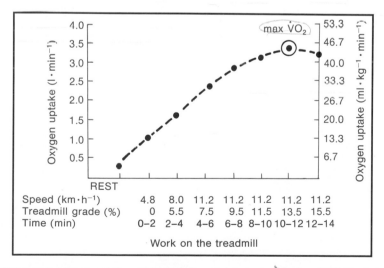

FIG. 11-7. *Peaking-over in oxygen uptake with increasing work output on the treadmill. Each point represents the average oxygen uptake of 18 sedentary male subjects. (From Physical Performance Research Laboratory, The University of Michigan.)*

ent of strength, speed, body size, and skill, with the exception of specialized tests such as swimming, rowing, and ice skating.

The max $\dot{V}O_2$ test may require a continuous 3- to 5-minute "supermaximal" effort, but it usually consists of increments in work (graded exercise) to the point at which the subject will no longer continue to exercise. Some researchers have perhaps imprecisely termed this end point "exhaustion." It should be kept in mind, however, that it is the performer who, for whatever reasons, terminates the test. This decision is often influenced by a variety of psychologic or motivational factors that may not necessarily reflect physiologic strain. We have found that it takes considerable urging and prodding to get subjects to the point where acceptable criteria can be demonstrated for the attainment of max $\dot{V}O_2$. Practical experience has shown that high motivation and a relatively large anaerobic output are generally required in order to demonstrate a plateau in oxygen consumption during the max $\dot{V}O_2$ test. This is especially the case with untrained people who are not normally exposed to strenuous exercise and its associated discomforts.

Maximal oxygen uptake tests are usually performed (1) continuously—with no rest periods between work increments, or (2) discontinuously—with the subject resting 5 or 10 minutes between work periods. The data in Table 11-3 show the results of a systematic comparison of max $\dot{V}O_2$ scores measured by six of the more common continuous and discontinuous treadmill and bicycle procedures.[40]

Although there was only a small 8-ml difference in maximal oxygen uptake between the continuous and discontinuous bicycle tests, the max $\dot{V}O_2$ during bicycle exercise averaged 6.4% to 11.2% below values on the treadmill. The largest difference between any of the three treadmill running tests was only 1.2%. The walking test, on the other hand, elicited max $\dot{V}O_2$ scores about 7% *above* values on the bicycle but 5% *below* the average for the three running tests.

A common complaint of subjects on both the continuous and discontinuous bicycle tests was a feeling of intense local discomfort in the thigh muscles during heavy work. Many subjects stated that this was the major factor limiting their ability to perform further work on the ergometer. In the walking test, the common complaint was severe local discomfort in the lower back and calf muscles, especially walking at the higher treadmill elevations. Local discomfort was not common in the running tests, and subjects complained more of a general fatigue that was usually categorized as feeling "winded." From a standpoint of ease of administration, the continuous treadmill run appears to be the test of preference for testing the aerobic capacity of large numbers of healthy subjects. The total time to administer the test averaged a little over 12 minutes, whereas discontinuous running tests averaged about 65 minutes. Subjects seemed to "tolerate" the continuous test well and preferred the shorter time period for testing.

Factors Affecting Maximal Aerobic Power

The maximal oxygen uptake score is influenced by many factors. Of these, the most important appear to be the mode of exercise and the person's heredity, state of training, age, sex, and body composition.

TABLE 11-3. *Average maximal oxygen uptakes for 15 college students during continuous and discontinuous tests on the bicycle and treadmill*[a]

VARIABLE	BIKE, DISCONTINUOUS	BIKE, CONTINUOUS	TREADMILL, DISCONTINUOUS WALK–RUN	TREADMILL, CONTINUOUS WALK	TREADMILL, DISCONTINUOUS RUN	TREADMILL, CONTINUOUS RUN
max $\dot{V}O_2$, ml · min⁻¹	3691 ± 453	3683 ± 448	4145 ± 401	3944 ± 395	4157 ± 445	4109 ± 424
max $\dot{V}O_2$, ml · kg⁻¹min⁻¹	50.0 ± 6.9	49.9 ± 7.0	56.6 ± 7.3	53.7 ± 7.5	56.6 ± 7.6	55.5 ± 6.8

Values are means ± standard deviation

[a] Adapted from McArdle, W.D. et al.: Comparison of continuous and discontinuous treadmill and bicycle tests for max $\dot{V}O_2$. Med. Sci. Sports. 5:156, 1973. Copyright 1973, the American College of Sports Medicine. Reprinted by Permission.

MODE OF EXERCISE. In various experiments where the max $\dot{V}O_2$ was determined on the same subjects during different forms of exercise, the highest max $\dot{V}O_2$ scores were obtained with treadmill exercise. However, bench-stepping generated max $\dot{V}O_2$ identical to values obtained on the treadmill and significantly higher than those obtained on the bicycle ergometer.[26] For skilled but untrained swimmers, the maximal oxygen uptake during swimming was generally about 20% below treadmill values.[32,41] However, a definite *test specificity* exists in this form of exercise, because trained collegiate swimmers achieved max $\dot{V}O_2$s swimming that were only 11% below their treadmill values,[38] and some elite competitive swimmers can equal or even exceed their treadmill max $\dot{V}O_2$ scores during a swimming test.[32]

In the laboratory, the treadmill is the apparatus of choice for determining max $\dot{V}O_2$ in healthy subjects. Work output is easily determined and regulated. Compared to other forms of exercise, the treadmill makes it easier for subjects to achieve one or more of the criteria for establishing that the max $\dot{V}O_2$ has in fact been attained. In field experiments or when funds are scarce, stepping or bicycle exercise is a suitable alternative. Stepping is a familiar form of exercise and is easily administered; benches are simple to construct, they do not require calibration, and can be easily transported.

HEREDITY. The question is frequently raised concerning the relative contribution of natural endowment to physiologic function and exercise performance.[3] For example, to what extent did heredity determine the extremely high aerobic capacities of the endurance athletes in Figure 11-6? Although the answer is far from complete, some researchers have focused on the question of the extent to which genetic variability accounts for differences between individuals in physiologic and metabolic capacity.

Studies were made of 15 pairs of identical twins (who presumably had the same heredity since they came from the same fertilized egg) and 15 pairs of fraternal twins (who do not differ from ordinary siblings because they result from the separate fertilization of two eggs) raised in the same city and whose parents were of similar socioeconomic backgrounds. It was concluded that heredity alone accounted for up to 93% of the observed differences in aerobic capacity as measured by the max $\dot{V}O_2$! In addition, the ca-

pacity of the short-term energy system of glycolysis and the maximum heart rate were shown to be genetically determined by about 81% and 86%, respectively.[30,31] Subsequent research indicates that the muscle-fiber composition of identical twins is similar whereas wide variations exist among fraternal twins.[48] It is possible that these estimates represent the upper limit of genetic determination, but the data do suggest that the aerobic systems are significantly influenced by factors related to heredity. Nevertheless, at any level of competition, it may be the effect of training that determines superior performance in aerobic activities.

STATE OF TRAINING. The max $\dot{V}O_2$ score must also be evaluated relative to the person's state of training at the time of measurement. Improvements in aerobic capacity with training generally range between 6% and 20%, although increases as large as 50% above pretraining levels have been reported. This subject is discussed further in Chapter 20.

SEX. Max $\dot{V}O_2$ values for men typically exceed scores for women by 15% to 30%; even among trained athletes, this difference ranges between 15% and 20%.[20] However, these differences are considerably larger if the max $\dot{V}O_2$ is expressed as an absolute value $(1 \cdot min^{-1})$ rather than relative to body weight $(ml \cdot kg^{-1} \cdot min^{-1})$.[14]

The apparent sex difference in max $\dot{V}O_2$ has generally been ascribed to differences in body composition and hemoglobin content. Untrained young adult women, for example, generally possess about 26% body fat whereas the corresponding value for men generally averages 15%.[27] Although trained athletes have a lower percentage of fat, women still possess significantly more body fat than their male counterparts. Thus, the male is generally able to generate more aerobic energy simply because he possesses a relatively larger muscle mass and less fat than the female.

For some unknown reason, men have a 10% to 14% greater concentration of hemoglobin than women.[1] This difference in the oxygen-carrying capacity of the blood potentially enables the male to circulate more oxygen during exercise and thus gives him a slight edge in aerobic capacity.

Although lower body fat and higher hemoglobin provide the male with some advantage in terms of aerobic power, we must look for other factors to explain fully the fairly large difference between the sexes. One possible explanation is the difference in the normal physical activity level between the "average" male and the "average" female. It can be convincingly argued that due to social constraints, the opportunities for women to exercise are considerably less than for men. Until recently, it was not socially acceptable for women to be physically active. Even for women desiring to compete in athletics, the opportunities for high-level training and coaching were limited. One can seriously question whether the "world class" female athlete is trained to the same extent as her male counterpart. Despite these possible limitations, however, the aerobic capacity of active females is generally higher than that of sedentary males. Female cross-country skiers, for example, have max $\dot{V}O_2$ scores 25% higher than the untrained male.[20] Even among the so-called normal population, considerable variability among the sexes is observed, and the max $\dot{V}O_2$ scores of many women exceed the values for the less-fit men.

BODY COMPOSITION. It is estimated that 69% of the differences in max $\dot{V}O_2$ scores among individuals can be explained simply by differences in body weight, 4% by differences in height, and 1% by variations in lean body weight.[52] Thus, it is usually not meaningful to compare exercise performance[11b] or the absolute value for oxygen consumption among individuals of different size or body composition. This has led to the common practice of expressing oxygen uptake in terms of body size—either in relation to surface area, body weight, or lean body weight. As can be seen from Table 11-4, for an untrained man and woman who differ considerably in body weight, the percent difference in the max $\dot{V}O_2$, expressed in liters per minute, is +75%. When the max $\dot{V}O_2$ is expressed in relation to body weight. $(ml \cdot kg^{-1} \cdot min^{-1})$, the man is still about 25% higher than the woman. When aerobic capacity is expressed in relation to lean body weight, however, the difference between

the two subjects is reduced still more. This is especially true when men and women of equal training status are compared.

AGE. The maximal oxygen uptake is not spared the effects of aging. Although inferences from cross-sectional studies of people of different ages are somewhat limited, the available data provide insight into the possible effects of aging on physiologic function. As shown in Figure 11-8, the maximal oxygen uptake in liters per minute rapidly increases during the growth stages of the early years and reaches its peak between 18 and 25 years of age. This apparent increase in aerobic capacity with age is essentially eliminated when the max $\dot{V}O_2$ is expressed relative to body weight, as $ml \cdot kg^{-1} \cdot min^{-1}$. *In other words, the maximal aerobic power of preteen girls and boys is no different from that of their adult counterparts.* After age 25, the max $\dot{V}O_2$ declines steadily so that by age 55 it is about 27% below values reported for 20-year-olds. The data in the insert graph indicate that while active adults retain a relatively high max $\dot{V}O_2$ at all ages, a progressive decline in this physiologic capacity occurs with advancing years. The age-related effects on physiologic function are discussed more fully in Chapter 29.

Tests to Predict max $\dot{V}O_2$

The direct measurement of max $\dot{V}O_2$ requires an extensive laboratory and considerable motivation on the part of the subject. Consequently, these tests are not suitable for measuring large groups of untrained subjects in a field situation. In addition, such heavy exercise could pose a potential hazard to adults who are not medically cleared or who are exercised without appropriate safeguards or supervision. In view of these considerations, a number of tests have been devised to *predict* the max $\dot{V}O_2$ from performance measures such as running endurance, or from easily obtained heart rates during or im-

TABLE 11-4. *Various ways of expressing oxygen uptake*

	FEMALE	MALE	% DIFFERENCE
Max $\dot{V}O_2$, $l \cdot min^{-1}$ (absolute)	2.00	3.50	+75
Body weight, kg	50	70	+40
Percent fat	25	15	−40
Lean body weight, kg	37.5	59.5	+59
Max $\dot{V}O_2$, $ml \cdot kg^{-1} \cdot min^{-1}$	40.0	50.0	+25
Max $\dot{V}O_2$, $ml \cdot kg\ LBW^{-1} \cdot min^{-1}$	53.3	58.8	+10.8

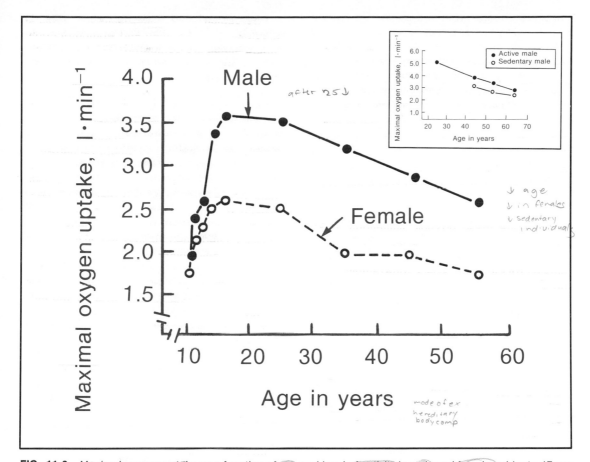

FIG. 11-8. *Maximal oxygen uptake as a function of age and level of activity in male and female subjects. (From Hermanson, L.: Individual differences. In Fitness, Health, and Work Capacity. International Standards for Assessment. Edited by L.A. Larson. New York, Macmillan Publishing Co., 1974. The inset graph was redrawn from tabled data of Åstrand, P.O., and Rodahl, K.R.: Textbook of Work Physiology. New York, McGraw-Hill Book Co., © 1970. Used with permission of McGraw-Hill Book Company.)*

mediately after exercise.[2,5,9,16,21,50,51] The tests are easy to administer, can be used with large groups of men or women, and usually require submaximal exercise.

ENDURANCE RUNS. Runs of various durations or distances are used routinely to evaluate aerobic fitness.[6,9,28,29] Such tests are based on the reasonable notion that the distance one is able to run in a specified time (in excess of 5 or 6 minutes) is determined by the ability to maintain a high steady-rate level of oxygen consumption. This, in turn, is largely based on one's maximum capacity to generate energy aerobically. Using this rationale, a field performance test was devised to evaluate aerobic fitness in military personnel.[6] The object of this test was to run as far as possible in 15 minutes. In 1968, Cooper shortened the run time to 12 minutes.[9]

In his original validation studies, Cooper observed an apparently strong correlation between the max $\dot{V}O_2$ of Air Force personnel and the distance they could run–walk in 12 minutes. A correlation coefficient of $r = 0.90$ was reported between the 12-minute run–walk distance and max $\dot{V}O_2$ in 47 men who varied considerably in age (17 to 54 years), body weight (52 to 123 kg), and max $\dot{V}O_2$ (31 to 59 ml · kg^{-1} · min^{-1}). This same correlation was also observed in 9 ninth-grade boys.[13] Other investigators, however, have been unable to demonstrate such a strong relationship between "Cooper test" scores and aerobic capacity. One study, for example, measured 11- to 14-year-old boys and reported a correlation of $r = 0.65$.[36] For a group of 26 female athletes, the correlation between the run–walk scores and max $\dot{V}O_2$ was $r = 0.70$,[36] whereas for 36 untrained college women a similar correlation of r = 0.67 was observed.[29]

We would like to point out that a simple correlation of run–walk scores with max $\dot{V}O_2$ does not take into account age and body-weight factors. These latter variables are in themselves related to the run–walk and max $\dot{V}O_2$ scores. To avoid spurious correlations, the proper statistical evaluation must be performed. In fact, when the original data of Cooper[9] were restricted to the same age range as those in the preceding study of 36 women,[29] the computed correlation was reduced significantly from r = 0.90 to r = 0.59!

The prediction of maximum aerobic capacity should be approached with caution when using running performance. The need to establish effective pacing for inexperienced subjects is critical. Some individuals may achieve an optimal pace so they do not run too fast in the early part of a run and are therefore forced to slow down or even stop due to lactic-acid buildup as the test progresses. Other individuals may begin too slowly and continue that way so that their final performance score reflects inappropriate pacing or motivation rather than physiologic and metabolic capacity. In addition, max $\dot{V}O_2$ is not the only variable that determines endurance running performance. Factors such as body weight and body fatness,[11a] running efficiency, and the percentage of one's aerobic capacity that can be sustained without lactic-acid buildup all contribute significantly to successful running.[10,29]

PREDICTIONS BASED ON HEART RATE. The most common tests for predicting max $\dot{V}O_2$ use the exercise or postexercise heart rate with a standardized regimen of submaximal exercise performed either on a bicycle, treadmill, or step test. These tests make use of the essentially linear relationship between heart rate and oxygen consumption for various intensities of light to moderately heavy exercise. The slope of this line (rate of heart rate increase) reflects the individual's aerobic fitness. The max $\dot{V}O_2$ can then be estimated by drawing a straight line through several submaximum points relating heart rate and oxygen consumption (or work intensity) and then extending this line to some assumed maximum heart rate for the particular age group.

Figure 11-9 illustrates the application of this "extrapolation" procedure for trained and untrained subjects. The heart rate–oxygen consumption line was drawn from four submaximal measures during bicycle exercise. Although each person's heart rate–oxygen consumption line tends to be linear, the slopes of the individual lines can differ considerably. Consequently, a person with relatively high aerobic fitness can do more work and achieve higher oxygen consumption before reaching a heart rate of 140 or 160 beats per minute than a less "fit" person. Also, since the heart rate increases linearly with the intensity of work, the person with the smallest increase in heart rate tends to have the largest work capacity and max $\dot{V}O_2$. For the two subjects illustrated in Figure 11-9, max $\dot{V}O_2$ was predicted by extrapolating the line to a heart rate of 195 beats per minute—the assumed maximum heart rate for subjects of college age.

The accuracy of predicting max $\dot{V}O_2$ from submaximal exercise heart rate is limited by the following assumptions underlying these procedures:

1. *Linearity of the heart rate–oxygen consumption (work intensity) relationship.* This assumption is met to a large degree, especially for various intensities of light to moderate exercise. In some subjects, however, the heart rate–oxygen consumption line curves or

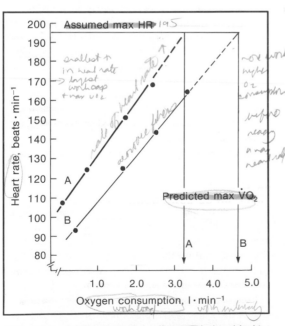

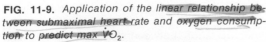

FIG. 11-9. *Application of the linear relationship between submaximal heart rate and oxygen consumption to predict max $\dot{V}O_2$.*

asymptotes at the heavier work loads in a direction that indicates a larger than expected increase in oxygen consumption per unit increase in heart rate. The oxygen consumption actually increases more than would be predicted through linear extrapolation of the heart rate–oxygen consumption line. Thus, the predicted max $\dot{V}O_2$ in these subjects would be considerably underestimated.

2. *Similar maximum heart rates for all subjects.* There is a standard deviation of approximately ±10 beats per minute about the average maximum heart rate of individuals of the same age. Therefore, the max $\dot{V}O_2$ of a person with an actual maximum heart rate of 185 beats per minute would be overestimated if the heart rate–oxygen consumption line were extrapolated to 195 or 200 beats per minute. The opposite would be true for a subject with an actual maximum heart rate of 210 beats per minute. Maximum heart rate also decreases with age. Unless this age effect is considered, older subjects will be consistently overestimated by assuming a maximum heart rate of 195 beats per minute, which is the appropriate heart rate maximum for 25-year-olds. More is said in Chapter 29 concerning the effect of age on maximum heart rate.

3. *Assumed constant mechanical efficiency.* In cases where submaximal oxygen consumption is not measured, but is instead estimated from work-load, the predicted max $\dot{V}O_2$ may be in error by the magnitude of variability in mechanical efficiency. A subject with poor mechanical efficiency (oxygen consumption at submaximal work higher than assumed) will be underestimated in terms of max $\dot{V}O_2$, because heart rate will be elevated due to the added oxygen cost of the inefficient work. The variation among individuals in oxygen consumption during walking, stepping, or cycling does not usually exceed ±6%.

4. *Day-to-day variation in heart rate.* Even under highly standardized conditions, the variation in submaximal heart rate is about ±5 beats per minute with day-to-day testing at the same exercise load.

Within the framework of these limitations, *the max $\dot{V}O_2$ predicted from submaximal heart rate is generally within 10% to 20% of the person's actual value.* Clearly, this is not acceptable accuracy for research purposes. However, these tests are well-suited for purposes of screening and classification in terms of aerobic fitness.

THE STEP TEST. The heart rate in recovery from a standardized bout of stepping is a practical and effective way to classify people in terms of aerobic fitness.[16,39] With the use of "prediction equations" applied to step-test results, the max $\dot{V}O_2$ can also be estimated with a reasonable degree of accuracy. Figure 11-10 illustrates the heart rate responses of three subjects of different fitness levels who perform 3 minutes of stepping to the cadence of a metronome.

In the first minute of exercise, there is a rapid increase in heart rate. Then heart rate levels off and remains fairly stable throughout the stepping period. The stress of 3 minutes of stepping brings about final exercise heart rates of 170, 142, and 120 beats per minute for a sedentary college student (subject C), physical education major (subject B), and varsity basketball player (subject A), respectively. On a relative scale, it certainly can be concluded that the cardiovascular efficiency (as reflected by heart rate) is least for the sedentary student, greater for the physical education major, and greatest for the athlete.

The recovery heart rate patterns shown in Figure 11-10 also provide valuable information concerning the cardiovascular response to exercise. In the first minute after stepping, heart rate decreases rapidly. Thereafter, the decline is more gradual, and within 2 minutes the heart rates have nearly returned to resting levels. By measuring heart rate in the early stages of recovery, it is still possible to discern noticeable differences in heart rate response to the previous exercise.

We have used a simple 3-minute step test to evaluate the heart-rate response of thousands of college men and women.[39] The test was developed using the gymnasium bleachers ($16\frac{1}{4}$ inches high) so that large numbers of students could be tested at the same time. Each stepping cycle was performed to a four-step cadence, "up-up-down-down." The women performed 22 complete step-ups per minute, which were regulated by a metronome at 88 beats per minute. Because the average man tended to be more fit for stepping exercise, the cadence was set at 24 steps per minute or 96 beats per minute on the metronome. After a brief demonstration and practice period, the step test was begun. At completion of stepping, the students remained standing, and pulse rate was measured for a 15-second period from 5 to 20 seconds into recovery. Recovery heart rate was

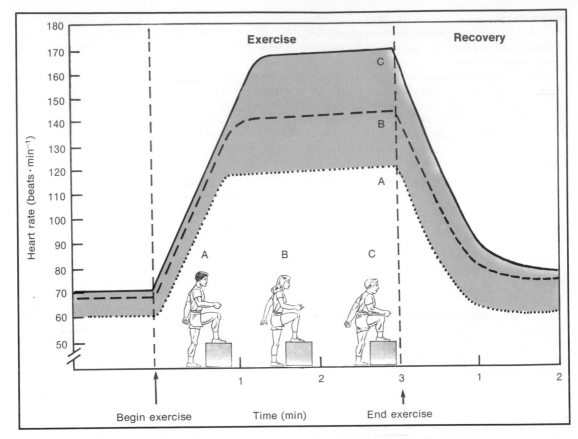

FIG. 11-10. *Heart rate response of three people during a stepping exercise and in recovery.*

converted to beats per minute (15 sec. HR × 4) and compared to the established percentile rankings presented in Table 11-5.

Based on our previous discussion of the essentially linear relationship between heart rate and oxygen consumption, one would expect a person with a low exercise heart rate and recovery step test score to be further away from maximal oxygen uptake than someone with a relatively high heart rate response. In other words, the lower the heart rate response to a standard work task, the higher is the max $\dot{V}O_2$. To evaluate the validity of the step test as a reflection of a person's aerobic capacity, we measured the max $\dot{V}O_2$ of a group of men and women who had also been evaluated by the step test. For the women in this group, the relationship between each subject's max $\dot{V}O_2$ and step-test score is shown in Figure 11-11. The results clearly indicated that knowledge of a person's max $\dot{V}O_2$ could be obtained from the score on the step test. Subjects with high recovery heart rates tended to have lower maximal oxygen uptakes, whereas a faster recovery

(lower heart rate) tended to be associated with a relatively high max $\dot{V}O_2$. To enable us to predict the max $\dot{V}O_2$ (ml · kg^{-1} · min^{-1}) from step-test results for similar groups of men and women, the following mathematical equations were written:

Men: max $\dot{V}O_2$ = 111.33 −
  (0.42 × step-test pulse rate, beats · min^{-1})
Women: max $\dot{V}O_2$ = 65.81 −
  (0.1847 × step-test pulse rate, beats · min^{-1})

To simplify these conversions, the last column of Table 11-5 also presents the predicted maximal oxygen uptake values for men and women determined from recovery heart rate scores. In terms of accuracy of prediction, one can be 95% confident that the predicted max $\dot{V}O_2$ will be within about ±16% of the true max $\dot{V}O_2$ of the person tested.

When a high degree of accuracy is required, the maximal oxygen uptake should be directly measured in the laboratory with an appropriate, graded exercise test. However, when this is impractical or when accuracy can be sacrificed

TABLE 11-5. *Percentile rankings for recovery heart rate (HR) and predicted maximal oxygen consumption for male and female college students*

PERCENTILE RANKING	RECOVERY HR, FEMALE	PREDICTED MAX $\dot{V}O_2$ $(ml \cdot kg^{-1} \cdot min^{-1})$	RECOVERY HR, MALE	PREDICTED MAX $\dot{V}O_2$ $(ml \cdot kg^{-1} \cdot min^{-1})$
100	128	42.2	120	60.9
95	140	40.0	124	59.3
90	148	38.5	128	57.6
85	152	37.7	136	54.2
80	156	37.0	140	52.5
75	158	36.6	144	50.9
70	160	36.3	148	49.2
65	162	35.9	149	48.8
60	163	35.7	152	47.5
55	164	35.5	154	46.7
50	166	35.1	156	45.8
45	168	34.8	160	44.1
40	170	34.4	162	43.3
35	171	34.2	164	42.5
30	172	34.0	166	41.6
25	176	33.3	168	40.8
20	180	32.6	172	39.1
15	182	32.2	176	37.4
10	184	31.8	178	36.6
5	196	29.6	184	34.1

From McArdle, W.D., et al.: Percentile norms for a valid step test in college women. Res Q Am Assoc Health Phys Educ, *44(4)*:498, 1973.

somewhat, the step test is extremely valuable for classification purposes. *This method gives as good an estimate of max $\dot{V}O_2$ as that obtained with other submaximal tests requiring treadmill or bicycle ergometer exercise, including the well-known Åstrand-Rhyming test.*[2]

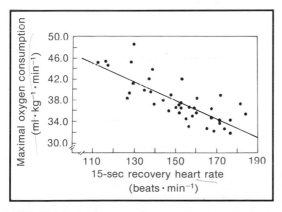

FIG. 11-11. *Scattergram and line of "best fit" relating step-test heart rate score and maximal oxygen consumption in college women. (From McArdle, W.D. et al.: Reliability and interrelationships between maximal oxygen uptake, physical work capacity, and step test scores in college women. Med. Sci. Sports, 4:182, 1972.)*

SUMMARY

1. The concepts of *individual differences* and *specificity* are important for understanding capacities for anaerobic and aerobic power. Individual differences refer to real differences among individuals in contrast to the instability of a measure for any one individual. Specificity refers to metabolic and physiologic function that is not a general factor but one that is dependent on a host of factors.

2. The contribution of anaerobic and aerobic energy transfer depends largely on the intensity and duration of exercise. During strength and power-sprint activities, the primary energy transfer involves the immediate and short-term systems. The long-term aerobic energy system becomes progressively more important in activities lasting longer than 2 minutes.

3. It is possible to estimate the capacity of each energy system using appropriate physiologic measurements and performance tests. These can be used to evaluate a capacity at a particular time or to show changes consequent to specific training programs.

4. Training status, motivation, and acid-base regulation are several of the factors that

may explain differences among individuals in the capacities of the immediate and short-term energy systems.

5. The maximal oxygen uptake provides important information on the power of the long-term energy system. The max $\dot{V}O_2$ has become a basic measure in exercise physiology. Consideration for type and amount of exercise performed and related physiologic functioning is required to assure that a "true" score has been attained. Under laboratory conditions, the max $\dot{V}O_2$ test gives very reproducible scores.

6. The maximal aerobic power is influenced by factors such as heredity, state of training, age, sex, and body composition. Each factor contributes uniquely to an individual's max $\dot{V}O_2$.

7. Field methods for predicting max $\dot{V}O_2$ should be viewed with caution. However, these tests can provide valuable information in the absence of more valid laboratory methods. Certain prediction tests are better than others.

References

1. Åstrand, P. O.: Human physical fitness with special reference to age and sex. Physiol. Rev., 36:307, 1956.
2. Åstrand, P. O., and Rhyming, I.: A nomogram for calculation of aerobic capacity (Physical Fitness) from pulse rate during submaximal work. J. Appl. Physiol., 7:218, 1954.
3. Åstrand, P. O., and Rodhal, K.: Textbook of Work Physiology. New York, McGraw-Hill, 1977.
4. Åstrand, P. O., and Saltin, B.: Maximal oxygen uptake and heart rate in various types of muscular activity. J. Appl. Physiol., 16:977, 1961.
5. Balke, B., and Ware, R. W.: An experimental study of fitness of Air Force personnel. U.S. Armed Forces Med. J., 10:675, 1959.
6. Balke, B.: A simple field test for the assessment of physical fitness. CARI Report. 63-18. Oklahoma City, Civil Aeromedical Research Institute, Federal Aviation Agency, 1963.
7. Bar-Or, O., and Zwiren, L. D.: Maximal oxygen consumption test during arm ergometry—reliability and validity. J. Appl. Physiol., 38:424, 1975.
8. Carey, P. et al.: Comparison of oxygen uptake during maximal work on the rowing ergometer. Med. Sci. Sports, 6:101, 1974.
9. Cooper, K.: Correlation between field and treadmill testing as a means for assessing maximal oxygen intake. J.A.M.A. 203:201, 1968.
10. Costill, D. L.: Physiology of marathon running. J.A.M.A. 221:1024, 1972.
11. Cunningham, D., and Faulkner, J. A.: The effect of training on aerobic and anaerobic metabolism during a short exhaustive run. Med. Sci. Sports, 1:65, 1969.
11a. Cureton, K. J. et al.: Effect of experimental alterations in excess weight on aerobic capacity and distance running performance. Med. Sci. Sports, 10:194, 1978.
11b. Cureton, K. J. et al.: Body fatness and performance differences between men and women. Res. Quart., 50:333, 1979.
12. Di Prampero, P. E. et al.: Maximal muscular power, aerobic and anaerobic, in 116 athletes performing in the XIXth Olympic games in Mexico. Ergonomics 13:665, 1970.
13. Doolittle, T. L., and Bigbee, R.: The twelve-minute run-walk: A test of cardiorespiratory fitness of adolescent boys. Res. Quart., 39:41, 1968.

14. Drinkwater, B.: Physiological responses of women to exercise. *In* Exercise and Sport Science Reviews, Vol. I. Edited by J. Wilmore. New York, Academic Press, 1973.

15. Ferguson, R. J. et al.: A maximal oxygen uptake test during ice skating. Med. Sci. Sports, *1:*207, 1969.

16. Fox, E. L.: A simple accurate technique for predicting maximal aerobic power. J. Appl. Physiol., *35:*914, 1973.

17. Full, F., and Herxheimer, H.: Ueber die Alkalireserve. *Klin. Wochenschr. 5:*228, 1926.

18. Gollnick, P. D. et al.: Glycogen depletion pattern in human skeletal muscle fiber after heavy exercise. J. Appl. Physiol., *34:*615, 1973.

19. Hermansen, L.: Individual differences. *In* Fitness, Health and Work Capacity: International Standard for Assessment. Edited by L. A. Larson. New York, Macmillan, 1974.

20. Hermansen, L. H., and Anderson, L.: Aerobic work capacity in young Norwegian men and women. J. Appl. Physiol., *20:* 425, 1965.

21. Hermiston, R., and Faulkner, J. A.: Prediction of maximal oxygen uptake by stepwide regression technique. J. Appl. Physiol., *30:*833, 1971.

22. Holmér, I. et al.: Maximal oxygen uptake during swimming and running by elite swimmers. J. Appl. Physiol., *36:*711, 1974.

23. Kalamen, J. L.: Measurement of maximum muscular power in man. Unpublished Ph.D. dissertation. The Ohio State University, 1968.

24. Karlsson, J., and Saltin, B.: Lactate, ATP, and CP in working muscles during exhaustive exercise in man. J. Appl. Physiol., *29:*598, 1970.

25. Karlsson, J. et al.: Muscle metabolites during submaximal and maximal exercise in man. Scand. J. Clin. Lab. Invest., *26:*385, 1971.

26. Kasch, F. W. et al.: A comparison of maximal oxygen uptake by treadmill and step test procedures. J. Appl. Physiol., *21:* 1387, 1966.

27. Katch, F. I., and McArdle, W. D.: Nutrition, Weight Control and Exercise. Boston, Houghton Mifflin, 1977.

28. Katch, F. I. et al.: Relationship between individual differences in steady pace endurance running performance and maximal oxygen intake. Res. Quart., *44:*206, 1973.

29. Katch, F. I. et al.: Maximal oxygen intake, endurance running performance, and body composition in college women. Res. Quart., *44:* 301, 1973.

30. Klissouras, V.: Heritability of adaptive variation. J. Appl. Physiol., *31:*338, 1971.

31. Klissouras, V. et al.: Adaptation to maximal effort: genetics and age. J. Appl. Physiol., *35:*288, 1973.

32. Magel, J. R., and Faulkner, J. A.: Maximum oxygen uptake of college swimmers. J. Appl. Physiol., *22:*929, 1967.

33. Magel, J. R. et al.: Specificity of swim training on maximum oxygen uptake. J. Appl. Physiol., *38:*151, 1975.

34. Magel, J. R. et al.: Metabolic and cardiovascular adjustment to arm training. J. Appl. Physiol.: Respirat. Environ. Exercise Physiol., *45:*75, 1978.

35. Maksud, M. G., and Coutts, K. D.: Application of the Cooper twelve-minute run-walk to young males. Res. Quart., *42:*54, 1971.

36. Maksud, M. G. et al.: Energy expenditure and $\dot{V}O_2$ max of female athletes during treadmill exercise. Res. Quart., *47:*692, 1976.

37. Margaria, R. et al.: Measurement of muscular power (anaerobic) in man. J. Appl. Physiol., *21:*1662, 1966.

38. McArdle, W. D. et al.: Metabolic and cardiorespiratory response during free swimming and treadmill walking. J. Appl. Physiol., *30:*733, 1971.

39. McArdle, W. D. et al.: Reliability and interrelationships between maximal oxygen intake, physical work capacity, and step-test scores in college women. Med. Sci. Sports, *4:*182, 1972.

40. McArdle, W. D. et al.: Comparison of continuous and discontinuous treadmill and bicycle tests for max $\dot{V}O_2$. Med. Sci. Sports, *5:*156, 1973.
41. McArdle, W. D. et al: Specificity of run training on $\dot{V}O_2$ max and heart rate changes during running and swimming. Med. Sci. Sports, *10:*16, 1978.
42. Mitchell, J. et al.: The physiological meaning of the maximal oxygen intake test. J. Clin. Invest., *37:*538, 1958.
43. Pechar, G. S. et al.: Specificity of cardiorespiratory adaptation to bicycle and treadmill training. J. Appl. Physiol., *36:*753, 1974.
44. Piehl, K.: Glycogen storage and depletion in human skeletal muscle fibers. Acta Physiol. Scand., Suppl. *402:*1, 1974.
45. Robinson, S., and Harmon, P. M.: The lactic acid mechanism and certain properties of the blood in relation to training. Am. J. Physiol., *132:*757, 1941.
46. Saltin, B.: Metabolic fundamentals in exercise. Med. Sci. Sports, *5:*137, 1973.
47. Sargent, D. A.: Physical test of man. Am. Phys. Ed. Rev., *26:*188, 1921.
48. Sjördin, B.: Lactate dehydrogenase in human skeletal muscle. Acta Physiol. Scand., Suppl. *436,* 1976.
49. Taylor, H. L. et al.: Maximal oxygen intake as an objective measure of cardiorespiratory performance. J. Appl. Physiol., *8:*73, 1955.
50. Wyndham, C. H.: Submaximal tests for estimating maximum oxygen uptake. Can. Med. Assoc. J., *96:*736, 1967.
51. Wyndham, C. H. et al.: Studies of the maximum capacity of men for physical effort. Part I. A comparison of methods of assessing the maximum oxygen intake. Int. Z. Angew. Physiol., *22:* 285, 1966.
52. Wyndham, C. H., and Hegns, A. J. A.: Determinants of oxygen consumption and maximum oxygen intake of caucasians and Bantu males. Int. Z. Angew. Physiol. *27:*51, 1969.

SECTION III.
Systems of Energy Delivery and Utilization

Most sport, recreational, and occupational activities require a moderately intense yet sustained energy release. This energy for the phosphorylation of ADP to ATP is provided by the *aerobic* breakdown of carbohydrates, fats, and proteins. Unless a steady rate can be achieved between oxidative phosphorylation and the energy requirements of the activity, an anaerobic-aerobic energy imbalance develops, lactic acid accumulates, tissue acidity increases, and fatigue quickly ensues. The ability to sustain a high level of physical activity without undue fatigue depends on two factors: (1) the capacity and integration of the various physiologic systems for oxygen delivery, and (2) the capacity of the specific muscle cells to generate ATP aerobically.

Understanding the role of the ventilatory, circulatory, and muscular systems during exercise enables us to appreciate individual differences in exercise capacity in essentially aerobic activities. Knowing the energy requirements of exercise and the corresponding physiologic adjustments also provides a sound basis for formulating a fitness program as well as for evaluating one's status before and during such a program.

Pulmonary Structure
and Function

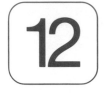

Chapters 12, 13, and 14 deal with the process of pulmonary ventilation and gas transport and elaborate the mechanisms whereby oxygen is supplied and extracted from the external environment and exchanged for almost equal quantities of carbon dioxide. This capability for pulmonary ventilation contributes significantly to the regulation of the internal environment at rest and during physical activity.

SURFACE AREA AND GAS EXCHANGE

If the oxygen supply of humans were dependent only on diffusion through the skin, it would be impossible to sustain the basal energy requirement, let alone the 3- to 4-liter gas exchange each minute necessary to run at a 5-minute per mile pace in a 26-mile marathon. Within the relatively compact human body, the needs for gas exchange are met by the remarkably effective *ventilatory system*. This system, depicted in Figure 12-1, regulates the gaseous state of the body's "external" environment in order to provide aeration of body fluids during rest and exercise.

ANATOMY OF VENTILATION

The process by which ambient air is brought into and exchanged with the air in the lungs is termed *pulmonary ventilation*. Air entering through the nose and mouth flows into the conductive portion of the ventilatory system where it is adjusted to body temperature, filtered, and almost completely humidified by the time it reaches the *trachea*. This air-conditioning

process continues as the inspired air passes into two *bronchi*, the large tubes that serve as primary conduits in each of the two lungs. The bronchi further subdivide into numerous *bronchioles* that conduct the inspired air via a tortuous and narrow route until it eventually mixes with the existing air in the *alveoli*, the terminal branches of the respiratory tract.

The Lungs

The lungs provide the surface between the blood and the external environment. Although the lung volume varies between 4 and 6 liters (about the amount of air contained in a basket-

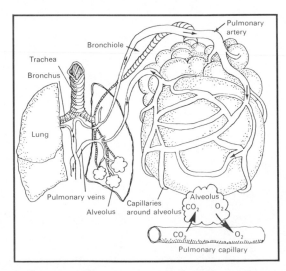

FIG. 12-1. *Air passages for pulmonary ventilation. (From* Nutrition, Weight Control, and Exercise *by Frank I. Katch and William D. McArdle. Copyright © 1977 by Houghton Mifflin Company. Reprinted by permission of the publisher.)*

154

ball), its moist surface area is considerable. The lungs of an average-sized man weigh about $2\frac{1}{2}$ lb, yet if spread out as in Figure 12-2, this tissue would cover a surface of 60 to 80 m². This is about 35 times greater than the surface of the man and would be sufficient to cover almost half a tennis court or an entire badminton court!

This highly vascularized, moist surface fits within the relatively small confines of the chest cavity by means of numerous infoldings so that lung membranes actually fold over onto themselves. The interface for the aeration of blood is considerable, because during any second of maximal exercise there is probably no more than one pint of blood in the fine network of blood vessels surrounding the lung tissue.

The Alveoli

There are more than 600 million alveoli. These elastic, thin-walled, membranous sacs provide the vital surface for gas exchange between the lungs and the blood. Alveolar tissue has the largest blood supply of any organ in the body.

Millions of short, thin-walled capillaries and alveoli lie side by side with air moving on one side and blood on the other. Diffusion occurs through the extremely thin barrier of these alveolar and capillary cells. Also, small pores within each alveolus enable the interchange of gas between adjacent alveoli. This provides for the indirect ventilation of some alveoli that may have been damaged or blocked as a result of disease.

During each minute at rest approximately 250 ml of oxygen leave the alveoli and enter the blood and about 200 ml of carbon dioxide diffuse in the reverse direction into the alveoli. During heavy exercise in trained endurance athletes, almost 25 times this quantity of oxygen is transferred across the alveolar membrane. The primary function of ventilation during rest and exercise is to maintain a fairly constant and favorable concentration of oxygen and carbon dioxide in the alveolar chambers. This assures effective gaseous exchange before the blood leaves the lungs to be transported throughout the body.

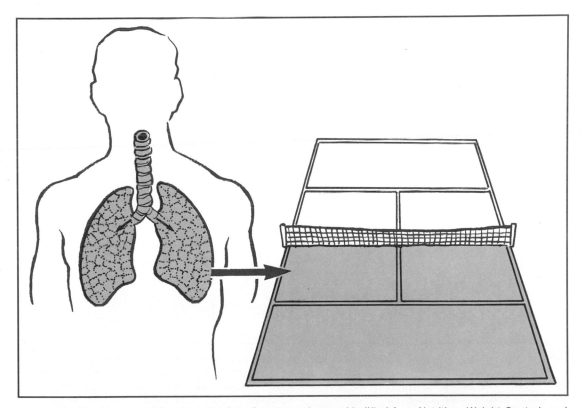

FIG. 12-2. *The lungs provide a large surface for gas exchange. Modified from* Nutrition, Weight Control, and Exercise *by Frank I. Katch and William D. McArdle. Copyright © 1977 by Houghton Mifflin Company. Reprinted by permission of the publisher.*

MECHANICS OF VENTILATION

Figure 12-3 illustrates the physical principle underlying the act of breathing. Two lung-shaped balloons are suspended in a jar whose glass bottom has been replaced by a thin rubber membrane. When the membrane is pulled down the jar's volume increases, the air pressure within the jar becomes less than the air outside the jar, and air rushes in causing the balloons to inflate. Conversely, if the elastic membrane is allowed to recoil, the pressure in the jar temporarily increases and air rushes out. A considerable volume of air can be exchanged within the balloons in a given time period if the depth and rate of the descent and ascent of the rubber membrane are increased. This is essentially how ambient air and alveolar air are exchanged in the lungs.

The lungs are not merely suspended in the chest cavity as in the example with the balloons. Rather, surface tension created by the natural moisture within the chest causes the lungs to adhere to the interior of the chest wall and literally follow its every movement. Thus, any change in the volume of the thoracic cavity causes a corresponding change in lung volume. The lungs depend on accessory means for altering their volume because they contain no muscles. The volume of the lungs is altered during *inspiration* and *expiration* by the action of voluntary muscles.

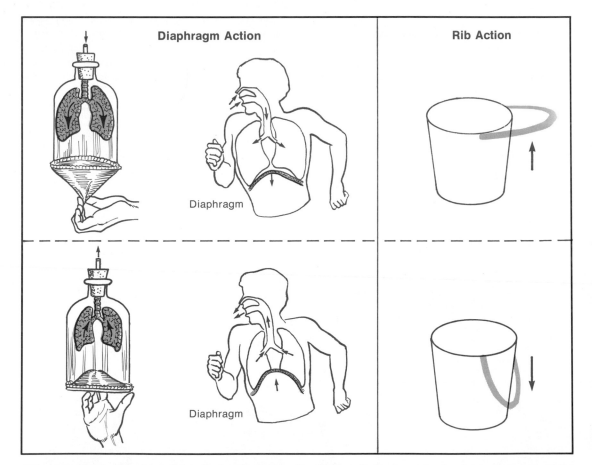

Diaphragm Action

Diaphragm

Diaphragm

Rib Action

FIG. 12-3. *Mechanics of breathing. During inspiration, the chest cavity increases in size due to the raising of the ribs and the lowering of the muscular diaphragm. During exhalation, the ribs swing down and the diaphragm returns to the relaxed position. This reduces the volume of the thoracic cavity and air rushes out. The movement of the rubber bottom of the jar simulates the action of the diaphragm and causes air to enter and leave the two balloons; the movement of the bucket handle simulates the action of the ribs. (Modified from* Nutrition, Weight Control, and Exercise *by Frank I. Katch and William D. McArdle. Copyright © 1977 by Houghton Mifflin Company. Reprinted by permission of the publisher.)*

Inspiration

A large dome-shaped sheet of muscle called the *diaphragm* serves the same purpose as the rubber membrane of the jar. This muscle makes an airtight separation between the abdominal and thoracic cavities. During inspiration, the diaphragm muscle contracts, flattens out, and moves downward toward the abdominal cavity by as much as 10 cm. This movement causes the chest cavity to enlarge and become elongated. Consequently, the air in the lungs expands and its pressure, referred to as *intrapulmonary pressure,* becomes reduced slightly below atmospheric pressure. The lungs inflate as air is literally sucked in through the nose and mouth, with the degree of filling depending on the magnitude of the inspiratory movements. Inspiration is completed when thoracic cavity expansion ceases and the intrapulmonary pressure increases to equal atmospheric pressure.

During exercise, the ribs and sternum also assist in the action of inspiration. The contraction of the *scaleni* and *intercostal* muscles between the ribs causes the ribs to rotate and lift up and away from the body. This action is similar to the movement of the handle lifted up-and-away from the side of the bucket at the right in Figure 12-3. The descent of the diaphragm, the upward swing of the ribs, and the outward thrust of the sternum all cause the volume of the chest cavity to increase with a subsequent inhalation of ambient air. It is not uncommon to see an athlete bend forward from the waist to facilitate breathing following an exhausting exercise. More than likely, this serves two purposes: (1) It facilitates the flow of blood to the heart, and (2) it minimizes the antagonistic effects of gravity on the usual upward direction of inspiratory movements.

Expiration

Expiration, the process of air movement from the lungs, is predominantly a passive process during rest and light exercise. It results from the recoil of the stretched lung tissue and the relaxation of the inspiratory muscles. This causes the sternum and ribs to swing down and the diaphragm to move back toward the thoracic cavity. These movements decrease the size of the chest cavity and compress alveolar gas so that air moves out through the respiratory tract into the atmosphere. Expiration is completed when the compressive forces of the expiratory musculature are no longer acting, and intrapulmonary pressure decreases to atmospheric pressure. During ventilation in heavy exercise, the internal intercostals and abdominal muscles act powerfully on the ribs and abdominal cavity, respectively to cause a reduction in thoracic dimensions. Thus, exhalation occurs more rapidly and to a more pronounced depth.

No major differences are observed in ventilatory mechanics between men and women or between people of different ages. At rest in the supine position, most people are abdominal, or diaphragmatic, breathers, whereas in the upright position, the action of the ribs and sternum becomes more apparent.[20] The rapid alterations in thoracic volume required during heavy exercise are accomplished mainly through the movement of the rib cage. This suggests that the muscles of the ribs are capable of more rapid action than the diaphragm and the abdominal muscles.

VALSALVA MANEUVER. The expiratory muscles play an important role in the ventilatory maneuvers of coughing and sneezing, as well as in the stabilization of the abdominal and chest cavities during the lifting of a heavy weight. During quiet breathing, the intrapulmonary pressure may fall only about 2 or 3 mm Hg during the inspiratory cycle and increase a similar amount above atmospheric pressure during exhalation. However, if the *glottis* is closed following a full inspiration and the expiratory muscles are maximally activated, the compressive forces of exhalation can increase the *intrathoracic* pressure by more than 100 mm Hg above atmospheric pressure. (The glottis is the narrowest part of the larynx through which air passes into and out of the trachea.) This forced exhalation against a closed glottis, termed the *Valsalva maneuver,* commonly occurs in weight lifting and in other activities that require a rapid and maximum application of force for a short duration. The fixation of the abdominal and chest cavities with this maneuver probably enhances the action of muscles that are attached to the chest.

PHYSIOLOGIC CONSEQUENCES OF THE VALSALVA. As illustrated in Figure 12-4, the increase in intrathoracic pressure during a Valsalva maneuver is transmitted through the thin walls of the veins that pass through the thoracic region. Because venous blood is under relatively low pressure, these veins are compressed, and blood flow into the heart is significantly reduced. This reduction in venous return can diminish the blood supply to the brain and frequently produces dizziness, "spots before the eyes," and even fainting with straining-type exercises. Once the glottis is opened and intrathoracic pressure is released, normal blood flow is reestablished.

With the onset of the Valsalva maneuver at the start of the lift (Figure 12-4C), there is an abrupt rise in blood pressure as the elevated intrathoracic pressure forces blood from the heart into the arterial system; blood pressure then falls sharply due to the reduced venous return from the thoracic veins. This temporary increase in blood pressure within the heart and arteries of the chest is probably compensated for by a proportionate pressure increase on their outside walls caused by the elevated intrathoracic pressure. Perhaps of more significance than the pressure changes within the vessels of the chest cavity is the fact that the Valsalva maneuver usually accompanies straining-type muscular exertion similar to that performed in isometric exercise and heavy weight training. Such exercise greatly increases resistance to blood flow in the active muscles during the sustained contraction. This causes a signifi-

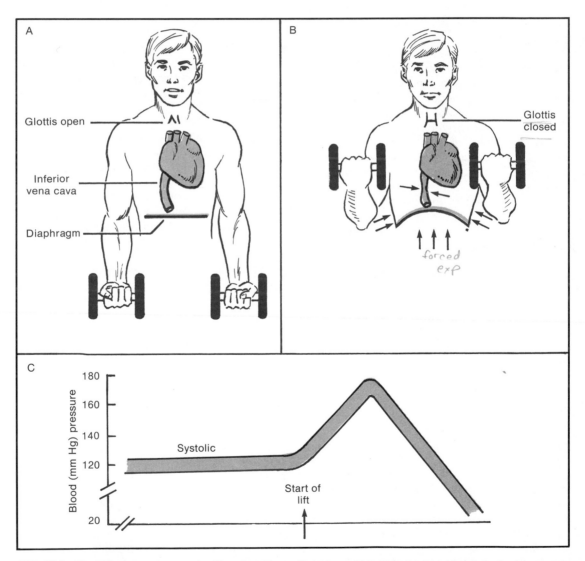

FIG. 12-4. *The Valsalva maneuver significantly reduces the return of blood to the heart because the increase in intrathoracic pressure collapses the vein that passes through the chest cavity. A, normal breathing, B, straining exercise with accompanying Valsalva, C, blood pressure response prior to and during straining-type exercise.*

cant *rise* both in arterial blood pressure and in the work load of the heart, even if the Valsalva maneuver is not performed. *This is one reason why individuals with heart and vascular disease should refrain from all-out straining exercises such as isometrics and should seek more rhythmic muscular activity that results in a steady flow of blood and only moderate increases in arterial blood pressure and strain on the heart.*

LUNG VOLUMES
AND CAPACITIES

The various lung volume measures that reflect one's ability to increase the depth of breathing are illustrated in Figure 12-5. The subject is breathing from a calibrated recording spirometer, similar to that described in Chapter 8 (Fig. 8-2), for measuring oxygen consumption by the closed-circuit method.

Static Lung
Volumes

The bell of the spirometer falls and subsequently rises as air is inhaled and exhaled from it. This provides a record of the ventilatory volume and breathing rate. The volume of air moved during either the inspiratory or expira-

tory phase of each breath is termed *tidal volume* (TV). It is indicated by the rise and fall of the spirometer in the first portion of the record. Under resting conditions, tidal volumes usually range between 0.4 and 1.0 liters of air per breath.

After several tracings of tidal volume are recorded, the subject is asked to inspire as deeply as possible following a normal inspiration. This additional volume of about 2.5 to 3.5 liters above the inspired tidal air represents one's reserve ability for inhalation and is termed the *inspiratory reserve volume* (IRV). After the measurement of IRV, the normal breathing pattern is once again established. Following a normal exhalation, the subject continues to exhale and forces as much air as possible from the lungs. This is the *expiratory reserve volume* (ERV), which ranges between 1.0 and 1.5 liters for an average-sized man. *During exercise, encroachment on both inspiratory and expiratory reserve volumes, particularly the inspiratory volume, provides for a considerable increase in tidal volume.*

The total volume of air that can be voluntarily moved in one breath, from full inspiration to maximum expiration, or vice versa, is termed the *vital capacity* (VC). This consists of the tidal volume plus the inspiratory and expiratory reserve volumes. Although values for vital capac-

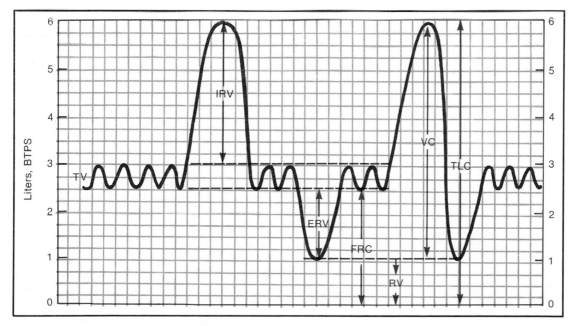

FIG. 12-5. *Static measures of lung volume.*

$FRC = ERV + RV$

ity vary considerably with body size as well as with the position of the body during the measurement, average values are usually 4 to 5 liters in healthy young men and 3 to 4 liters in young women. Vital capacities of 6 to 7 liters are not uncommon for tall individuals and values of 7.6 and 8.1 liters have been reported for a professional football player and an Olympic gold medalist in cross-country skiing, respectively.[3,24]. The large lung volumes of such athletes probably reflect genetic influences, because it is questionable whether static lung volumes can be changed significantly with training.[1] However, it should be noted that temporary changes in vital capacity are possible in healthy individuals as it has been demonstrated that this measure is significantly reduced as a result of prolonged exercise such as marathon running.[8,16a] This change (which is reversed within 24 hours) is probably due to a closure of the small airways in the lung, thus preventing a person from achieving a complete exhalation.[16a]

RESIDUAL LUNG VOLUME. When one exhales as deeply as possible, there is still a volume of air that remains in the lungs. This volume that cannot be exhaled is the *residual lung volume* (RV). It averages between 1.0 and 1.2 liters for women and 1.2 and 1.4 liters for men, although values of 0.96 to 2.46 liters have been reported for apparently healthy professional football players.[24] Residual lung volume tends to increase with age, whereas the inspiratory and expiratory reserve volumes become proportionally smaller. The loss in breathing reserve and the concomitant increase in residual volume are generally attributed to a decrease in the elastic components of the lung tissue with aging.[22]

The residual lung volume serves an important physiologic function in that it allows for an uninterrupted exchange of gas between the blood and alveoli and thus prevents fluctuations in blood gases during phases of the breathing cycle, including deep breathing. The residual lung volume plus the vital capacity constitutes *the total lung capacity* (TLC).

The residual lung volume cannot be measured directly from spirographic tracings but can be determined by several techniques that involve rebreathing a known volume of gas containing either helium or pure oxygen.

With the *helium method,* the subject expires normally. The air remaining in the lungs at this end-normal expiration position is called the *functional residual capacity* (FRC) and includes the known expiratory reserve volume and the unknown residual volume. The subject then rebreathes a known helium mixture for about 5 minutes. Expired carbon dioxide is absorbed and the exact amount of oxygen consumed is continuously replaced in order to maintain a constant rebreathing volume. The functional residual lung volume can be easily computed from the dilution of the original helium mixture. This volume minus the expiratory reserve volume is equal to the residual lung volume.

The *oxygen dilution method* is considerably more rapid than the helium method although it is similar in principle.[23] With this technique, the functional residual volume is determined from the dilution of the lung's original nitrogen concentration. Dilution is achieved by the rapid rebreathing of a volume of about 5 liters of pure oxygen.

LUNG VOLUME AVERAGES FOR MEN AND WOMEN. As is the case with many anatomic and physiologic measures, lung volumes vary with age, sex, and body size, especially height. *For this reason, lung volumes should only be evaluated in relation to norms based on age, sex, and size.* Average values for various lung volumes for men and women are presented in Table 12-1.

Dynamic Lung Volumes

In appraising the adequacy of ventilation, the important consideration is the individual's ability to sustain high levels of airflow, rather than the quantity of air that can be brought into the lungs in one breath. Dynamic ventilation depends on two factors: (1) the maximum "stroke volume" of the lungs, or the vital capacity, and (2) the speed with which this volume can be moved. The velocity of airflow, in turn, is dependent upon the resistance offered by the respiratory passages to the smooth flow of air and upon the resistance offered by both the chest and lung tissue to a change in shape during breathing.

Normal values for vital capacity can be achieved by individuals with severe lung disease if no time limit is placed on the ventilatory maneuver. For this reason, physicians usually obtain a more "dynamic" measure of lung function such as the percentage of the vital capacity that can be expired in 1 second. This measure, termed *forced expiratory volume* ($FEV_{1.0}$), provides an indication of expiratory power and overall resistance to air movement in the lungs. Normally, about 80% of the vital capacity can be expelled in 1 second. With severe obstructive lung disease such as emphysema or bronchial asthma, however, the $FEV_{1.0}$ is considerably reduced and may represent only about 28% of the vital capacity.[7]

Another dynamic test of ventilatory capacity requires rapid and deep breathing for 15 seconds. This 15-second volume is then extrapolated to the volume that would have been breathed had the subject continued for 1 minute, and represents the *maximum voluntary ventilation* (MVV). The MVV is usually about 25% higher than the ventilation volume observed during maximal exercise.[7] This is because the ventilatory system is not stressed maximally in exercise. The MVV of healthy, college-aged men is usually 140 to 180 liters of air per minute, whereas values for women are 80 to 120 liters per minute. Male members of the 1972 United States Nordic Ski Team averaged 192 liters per minute with an individual high MVV of 239 liters per minute.[12] Patients with obstructive lung disease, on the other hand, can only achieve about 40% of the MVV predicted normal for their age and size.[15] Specific exercise therapy may be beneficial for such patients, because it has been demonstrated that the strength and endurance of the respiratory muscles and the MVV can be increased by exercises that train the breathing musculature.[14]

Lung Function and Exercise Performance

Although some measures of lung function are sensitive indices of the severity of obstructive lung disease, they are of little use in predicting fitness or performance, provided that the values fall within the normal range. For example, no difference was noted in the average vital capacity values of Olympic wrestlers[19] and trained middle-distance athletes,[18] and in those of untrained, healthy subjects. Surprisingly, players from a professional football team averaged only 94% of their predicted vital capacity, with the defensive backs achieving only 83% of values predicted "normal" for their body size![24]

Swimming and diving may be more conducive to the development of larger than normal vital capacities. In these sports, the inspiratory muscles are probably strengthened as they work against additional resistance caused by the weight of water compressing the thoracic cage. Relatively large vital capacities have been reported for skindivers[5,21] and competitive swimmers.[18] Significant improvement in vital capacity following swim training has also been reported.[4] The increased vital capacity was attributed to an improved inspiratory capacity as well as to a reduced residual lung volume due to more complete exhalation. However, similar results were not shown for 10-year-old female competitive swimmers who were compared with swimmers who did not make the team and with untrained girls who had no interest in com-

TABLE 12-1. *Average lung volumes and capacities in healthy recumbent subjects*[a,b]

MEASURE	MALES (20–30 years)	FEMALES (20–30 years)	MALES (50–60 years)
Tidal volume	600	500	500
Inspiratory capacity	3600	2400	2600
Inspiratory reserve volume	3000	1900	2100
Expiratory reserve volume	1200	800	1000
Vital capacity	4800	3200	3600
Residual volume	1200	1000	2400
Functional residual capacity	2400	1800	3400
Total lung capacity	6000	4200	6000
RV/TLC $\times$ 100	20%	24%	40%

[a] Volumes are averages in milliliters for male and female subjects with surface areas of 1.7 m^2 and 1.6 m^2, respectively.
[b] Modified and reproduced with permission from Comroe, J.H., Jr. et al.: The Lung, 2nd edition. Copyright © 1962 by Year Book Medical Publishers, Inc., Chicago.

petition.[17] No differences were demonstrated between groups in either static or dynamic measures of lung function, although the cardiovascular response to exercise was significantly more efficient in the trained swimmers. In another study,[16] the lung volumes of Olympic speed skaters tended to be larger than those of untrained, healthy subjects, yet these measures were of little value in distinguishing those skaters who made the 1968 United States Olympic squad and those who did not.

The inability to predict exercise performance of healthy individuals from lung function measures was further demonstrated with a large group of teenage boys and girls following summer camp.[6] When lung volumes and capacities were normalized for body size, there was essentially no relationship between the lung function and various track performances, including a distance run. Similarly, in a study of marathon runners,[13] essentially no difference existed between the athletes' actual values for eight lung function measures and the values predicted normal for their body size. These observations, which are summarized in Table 12-2, are further supported by the fact that several of the top finishers in the Boston Marathon had below "normal" vital capacities.[8] Also, when variations in body size are considered, no relationship is demonstrated between maximal oxygen uptake and either vital capacity or maximum ventilation volume for healthy, untrained subjects.[11]

Although the feelings of fatigue in strenuous exercise are frequently related to feeling "out of breath" or "winded," it appears that the normal capacity for pulmonary ventilation does not limit exercise performance. The larger-than-normal lung volumes and breathing capacities of *some* athletes have generally been attributed to differences in genetic endowment[10] and may reflect strengthened respiratory muscles as a result of specific exercise training.

PULMONARY VENTILATION

Minute Ventilation

During quiet breathing at rest, the breathing rate may average 12 breaths per minute whereas the tidal volume averages about 0.5 liters of air per breath. Under these conditions, the volume of air breathed each minute, or *minute ventilation* ($\dot{V}_E$), is 6 liters.

$$\begin{array}{ccc} \text{Minute} & \text{Breathing} & \text{Tidal} \\ \text{ventilation } (\dot{V}_E) = & \text{rate} \times & \text{volume} \\ 6 \text{ liters} \cdot \text{min}^{-1} = & 12 \quad \times & 0.5 \end{array}$$

Significant increases in minute ventilation result from an increase in either the depth or rate of breathing, or both. During strenuous exercise, the breathing rate of healthy young adults usually increases to 35 to 45 breaths per minute (although breathing frequencies as high as 60 and 76 breaths per minute have been reported during maximal exercise for a male and female Olympic speed-skating candidate, respectively[16]). Tidal volumes of 2.0 liters and larger are common during exercise. Consequently, with increases in breathing rate and tidal volume, the minute ventilation can easily reach 100 liters, or about 17 times the resting value. In well-conditioned male endurance athletes, ventilation may increase to 160 liters per

TABLE 12-2. *Comparison of mean pulmonary function measures of 11 marathon runners with values predicted normal for their body size*[a]

MEASURE	PREDICTED AVERAGE	OBSERVED AVERAGE	DIFFERENCE[b]
VC (liters)	5.10	5.92	−0.82
$FEV_{1.0}$ (liters)	4.21	4.78	−0.56
$FEV_{1.0}/VC$ (%)	81.3	81.6	−0.28
TLC (liters)	7.06	8.07	−1.01
FRC (liters)	3.90	3.64	0.26
FRC/TLC (%)	49.3	45.3	4.0
RV (liters)	1.87	2.15	−0.28
RV/TLC (%)	26.3	26.3	0.0

[a] From Kaufman, D.A. et al.: Pulmonary function of marathon runners. Med. Sci. Sports, 6:114, 1974. Copyright 1974, the American College of Sports Medicine. Reprinted by permission.
[b] Differences are not statistically significant.

minute in response to maximal exercise. In fact, ventilation volumes of 200 liters per minute have been reported in several research studies, and a high of 208 liters was observed for a professional football player during maximal bicycle exercise.[24] Even with these large minute ventilations, the tidal volume rarely exceeds 55% of the vital capacity.

Alveolar Ventilation

A portion of the air in each breath does not enter the alveoli and thus is not involved in gaseous exchange with the blood. This air, which fills the nose, mouth, trachea, and other non-diffusable conducting portions of the respiratory tract, is contained within the *anatomic dead space*. In healthy subjects, this volume averages 150 to 200 ml or about 30% of the resting tidal volume. The composition of dead-space air is almost identical to that of ambient air except that it is fully saturated with water vapor.

Because of the dead-space volume, approximately 350 ml of the 500 ml of ambient air inspired in the tidal volume at rest enters into and mixes with the existing alveolar air. This does not mean that only 350 ml of air enters and leaves the alveoli with each breath. On the contrary, if the tidal volume is 500 ml, 500 ml of air enters the alveoli but only 350 ml is fresh air. This represents about one-seventh of the total air in the alveoli. Such a relatively small and seemingly inefficient *alveolar ventilation* prevents drastic changes in the composition of alveolar air and assures a consistency in arterial blood gases throughout the entire breathing cycle.

The minute ventilation does not always reflect the actual alveolar ventilation. This is shown in Table 12-3. In the first example of shallow breathing, the tidal volume is reduced to 150 ml, yet it is still possible to achieve a 6-liter minute ventilation if the breathing rate is increased to 40 breaths per minute. The same 6-liter minute volume can also be achieved by decreasing the breathing rate to 12 breaths per minute and increasing the tidal volume to 500 ml. On the other hand, by doubling this tidal volume and halving the ventilatory rate, as in the example of deep breathing, the 6-liter minute ventilation is again achieved. However, each of these ventilatory adjustments drastically affects alveolar ventilation. In the example of shallow breathing, all that has been moved is the dead-space air: No alveolar ventilation has taken place. In the other examples, the breathing is deeper, and a larger portion of each breath enters into and mixes with the existing alveolar air. It is this alveolar ventilation that determines the gaseous concentrations at the alveolar–capillary membrane.

DEAD SPACE VERSUS TIDAL VOLUME. The preceding examples for alveolar ventilation were overly simplified in that a constant dead space was assumed despite changes in tidal volume. Actually, the anatomic dead space increases as tidal volume gets larger; it may actually be doubled during deep breathing due to some stretching of the respiratory passages with a fuller inspiration[2] This increase in dead space, however, is still proportionately less than the increase in tidal volume. Consequently, deeper breathing provides for more effective alveolar ventilation than does similar minute ventilation achieved only through an increase in breathing rate.

PHYSIOLOGIC DEAD SPACE. Adequate gas exchange between the alveoli and the blood requires ventilation that is well matched to the quantity of blood perfusing the pulmonary cap-

TABLE 12-3. *Interrelationship between tidal volume, breathing rate, and pulmonary ventilation*

CONDITION	TIDAL VOLUME (ml)	×	BREATHING RATE (breaths · min⁻¹)	=	MINUTE VENTILATION (ml · min⁻¹)	−	DEAD SPACE VENTILATION (ml · min⁻¹)	=	ALVEOLAR VENTILATION (ml · min⁻¹)
Shallow breathing	150		40		6000		(150 ml × 40)		0
Normal breathing	500		12		6000		(150 ml × 12)		4200
Deep breathing	1000		6		6000		(150 ml × 6)		5100

illaries. For example, at rest, approximately 4.2 liters of air ventilate the alveoli each minute, whereas an average of 5.0 liters of blood flow through the pulmonary capillaries. In this instance, the ratio of alveolar ventilation to pulmonary blood flow, termed the *ventilation-perfusion ratio*, is approximately 0.8 (4.2 ÷ 5.0). This ratio indicates that each liter of pulmonary blood is matched by an alveolar ventilation of 0.8 liters. In light exercise, the ventilation-perfusion ratio is maintained at about 0.8, whereas in heavy exercise there is a disproportionate increase in alveolar ventilation. In such exercise in healthy subjects, the ventilation-perfusion ratio may increase above 5.0 in order to assure adequate aeration of the blood returning in the venous circulation.

In certain instances, a portion of the alveoli may not function adequately in gas exchange due to either (1) an underperfusion of blood or (2) an inadequate ventilation relative to the size of the alveoli. This portion of the alveolar volume with a poor ventilation-perfusion ratio has been termed the *physiologic dead space*. As illustrated in Figure 12-6, the physiologic dead space in the healthy lung is small and can be considered negligible. However, physiologic dead space can increase to as much as 50% of the tidal volume with *inadequte perfusion* during hemorrhage or blockage of the pulmonary circulation or with *inadequate ventilation* that occurs in emphysema, asthma, and pulmonary fibrosis. When the total dead space of the lung exceeds 60% of the lung volume, adequate gas exchange becomes impossible.

DEPTH VERSUS RATE. During exercise, alveolar ventilation is maintained through an increase in both the rate and depth of breathing. In moderate exercise, well-trained athletes achieve adequate alveolar ventilation by increasing tidal volume with only a small increase in breathing rate.[9] Due to this deeper breathing, alveolar ventilation may increase from 70% of the minute ventilation at rest to over 85% of the total exercise ventilation. Figure 12-7 shows that the increase in tidal volume in exercise is due largely to encroachment on the inspiratory reserve volume with an accompanying but smaller decrease in the end-expiratory level. This adjustment occurs unconsciously, so each individual develops a "style" of breathing in which the respiratory frequency and tidal volume are blended to provide effective alveolar ventilation. Conscious attempts to modify breathing during general physical activities such as running are usually doomed to failure and probably are of no benefit in terms of performance. In fact, conscious manipulation of breathing would be detrimental to the exquisitely regulated physiologic adjustments to exercise. *At rest and in exercise, each individual should breathe in the manner that seems most natural.*

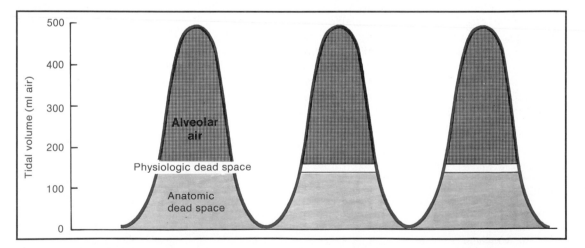

FIG. 12-6. *Distribution of tidal volume in healthy subject at rest. This tidal volume includes about 350 ml of ambient air that mixes with alveolar air, about 150 ml of air in the larger air passages (anatomic dead space), and a small portion of air distributed to either poorly ventilated or perfused alveoli (physiologic dead space).*

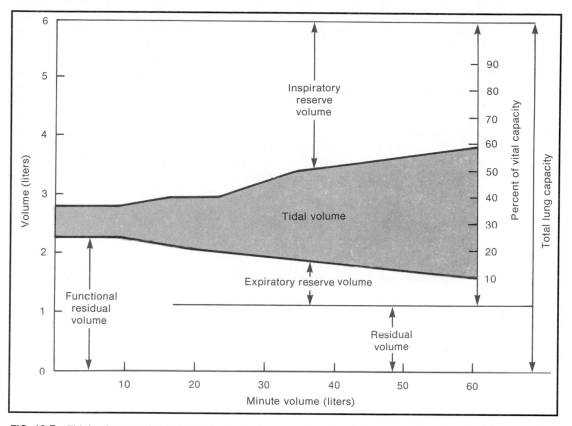

FIG. 12-7. *Tidal volume and subdivisions of pulmonary air at rest and during exercise. (Modified from Lambert-sen, C.J.: Physical and mechanical aspects of respiration.* In *Medical Physiology. Edited by V.B. Mountcastle, St. Louis, C.V. Mosby Co., 1968.)*

SUMMARY

1. The lungs provide a large interface between the body's internal fluid environment and the gaseous external environment. At any one second, there is probably no more than a pint of blood in the pulmonary capillaries.

2. Pulmonary ventilation is geared to maintain favorable concentrations of alveolar oxygen and carbon dioxide to assure adequate aeration of the blood flowing through the lungs.

3. Pulmonary air flow depends upon small pressure differences between ambient air and air within the lungs. These differences are brought about by the action of various muscles that act to alter the dimensions of the chest cavity.

4. A forced exhalation against a closed glottis is called a Valsalva maneuver. It can cause a large increase in pressure within the chest cavity that compresses the thoracic

veins, thereby significantly reducing venous return to the heart. The straining-type muscular effort usually accompanying the Valsalva maneuver temporarily elevates blood pressure and places an added work load on the heart. Thus, individuals with heart and vascular disease should refrain from straining exercises such as isometrics.

5. Lung volumes vary with age, sex, and body size, especially height, and should only be evaluated in relation to norms based on these factors.

6. Tidal volume is increased during exercise by encroachment on both the inspiratory and expiratory reserve volumes. Even when a person breathes to vital capacity there is still air remaining in the lungs at maximal exhalation. This residual lung volume allows for an uninterrupted exchange of gas during all phases of the breathing cycle.

7. Forced expiratory volume and maximum voluntary ventilation give a dynamic picture of one's ability to sustain high levels of airflow. They serve as excellent screening tests to detect possible lung disease.

8. Tests of static and dynamic lung function are of little use in predicting fitness and exercise performance, provided that the values fall within a normal range.

9. Minute ventilation is a function of breathing rate and tidal volume. Minute ventilation averages 6 to 10 liters at rest, whereas in maximum exercise, increases in breathing rate and depth may result in ventilations as high as 200 liters per minute.

10. Alveolar ventilation is the portion of the minute ventilation entering the alveoli to be involved in gaseous exchange with the blood.

11. The ratio of alveolar ventilation to pulmonary blood flow is termed the ventilation-perfusion ratio. At rest and in light exercise, this ratio is maintained at about 0.8. This indicates that each liter of pulmonary blood is matched by an alveolar ventilation of 0.8 liters. In heavy exercise, alveolar ventilation in healthy people increases disproportionately, so this ratio may reach 5.0.

12. At rest and in exercise, a healthy person should breathe in a manner that seems most natural.

References

1. Adams, W.C.: Effect of a season of varsity track and field on selected anthropometric, circulatory and pulmonary function parameters. Res. Quart., *39:*5, 1968.
2. Asmussen, E., and Nielsen, M.: Physiological dead-space and alveolar gas pressures at rest and during muscular exercise. Acta Physiol. Scand., *38:*1, 1956.
3. Åstrand, P-O., and Rodahl, K.: Textbook of Work Physiology. New York, McGraw-Hill, 1977.
4. Bachman, J.C., and Horvath, S.M.: Pulmonary function changes which accompany athletic training programs. Res. Quart., *39:*235, 1968.
5. Carey, C.R. et al.: Effects of skin diving on lung volumes. J. Appl. Physiol., *8:*519, 1955.
6. Cummings, G.R.: Correlation of athletic performance with pulmonary function in 13 to 17 year old boys and girls. Med. Sci. Sports, *1:*140, 1969.
7. Gaensler, E.A.: Analysis of ventilatory defect by timed capacity measurements. Am. Rev. Tuberc., *64:*256, 1951.
8. Gordon, B. et al.: Observations on a group of marathon runners with special reference to the circulation. Arch. Intern. Med., *33:*425, 1924.
9. Grimby, G.: Respiration in exercise. Med. Sci. Sports, *1:*9, 1969.
10. Grimby, G., and Saltin, B.: Physiological effects of physical training in different ages. Scand. J. Rehabil. Med., *3:*6, 1971.
11. Grimby, G., and Soderholm, B.: Spirometric studies in normal subjects. 111. Acta Med. Scand., *173:*199, 1963.
12. Hanson, J.S.: Maximal exercise performance in members of the U.S. Nordic Ski Team. J. Appl. Physiol., *33:*592, 1973.
13. Kaufmann, D.A. et al.: Pulmonary function of marathon runners. Med. Sci. Sports, *6:*114, 1974.
14. Leith, D.E., and Bradley, M.: Ventilatory muscle strength and endurance training. J. Appl. Physiol., *41:*508, 1976.
15. Levison, H., and Cherniack, R.: Ventilatory cost of exercise in chronic obstructive pulmonary disease. J. Appl. Physiol., *25:*21, 1968.

16. Maksud, M.G. et al.: Maximal $\dot{V}O_2$, ventilation, and heart rate of Olympic speed skating candidates. J. Appl. Physiol., *29:*186, 1970.

16a. Maron, M.B. et al.: Alterations in pulmonary function consequent to competitive marathon running. Med. Sci. Sports., *11:*244, 1979.

17. Ness, G.E. et al.: Cardiopulmonary function in prospective competitive swimmers and their parents. J. Appl. Physiol., *37:*27, 1974.

18. Newman, F. et al.: A comparison between body size and lung function of swimmers and normal school children. J. Physiol., *156:*9, 1961.

19. Rasch, P.J., and Brandt, J.W.A.: Measurement of pulmonary function in United States Olympic free style wrestlers. Res. Quart., *28:*279, 1957.

20. Sharp, J.T. et al.: Relative contributions of rib cage and abdomen to breathing in normal subjects. J. Appl. Physiol., *39:*608, 1975.

21. Tatai, K.: Comparisons of ventilatory capacities among fishing divers, nurses, and telephone operators in Japanese females. Jpn. J. Physiol., *7:*37, 1957.

22. Turner, J.M. et al.: Elasticity of human lungs in relation to age. J. Appl. Physiol., *25:*664, 1968.

23. Wilmore, J.H.: A simplified method for the determination of residual lung volume. J. Appl. Physiol., *27:*96, 1969.

24. Wilmore, J.H., and Haskell, W.L.: Body composition and endurance capacity of professional football players. J. Appl. Physiol., *33:*564, 1972.

Gas Exchange
and Transport

Our supply of oxygen depends on the oxygen *concentration* in ambient air and its *pressure*. Ambient or atmospheric air remains relatively constant in terms of composition. It is composed of approximately 20.93% oxygen, 79.04% nitrogen (this includes small quantities of other inert gases that behave physiologically like nitrogen), 0.03% carbon dioxide, and usually small quantities of water vapor. The gas molecules move at relatively great speeds and exert a pressure against any surface with which they come in contact. At sea level, the pressure of the gas molecules in air is sufficient to raise a column of mercury to a height of 760 mm, or 29.9 inches. These barometric readings vary somewhat with changing weather conditions and are considerably lower at altitude (see Chapter 23).

PART 1

Gaseous Exchange in the Lungs and Tissues

CONCENTRATIONS AND PARTIAL PRESSURES OF RESPIRED GASES

The molecules of a specific gas in a mixture of gases exert their own *partial pressure*. The total pressure of the mixture is simply the sum of the partial pressures of the individual gases. Partial pressure is computed as:

$$\frac{\text{Partial}}{\text{pressure}} = \frac{\text{Percent}}{\text{concentration}} \times \frac{\text{Total pressure of}}{\text{gas mixture}}$$

Ambient Air

The volume, percentage, and partial pressure of the gases in dry, ambient air at sea level are presented in Table 13-1. The partial pressure of oxygen is 20.93% of the total pressure of 760 mm Hg exerted by air, or 159 mm Hg

(.2093 × 760 mm Hg); the random movement of the minute quantity of carbon dioxide exerts a pressure of only 0.2 mm Hg (.0003 × 760 mm Hg), whereas the molecules of nitrogen exert a pressure that would raise the mercury in a manometer about 600 mm (.7094 × 760 mm Hg). Partial pressure is usually denoted by a P in front of the gas symbol; the P_{O_2}, P_{CO_2}, and P_{N_2} in ambient air at sea level are 159, 0.2, and 600 mm Hg, respectively.

Tracheal Air

Air becomes completely saturated with water vapor as it enters the nose and mouth and passes down the respiratory tract. This vapor dilutes the inspired air mixture somewhat. At a body temperature of 37°C, for example, the pressure of water molecules in humidified air is

TABLE 13-1. *Partial pressure and volume of the gases in dry ambient air at sea level*

GAS	PERCENTAGE	PARTIAL PRESSURE (AT 760 mm Hg)	VOLUME OF GAS (ml · l⁻¹)
Oxygen	20.93	159 mm Hg	209.3
Carbon dioxide	0.03	0.2 mm Hg	0.4
Nitrogen	79.04[a]	600 mm Hg	790.3

[a]Includes 0.93% argon and other trace rare gases.

47 mm Hg; this leaves 713 mm Hg (760 − 47) as the total pressure exerted by the inspired dry air molecules. Consequently, the effective P_{O_2} in *tracheal air* is lowered by about 10 mm Hg from its ambient value of 159 mm Hg to 149 mm Hg [.2093(760 − 47 mm Hg)]. Because carbon dioxide is almost negligible in inspired air, the humidification process has little effect on the inspired P_{CO_2}.

Alveolar Air

The composition of alveolar air differs considerably from that of the incoming breath of moist ambient air because carbon dioxide is continually entering the alveoli from the blood, whereas oxygen is leaving the lungs to be carried throughout the body. As shown in Table 13-2, alveolar air contains approximately 14.5% oxygen, 5.5% carbon dioxide, and about 80.0% nitrogen. After subtracting the vapor pressure of moist alveolar gas, the average alveolar P_{O_2} and P_{CO_2} is 103 mm Hg [.145 (760 − 47 mm Hg)] and 39 mm Hg [.055 (760 − 47 mm Hg)], respectively. *These values represent the average pressures exerted by oxygen and carbon dioxide molecules against the alveolar side of the alveolar-capillary membrane.* They are not physiologic constants but vary somewhat with the phase of the ventilatory cycle as well as with the adequacy of ventilation in various portions of the lung. It should be recalled, however, that a relatively large volume of air remains in the lungs after each normal exhalation. This *func-*

tional residual volume serves as a damper so that each incoming breath of air has only a small effect on the composition of alveolar air. *Thus, the partial pressure of gases in the alveoli remains relatively stable.*

MOVEMENT OF GAS IN AIR AND FLUIDS

In accordance with *Henry's Law,* the amount of gas that dissolves in a fluid is a function of two factors: (1) the *pressure* of the gas above the fluid, and (2) the *solubility* of the gas.

Pressure

Oxygen molecules continually strike the surface of the water in the three chambers illustrated in Figure 13-1. Because the pure water in container A contains no oxygen, a large number of oxygen molecules enter the water and become dissolved. Because dissolved gas molecules are also in random motion, some oxygen molecules leave the water. In chamber B, the net movement of oxygen is still into the fluid from the gaseous state. Eventually, the number of molecules entering and leaving the fluid becomes equal as in chamber C. When this occurs, the gas pressures are in *equilibrium,* and no net diffusion of oxygen occurs. Conversely, if the pressure of dissolved oxygen molecules exceeds the pressure of the free gas in the air, oxygen will leave the fluid until a new pressure equilibrium is reached.

TABLE 13-2. *Partial pressure and volume of dry alveolar gases at sea level (37°C)*

GAS	PERCENTAGE	PARTIAL PRESSURE (AT 760−47 mm Hg)	VOLUME OF GAS (ml · l⁻¹)
Oxygen	14.5	103 mm Hg	145
Carbon dioxide	5.5	39 mm Hg	55
Nitrogen	80.0	571 mm Hg	800
Water Vapor		47 mm Hg	

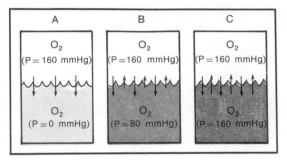

FIG. 13-1. *Solution of oxygen in water: A, when oxygen first comes in contact with pure water, B, after the dissolved oxygen is halfway to equilibrium with gaseous oxygen, and C, after equilibrium has been established.*

Solubility

For two different gases at identical pressures, the number of molecules moving into or out of a fluid is determined by the solubility of each gas. For each unit of pressure favoring diffusion, for example, approximately 25 times more carbon dioxide than oxygen will move into (or from) a fluid. Viewed another way, equal quantities of oxygen and carbon dioxide will enter or leave a fluid under significantly different pressure gradients for each gas.

GAS EXCHANGE IN THE LUNGS AND TISSUES

The exchange of gases between the lungs and the blood as well as their movement at the tissue level is due entirely to the passive process of diffusion. Figure 13-2 illustrates the pressure gradients favoring gas transfer in the body.

Gas Exchange in the Lungs

At rest, the pressure of oxygen molecules in the alveoli is about 60 mm Hg greater than that in the venous blood entering the pulmonary capillaries. Consequently, oxygen dissolves and diffuses through the alveolar membrane *into the blood.* Carbon dioxide, on the other hand, exists under a slightly greater pressure in returning venous blood than it does in the alveoli. The net diffusion of carbon dioxide is, therefore, from the blood *into the lungs.* Although the pressure gradient of 6 mm Hg for carbon dioxide diffusion is small compared to that for

oxygen, adequate transfer of this gas is achieved rapidly due to its high solubility. Nitrogen, which is neither utilized nor produced in metabolic reactions, remains essentially unchanged in alveolar-capillary gas.

The process of gas exchange is so rapid in the healthy lung that an equilibrium between blood and alveolar gas occurs in less than 1 second, or at about the midpoint of the blood's transit through the lungs. Thus, the blood leaving the lungs to be delivered throughout the body contains oxygen at a pressure of approximately 100 mm Hg and carbon dioxide at 40 mm Hg.*

Gas Transfer in the Tissues

In the tissues, where oxygen is consumed in energy metabolism and an almost equal amount of carbon dioxide is produced, gas pressures can differ considerably from those in arterial blood. At rest, the average P_{O_2} in the fluid immediately outside a muscle cell rarely drops below 40 mm Hg, and the cellular P_{CO_2} averages about 46 mm Hg. In heavy exercise, however, the pressure of oxygen molecules in the muscle tissue may fall to about 3 mm Hg,[7] whereas the pressure of carbon dioxide approaches 90 mm Hg. *It is the pressure differences between gases in the plasma and tissues that establishes the gradients for diffusion.* Oxygen leaves the blood and diffuses toward the metabolizing cell while carbon dioxide flows from the cell to the blood. The blood then passes into the veins and is returned to the heart to be subsequently pumped to the lungs. As the blood enters the dense capillary network of the lungs, diffusion rapidly begins once again.

The body does not attempt to rid itself completely of carbon dioxide. On the contrary, as the blood leaves the lungs with a P_{CO_2} of 40 mm Hg, it still contains about 50 ml of carbon dioxide in each 100 ml of blood. As can be seen in

---

*The P_{O_2} of arterial blood is usually slightly lower than the alveolar P_{O_2} because some blood in the alveolar capillaries may pass through poorly ventilated alveoli. Also, the blood leaving the lungs is joined by venous blood from the bronchial and cardiac circulations. This small amount of poorly oxygenated blood has been termed *venous admixture.* Although its effect is small in healthy individuals, it does reduce the arterial P_{O_2} slightly below that existing in pulmonary end-capillary blood.

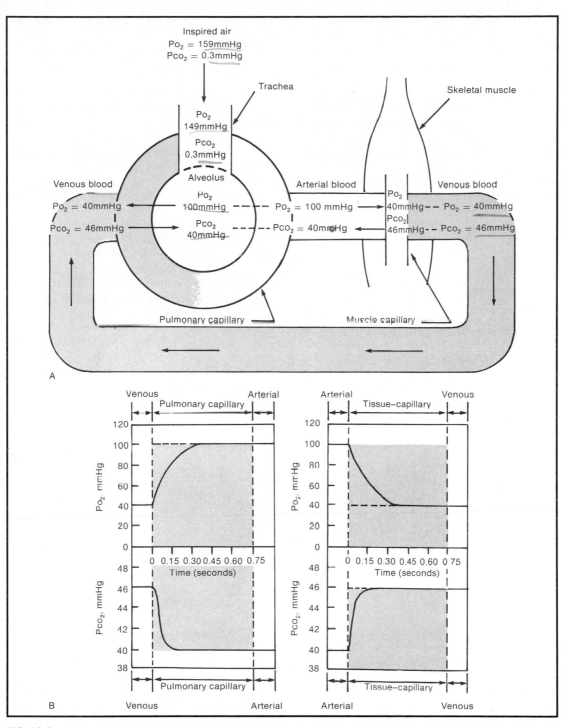

FIG. 13-2. *Pressure gradients for gas transfer in the body at rest. In A, the Po₂ and Pco₂ of ambient, tracheal, and alveolar air are shown as well as the gas pressures in venous and arterial blood and muscle tissue. Movement of gases at the alveolar–capillary and tissue–capillary membranes is always from an area of higher partial pressure to one of lower partial pressure. The time required for gas exchange is shown in B. At rest, blood remains in the pulmonary and tissue capillaries for about 0.75 s. During maximal exercise, the transit time is reduced to about 0.4 s, but this is still adequate for complete aeration of the blood. (From Mathews, D.K., and Fox, E.L.: The Physiological Basis of Physical Education and Athletics. Philadelphia, W.B. Saunders Co., 1976.)*

the next chapter, this "background level" of carbon dioxide is vital because it provides chemical input for the control of breathing through its effect on the respiratory center in the brain.

If it were not for our capacity to breathe, some average pressure would be reached between alveolar and blood gases and diffusion would cease. By bringing in another breath of air, however, the oxygen content of the alveoli is increased whereas the carbon dioxide is diluted. *By adjusting alveolar ventilation to metabolic demands, the composition of alveolar gas remains remarkably constant, even during strenuous exercise that can increase oxygen uptake and carbon dioxide output by as much as 25 times.*

SUMMARY

1. At the lungs and tissues, gas molecules diffuse down their concentration gradients from an area of higher concentration (higher pressure) to one of lower concentration (lower pressure).

2. The partial pressure of a specific gas in a mixture of gases is proportional to the concentration of the gas and the total pressure exerted by the mixture.

3. The quantity of gas that dissolves in a fluid is determined by pressure and solubility. Because carbon dioxide is about 25 times more soluble in plasma than oxygen, large amounts of this gas move into and out of body fluids down a relatively small diffusion (pressure) gradient.

4. At rest and during exercise, adjustments in alveolar ventilation occur; thus, the composition of alveolar gas remains constant. Oxygen and carbon dioxide pressures are maintained at about 100 mm Hg and 40 mm Hg, respectively. Because venous blood contains oxygen at lower and carbon dioxide at higher pressure than alveolar gases, oxygen diffuses into the blood and carbon dioxide diffuses into the lungs.

5. Gas exchange is so rapid in the healthy lung that equilibrium occurs at about the midpoint of the blood's transit through the pulmonary capillaries.

6. At the tissues, the diffusion gradient favors the movement of oxygen from the capillary to the tissues and carbon dioxide from the cells into the blood. In exercise, these gradients are expanded, and oxygen and carbon dioxide diffuse rapidly.

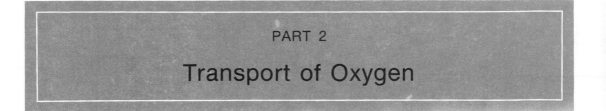

PART 2

Transport of Oxygen

OXYGEN TRANSPORT IN THE BLOOD

Oxygen is carried in the blood in two ways: (1) in physical solution dissolved in the fluid portion of the blood, and (2) in loose combination with hemoglobin, the iron–protein molecule in the red blood cell.

Oxygen in Solution

Oxygen is not particularly soluble in fluids. In fact, at an alveolar Po_2 of 100 mm Hg, only about 0.3 ml of gaseous oxygen dissolves in each 100 ml of plasma; this is equivalent to 3 ml

of oxygen per liter of plasma. Because the average blood volume is about 5 liters, 15 ml of oxygen are carried dissolved in the fluid portion of the blood (3 ml per liter × 5). This is enough oxygen to sustain life for about 4 seconds!

The small quantity of oxygen transported in physical solution, however, does serve several important physiologic functions. The random movement of dissolved oxygen molecules establishes the Po_2 of the blood and tissue fluids. This pressure of dissolved oxygen plays a role in the regulation of breathing; it also determines the loading and subsequent release of oxygen from hemoglobin in the lungs and tissues, respectively.

Oxygen Combined with Hemoglobin

Metallic compounds are present in the blood of many species of animals and serve to augment the blood's oxygen-carrying capacity. In humans, this compound is *hemoglobin,* an iron-containing protein pigment. Hemoglobin, a main component of the body's 5 billion red blood cells, increases the blood's oxygen-carrying capacity 65 to 70 times above that normally dissolved in plasma. Thus, for each liter of blood, about 197 ml of oxygen are temporarily "captured" by hemoglobin. Each of the four iron atoms in the hemoglobin molecule can loosely bind one molecule of oxygen in the reversible reaction:

$$Hb_4 + 4O_2 \rightleftharpoons Hb_4O_8$$

This reaction requires no enzymes, and it occurs without a change in the valance of Fe^{2+}, which would occur in the more permanent process of oxidation. *The oxygenation of hemoglobin to oxyhemoglobin depends entirely on the partial pressure of oxygen in solution.*

OXYGEN-CARRYING CAPACITY OF HEMOGLOBIN. In men, there are approximately 15 to 16 g of hemoglobin in each 100 ml of blood. The value is somewhat less for women and averages about 14 g per 100 ml of blood. This apparent "sex difference" may account to some degree for the lower maximal aerobic capacity of women, even after differences in body weight and body fat are considered.

Each gram of hemoglobin can combine loosely with 1.34 ml of oxygen. Thus, if the hemoglobin content of the blood is known, its oxygen-carrying capacity can easily be calculated as follows:

Blood's oxygen capacity (ml · 100 ml⁻¹ blood)	=	Hemoglobin (g · 100 ml⁻¹ blood)	×	Oxygen capacity of hemoglobin (ml O_2 · g⁻¹)
20 ml O_2	=	15	×	1.34

On the average, approximately 20 ml of oxygen would be carried with the hemoglobin in each 100 ml of blood when the hemoglobin is fully saturated with oxygen; that is, when all of the hemoglobin is converted to HbO_2.

The blood's oxygen transport capacity changes only slightly with normal variations in hemoglobin content. However, a significant decrease in the iron content of the red blood cell, such as that which occurs in *iron defi-* ciency anemia, causes a corresponding decrease in the blood's oxygen-carrying capacity.

Individuals who suffer from iron deficiency anemia and associated low hemoglobin levels have a reduced capacity for sustaining even mild aerobic exercise.[1] This is shown in Table 13-3. Twenty-nine iron-deficient-anemic subjects (13 men, 16 women) with low hemoglobin levels were placed in one of two groups; one group received intramuscular injections of iron over an 80-day period, whereas the placebo group received similar intramuscular injections of colored salt solution. A third group with normal levels of hemoglobin served as controls. All groups were tested during exercise prior to the experiment and after 80 days of either iron therapy or placebo treatment. The results clearly show that the anemic group given the iron sup-

TABLE 13-3. *Hematologic and exercise heart rate responses of anemic subjects to iron treatment*

SUBJECTS	Hb (g per 100 ml blood) (AVERAGE)	PEAK EXERCISE HEART RATE (AVERAGE)
Normal		
Men	14.3	119
Women	13.9	142
Iron-Deficient Men		
Pretreatment	7.1	155
Post-treatment	14.0	113
Iron-Deficient Women		
Pretreatment	7.7	155
Post-treatment	12.4	123
Iron-Deficient Men		
Preplacebo	7.7	146
Postplacebo	7.4	137
Iron-Deficient Women		
Preplacebo	8.1	154
Postplacebo	8.4	144

[a] From Gardner, G.W., et al.: Cardiorespiratory, hematological, and physical performance responses of anemic subjects to iron treatment. *Am. J. Clin. Nutr., 28:982, 1975.*

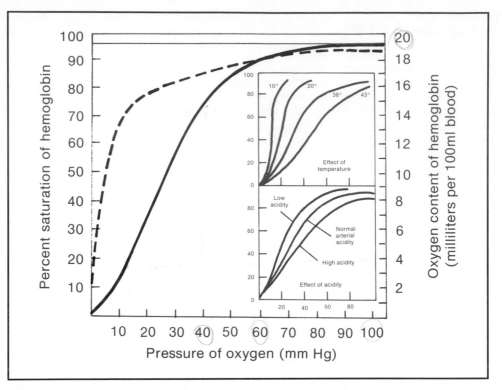

FIG. 13-3. *Percent saturation of hemoglobin (solid line) and myoglobin (dashed line) in relation to oxygen pressure. The quantity of oxygen carried in each 100 ml of blood under normal conditions is shown on the right ordinate. The insert curves indicate the effects of temperature and acidity in altering the affinity of hemoglobin for oxygen.*

plement improved significantly in exercise response compared to their non-supplemented counterparts. Peak heart rate as measured during a 5-minute stepping performance decreased from 155 to 113 beats per minute for men and from 152 to 123 beats per minute for women. This translates into an average of 15% more oxygen delivered per heart beat.

PO₂ AND HEMOGLOBIN SATURATION. Thus far, we have assumed that the hemoglobin becomes fully saturated with oxygen when exposed to alveolar gas. Figure 13-3 illustrates the *oxyhemoglobin dissociation* curve, which shows the saturation of hemoglobin with oxygen at various P_{O_2} including that of normal alveolar-capillary gas (P_{O_2} = 100 mm Hg). Dissociation curves are usually established by exposing a small amount of blood in a sealed glass vessel to various pressures of oxygen. Once the blood-gas mixture has equilibrated in a water bath at a known temperature, the oxygen content and percent saturation of the blood are determined. Percent saturation is calculated as:

$$\text{Percent saturation} = \frac{\text{O}_2 \text{ combined with hemoglobin}}{\text{O}_2 \text{ capacity of hemoglobin}} \times 100$$

Percent saturation in this case does not mean that a certain percentage of hemoglobin molecules are fully saturated and the remaining molecules carry no oxygen. On the contrary, 50% saturation means that an average of two out of the four iron atoms in each hemoglobin molecule have combined with oxygen. Shown on the right ordinate of this dissociation curve is the quantity of oxygen carried in each 100 ml of normal blood at a particular plasma P_{O_2}.

Po₂ in the Lung. Hemoglobin is about 98% saturated with oxygen at the normal alveolar P_{O_2} of 100 mm Hg. By applying this partial pressure value to the right ordinate of Figure 13-3, it is seen that for each 100 ml of blood leaving the lungs, hemoglobin carries about 19.7 ml of oxygen. Clearly, any additional increase in alveolar

Po_2 contributes little to the quantity of oxygen already combined with hemoglobin. In addition to the oxygen bound to hemoglobin, the plasma of each 100 ml of arterial blood contains about 0.3 ml of oxygen in solution. This dissolved gas exerts a pressure of about 100 mm Hg when one breathes ambient air at sea level; this plasma Po_2 regulates the loading and unloading of hemoglobin. Thus, for healthy individuals breathing ambient air at sea level, approximately 20.0 ml of oxygen are carried in each 100 ml of blood leaving the lungs; 19.7 ml are bound to hemoglobin, and 0.3 ml are dissolved in plasma.

Figure 13-3 shows that the saturation of hemoglobin changes little until the pressure of oxygen falls to about 60 mm Hg. This flat, upper portion of the oxyhemoglobin curve provides a margin of safety to assure that the blood is adequately loaded with oxygen. Even if the alveolar Po_2 is reduced to 75 mm Hg, as could occur with certain lung diseases or when one travels to a higher altitude, the saturation of hemoglobin is only lowered about 6%. At an alveolar Po_2 of 60 mm Hg, hemoglobin is still 90% saturated with oxygen! Below this pressure, however, there is a sharp drop in the quantity of oxygen that will combine with hemoglobin.

Po_2 in the Tissues. At rest, the Po_2 in the cell fluids is approximately 40 mm Hg. Dissolved oxygen from the plasma diffuses across the capillary membrane through the tissue fluids into the cells. This reduces the plasma Po_2 below the Po_2 in the red blood cell, and hemoglobin is unable to maintain its high oxygen saturation. The released oxygen ($HbO_2 \rightarrow Hb + O_2$) moves out of the blood cells through the capillary wall and into the tissues.

At the tissue-capillary Po_2 at rest ($Po_2 = 40$ mm Hg), hemoglobin holds about 70% of its total oxygen (Fig. 13-3). Blood leaving the tissues, therefore, carries about 15 ml of oxygen in each 100 ml of blood; nearly 5 ml of oxygen have been released to the tissues. This difference in the oxygen content of arterial and mixed venous blood is termed the *arteriovenous oxygen difference,* or a-$\bar{v}O_2$ *difference.*

The a-$\bar{v}O_2$ difference at rest normally averages 4 to 5 ml of oxygen per 100 ml of blood. The large quantity of oxygen still remaining with hemoglobin provides an "automatic" reserve by which cells can immediately obtain oxygen should the metabolic demands suddenly increase. As the cell's need for oxygen increases

in exercise, the tissue Po_2 becomes reduced and a larger quantity of oxygen is rapidly released. During vigorous exercise, for example, when the extracellular Po_2 decreases to about 15 mm Hg, only about 5 ml of oxygen remain bound to hemoglobin. As a result, the a-$\bar{v}O_2$ difference increases to 15 ml of oxygen per 100 ml of blood. When tissue Po_2 falls to 3 mm Hg during exhaustive exercise, virtually all of the oxygen is released from the blood perfusing the active tissues.[7] Clearly, then, without any increase in local blood flow, the amount of oxygen released to the muscles can increase almost three times above that normally supplied at rest—just by a more complete unloading of hemoglobin.

THE BOHR EFFECT. The solid line in Figure 13-3 shows the oxyhemoglobin dissociation curve under resting physiologic conditions at an arterial pH of 7.4 and tissue temperature of 37°C. The insert curves depict other important characteristics of hemoglobin. Any increase in acidity, temperature, or concentration of carbon dioxide causes the dissociation curve to shift significantly downward and to the right. This phenomenon is called the *Bohr effect* and is a consequence of an alteration in the molecular structure of hemoglobin. The Bohr effect describes the reduced effectiveness of hemoglobin to hold oxygen, especially in the Po_2 range of 20 to 50 mm Hg. This is particularly important in vigorous exercise, because even more oxygen is released to the tissues with the accompanying increase in metabolic heat, carbon dioxide, and lactic acid. The Bohr effect in pulmonary capillary blood is negligible during maximal exercise. This is important because it allows hemoglobin to load completely with oxygen as blood passes through the lungs.

RED-BLOOD-CELL 2,3-DPG. The substance *2,3-diphosphoglycerate,* or 2,3-DPG, is produced within the red blood cell during the anaerobic reactions of glycolysis. This compound appears to bind loosely with subunits of the hemoglobin molecule, reducing its affinity for oxygen. For a given decrease in Po_2, therefore, more oxygen is released to the tissues. It has been reported that individuals with cardiopulmonary disorders and those who live at high altitudes have an increased level of red blood cell 2,3-DPG.[2] This apparently provides a compensatory adjustment to facilitate oxygen release to the cells.

TABLE 13-4. *Red-blood-cell 2,3-DPG in sedentary and athletic subjects and after short-term maximal and prolonged endurance exercise*[a]

	2,3-DPG (μ mols per g of hemoglobin)		
	REST	ALL-OUT RUN 5 min, 45 s	ENDURANCE RUN 51 min, 36 s
Sedentary men	13.75		
Middle-distance athletes	16.82	19.85	
Endurance athletes	16.23		15.20

[a] From Taunton, J.E. et al.: Alterations in 2,3-dpg and P_{50} with maximal and submaximal exercise. *Med. Sci. Sports,* 6:238, 1974. Copyright 1974, the American College of Sports Medicine. Reprinted by permission.

The presence of 2,3-DPG would also aid in oxygen transfer to the muscles during strenuous exercise. Conflicting results have been reported in comparing the 2,3-DPG level of trained and untrained subjects. In one study,[5] no difference in 2,3-DPG was observed between 46 world-class athletes and healthy, sedentary controls. In contrast, as illustrated in Table 13-4, significantly higher resting levels of this metabolic intermediate were observed in two groups of athletes than in untrained subjects.[8] The researchers also observed that the level of 2,3-DPG increased by 15% for the middle-distance runners following maximal exercise of short duration. Prolonged steady-rate exercise, on the other hand, resulted in a small decrease in 2,3-DPG in endurance athletes. More than likely, this difference in the effects of exercise on hemoglobin's affinity for oxygen is due to the specific metabolic demands of exercise. More research is needed before the effects of *exercise* and *training* on the affinity of hemoglobin for oxygen can be precisely evaluated.

Myoglobin, the Muscle's Oxygen Store

Myoglobin is an iron–protein compound found in skeletal and cardiac muscle. Reddish muscle fibers have a high concentration of this respiratory pigment, whereas fibers deficient in myoglobin appear pale or white. Myoglobin is similar to hemoglobin in that it also combines reversibly with oxygen; however, each myoglobin molecule contains only one iron atom in contrast to hemoglobin, which contains four atoms. Myoglobin adds additional oxygen to the muscle in the reaction:

$$Mb + O_2 \longrightarrow MbO_2$$

Aside from its function as an "extra" source of oxygen in muscle, myoglobin probably acts to facilitate the transfer of oxygen to the mitochondria, especially during exercise when there is a considerable drop in cellular Po_2. It can be noted from the dissociation curve for myoglobin shown in Figure 13-3 (dashed line) that the line is not s-shaped, as was the case with hemoglobin, but forms a rectangular hyperbola. This shows that myoglobin binds and retains oxygen at low pressures much more readily than hemoglobin. During rest and moderate levels of exercise, myoglobin retains a high saturation with oxygen. For example, at a Po_2 of 40 mm Hg, myoglobin contains 95% of its oxygen; at 20 mm Hg, it is still about 75% saturated. The greatest quantity of oxygen is released from MbO_2 when the tissue Po_2 drops to 5 mm Hg or less. Unlike hemoglobin, myoglobin does not demonstrate a "Bohr effect."

As might be expected, slow-twitch fibers that have a high capacity to generate ATP aerobically contain relatively large quantities of myoglobin. The myoglobin level of muscle also appears to be related to an animal's level of physical activity. The leg muscles of active hunting dogs contain more myoglobin than the muscles of sedentary house pets[9]; this is also the case for grazing cattle compared to cattle that are penned.[6] It has also been clearly demonstrated that endurance-type exercise programs enhance myoglobin storage.[3,4] In one study, rats were exercised by treadmill running for 15 weeks. As seen in Table 13-5, the myoglobin content of the quadriceps and hamstring muscles was about 80% higher in the exercising group than the sedentary animals. This improvement occurred only in the specifically exercised muscles, because the myoglobin content of the untrained abdominal muscles was unaffected. This is another of the many examples in which specific training brings about specific adaptations that improve subsequent performance in exercise.

SUMMARY

1. Hemoglobin, the iron–protein pigment in the red blood cell, increases the oxygen-carrying capacity of whole blood about 65 times that carried in physical solution dissolved in the plasma.

2. The small amount of oxygen dissolved in plasma exerts molecular movement and establishes the partial pressure of oxygen in the blood. This determines the loading (oxygenation) and unloading (deoxygenation) of hemoglobin at the lungs and tissues, respectively.

3. The blood's oxygen transport capacity varies only slightly with normal variations in hemoglobin content. However, iron deficiency anemia significantly decreases the blood's oxygen-carrying capacity and consequently reduces aerobic exercise performance.

4. The s-shaped nature of the oxyhemoglobin dissociation curve shows that hemoglobin saturation changes very little until the P_{O_2} falls below 60 mm Hg. Because this low pressure occurs in the tissues, there is a sharp drop in the quantity of oxygen bound to hemoglobin. Thus, oxygen is rapidly released from capillary blood and flows into the tissues in response to the cells' metabolic demands.

5. At rest, only about 25% of the blood's total oxygen is released to the tissues; the remaining 75% returns to the heart in the venous blood. This is the arteriovenous oxygen differ-

ence and indicates that an "automatic" reserve of oxygen exists so cells can rapidly obtain oxygen should the metabolic demands increase suddenly.

6. Increases in acidity, temperature, carbon dioxide concentration, and red-blood-cell 2, 3-DPG cause an alteration in the molecular structure of hemoglobin, thereby reducing its effectiveness to hold oxygen. Because these factors are accentuated in exercise, the release of oxygen to the tissues is further facilitated.

7. In skeletal and cardiac muscle, the iron–protein pigment myoglobin acts as an "extra" oxygen store. It releases its oxygen at low oxygen pressures and probably facilitates oxygen transfer to the mitochondria, especially during strenuous exercise when cellular P_{O_2} decreases considerably.

TABLE 13-5. *Effects of 15 weeks of run training on the average myoglobin content of various skeletal muscles of rats*[a]

	Myoglobin Content ($mg \cdot g^{-1}$ wet muscle)		
GROUP	HAMSTRINGS	QUADRICEPS	RECTUS ABDOMINIS
Exercised group	1.90	2.17	0.73
Sedentary group	1.05	1.20	0.70
Difference	0.85[b]	0.97[b]	0.03

[a]From Pattengale, P.K., and Holloszy, J.O.: Augmentation of skeletal muscle myoglobin by a program of treadmill running. *Am. J. Physiol.,* 213:783, 1967.
[b]Difference is statistically significant.

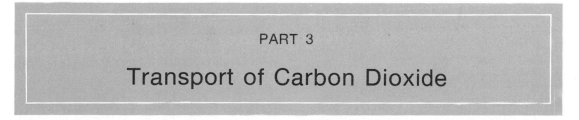

PART 3

Transport of Carbon Dioxide

CARBON DIOXIDE TRANSPORT IN THE BLOOD

Once carbon dioxide is formed in the cell, its only means for "escape" is via the process of diffusion and subsequent transport to the lungs

in the venous blood. As with oxygen, a small amount of carbon dioxide is carried in physical solution in the plasma of the blood. Carbon dioxide is also transported combined with hemoglobin, and a large fraction combines with water and is delivered to the lung in the form of *bicarbonate.* Figure 13-4 illustrates the various

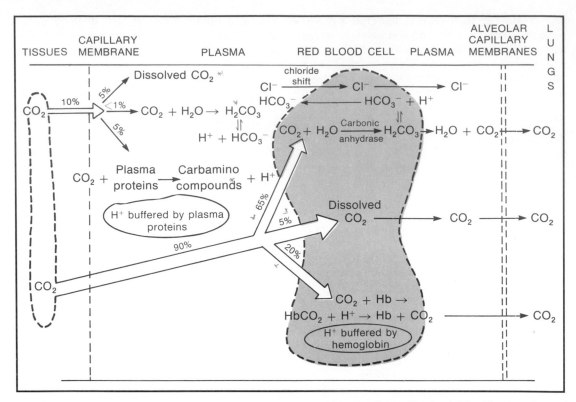

FIG. 13-4. *Transport of carbon dioxide in the plasma and red blood cells as dissolved CO₂, bicarbonate, and carbamino compounds.*

means for transport of carbon dioxide from the tissues to the lungs.

Carbon Dioxide Transport in Solution

Approximately 5% of the carbon dioxide produced during energy metabolism is carried as free carbon dioxide in solution in the plasma. Although this quantity is relatively small, it is the random movement of dissolved carbon dioxide molecules that establishes the P_{CO_2} of the blood.

Carbon Dioxide Transport As Bicarbonate

Carbon dioxide in solution combines with water in a reversible reaction to form *carbonic acid.*

$$CO_2 + H_2O \rightleftharpoons H_2CO_3$$

This reaction is slow, and little carbon dioxide would be carried in this form if it were not for the action of *carbonic anhydrase,* a zinc-containing enzyme in the red blood cell. This cata-

lyst accelerates the interaction of CO_2 and water about 5000 times. In fact, the reaction reaches equilibrium while the blood cell is still moving through the tissue's capillary.

Once carbonic acid is formed in the tissues, most of it ionizes to hydrogen ions (H^+) and bicarbonate ions (HCO_3^-) as follows:

In Tissues

$$CO_2 + H_2O \xrightarrow[\text{anhydrase}]{\text{Carbonic}} H_2CO_3 \longrightarrow H^+ + HCO_3$$

The H^+ is then buffered by the protein portion of hemoglobin to maintain the pH of the blood within relatively narrow limits (see "Acid-Base Regulation," Chap. 14). Because HCO_3^- is quite soluble in blood, it diffuses from the red blood cell into the plasma in exchange for the chloride ion (Cl^-) that moves into the blood cell to maintain ionic equilibrium. This "chloride shift" causes the Cl^- content of the erythrocytes in venous blood to be higher than the arterial blood cells, especially during exercise.

Sixty to eighty percent of the total carbon dioxide is carried as plasma bicarbonate. The bicarbonate is formed in accordance with the law of mass action; as tissue P_{CO_2} increases, carbonic acid is rapidly formed. Conversely, in the lungs, carbon dioxide leaves the blood and plasma P_{CO_2} is lowered. This disturbs the equilibrium between carbonic acid and the formation of bicarbonate ions. As a result, H^+ and HCO_3^- recombine to form carbonic acid. In turn, carbon dioxide and water re-form and carbon dioxide exits through the lungs as follows:

In Lungs

$$H^+ + HCO_3^- \longrightarrow H_2CO_3 \xrightarrow[\text{anhydrase}]{\text{Carbonic}} CO_2 + H_2O$$

Because the plasma bicarbonate is lowered in the pulmonary capillaries, the Cl^- moves from the red blood cell back into the plasma.

Carbon Dioxide Transport as Carbamino Compounds

At the tissue level, carbon dioxide reacts directly with the amino acid molecules of blood proteins to form *carbamino compounds*. This is especially true for the *globin* portion of hemoglobin that carries about 20% of the body's carbon dioxide as follows:

$$CO_2 + NbNH \longrightarrow NbNHCOOH$$
$$\text{(Hemoglobin)} \qquad \text{(Carbaminohemoglobin)}$$

The formation of carbamino compounds is reversed as the plasma P_{CO_2} is lowered in the lungs. This causes carbon dioxide to move into solution and enter the alveoli. Concurrently, the oxygenation of hemoglobin reduces its binding ability for carbon dioxide. The interaction between oxygen loading and carbon dioxide release is termed the *Haldane effect*. This phenomenon facilitates the removal of carbon dioxide in the lung.

SUMMARY

1. A small amount of carbon dioxide is carried as free carbon dioxide in solution in the plasma. This dissolved carbon dioxide establishes the P_{CO_2} of the blood.

2. The major quantity of carbon dioxide is transported in chemical combination with water and is ultimately carried as bicarbonate as follows:

$$CO_2 + H_2O \rightarrow H_2CO_3 \rightarrow H^+ + HCO_3^-$$

In the lungs, this reaction is reversed and carbon dioxide leaves the blood and moves into the alveoli.

3. About 25% of the body's carbon dioxide combines with blood proteins, including hemoglobin, to form carbamino compounds.

References

1. Gardner, G.W. et al.: Cardiorespiratory, hematological and physical performance responses of anemic subjects to iron treatment. Am. J. Clin. Nutr., 28:982, 1975.
2. Lenfant, C. et al.: Effect of altitude on oxygen binding by hemoglobin and on organic phosphate levels. J. Clin. Invest., 47:2652, 1968.
3. Lawrie, R.A.: Effect of enforced exercise on myoglobin in muscle. Nature, 171:1069, 1953.
4. Pattengale, P.K., and Holloszy, J.O.: Augmentation of skeletal muscle myoglobin by a program of treadmill running. Am. J. Physiol., 213:783, 1967.
5. Rand, P.W. et al.: Influence of athletic training on hemoglobin-oxygen affinity. Am. J. Physiol., 224:1334, 1973.
6. Shenk, J.H. et al.: Spectrophotometric characteristics of hemoglobins. J. Biol. Chem., 105:741, 1934.
7. Stainsby, W.N., and Otis, A.B.: Blood flow, blood oxygen tension, oxygen uptake and oxygen transport in skeletal muscle. Am. J. Physiol., 206:858, 1964.
8. Taunton, J.E. et al.: Alterations in 2,3-dpg and P_{50} with maximal and submaximal exercise. Med. Sci. Sports 6:238, 1974.
9. Whipple, G.H.: The hemoglobin of striated muscle. I. Variations due to age and exercise. Am. J. Physiol., 76:693, 1926.

Dynamics of
Pulmonary Ventilation

14

CONTROL OF VENTILATION

The rate and depth of breathing are exquisitely adjusted in response to the body's metabolic needs. In healthy individuals, the arterial pressures of oxygen and carbon dioxide and pH are essentially regulated at the resting value regardless of the exercise intensity. The mechanisms for this regulation, however, are complex and not fully understood. Intricate neural circuits relay information from higher centers in the brain, from the lungs themselves, and from other sensors throughout the body to contribute to the control of ventilation. In addition, the gaseous and chemical state of the blood, especially that bathing the sensitive neurons in the medulla and chemoreceptors in the aorta and carotid arteries act to mediate alveolar ventilation. As a result, relatively constant alveolar gas pressures are maintained even during exhaustive exercise. A schematic representation of the input for ventilatory control is shown in Figure 14-1.

Neural Factors

The normal respiratory cycle results from the inherent and automatic activity of inspiratory neurons whose cell bodies are located in the medial portion of the medulla. These neurons activate the diaphragm and intercostal muscles and the lungs inflate. The inspiratory neurons cease firing due to their own self-limitation as well as to the inhibitory influence from expiratory neurons also located in the medulla. As the lungs inflate, stretch receptors in lung tissue, especially in the bronchioles, are also stimulated. These receptors act through afferent fibers to inhibit inspiration and stimulate expiration.

As the inspiratory muscles relax, exhalation occurs by the passive recoil of the stretched lung tissue and raised ribs. The activation of expiratory neurons and associated muscles that further facilitate expiration are synchronized with this passive phase. As expiration proceeds, the inspiratory center is progressively released from inhibition and once again becomes active.

The inherent activity of the respiratory center cannot itself account for the smooth pattern of breathing in response to metabolic demands. The controlling influence of neurons in the cerebral hemispheres, the pons, and other regions of the brain also plays an important role in establishing the duration and intensity of the inspiratory cycle. For example, activation of the inspiratory center stimulates the pons region of

180

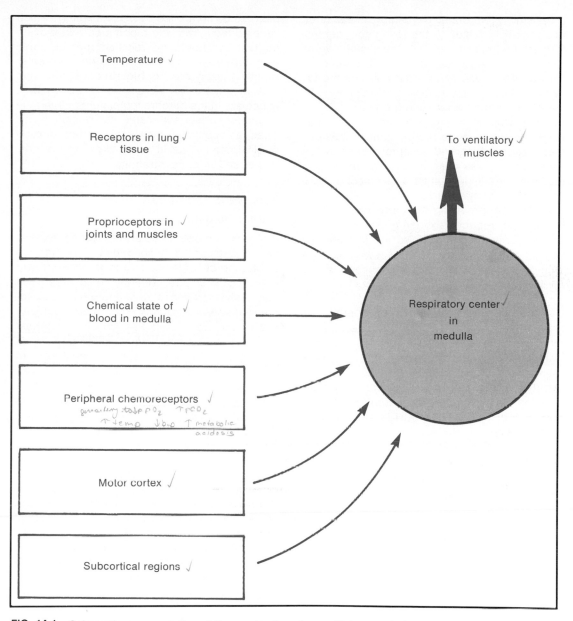

FIG. 14-1. *Schematic representation of the mechanisms for ventilatory control.*

the hindbrain, especially during labored breathing. The pons, in turn, relays excitatory impulses to the expiratory center, which hastens the exhalation phase of the breathing cycle.

Humoral Factors

Pulmonary ventilation at rest is largely regulated by the chemical state of the blood. Variations in arterial P_{O_2}, P_{CO_2}, and acidity and temperature activate sensitive neural units in the medulla and arterial system that adjust ventila-

tion to maintain arterial blood chemistry within narrow limits.

PLASMA P_{O_2} AND CHEMORECEPTORS. Inhalation of a gas mixture containing 80% oxygen greatly increases alveolar P_{O_2} and causes about a 20% reduction in minute ventilation. Conversely, if the inspired oxygen concentration is reduced, ventilation increases, especially if the alveolar P_{O_2} falls below 60 mm Hg. It should be recalled that it is at this P_{O_2} that hemoglobin saturation begins to fall considerably.

Sensitivity to reduced oxygen pressures does not appear to reside in the respiratory center. Rather, it is more a result of the stimulation of peripheral *chemoreceptors*. As illustrated in Figure 14-2, these specialized neurons are located in the arch of the aorta and at the branching of the carotid arteries in the neck.

A decrease in arterial P_{O_2}, as would occur when one ascends to high altitudes, activates the aortic and carotid receptors to increase ventilation. These chemoreceptors alone protect the organism against a reduced oxygen pressure in inspired air.

Aside from providing the early warning system against reduced oxygen pressure, the peripheral chemoreceptors also act to stimulate ventilation in response to increases in carbon dioxide, temperature, metabolic acidosis, and a fall in blood pressure.[31]

PLASMA P_{CO_2} AND HYDROGEN ION CONCENTRATION. At rest, the most important respiratory stimulus is the carbon dioxide pressure in arterial plasma. Small increases in P_{CO_2} in the inspired air cause large increases in minute ventilation. The resting ventilation is almost doubled, for example, by increasing the inspired P_{CO_2} to just 1.7 mm Hg (0.22% CO_2 in inspired air).

The regulation of ventilation by arterial P_{CO_2} is probably not mediated by the action of molecular carbon dioxide. Rather, ventilation appears to be controlled by plasma acidity, which varies directly with the blood's carbon dioxide content. It should be recalled that carbonic acid formed from carbon dioxide and water rapidly dissociates to bicarbonate ions and hydrogen ions. The increase in hydrogen ions, especially in the cerebrospinal fluid bathing the respiratory areas, stimulates inspiratory activity. Then, as ventilation increases, carbon dioxide is eliminated. This in turn lowers the arterial hydrogen ion concentration.

Hyperventilation and Breath-Holding

If a person breathholds after a normal exhalation, it takes about 40 seconds before the urge to breathe becomes so strong that the subject is forced to inspire. The desire to breathe is due mainly to the stimulating effects of increased arterial P_{CO_2} and H^+ concentration and *not* to the decreased P_{O_2} in the breathhold condition.[6a] The breaking point for breathhold corresponds to an increase in arterial P_{CO_2} to about 50 mm Hg.

If this same person prior to breathhold consciously increases ventilation above the normal level, the composition of alveolar air will change and become more like that of ambient air. As a result of this overbreathing, or *hyperventilation,* alveolar P_{CO_2} may decrease to 15 mm Hg. This creates a considerable diffusion gradient for the run-off of carbon dioxide from the venous blood entering the pulmonary capillaries. Consequently, a larger than normal quantity of carbon dioxide leaves the blood, and arterial P_{CO_2} becomes reduced significantly below normal levels. This extends the breathhold until the arterial P_{CO_2} and/or the H^+ concentration rise to the level to stimulate ventilation.

The effects of hyperventilation on arterial P_{CO_2} and subsequent breathhold time have been used by swimmers and divers in an attempt to improve performance. In sprint swimming, for example, it is undesirable from a mechanical viewpoint to roll the body and turn the head during the breathing phase of the stroke. Consequently, many swimmers hyperventilate on the starting blocks to prolong breathhold time during the swim. In sport diving, the intention of hyperventilation is the same as in competitive swimming—to extend breathhold time. In this sport, however, the results can be tragic.[6] As the length and depth of the dive increase,

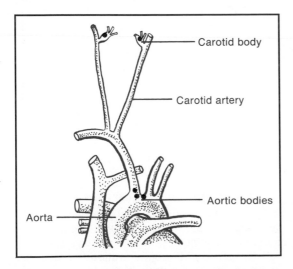

FIG. 14-2. *Cell bodies sensitive to a reduced plasma P_{O_2} are located in the aortic arch and bifurcation of the carotid arteries, and provide the body's first line of defense against arterial hypoxia.*

Labels in figure: Carotid body, Carotid artery, Aortic bodies, Aorta the oxygen content of the blood may be reduced to critically low values before arterial Pco_2 reaches the level to stimulate breathing and signal ascent to the surface. This can cause the diver to lose consciousness before reaching the surface. Hyperventilation and other factors related to diving are discussed in Chapter 25.

REGULATION OF VENTILATION IN EXERCISE

Chemical Control

Chemical stimuli probably cannot entirely explain the increased ventilation, or *hyperpnea*, during physical activity. For example, even when artificial changes are made in Po_2, Pco_2, and acidity, increases in minute ventilation are not nearly as large as those observed in vigorous exercise.

During exercise, arterial Po_2 is *not* reduced to an extent that would increase ventilation due to chemoreceptor stimulation. In fact, in vigorous exercise, the large breathing volumes may cause the alveolar Po_2 to rise above the average resting value of 100 mm Hg. This is illustrated in Figure 14-3 in which venous and alveolar Pco_2 and alveolar Po_2 are plotted in relation to oxygen consumption during a progressive exercise test. The slight *increase* in alveolar Po_2 in heavy exercise may even facilitate the oxygenation of blood in the alveolar capillaries.

During light and moderate exercise, the alveolar (and arterial) Pco_2 is generally maintained at about 40 mm Hg. In strenuous exercise, the ventilatory adjustments usually *reduce* alveolar Pco_2 below this value, sometimes to as low as 25 mm Hg. This would actually result in a decrease in arterial Pco_2 and in a corresponding

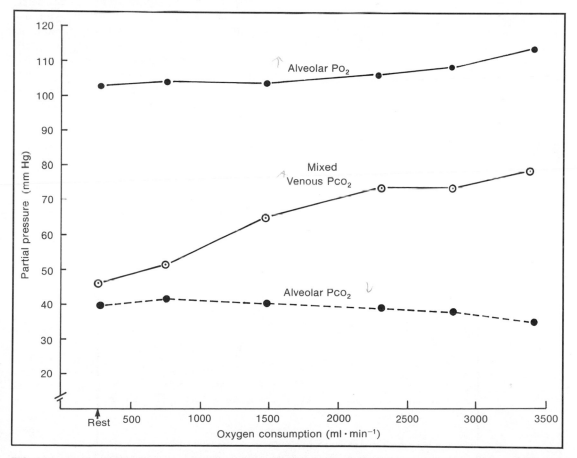

FIG. 14-3. *Values for the Pco_2 of mixed venous blood entering the lungs and the alveolar Po_2 and Pco_2 in relation to oxygen consumption during exercise. (Courtesy of Applied Physiology Laboratory, Queens College.)*

reduction in the ventilatory drive from carbon dioxide during exercise.

Then, one might ask, how do the peripheral chemoreceptors exert their influence on ventilation during exercise? A possible explanation lies in the pattern of ventilation that causes the alveolar and capillary P_{CO_2} to be slightly lower at the end of inhalation and higher at the end of exhalation. Consequently, even though the *average* levels of arterial oxygen, carbon dioxide, and pH are well regulated in moderate exercise, the amplitude of cyclic changes or oscillations in these chemical factors during the breathing cycle may be detected by the chemoreceptors to influence breathing during exercise. This detection may also be facilitated by an increase in the sensitivity of the chemoreceptors as well as by other changes that affect the equilibrium of blood chemistry in exercise.[31]

Nonchemical Control

The changes in minute ventilation at the onset, during, and at the end of moderate exercise are shown in Figure 14-4. As exercise begins, ventilation increases so rapidly that it occurs almost within a single ventilatory cycle.* This immedi-

---

*Some variation has been demonstrated in the rapidity of this initial ventilatory adjustment to exercise. Thus, the response should probably not be considered general, but rather a characteristic pattern of many people.[4,32]

ate change is followed by a plateau that lasts about 30 seconds and then by a gradual increase as the ventilation approaches a steady state. When exercise is terminated, ventilation decreases exponentially to a point about 40% of the steady-state value and then gradually returns to the resting level. The rapidity of the ventilatory response at the onset and at the cessation of exercise strongly suggests that this portion of exercise hyperpnea is mediated by input other than changes in arterial P_{CO_2} and H^+ content.

NEUROGENIC FACTORS. These include both cortical and peripheral influences: (1) *cortical influence*—Neural outflow from regions of the motor cortex as well as cortical activation in anticipation of exercise stimulate the respiratory neurons in the medulla. This cortical outflow may act in concert with the demands of work to contribute to the abrupt increase in ventilation at the start of exercise. (2) *Peripheral influence*—A strong argument has been raised that sensory input from joints, tendons, or muscles influences the ventilatory adjustments to exercise. Although such peripheral receptors have not been identified, experiments involving passive limb movements, electrical stimulation of muscles, and voluntary exercise with the muscle's blood flow occluded support the existence of such *mechanoreceptors* in producing a reflex hyperpnea. In one interesting experiment,[2] the circulation to and from the legs was blocked by pneumatic cuffs during

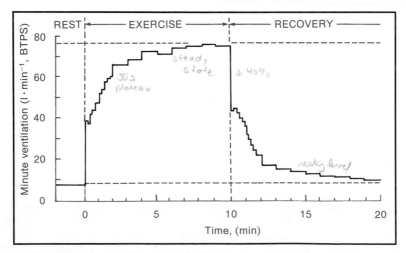

FIG. 14-4. *Rapid and slower components of ventilatory response during and in recovery from steady-rate exercise. (From Dejours, P.: Neurogenic factors in the control of ventilation during exercise. Circ. Res., XX, XXI (Suppl.1), 146-153, 1967. Reprinted by permission of the American Heart Association, Inc.)*

steady-rate bicycle exercise. The carbon dioxide in inspired air was adjusted to maintain a constant arterial P_{CO_2}. The results showed that ventilation increased with exercise, even though the subject's oxygen consumption actually decreased due to the occlusion of muscle blood flow. At the same time, the cuff eliminated the possibility that metabolites from the working muscles might be carried via the circulation to stimulate central chemoreceptors. It was speculated that mechanical factors increased the outflow from peripheral receptors, which in turn modified the activity of the respiratory center.

INFLUENCE OF TEMPERATURE. An increase in body temperature has a direct stimulating effect on the neurons of the respiratory center. This probably exerts some control over ventilation in prolonged exercise. However, the changes in ventilation at the beginning and end of exercise are much more rapid than can be accounted for by changes in core temperature.

Integrated Regulation

The control of breathing in exercise is not the result of a single factor but rather is the combined and perhaps simultaneous result of several chemical and neural stimuli.[17a,25a] The model for respiratory control illustrated in Figure 14-5 suggests that neurogenic stimuli from the cerebral cortex and/or the exercising limbs cause the initial, abrupt increase in breathing at the beginning of exercise. After this initial change, minute ventilation gradually rises to a steady level that adequately meets the demands for metabolic gas exchange. Then, the regulation of alveolar gas pressures is probably maintained by central and reflex chemical stimuli, especially those provided by temperature, carbon dioxide, and hydrogen ions.[25a]

Recent research provides some challenge to this current theory of ventilatory control in exercise. It has been observed in dogs that ventila-

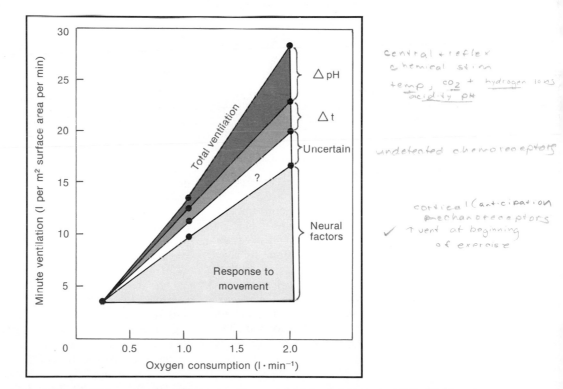

central + reflex
chemical stim
temp, CO_2 + hydrogen ions
acidity pH

undetected chemoreceptors

cortical (anticipation
mechanoreceptors
↑ vent at beginning
of exercise

FIG. 14-5. *Composite of the ventilatory response to exercise. The contribution of changes in acidity (ΔpH) and temperature (Δt), as well as the effects of neurogenic stimuli from the cerebral regions and/or joints and muscles is estimated. The unshaded wedge (?) represents the ventilatory change not quantitatively accounted for by the other three factors. (From Lambertsen, C.J.: Interactions of physical, chemical, and nervous factors in respiratory control. In Medical Physiology. Edited by V.B. Mountcastle, St. Louis, C.V. Mosby Co., 1974.)*

tion increases immediately following an artificially induced, abrupt increase in blood flow through the heart, similar to that which occurs at the onset of exercise.[29] The rapidity of this ventilatory increase due to a surge in cardiac output suggests the presence of previously undetected chemoreceptors. The existence of such chemoreceptors would help explain the effective linkage between the cardiovascular and respiratory systems, as well as the rapid changes in breathing at the start and cessation of exercise.[13]

SUMMARY

1. The normal respiratory cycle results from the inherent activity of neurons in the medulla. Superimposed on this neural output are intricate neural circuits that relay information from higher brain centers, from the lungs themselves, and from other sensors throughout the body.

2. At rest, several chemical factors act directly on the respiratory center or modify its activity reflexly via chemoreceptors to control alveolar ventilation. The most important factors are the level of arterial P_{O_2}, P_{CO_2}, and acidity.

3. Hyperventilation significantly lowers arterial P_{CO_2} and H^+ concentration. This prolongs breathhold time until normal levels of carbon dioxide and acidity are reached to stimulate breathing. Extended breathhold by hyperventilation should not be practiced during underwater swimming: The consequences can be tragic.

4. Ventilatory adjustments to exercise are augmented by nonchemical regulatory factors. These include (a) cortical activation in anticipation of exercise as well as outflow from the motor cortex when exercise begins, (b) peripheral sensory input from mechanoreceptors in joints and muscles, and (c) increases in body temperature.

5. Effective alveolar ventilation in exercise is the result of many neural and chemical factors operating singularly and in combination. Each factor probably takes on greater importance at a particular phase of the adjustment to exercise.

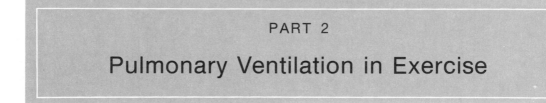

PART 2

Pulmonary Ventilation in Exercise

VENTILATION AND ENERGY DEMANDS

Physical activity affects oxygen consumption and carbon dioxide production more than any other form of metabolic stress. With exercise, large amounts of oxygen diffuse from the alveoli into the venous blood returning to the lungs. Conversely, considerable quantities of carbon dioxide move from the blood into the alveoli. Concurrently, ventilation increases to maintain the proper alveolar gas concentrations to allow for this increased oxygen and carbon dioxide exchange.

Ventilation in Steady-Rate Exercise

The relationship between oxygen consumption and minute ventilation during various levels of exercise up to the maximal oxygen uptake is illustrated in Figure 14-6. During light and moderate steady-rate exercise, ventilation increases linearly with oxygen uptake and averages between 20 and 25 liters of air for each liter of oxygen consumed. With this adjustment in ventilation, there is complete aeration of blood because the alveolar P_{O_2} and P_{CO_2} remain at near resting values.[9]

The ratio of minute ventilation to oxygen consumption is termed the *ventilatory equivalent* and is symbolized $\dot{V}_E/\dot{V}_{O_2}$. In healthy young adults, this ratio is usually maintained at about 25 to 1 (that is, 25 liters of air breathed per liter of oxygen consumed) during submaximal exercise up to about 55% of the maximal oxygen uptake.[19,28,30] The ventilatory equivalent is progressively higher in younger children and averages about 32 liters in children 6 years old.[3]

During prone *swimming*, the ventilatory equivalents are significantly *lower* at all levels of energy expenditure.[11,18] More than likely, this is

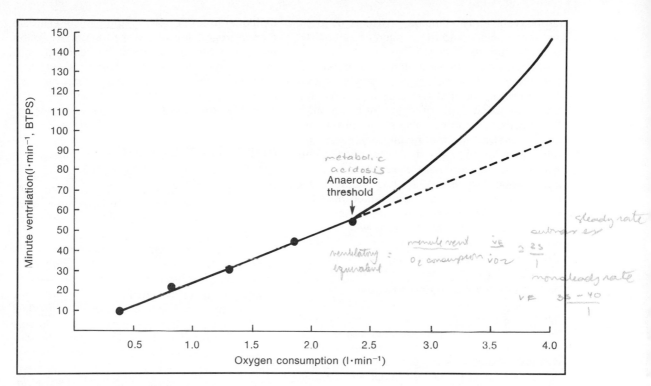

FIG. 14-6. *Pulmonary ventilation and oxygen consumption during incremental exercise to the maximal oxygen uptake. The dashed line represents the extrapolation of the linear relationship between $\dot{V}_E$ and $\dot{V}o_2$ observed during submaximal exercise. The "anaerobic threshold" indicates the onset of metabolic acidosis and is detected by the point at which the relationship between ventilation and oxygen consumption deviates from linearity (see "Anaerobic Threshold").*

due to the restrictive nature of swimming on breathing. This restriction may pose a problem in providing for adequate gas exchange at maximal swimming and may partly contribute to the generally lower maximal oxygen uptake during swimming than during running.[17,18]

Ventilation in Non-Steady-Rate Exercise

In more intense submaximal exercise, the minute ventilation takes a sharp upswing and increases disproportionately with increases in oxygen consumption. As a result, the ventilatory equivalent is greater than that during steady-rate exercise and may increase to 35 or 40 liters of air per liter of oxygen consumed.

ANAEROBIC THRESHOLD. During steady-rate exercise, sufficient oxygen is supplied to and utilized by the working muscles. Under these conditions, lactic acid does not exceed resting values. However, if aerobic metabolism is insufficient, anaerobic glycolysis contributes to the energy requirements and lactic acid is formed.

The onset of this anaerobiosis normally occurs between 55% and 65% of the maximal oxygen uptake in healthy, untrained subjects.[7,25,30] Almost all of the lactic acid generated during anaerobic metabolism is buffered in the blood by sodium bicarbonate in the following reaction:

$$\text{Lactic acid} + \text{NaHCO}_3 \longrightarrow \text{Na lactate} + \text{H}_2\text{CO}_3$$

$$\Downarrow$$

$$\text{H}_2\text{O} + \text{CO}_2$$

The carbon dioxide released in this buffering reaction is exhaled into the atmosphere as the venous blood enters the lungs.

In exercise, the onset of metabolic acidosis, or the *anaerobic threshold,* can be detected in one of several ways: (1) an increase in blood lactic acid, (2) a corresponding decrease in blood pH and bicarbonate, (3) an increase in the respiratory exchange ratio (R) due to a release of "excess" carbon dioxide in the buffering process outlined previously, and (4) a deviation from linearity in the relationship between oxygen consumption and ventilation due to the strong ventilatory stimulus provided by both increased acidity and the release of carbon dioxide through buffering.[21,27,28]

Although all of these methods for detecting the anaerobic threshold require only submaximal exercise, the first two techniques involve blood sampling. The third method, although "bloodless," requires almost a breath-by-breath analysis of the respiratory exchange ratio. The fourth method simply involves the continuous measurement of ventilation during incremental exercise. With this method, the anaerobic threshold can be detected because it represents the point where ventilation deviates from its linear relationship with oxygen consumption (or exercise intensity) (Fig. 14-6). It is at this point that lactic acid buildup and associated changes in bicarbonate, pH, and respiratory exchange ratio occur.[7,30]

Because the anaerobic threshold is reached during submaximal exercise, the test can be terminated well before the subject incurs a significant degree of metabolic acidosis or cardiovascular strain. The anaerobic threshold test has many advantages in clinical evaluations, because maximal test procedures may be contraindicated for some individuals. Although this test "makes sense" from a metabolic standpoint, considerably more research is needed to determine the reliability and objectivity of the test scores and of its applicability and precise meaning as a fitness measure.

SPECIFICITY OF ANAEROBIC THRESHOLD. As with many measures of physiologic function, the ventilatory response in exercise is specific to the exercise task. Greater ventilatory equivalents have been observed in bicycle than in treadmill exercise at all levels of oxygen consumption.[15] This difference was due to relatively greater metabolic acidosis during all submaximal work levels on the bicycle. Consequently, the anaerobic threshold became manifested at a lower level of oxygen uptake in bicycle exercise. The influence of the specific form of exercise on the anaerobic threshold has also been shown for arm-cranking exercise when this type of work is compared to bicycle and treadmill exercises.[7] More than likely, these differences in ventilatory response are the result of variations in the muscle mass activated in specific exercises. At a particular rate of submaximal oxygen consumption, for example, the metabolic rate per unit of muscle mass would

be higher in arm cranking and bicycle exercise than in treadmill walking or running. Thus, the anaerobic threshold would be reached at a lower oxygen uptake. *It certainly appears that different forms of exercise should not be used interchangeably to determine and quantify the anaerobic threshold*.

DOES VENTILATION LIMIT AEROBIC POWER?

If one's ability to breathe during exercise is inadequate, then the line relating pulmonary ventilation and oxygen consumption would curve in a direction opposite to that indicated in Figure 14-6, and the ventilation equivalent would decrease. Such a response would indicate a *failure* for ventilation to keep pace with oxygen consumption; in this instance, we would truly "run out of wind!" Actually, a healthy individual overbreathes during heavy exercise. This was clearly illustrated in Figure 14-3, which demonstrated that the ventilatory adjustment to strenuous exercise generally results in a *decrease* in alveolar P_{CO_2} with a concomitant small *increase* in alveolar P_{O_2}.

ENERGY COST OF BREATHING

Figure 14-7 shows the relationship between pulmonary ventilation and oxygen consumption during rest and submaximal exercise and its division into ventilatory and nonventilatory components.[16] At rest and in light exercise in healthy subjects, the oxygen requirement of breathing is small, averaging 1.9 to 3.1 ml of oxygen per liter of air breathed, or about 2% of the total energy expenditure. As the rate and depth of breathing increase, the cost of breathing rises to about 4 ml of oxygen per liter of ventilation.

The contribution of the oxygen cost of ventilation to the oxygen deficit and recovery oxygen consumption has been estimated during steady-rate exercise.[13] As shown in Figure 14-8 A, the cost of breathing accounted for about 19% of the oxygen deficit and 11% of the recovery oxygen consumption. These results indicate that the oxygen cost of ventilation has approximately a twofold greater influence on oxygen deficit than on recovery oxygen consumption. The reason for the smaller contribution of ventilation cost to the total cost of recov-

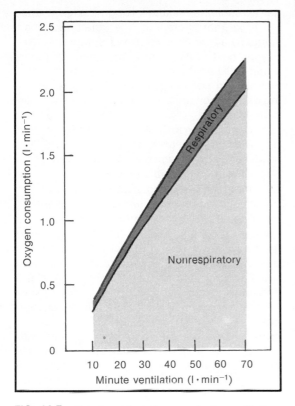

FIG. 14-7. *Relationship between minute ventilation and total oxygen consumption and its respiratory and nonrespiratory components during submaximal exercise in healthy subjects. (From Levison, H., and Cherniack, R.: Ventilatory cost of exercise in chronic obstructive pulmonary disease. J. Appl. Physiol., 25:21, 1968.)*

ery is because minute ventilation volume declines exponentially at the end of exercise in the same fashion as recovery oxygen intake (Fig. 14-8 B). This is clearly not the case in the beginning of exercise, where ventilation increases at a much greater rate than does oxygen consumption.

Respiratory Disease

In respiratory disease, the work of breathing in itself may become an exhaustive exercise. In patients with obstructive lung disease, the cost of ventilation at rest may be three times that of normals, and in light exercise it may increase to as much as 10 ml of oxygen for each liter of air breathed.[16] In severe pulmonary disease, the cost of breathing may easily reach 40% of the total exercise oxygen consumption. This would

encroach on the oxygen available to the exercising, nonrespiratory muscles and seriously limit the exercise capabilities of these patients.

Cigarette Smoking

The research relating smoking habits to exercise performance is meager, although the majority of endurance athletes avoid cigarettes for fear of hindering performance due to a "loss of wind." The chronic cigarette smoker tends to show a decrease in dynamic lung function that, in severe instances, is manifested in obstructive lung disorders. Such pathologic processes,

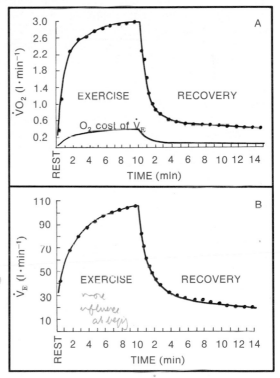

FIG. 14-8. *A, Estimated oxygen cost of ventilation on oxygen deficit and recovery oxygen consumption. For the 33 subjects, the steady-rate oxygen uptake averaged 2.90 liters · min⁻¹ during the 10-minute exercise on a bicycle ergometer (60 rpm at 3.0 kg; 1080 kgm · min⁻¹). B, Two-component exponential curve form for exercise and recovery ventilation. Mean ventilation volume averaged 108 liters · min⁻¹, BTPS. (From Katch, F.I. et al.: The influence of the estimated oxygen cost of ventilation on oxygen deficit and recovery oxygen intake for moderately heavy bicycle ergometer exercise. Med. Sci. Sports, 4:71, 1972. Copyright 1972, the American College of Sports Medicine. Reprinted by Permission.)*

however, usually take some time to develop. Thus, with young smokers, chronic alterations in lung function may be minimal and insignificant in terms of their effect on physical performance. Other more *acute effects* of cigarette smoking may adversely affect exercise capacity.

Airway resistance at rest is increased as much as threefold in both chronic smokers and nonsmokers following 15 puffs on a cigarette during a 5-minute period.[20] This added resistance to breathing lasts an average of 35 minutes and probably has only a minor effect in light exercise where the oxygen cost of breathing is small. In vigorous exercise, however, this residual effect of smoking could be detrimental because the additional cost of breathing might become prohibitive. In this situation, the total oxygen available for muscular exercise would be reduced. Apparently, the bronchorestriction from smoking is not due to the nicotine in cigarettes but to a constrictive reflex triggered from sensory stimulation by minute particles in the cigarette smoke.

The oxygen cost of breathing was studied in six habitual smokers immediately after they smoked two cigarettes and one day after abstinence from tobacco.[24] The subjects ran on the treadmill at a speed and grade that required approximately 80% of the individual's max $\dot{V}O_2$. Ventilation during the "smoking" and "nonsmoking" runs was then increased in two ways: (1) Subjects voluntarily hyperventilated during the run (Voluntary HV), and (2) hyperventilation was induced by increasing alveolar PCO_2 by having subjects breathe through a large-diameter tube that increased the anatomic dead space by about 1400 ml (Dead Space HV). The oxygen cost of the "extra" breathing was then determined as the difference between the normal oxygen consumption and the corresponding oxygen consumption in the hyperventilation experiments.

As can be seen in Table 14-1, the oxygen cost of breathing decreased between 13% and 79% as a result of abstinence. During exercise at 80% of maximal aerobic power, the energy requirement of breathing averaged 14% of the exercise oxygen consumption after smoking and only 9% in the "nonsmoking" trials for the heaviest smokers. Also, heart rates averaged 5% to 7% lower during exercise following one day of cigarette abstinence, and all subjects reported that they felt better exercising in the nonsmoking condition. It appears that a substantial reversibility of the increased oxygen cost of breathing with smoking can occur in chronic smokers with *only one day of abstinence*. Thus, if an athlete is unable to eliminate smoking completely, he should at least stop on the day of competition.

ADAPTATIONS IN BREATHING WITH TRAINING

Aerobic training brings about several changes in pulmonary ventilation during maximal and submaximal exercise.

TABLE 14-1.   *The oxygen cost of hyperventilation (HV) in "smoking" and "nonsmoking" exercise that represented approximately 80% of each subject's max $\dot{V}O_2$[a]*

	SMOKING				NONSMOKING			
	VOLUNTARY HV		DEAD SPACE HV		VOLUNTARY HV		DEAD SPACE HV	
SUBJECT	$\dot{V}_E$ (l·min⁻¹)	COST (ml·l⁻¹)	$\dot{V}_E$ (l·min⁻¹)	COST (ml·l⁻¹)	$\dot{V}_E$ (l·min⁻¹)	COST (ml·l⁻¹)	$\dot{V}_E$ (l·min⁻¹)	COST (ml·l⁻¹)
1	26.4	15.1	18.9	12.7	22.7	11.4	23.0	6.5
2	39.0	10.3	28.1	5.9	42.6	11.3	41.3	4.8
3	22.8	7.9	27.2	7.0	23.8	7.2	22.8	5.7
4	36.3	5.0	28.7	5.6	44.7	3.8	18.6	−1.6[b]
5	52.7	13.5	26.7	12.4	75.2	6.1	22.8	5.7
6	22.4	8.5	27.3	1.1	23.2	3.4	30.1	3.0
Average	32.6	10.1	26.2	7.4	38.7	7.2	26.5	4.0

[a] From Rode, A., and Shephard, R.J.: The influence of cigarette smoking upon the oxygen cost of breathing jn near-maximal exercise. *Med. Sci. Sports,* 3:51, 1971. Copyright 1971, the American College of Sports Medicine. Reprinted by Permission.
[b] The implication of the "negative" cost of $\dot{V}_E$ in this subject is that the added dead space reduced the cost of the normal exercise ventilation.

1. *Maximal exercise.* As might be expected, maximal exercise ventilation increases with improvements in maximal oxygen uptake. This makes sense physiologically, since any increase in aerobic capacity results in a larger oxygen requirement and in the correspondingly larger production of carbon dioxide, which must be eliminated through increased alveolar ventilation.

2. *Submaximal exercise.* Following only 4 weeks of training, a considerable *reduction* in the ventilatory equivalent is observed in submaximal exercise.[1] Consequently, there is a smaller amount of air breathed at a particular rate of submaximal oxygen consumption; this reduces the percentage of the total oxygen cost of exercise attributable to breathing. Theoretically, this would be of considerable importance in performing prolonged, vigorous exercise, because any oxygen freed from use by the respiratory muscles becomes available to the exercising muscles.

The mechanism for the training adaptations in ventilation in submaximal exercise is unknown. However, these changes have been consistently observed in studies of adolescents and in both young and older men and women.[5,8,12,14,26] In general, the tidal volume becomes larger and breathing frequency is considerably reduced. Air remains in the lungs for a longer period of time between breaths. This results in an increase in the amount of oxygen extracted from the inspired air. The exhaled air of trained individuals often contains only 14% to 15% oxygen during submaximal exercise, whereas the expired air of untrained persons may contain 18% oxygen at the same work level. Obviously, the untrained person must ventilate proportionately more air to achieve the same submaximal oxygen uptake.

Ventilatory adaptations appear to be highly *specific* to the type of exercise used in training. When subjects performed either arm or leg exercise, the ventilation equivalent was always greater during arm exercise than during leg work (Fig. 14-9).[23] After training, there was a significant reduction in the ventilatory equivalent. However, this was noted *only* during exercise that used the specifically trained muscle groups. For the group trained by arm ergometry, the ventilation equivalent was reduced only in arm exercise and vice-versa for the leg-trained group. This training adaptation was closely re-

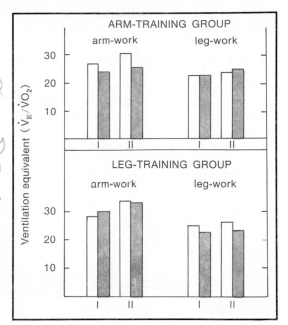

FIG. 14-9. *Ventilatory equivalents during light (I) and heavy (II) submaximal arm and leg exercise before and after arm training (top) and leg training (bottom). Shaded bars indicate post-training values. (From Rasmussen, B. et al.: Pulmonary ventilation, blood gases, and blood pH after training of the arms and the legs. J. Appl. Physiol., 38:250, 1975.)*

lated to a less pronounced rise in blood lactic acid and heart rate in the specific training exercise. It is likely that the ventilatory adjustment to training results from local neural or chemical adaptations in the specific muscles trained through exercise.

SUMMARY

1. In light to moderate exercise, ventilation increases linearly with oxygen consumption. The ventilatory equivalent is maintained at 20 to 25 liters of air breathed per liter of oxygen consumed.

2. In non-steady-rate exercise, ventilation increases disproportionately with increases in oxygen consumption, and the ventilatory equivalent may reach 35 or 40 liters.

3. The sharp upswing in ventilation during incremental exercise provides an effective, simple means for establishing a person's *anaerobic threshold.* This measure relates closely to the onset of anaerobiosis and the subsequent accumulation of lactic acid. Thus, one aspect

of aerobic fitness can be evaluated without a significant degree of metabolic acidosis or cardiovascular strain.

4. For healthy people, the oxygen cost of breathing is relatively small, even during the most severe exercise. In respiratory disease, however, the work of breathing becomes excessive, and alveolar ventilation often becomes inadequate.

5. Airway resistance is greatly increased following cigarette smoking. This increases the oxygen cost of breathing, which could be detri-

mental during prolonged, vigorous exercise. Substantial reversibility of these smoking effects can occur with one day of abstinence.

6. Training generally reduces the ventilatory equivalent in submaximal exercise. This "conserves" oxygen because the cost of breathing for a particular work task is lowered.

7. Ventilatory adjustments with training follow the principle of training specificity. A more efficient breathing pattern is generally observed *only* during the type of exercise used in training.

PART 3

Acid–Base Regulation

BUFFERING

Substances that dissociate and release H^+ are called *acids,* whereas a compound that can pick up or accept H^+ is a *base*. The term *buffering* is used to designate reactions that minimize changes in H^+ concentration, and the chemicals involved in preventing this change are termed buffers.

The acid–base quality of body fluids must be regulated within narrow limits because metabolism is highly sensitive to the H^+ concentration (pH) of the reacting medium. Blood pH is normally regulated on the slightly alkaline side of neutrality at a pH value of 7.4; this means that slightly more negative hydroxyl ions (OH^-) are present than H^+. An increase in pH above the normal average of 7.4 is the direct result of a decrease in H^+ concentration and is termed *alkalosis.* Conversely, an increase in H^+ concentration (decrease in pH) is referred to as *acidosis.*

A buffering system consists of a weak acid and the salt of that acid. The bicarbonate buffer, for example, is made up of the weak acid, *carbonic acid,* and the salt of that acid, *sodium bicarbonate.* Carbonic acid is formed when bicarbonate binds H^+. As long as the H^+ concentration remains elevated, the reaction produces the weak acid because the excess H^+ ions are bound in accordance with the general reaction:

$$H^+ + Buffer \longrightarrow H\text{–}Buffer$$

However, if the concentration of H^+ decreases (as would occur during hyperventilation when plasma carbonic acid decreases because carbon dioxide is eliminated from the blood), the buffering reaction moves in the opposite direction:

$$H^+ + Buffer \longleftarrow H\text{–}Buffer$$

In the process, H^+ ions are released and acidity increases.

Much of the carbon dioxide generated in energy metabolism reacts with water to form the relatively weak carbonic acid. This then dissociates to H^+ and HCO_3^-. Likewise, lactic acid, a stronger acid, reacts with sodium bicarbonate to form sodium lactate and carbonic acid; in turn, carbonic acid dissociates and increases the H^+ concentration of the extracellular fluids. Other organic acids such as fatty acids dissociate and liberate H^+, as do the sulfuric and phosphoric acids produced during protein breakdown.

Three mechanisms control the acid-base quality of the internal environment: (1) chemical buffers, (2) pulmonary ventilation, and (3) kidney function.

CHEMICAL BUFFERS

Bicarbonate, phosphate, and protein chemical buffers provide the rapid first line of defense to maintain a consistency in the acid-base quality of the internal environment.

Bicarbonate Buffer

The bicarbonate buffer system consists of carbonic acid and sodium bicarbonate in solution. In the buffering process, for example, hydrochloric acid (a strong acid) is changed into a much weaker acid by combining with sodium bicarbonate in the reaction:

$$HCl + Na\ HCO_3 \longrightarrow Na\ Cl + H_2CO_3$$

$$\Updownarrow$$

$$H^+ + HCO^-_3$$

Buffering by sodium bicarbonate, therefore, produces only a slight reduction in pH. As mentioned previously, sodium bicarbonate in the plasma exerts a strong buffering action on lactic acid, the anaerobic metabolite. This causes the formation of sodium lactate and carbonic acid; consequently, a change in pH is minimized. Any additional increase in H$^+$ concentration (acidity) brought about by carbonic acid dissociation causes the dissociation reaction to move back in the opposite direction. In this situation, carbon dioxide is released into solution as follows:

Acidosis

$$H_2O + CO_2 \longleftarrow H_2CO_3 \longleftarrow H^+ + HCO_3^-$$

An increase in plasma carbon dioxide or acidity immediately stimulates ventilation, and the "excess" carbon dioxide is eliminated. Conversely, if the H$^+$ concentration is reduced and the body fluids become more alkaline, the ventilatory drive is inhibited, carbon dioxide is retained to combine with water, and the acidity is normalized as follows:

Alkalosis

$$H_2O + CO_2 \longrightarrow H_2CO_3 \longrightarrow H^+ + HCO_3^-$$

Phosphate Buffer

This buffer system consists of phosphoric acid and sodium phosphate. These chemicals act in a manner similar to that of the bicarbonate system. The phosphate buffer is particularly important in regulating the acid–base balance in the kidney tubules and intracellular fluids where there is a relatively high concentration of phosphates.

Protein Buffer

Although carbonic acid produced from the union of water and carbon dioxide is a relatively weak acid, the H$^+$ released when it dissociates must be buffered in the venous blood. By far, the most important H$^+$ acceptor for this function is hemoglobin. Its potency for regulating acidity is almost six times greater than that of the other plasma proteins. In addition, when hemoglobin releases its oxygen to the cells, it becomes a weaker acid. This, in turn, increases its affinity for binding with H$^+$. The H$^+$ generated from the formation of carbonic acid in the erythrocyte combines readily with deoxygenated hemoglobin (Hb$^-$) in the reaction:

$$H^+ + Hb^-\ (Protein) \longrightarrow HHb$$

Intracellular tissue proteins also contribute to the regulation of plasma pH. Some amino acids have free acidic radicals that, when dissociated, form OH$^-$ that can react with H$^+$ to form water.

Relative Power of Chemical Buffers

Table 14-2 shows the relative power of the different chemical buffers in the blood, as well as blood plus interstitial fluids combined. As a frame of reference, the buffering power of the bicarbonate system is assumed to be 1.00.

TABLE 14-2. Relative buffering power of chemical buffers[a]

CHEMICAL BUFFER	BLOOD	BLOOD PLUS INTERSTITIAL FLUIDS
Bicarbonate	1.0	1.0
Phosphate	0.3	0.3
Proteins (excluding hemoglobin)	1.4	0.8
Hemoglobin	5.3	1.5

[a]Modified from Guyton, A.C.: Medical Physiology. Philadelphia, W.B. Saunders Co., 1971.

PHYSIOLOGIC BUFFERS

The second line of defense in acid–base regulation is the ventilatory and renal systems. These provide buffering function only when a change in pH has already occurred.

Ventilatory Buffer

Any increase in the quantity of free H^+ in extracellular fluids and plasma directly stimulates the respiratory center and causes an immediate increase in alveolar ventilation. This adjustment rapidly reduces alveolar P_{CO_2} and causes carbon dioxide to be "blown-off" from the blood. The reduction in plasma carbon dioxide facilitates the recombining of H^+ and HCO_3^-, thus lowering the free H^+ in the plasma. For example, if alveolar ventilation at rest is doubled by hyperventilation, the blood becomes more alkaline and pH increases by 0.23 units from 7.40 to 7.63. Conversely, reducing normal ventilation by one-half causes the blood to become more acidic by about 0.23 pH units. The potential magnitude of the ventilatory buffer has been estimated to be about twice that of the combined effect of all the chemical buffers.

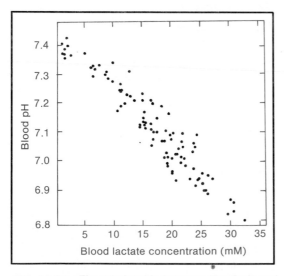

FIG. 14-10. *The relationship between blood pH and blood lactate concentration at rest and in maximal intermittent exercise of short duration. (From Osnes, J.B., and Hermansen, L.: Acid-base balance after maximal exercise of short duration. J. Appl. Physiol., 32:59, 1972.)*

Renal Buffer

The chemical buffers nullify the effects of excess acid only temporarily. The excretion of H^+ by the kidneys, although more time-consuming than the action of the chemical and ventilatory buffers, is of utmost importance if the buffer reserve, or *alkaline reserve*, of the body is to be maintained. To this end, the kidneys stand as final sentinels. Acidity can be controlled by the renal buffer through complex chemical reactions in the renal tubules that involve alterations in the amounts of ammonia and H^+ secreted into the urine and in the amounts of alkali, chloride, and bicarbonate reabsorbed.

EFFECTS OF EXERCISE AND TRAINING

The regulation of pH becomes progressively more difficult in strenuous exercise where there is an increase in H^+ from both carbon dioxide and lactic acid formation. This occurs particularly in the case of maximal, intermittent exercise of short duration, when blood lactate values can reach 30 millimols (mmol) (about 270 mg of lactate per 100 ml of blood), or more.[10]

As seen in Figure 14-10, a generally linear relationship exists at rest and in various levels of intermittent exercise between blood lactate concentration and blood pH.[22] In these experiments, blood lactate varied between 0.8 mmol at rest (pH 7.43) and 32.1 mmol, or approximately 290 mg of lactate per 100 ml of blood during exhaustive exercise (pH 6.80).

These results indicate that humans are able *temporarily* to tolerate pronounced disturbances in the acid–base balance, at least as low as a pH of about 6.80 (which is one of the lowest values ever reported for a human subject). The degree of acidosis at pH values of 7.00 and lower is not without consequence, however; many subjects experienced nausea, headache, and dizziness, as well as pain in the muscle groups involved in exercise.

Does training improve buffering capacity? It is well known that vigorous anaerobic training enables a person to tolerate higher lactic acid levels and lower plasma pH values than were possible before training. It is tempting to speculate that such training may have some positive effect on the body's capability for acid–base regulation, perhaps through an enhancement of the chemical buffers or the alkaline reserve. However, it has never been shown that buffering capacity becomes enhanced through specific modes of training. Improved anaerobic tolerance following a training program may be due to motivational influences; the repeated stress of vigorous training probably modifies one's mental attitude for tolerating the extreme discomforts of the acid condition.

SUMMARY

1. The acid–base quality of the body fluids is normally regulated within narrow limits by chemical and physiologic buffer systems.

2. The bicarbonate, phosphate, and protein chemical buffers provide the rapid first line of defense in acid–base regulation. These buffers consist of a weak acid and the salt of that acid. In an acidic condition, their action converts strong acids to weaker acids and neutral salts.

3. The lungs and kidneys regulate pH when the chemical buffer system is stressed. Changes in alveolar ventilation can rapidly and significantly alter the free H^+ in extracellular fluids. In response to increased acidity, the renal tubules act as final sentinals and secrete H^+ into the urine and reabsorb bicarbonate.

4. Vigorous exercise creates a great demand for buffering; thus the regulation of pH becomes progressively more difficult. From available evidence, however, it does not appear that training enhances the body's buffering capacity.

References

1. Andrew, G.M. et al.: Effect of athletic training on exercise cardiac output. J. Appl. Physiol., *21:*603, 1966.
2. Asmussen, E., and Nielsen, M.: Experiments on nervous factors controlling respiration and circulation during exercise employing blocking of blood flow. Acta Physiol. Scand., *60:*103, 1964.
3. Åstrand, P.O.: Experimental studies of physical working capacity in relation to sex and age. Copenhagen, Munksgaard, 1952.
4. Beaver, W.L., and Wasserman, K.: Transients in ventilation at the start and end of exercise. J. Appl. Physiol., 25:330, 1968.
5. Clausen, J.P. et al.: The effects of training on the heart rate during arm and leg exercise. Scand. J. Clin. Lab. Invest., 26:295, 1970.
6. Craig, A.B., Jr.: Summary of 58 cases of loss of consciousness during underwater swimming and diving. Med. Sci. Sports, 8:171, 1976.
6a. Craig, A.B., Jr.: Principles and problems of underwater diving. The Physician and Sports Medicine, 8:72, 1980.
7. Davis, J.A. et al.: Anaerobic threshold and maximal aerobic power for three modes of exercise. J. Appl. Physiol., *41:* 544, 1976.
8. Fringer, M.N., and Stull, G.A.: Changes in cardiorespiratory parameters during periods of training and detraining in young adult females. Med. Sci. Sports, 6:20, 1974.
9. Grimby, G.: Respiration in exercise. Med. Sci. Sports *1:*9, 1969.
10. Hermansen, L.: Lactate production during exercise. *In* Muscle Metabolism During Exercise. Edited by B. Pernow and B. Saltin. New York, Plenum, 1971.
11. Holmér, I. et al.: Hemodynamic and respiratory responses compared in swimming and running. J. Appl. Physiol., *37:*48, 1974.
12. Jirka, Z., and Adamus, M.: Changes of ventilation equivalents in young people in the course of three years of training. J. Sports Med., *5:*1, 1965.
13. Katch, F. I. et al.: The influence of the estimated oxygen cost of ventilation on oxygen deficit and resting oxygen intake for moderately heavy bicycle ergometer exercise. Med. Sci. Sports, *4:*71, 1972.

14. Kilbom, A.: Physical training in women. Scand. J. Clin. Invest., *28:* Suppl. 119, 1971.
15. Koyal, S. N. et al.: Ventilatory responses to the metabolic acidosis of treadmill and cycle ergometry. J. Appl. Physiol., *40:*864, 1976.
16. Levison, H., and Cherniack, R.: Ventilatory cost of exercise in chronic obstructive pulmonary disease. J. Appl. Physiol. *25:*21, 1968.
17. Magel, J. R. et al.: Specificity of swim training on maximum oxygen uptake. J. Appl. Physiol., *38:*151, 1975.
17a. Mahler, M.: Neural and humoral signals for pulmonary ventilation arising in exercising muscle. Med. Sci. Sports, *11:*191, 1979.
18. McArdle, W.D. et al.: Metabolic and cardiorespiratory response during free swimming and treadmill walking. J. Appl. Physiol., *30:* 733, 1971.
19. McArdle, W.D. et al.: Metabolic and cardiovascular adjustment to work in air and water at 18, 25 and 33°C. J. Appl. Physiol., *40:*85, 1976.
20. Nadel, J.A., and Comroe, J.H.: Acute effects of inhalation of cigarette smoke on airway resistance. J. Appl. Physiol., *16:*713, 1961.
21. Naimark, A. et al.: Continuous measurement of ventilatory exchange ratio during exercise. J. Appl. Physiol., *19:* 644, 1964.
22. Osnes, J. B., and Hermansen, L.: Acid-base balance after maximal exercise of short duration. J. Appl. Physiol., *32:* 59, 1972.
23. Rasmussen, R. et al.: Pulmonary ventilation, blood gases and blood pH after training of the arms and the legs. J. Appl. Physiol., *38:* 250, 1975.
24. Rode, A., and Shephard, R. J.: The influence of cigarette smoking upon the oxygen cost of breathing in near-maximal exercise. Med. Sci. Sports, *3:* 51, 1971.
25. Shephard, R. J. et al.: Standardization of submaximal exercise tests. Bull. WHO, *38:* 765, 1968.
25a. Sutton, J.R., and Jones, N.L.: Control of pulmonary ventilation during exercise and mediators in the blood: CO_2 and hydrogen ion. Med. Sci. Sports, *11:*198, 1979.
26. Tzankoff, S.P. et al.: Physiological adjustments to work in older men as affected by physical training. J. Appl. Physiol., *33:* 346, 1972.
27. Wasserman, K., and McIlroy, M. B.: Detecting threshold of anaerobic metabolism in cardiac patients during exercise. Am. J. Cardiol., *14:* 844, 1964.
28. Wasserman, K. et al.: Interactions of physiological mechanisms during exercise. J. Appl. Physiol., *22:* 71, 1967.
29. Wasserman, K. et al.: Cardiodynamic hyperpnea: hyperpnea secondary to cardiac output increase. J. Appl. Physiol., *36:* 457, 1974.
30. Wasserman, K. et al.: Anaerobic threshold and respiratory gas exchange during exercise. J. Appl. Physiol., *35:* 236, 1973.
31. Whipp, B. J., and Davis, J. A.: Peripheral chemoreceptors and exercise hyperpnea. Med. Sci. Sports, *11:* 204, 1979.
32. Whipp, B.J., and Wasserman, K.: The effect of work intensity on the transient respiratory response immediately following exercise. Med. Sci. Sports, *5:* 14, 1973.

The Cardiovascular System

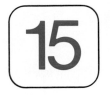

The *cardiovascular system,* which serves to integrate the body as a unit, provides the muscles with a continuous stream of nutrients and oxygen so that a high energy output can be maintained for a considerable period of time. Conversely, by-products of metabolism are rapidly removed from the site of energy release via the circulation.

In Chapters 15, 16, and 17, we explore the process of circulation, especially its role in oxygen delivery during exercise, and examine the basic differences in cardiovascular function between physically trained and untrained individuals. Oxygen transport, coupled with the capability of specific muscles to generate ATP aerobically, ultimately sets the maximum level of aerobic energy release during strenuous physical activity.

COMPONENTS OF THE CARDIOVASCULAR SYSTEM

The cardiovascular system is a continuous vascular circuit consisting of a pump, a high-pressure distribution circuit, exchange vessels, and a low-pressure collection and return circuit. A schematic view of this system is presented in Figure 15-1.

The Heart

The heart provides the impetus for blood flow. It is situated in the midcenter of the chest cavity with about two-thirds of its mass to the left of the body's midline. Although this four-chambered muscular organ weighs less than a pound, it beats so steadily and powerfully that the force generated during its 40 million beats per year could lift its owner 100 miles above the earth. Even for a person of average fitness, the maximum output of blood from this remarkable organ is greater than the fluid output from a household faucet turned wide open.

The heart muscle, or *myocardium,* is a form of striated muscle similar to skeletal muscle. The individual fibers, however, are multinucleated cells interconnected in a latticework fashion. Consequently, when one cell is stimulated or depolarized, the action potential speeds through the myocardium to all cells, causing the heart to function as a unit.

Figure 15-2 shows the details of the heart as a pump. Functionally, the heart may be viewed as two separate pumps. The hollow chambers that comprise the right side of the heart (right heart) perform two important functions: (1) receive blood returning from all parts of the body, and (2) pump blood to the lungs for aeration via the pulmonary circulation. The left heart receives oxygenated blood from the lungs and pumps it into the thick-walled, muscular *aorta* for distribution throughout the body in the systemic circulation. A thick, solid muscular wall or *septum* separates the left and right sides of the heart.

The *atrioventricular valves* situated in the heart provide for a one-way passage of blood from the right atrium to the right ventricle (*tricuspid valve*) and from the left atrium to the left ventricle (*mitral* or *bicuspid valve*). The *semilunar valves* located in the arterial wall just outside the heart prevent blood from flowing back into the heart between contractions.

The relatively thin-walled, saclike atrial chambers serve as primer pumps to receive and store blood during the period of ventricular contraction. About 70% of the blood returning to the atria flows directly into the ventricle be-

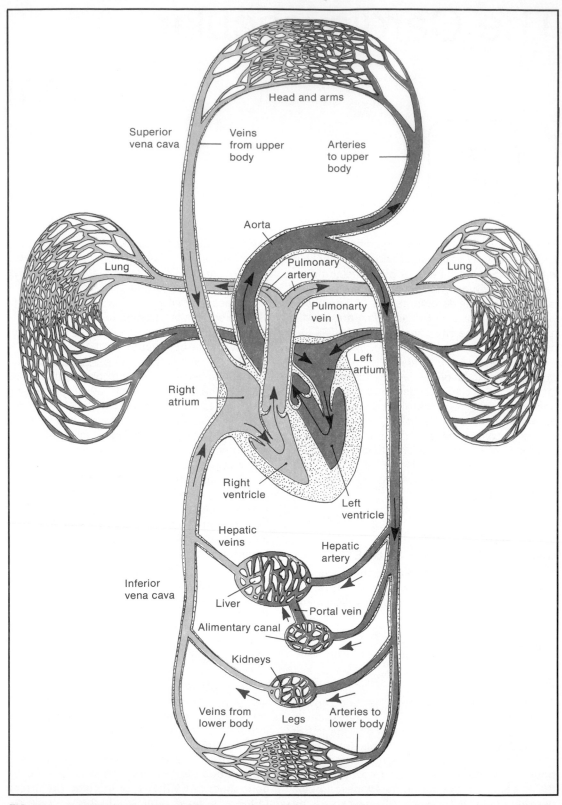

FIG. 15-1. *Schematic view of the cardiovascular system consisting of the heart and the pulmonary and systemic vascular circuits. The dark shading indicates the oxygen-rich arterial blood, whereas the deoxygenated venous blood is somewhat paler. In the pulmonary circuit, the situation is reversed, and oxygenated blood returns to the heart in the right and left pulmonary veins.*

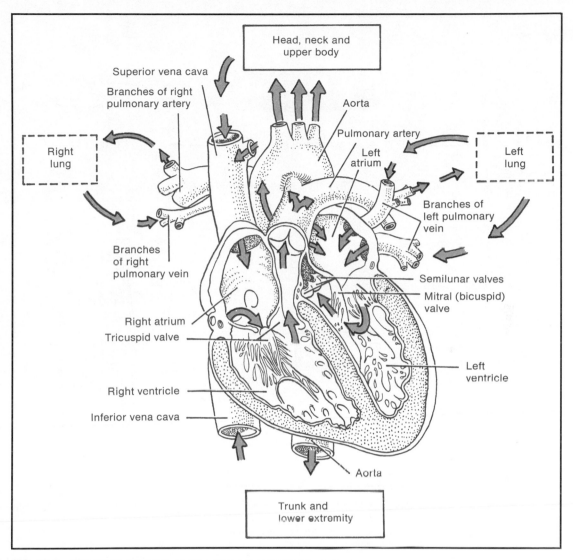

FIG. 15-2. *The heart: Direction of blood flow is indicated by arrows.*

fore the atria contract. The simultaneous contraction of both atria then forces the remaining blood into their respective ventricles directly below. Almost immediately following atrial contraction, the ventricles contract and force blood into the arterial system.

At the onset of ventricular contraction, the heart valves remain closed for 0.02 to 0.06 seconds. This brief interval of rising ventricular tension during which the heart volume and fiber length remain unchanged represents the heart's *isometric contraction period.* As ventricular pressure builds, the atrioventricular valves snap closed. Blood is ejected from the

heart when the ventricular pressure exceeds arterial pressure. By the nature of the spiral and circular arrangement of bands of cardiac muscle, blood is virtually "wrung out" of the heart with each contraction.

The Arterial System

THE ARTERIES. The arteries are the high-pressure tubing that conducts oxygen-rich blood to the tissues. As depicted in Figure 15-3, the arteries are composed of layers of connective tissue and smooth muscle. The walls of these ves-

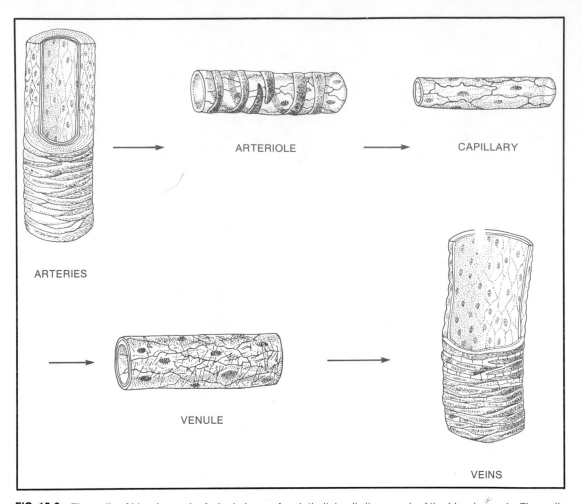

FIG. 15-3. *The walls of blood vessels. A single layer of endothelial cells lines each of the blood vessels. The walls of arteries are surrounded by fibrous tissue and wrapped in several layers of smooth muscle cells. The arterioles are similar but are sheathed in a single layer of muscle cells, whereas the capillaries consist only of a layer of endothelial cells. In the venule, the endothelial cells are sheathed in fibrous tissues whereas the veins also possess a layer of smooth muscle.*

sels are so thick that no gaseous exchange takes place between arterial blood and the surrounding tissues. Blood pumped from the left ventricle into the highly muscular yet elastic *aorta* is eventually distributed throughout the body via smaller arterial branches called *arterioles*. The walls of arterioles are composed of circular layers of smooth muscle that either constrict or relax to regulate peripheral blood flow. As is discussed in a following section, it is the capacity of these "resistance vessels" to alter dramatically their internal diameter that provides a rapid and effective means for regulating blood flow through the vascular circuit. This redistribution function is especially impor-

tant during exercise because blood can be diverted to working muscles from areas that can temporarily compromise their blood supply.

BLOOD PRESSURE. A surge of blood enters the aorta with each contraction of the left ventricle. Because the peripheral vessels do not permit blood to be "run-off" from the arterial system as rapidly as it is ejected from the heart, a portion of the blood pumped from the heart is "stored" in the aorta. This creates pressure within the entire arterial system and causes a pressure wave to travel down the aorta to the remote branches of the arterial tree. This stretch and subsequent recoil of the arterial wall during a cardiac cycle can readily be felt as the characteristic "pulse" in any superficial artery of the body. In healthy individuals, the pulse rate and heart rate are identical.

At rest, the highest pressure generated by the heart is usually about 120 mm Hg during the contraction, or *systole,* of the left ventricle. The point of reference for this measurement is usually the brachial artery at the level of the right atrium. *Systolic pressure* provides an estimate of the work of the heart and of the strain against the arterial walls during ventricular contraction. As the heart relaxes and the aortic valves close, the natural elastic recoil of the arterial system provides for a continuous head of pressure to maintain a steady flow of blood into the periphery, until the next surge of blood.

During *diastole,* or the relaxation phase of the cardiac cycle, arterial blood pressure decreases to 70 to 80 mm Hg. Diastolic pressure provides an indication of *peripheral resistance* or of the ease with which blood flows from the arterioles into the capillaries. When peripheral resistance is high, the pressure within the arteries after systole is not dissipated and remains elevated for a large portion of the cardiac cycle.

The average systolic and diastolic blood pressure for young adults at rest is about 120 and 80 mm Hg, respectively. Because the heart remains in diastole longer than it does in systole, the average or *mean arterial pressure* is slightly less than simply the average of the systolic and diastolic pressures. Thus, the mean arterial pressure of healthy young adults at rest is about 96 mm Hg. This pressure represents the average force exerted by the blood against the walls of the arteries during the entire cardiac cycle.

The Capillaries

The arterioles continue to branch forming smaller and less muscular vessels called *metarterioles.* These end in a network of microscopic blood vessels called *capillaries.* As was shown in Figure 15-3, the capillary wall consists of only a single layer of endothelial cells. Some capillaries are so narrow that they provide room for only one blood cell to squeeze through, single file. In many instances, the proliferation of capillaries is so extensive that the walls of these blood vessels actually abut the membranes of the surrounding cells. It is likely that the capil-

lary density of human skeletal muscle is between 2000 and 3000 capillaries per square millimeter of tissue.[11] This density is even greater in heart muscle; thus, no cell lies further away than .008 mm from its nearest capillary.

The diameter of the capillary opening is controlled by a ring of smooth muscle, the *precapillary sphincter,* that encircles the vessel at its origin. The action of this sphincter is extremely important in exercise, because it provides a local means for regulating capillary blood flow within a specific tissue to meet its metabolic requirements.

Branching of the microcirculation results in an increase in the cross-sectional area of these peripheral vessels that is about 800 times greater than that of the 1-inch diameter aorta. Because the velocity of blood flow is inversely proportional to the cross section of the vasculature, there is a progressive decrease in velocity as blood moves toward and into the capillaries. Thus, about $1\frac{1}{2}$ seconds are required for a blood cell to pass through an average capillary. The total surface of the capillary walls is more than 100 times greater than the external surface of an average male adult. When this tremendous surface is combined with a slow rate of blood flow, an extremely effective means for exchange between the blood and tissues exists.

The Veins

The continuity of the vascular system is maintained as the capillaries feed deoxygenated blood at almost a trickle into the venules or small veins with which they merge. Blood flow then increases somewhat because the cross-sectional area of the venous system is now less than that of the capillaries. The smaller veins in the lower portion of the body eventually empty into the body's largest vein, the *inferior vena cava,* which travels through the abdominal and chest cavities toward the heart. Venous blood coming from the head, neck, and shoulder regions empties into the *superior vena cava* and moves downward to join the inferior vena cava at heart level. This mixture of blood from the upper and lower body then enters the right atrium where it descends into the right ventricle to be pumped through the pulmonary artery to the lungs. Gas exchange takes place in the alveolar–capillary network of the lungs, and the blood returns in the pulmonary vein to the left side of the heart to once again begin its passage around the body.

As illustrated in Figure 15-4, the pressure in the systemic circulation varies considerably. In the aorta and the large arteries, blood pressure fluctuates between 120 and 80 mm Hg during the cardiac cycle. The pressure then falls in direct proportion to the resistance encountered in the vascular circuit. The blood at the arteriole end of the capillaries exerts an average pressure of only 30 mm Hg. As blood enters the venules, the impetus for blood flow is almost entirely lost. By the time blood reaches the right atrium, the pressure has fallen to approximately zero. Because the venous system operates under relatively low pressure, the walls of the veins are much thinner and less muscular than the thicker-walled and less distensible arteries (see Fig. 15-3).

VENOUS RETURN. The low pressure of venous blood poses a special problem that is partly solved by a unique characteristic of veins. Figure 15-5 shows that thin, membranous, flaplike valves spaced at short intervals within the vein permit a one-way blood flow back to the heart. Because venous blood is under relatively low pressure, veins are easily compressed by the smallest muscular contractions or even by minor pressure changes within the chest cavity

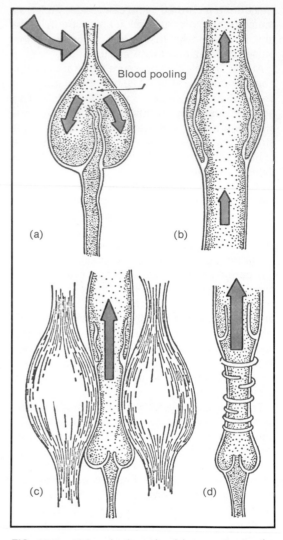

FIG. 15-5. *Valves in the veins (a) prevent returning flow but (b) do not hinder the normal flow very much. Blood can be pushed through veins (c) by nearby active muscle or (d) by the action of smooth muscle bands. (From Elias, H., and Pauly, J. E.: Human Microanatomy. Philadelphia, F. A. Davis, 1966.)*

during the act of breathing. This alternate compression and relaxation of the veins, as well as the one-way action of their valves, provides a "milking" action similar to the action of the heart. Compression of the veins imparts considerable energy for blood flow, whereas the "diastole" of these vessels enables them to refill as blood moves toward the heart. If valves were not present in these vessels, the blood would tend to pool, as it sometimes does in the veins of the extremities, and people would faint

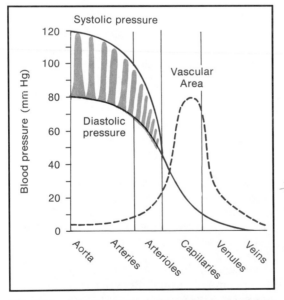

FIG. 15-4. *Blood pressure in the systemic circulatory system. The fall in pressure is in direct relation to the resistance offered in each portion of the vascular tree.*

every time they stood up due to a reduction in cerebral blood flow.

The veins are *not* merely passive conduits. The vessel walls contain a thin layer of smooth muscle that is regulated by nerves and hormones. Contraction and relaxation of these muscular bands alter the diameter of the venous tree, thereby altering the quantity of blood contained within this vascular compartment. At rest, the venous system normally contains about 65% of the total blood volume; hence, the veins are considered capacitance vessels and serve as *blood reservoirs*. A slight increase in the tension or tone of the smooth muscle layer produces a significant redistribution of blood from the peripheral venous circulation toward the central blood volume returning to the heart. This gives the venous system a very important role as an active blood reservoir to either retard or deliver blood to the systemic circulation.

VARICOSE VEINS. Sometimes the valves within a vein become defective and fail to maintain the one-way flow of blood. This condition is called *varicose veins* and usually occurs in the superficial veins of the lower extremities due to the force of gravity retarding blood flow in an upright posture. Blood gathers in these veins, they become excessively distended and painful, and circulation from the affected area is actually impaired. In severe cases, the venous wall may degenerate and the vessel must be surgically removed.

Individuals with varicose veins should probably avoid straining exercises such as those often used in strength training. During such sustained, nonrhythmic muscular contractions, both the muscle and ventilatory "pumps" are unable to contribute significantly to venous return. The increased abdominal pressure associated with straining also impedes venous return. All of these factors act to cause blood to pool in the veins of the lower body and could aggravate an existing varicose vein condition.

VENOUS POOLING. The rhythmic action of muscular contraction is so important to venous return that many people faint when forced to maintain an upright posture without movement. The classic "tilt table" experiment demonstrates this point. The subject is strapped to a table that can pivot to different positions. The heart rate and blood pressure are stable as long as the subject remains horizontal. Once the table is tilted vertically, an uninterrupted column of blood exists from the subject's heart to toes. This creates a hydrostatic force of about 80 to 100 mm Hg and causes blood to pool in the lower extremities. This results in a backup of fluid in the capillary bed that then seeps into the surrounding tissues and causes swelling, or *edema*. Consequently, venous return is reduced and blood pressure declines; at the same time, heart rate accelerates and venoconstriction occurs in an attempt to counter the effects of venous pooling. If the upright position is still maintained, the subject eventually faints due to insufficient cerebral blood supply. Tilting the person either horizontally or head down immediately restores circulation and consciousness is quickly regained.

The change in heart rate and blood pressure in moving from either a recumbent or seated position to standing has been used as the basis of some "fitness" tests. It was assumed that venous return would be maintained with little change in heart rate and blood pressure as the fit person adjusted to a stationary, upright position. Although this may be the case at the extremes of cardiovascular fitness, scores from these tests are of little value for the majority of people in terms of predicting their aerobic power and exercise capacity.

The preceding discussion of venous pooling can be used to justify the action of those who continue to walk about or jog at a slow pace after strenuous exercise. Such moderate exercise, or "cooling down," would certainly facilitate blood flow through the vascular circuit (including the heart) during recovery. (It should be recalled from Chapter 7 that this "active recovery" also aids in removing lactic acid from the blood.) The pressurized suits worn by test pilots and special support stockings also aid in reducing the hydrostatic shift of blood to the veins of the lower extremities in the upright position. A similar supportive effect can be achieved in upright exercise in a swimming pool, because the external support of the water facilitates the return of blood to the heart.

HYPERTENSION: EFFECTS OF TRAINING

For individuals whose arteries have become "hardened" because fatty materials have deposited within their walls (or because the vessel's connective tissue layer has thickened) or whose arterial system offers excessive resistance to blood flow in the periphery due to nervous strain or kidney malfunction, systolic pressure at rest may be as high as 250 or even 300 mm Hg. The diastolic or run-off pressure may also be elevated above 90 mm Hg. Such high blood pressure, called hypertension, imposes a chronic, excessive strain on the normal functioning of the cardiovascular system.

It has been estimated that one out of every five persons will have abnormally high blood pressure sometime during their lives. Presently, more than 20 million Americans have systolic pressures over 140 mm Hg or diastolic pressures over 90 mm Hg. Uncorrected chronic hypertension can lead to heart failure or stroke. Because elevated blood pressure can progress unnoticed for many years, yet can be effectively treated by medications that reduce extracellular fluid volume, it is prudent to recommend that blood pressure be checked at periodic intervals.

Both systolic and diastolic blood pressure can be significantly lowered with a regular program of exercise. These results have been observed with normotensive[5,10,13,15] and hypertensive[3,5,8,13] subjects at rest. A reduction in mean arterial pressure during submaximal exercise testing has also been observed in healthy middle-aged men following endurance training.[9,14]

In patients with documented coronary artery disease[4,12] and in "borderline" hypertensive patients,[5] the effects of exercise training on blood pressure are even more impressive. As indicated in Table 15-1, the average resting systolic pressure of seven middle-aged male patients decreased from 139 to 133 mm Hg following 4 to 6 weeks of interval training. In addi-

tion, at similar submaximal exercise levels, systolic pressure fell from 173 to 155 mm Hg, whereas diastolic pressure was also reduced from 92 to 79 mm Hg. Consequently, mean arterial blood pressure during exercise was reduced by approximately 14% following training. Similar findings were observed for an apparently healthy yet borderline hypertensive group of 37 middle-aged men following a 6-month exercise program.[5] Based on available evidence, a prudent recommendation is to include exercise in most therapeutic progams to manage hypertension.

BLOOD PRESSURE AND EXERCISE.

Static Exercise

Straining-type exercises compress the peripheral arterial system, which brings about a significant increase in resistance to blood flow. This causes a large and rapid rise in blood pressure with a corresponding increase in the workload of the heart. This cardiovascular strain can be harmful for individuals with heart and vascular disease. For these people more rhythmic forms of moderate exercise are desirable and beneficial.

Steady-Rate Exercise

In rhythmic muscular activity such as jogging, swimming, and bicycling, the dilation of the blood vessels in the working muscles enhances the flow of blood through large portions of the peripheral vasculature. The alternate contrac-

TABLE 15-1. Measures of blood pressure at rest and during submaximal exercise prior to and following 4 to 6 weeks of training in seven middle-aged patients with coronary heart disease[a]

MEASURE[b]	REST MEAN VALUE			SUBMAXIMAL EXERCISE MEAN VALUE		
	BEFORE	AFTER	DIFFERENCE (%)	BEFORE	AFTER	DIFFERENCE (%)
Systolic blood pressure (mm Hg)	139	133	−4.3	173	155	−10.4
Diastolic blood pressure (mm Hg)	78	73	−6.4	92	79	−14.1
Mean blood pressure (mm Hg)	97	92	−5.2	127	109	−14.3

[a]Modified from Clausen, J.P. et al.: Physical training in the management of coronary artery disease. Circulation XL: 143, 1969. Reproduced by permission of the American Heart Association, Inc.
[b]Blood pressure was measured directly by means of pressure transducer inserted into brachial artery.

tion and relaxation of the muscles themselves also provide a significant pumping force to propel blood through the vascular circuit and return it to the heart. The increased blood flow during moderate, rhythmic exercise causes systolic pressure to rise rapidly in the first few minutes of exercise. The blood pressure then levels off at 140 to 160 mm Hg.[6] As steady-rate exercise continues, systolic pressure may gradually fall as the arterioles in the muscles continue to dilate and peripheral resistance to blood flow becomes reduced. During this exercise, the diastolic blood pressure remains relatively unchanged.

Graded
Exercise

The blood pressure response as measured directly by pressure transducers inserted into the brachial artery during progressive exercise of increasing severity is illustrated in Figure 15-6. In this situation, systolic, diastolic, and mean arterial pressure are plotted as a function of the quantity of blood ejected into the arterial circuit each minute, the *cardiac output.*

As can be seen, arterial blood pressure increases linearly with cardiac output. The greatest increases in exercise blood pressure are observed during cardiac systole whereas the diastolic pressure increases by only about 12% during the full range of exercise. This response is similar for both physically conditioned and sedentary subjects. However, during maximum exercise performed by healthy endurance athletes, the systolic blood pressure may increase to 200 mm Hg, a response apparently due to the large cardiac outputs of these athletes.[2]

Blood Pressure in
Arm Exercise

As shown in Table 15-2, at a given percentage of the maximal oxygen consumption, systolic and diastolic blood pressures are considerably higher when work is performed with the arms than when performed with the legs.

It is likely that the smaller muscle mass and vasculature of the arms offer greater resistance to blood flow than the larger muscle mass and vasculature of the legs.[1] Blood flow to the arms during exercise would therefore require a much larger systolic head of pressure. Clearly, this form of exercise represents greater cardiovascular strain because the work of the heart is

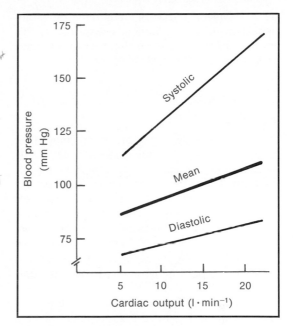

FIG. 15-6. *The relationship between blood flow during exercise and systemic arterial pressures measured at the brachial artery. (From Ekelund, L. G., and Holmgren, A.: Central hemodynamics during exercise. Am. Heart Assoc. Monogr., No. 15: 33, 1967. Reprinted by permission of the American Heart Association, Inc.)*

increased considerably. For individuals with cardiovascular dysfunction, these observations support the use of exercise requiring large muscle groups, such as walking, bicycling, and running, in contrast to exercises that engage a rather limited muscle mass such as shoveling, overhead hammering, or even arm ergometry. If a systematic program of arm exercise is uti-

TABLE 15-2. *Comparison of systolic and diastolic blood pressure during arm and leg exercise at similar percentages of the maximal oxygen intake[a]*

PERCENT OF MAX $\dot{V}O_2$	SYSTOLIC PRESSURE (mm Hg)		DIASTOLIC PRESSURE (mm Hg)	
	ARMS	LEGS	ARMS	LEGS
25	150	132	90	70
40	165	138	93	71
50	175	144	96	73
75	205	160	103	75

[a]From Åstrand, P.-O. et al.: Intra-arterial blood pressure during exercise with different muscle groups. *J. Appl. Physiol., 20:253, 1965.*

lized, however, the work loads must be established based on the person's response to this form of exercise and *not* from some exercise stress test using bicycling or running.

THE HEART'S
BLOOD SUPPLY

Although literally tons of blood may flow through the heart's chambers each day, none of its nourishment passes directly into the myocardium. This is because there are no direct circulatory channels within the heart's chambers leading to its tissues. Instead, the heart muscle has an elaborate circulatory network of its own. As shown in Figure 15-7, these vessels form an especially visible, crownlike network arising from the top portion of the heart called the *coronary circulation.*

The openings for the left and right coronary arteries are situated in the aorta just above the semilunar valves at a point where the oxygenated blood leaves the left ventricle. These arteries then curl around the heart's surface; the right coronary supplies predominantly the right atrium and ventricle whereas the greatest volume of blood flows in the left coronary artery to supply the tissue of the left atrium and ventricle and a small part of the right ventricle. These vessels divide and eventually form a dense capillary network within the heart muscle. Blood then leaves the tissues of the left ventricle via the coronary *sinus;* blood from the right ventricle exits via the *anterior cardiac veins,* which empty directly into the right atrium.

With each heart beat, the driving force of the heart pushes a portion of blood into the coronary arteries. At rest, normal blood flow to the myocardium is 200 to 250 ml per minute, which is about 5% of the total cardiac output.

Myocardial Oxygen
Utilization

Even at rest, the oxygen utilization of the myocardium is high in relation to its blood flow. About 70% to 80% of the oxygen is extracted from the blood flowing in the coronary vessels. This is in contrast to most other tissues at rest, which use as little as one-fourth of the available oxygen. The increased myocardial oxygen demands during exercise can only be met therefore by a proportionate increase in coronary blood flow. In vigorous exercise, coronary

blood flow may increase four to five times above the resting level. This is achieved in two ways: (1) Increased myocardial metabolism during exercise has a direct effect on the coronary vessels, causing them to dilate. For example, hypoxia has an extremely potent effect for increasing blood flow through the myocardium. In addition to local factors, hormones of the sympathetic nervous system are released during exercise and cause coronary dilitation. (2) During exercise, the increased aortic pressure forces a proportionately greater quantity of blood into the coronary circulation. The ebb and flow of blood in the coronary vessels fluctuates with each phase of the cardiac cycle. On the average, coronary blood flow is about 2.5 times greater during diastole than during systole.[7]

An adequate oxygen supply is critical for the myocardium, because unlike skeletal muscle, this tissue has an extremely limited ability to generate energy anaerobically. The blood supply to the heart is so profuse that at least one capillary supplies each of the heart's muscle fibers. Impairment in coronary blood flow usually results in chest pains, or *angina pectoris.* These pains become especially pronounced during exercise. In fact, the stress of exercise is often used to document or evaluate this condition. A blood clot, or *thrombus,* lodged in one of the coronary vessels may severely impair normal heart function. Although this form of ''heart attack,'' or more specifically *myocardial infarction,* may be mild, a more complete blockage causes severe damage to the myocardium and could result in death. A more complete discussion of coronary heart disease, stress testing, and the possible role of exercise as preventive medicine is presented in Chapter 29.

Myocardial Metabolism

As with all tissue, the heart utilizes the chemical energy stored in food nutrients to power its work. The heart, however, relies almost totally on energy released in aerobic reactions. As such, myocardial fibers have the greatest mitochondrial concentration of all tissues.

Figure 15-8 shows the substrate utilization by the heart at rest and during exercise and recovery. Glucose, fatty acids, and the lactic acid formed in skeletal muscle during glycolysis provide the energy for proper myocardial functioning. At rest, these three substrates are utilized in approximately equal percentages to synthe-

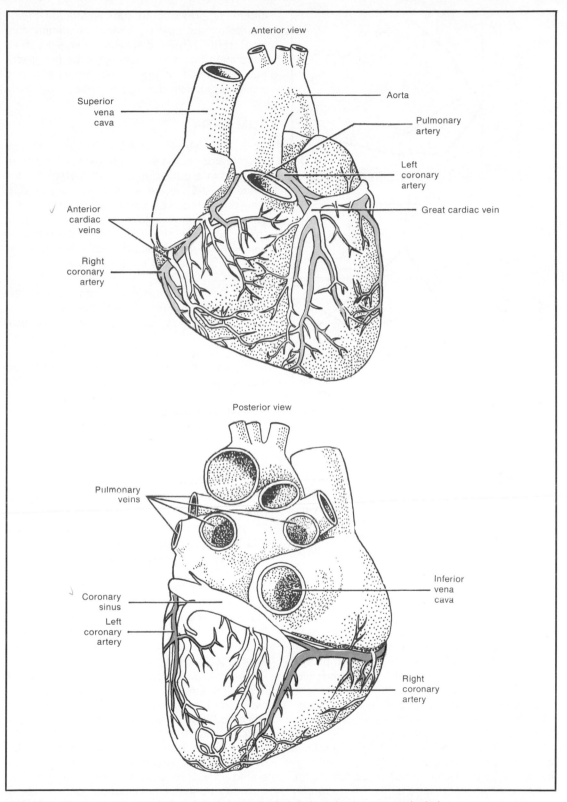

FIG. 15-7. *The coronary circulation. Arteries are shaded dark and veins are unshaded.*

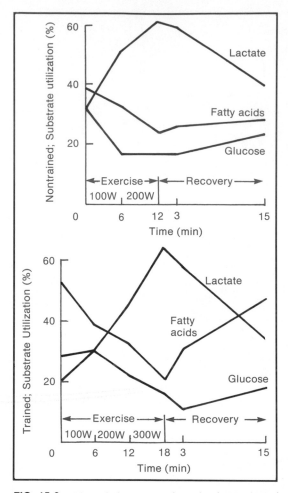

FIG. 15-8. *The relative proportion of substrate used by the heart at various work loads (W-watts) and during recovery in trained and nontrained subjects. (From Keul, J., Doll, E., and Keppler, D.: Medicine and Sport, Vol. 7, Energy Metabolism of Human Muscle. Basel, Karger, 1972.)*

size ATP. With exercise, however, the heart's utilization of circulating lactic acid increases, and during strenuous exercise, the energy derived from circulating lactate nearly triples in relation to the energy contribution from glucose and free fatty acids. During prolonged submaximal activity that occurs in distance running, skiing, or swimming, the myocardial metabolism of free fatty acids rises to almost 70% of the total energy requirement. This metabolic pattern is similar for trained and untrained subjects, *although the contribution of fats to the total energy requirement is considerably greater among trained endurance athletes.* This

difference provides another illustration of the "carbohydrate sparing effect" of training that also occurs in trained skeletal muscle. Such an adaptation helps to preserve the body's glycogen reserves that are crucial to muscle and brain metabolism during prolonged exercise.

SUMMARY

1. The striated fibers of the myocardium are interconnected so that portions of the heart contract in a unified manner. Functionally, the heart may be viewed as two separate pumps: One pump receives blood returning from the body and pumps it to the lungs for aeration (pulmonary circulation), whereas the other receives oxygenated blood from the lungs and pumps it throughout the body (systemic circulation).

2. Pressure changes created during the cardiac cycle act on the heart's valves to provide for a one-way flow of blood into the vascular circuit.

3. The surge of blood with the contraction of the ventricles (and subsequent run-off during relaxation) creates pressure changes within the arterial vessels. The systolic pressure, or highest pressure generated during the cardiac cycle, occurs during ventricular contraction. The diastolic pressure is the lowest pressure reached before the next ventricular contraction.

4. Hypertension imposes a chronic stress on cardiovascular function. Regular aerobic training can bring about significant reductions in systolic and diastolic blood pressure at rest and during submaximal exercise.

5. Systolic blood pressure increases in proportion to oxygen consumption and cardiac output during graded exercise, whereas diastolic pressure remains relatively unchanged or increases slightly. At the same relative work load, systolic pressures are greater when work is performed with the arms than when performed with the legs.

6. The dense capillary network provides a large and effective surface for exchange between the blood and tissues. These vessels adjust blood flow in response to the tissue's metabolic activity.

7. Compression and relaxation of the veins by the action of skeletal muscles impart considerable energy to facilitate venous return. This provides aditional justification' for the use of active recovery following vigorous exercise.

8. Nerves and hormones act on the smooth muscle layer in the venous walls, causing them to constrict or stiffen. This alteration in venous tone can have a profound effect on the distribution of total blood volume.

9. The hemodynamic adjustments with postural changes are of little value in predicting one's exercise capability.

10. At rest, about 80% of the oxygen flowing through the coronary arteries is extracted by the myocardium. This high extraction means that the increased myocardial oxygen demands in exercise can only be met by a proportionate increase in coronary blood flow.

11. Because the myocardium is essentially aerobic tissue, it must continually be supplied with oxygen. Impairment of coronary blood flow causes anginal pains, and blockage of a coronary artery (myocardial infarction) rapidly causes irreversible damage to the heart muscle.

12. The main substrates used by the heart for energy are glucose, fatty acids, and lactic acid. The percentage utilization of these substrates varies with the severity and duration of exercise.

References

1. Åstrand, P. O. et al.: Intra-arterial blood pressure during exercise with different muscle groups. J. Appl. Physiol., *20:*253, 1965.
2. Bevegård, S. et al.: Circulatory studies in well-trained athletes at rest and during heavy exercise, with special reference to stroke volume and the influence of body position. Acta Physiol. Scand. *57:*26, 1963.
3. Boyer, J. L. and Kasch, F. W.: Exercise therapy in hypertensive men. J.A.M.A. *211:* 1668, 1970.
4. Clausen, J. P. et al.: Physical training in the management of coronary artery disease. Circulation, *30:*143, 1969.
5. Choquette, G., and Ferguson, R. J.: Blood pressure reduction in "borderline" hypertensives following physical training. Can. Med. Assoc. J., *108:*699, 1973.
6. Ekelund, L. G., and Holmgren, A · Central hemodynamics during exercise. Circ. Res., *20* (Suppl. 1):33, 1967.
7. Gregg, D. E., and Coffman, J. D.: Coronary circulation. *In* Blood Vessels and Lymphatics. Edited by D. S. Abramson. New York, Academic Press, 1962.
8. Hanson, J. S., and Nedde, W. H.: Preliminary observations on physical training for hypertensive males. Circ. Res., *27* (Suppl. 1):49, 1970.
9. Hartley, L. H. et al.: Physical training in sedentary middle-aged and older men. III. Cardiac output and gas exchange at submaximal and maximal exercise. Scand. J. Clin. Lab. Invest., *24:*335, 1969.
10. Kasch, F. W., and Boyer, J. L.: Changes in maximum work capacity resulting from six months training in patients with ischemic heart disease. Med. Sci. Sports, *1:*156, 1969.
11. Krough, A.: *The Anatomy and Physiology of Capillaries.* New Haven, Conn., Yale University Press, 1929.
12. Redwood, D. R. et al.: Circulatory and symptomatic effects of physical training in patients with coronary-artery disease and angina pectoris. N. Engl. J. Med., *286:* 959, 1972.
13. Terjung, R. I. et al.: Cardiovascular adaptation to twelve minutes of mild daily exercise in middle-aged sedentary men. J. Am. Geriatr. Soc., *21:*164, 1973.
14. Tzankoff, S. P. et al.: Physiological adjustments to work in older men as effected by physical training. J. Appl. Physiol., *33:*346, 1972.
15. Wilmore, J. H. et al.: Physiological alterations resulting from a 10-week program of jogging. Med. Sci. Sports, *2:*7, 1970.

Cardiovascular Regulation and Integration

16

In humans, a "closed" circulatory system has evolved in which the blood cells remain trapped within the confines of a continuous vascular circuit. Nerves and chemicals regulate both the speed of the pumping heart and the internal opening of various blood vessels. This provides for rapid and effective control of the heart as well as for the distribution of blood throughout the body. When a person is resting comfortably, about 5% of the 5 liters of blood pumped each minute from the heart goes to the skin. This is in contrast to exercise performed in a hot, humid environment where as much as 20% of the total blood flow is diverted to the body's surface for the purpose of heat dissipation. This "shunting" can occur only within a closed vascular system that has the capability for immediate redistribution of blood depending on the body's metabolic and physiologic needs.[7a]

REGULATION OF HEART RATE

Cardiac muscle is unique in that it has the capability of maintaining its own rhythm. If left to this inherent rhythmicity, the heart would beat steadily between 70 and 80 times each minute. However, nerves that go directly to the heart, as well as chemicals circulating in the blood, can change the heart rate rapidly. These *extrinsic* controls of cardiac function cause the heart to speed up in "anticipation," even before the start of exercise. To a large extent, extrinsic regulation provides for heart rates that may be as slow as 30 beats per minute in highly trained endurance athletes at rest, and as fast as 220 beats per minute in maximum exercise.

Intrinsic Regulation of Heart Rate

Situated within the posterior wall of the right atrium is a mass of specialized muscle tissue called the *sinoatrial node* or *S-A node*. This node spontaneously depolarizes and repolarizes to provide the "innate" stimulus to the heart. For this reason, the S-A node is referred to as the "pacemaker." The normal route for the transmission of the impulse across the myocardium is shown in Figure 16-1.

THE HEART'S ELECTRIC IMPULSE. Rhythms originating at the S-A node spread across the atria to another small knot of tissue, the *atrioventricular node* or *A-V node*. Here the impulse is delayed about 0.10 second to provide sufficient time for the atria to contract and force blood into the ventricles. The A-V node gives rise to the *A-V bundle* (bundle of His) that transmits the impulse rapidly through the ventricles over specialized conducting fibers often referred to as the *Purkinje system.* These fibers form distinct branches that penetrate the right and left ventricles. Each ventricular cell is stimulated within about 0.06 second from the passage of the impulse into the ventricles; this permits a unified and simultaneous contraction of the entire musculature of both ventricles. The transmission of the cardiac impulse can be summarized as follows:

S-A node → Atria → A-V node → A-V bundle (Purkinje fibers) → Ventricles

ELECTROCARDIOGRAPHY. Like all nerve and muscle tissue, the outer surface of the myocardial cells is electrically more positive than the

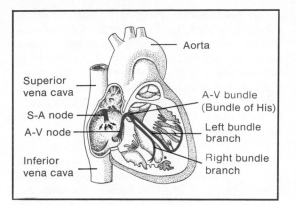

FIG. 16-1. *Excitation and conduction of cardiac impulse from the S-A node.*

inside. This polarity is reversed just prior to contraction, when the heart is stimulated and the inside of the cell actually becomes more positive than the outside. During the diastolic phase of the cardiac cycle, the membranes repolarize and the resting membrane potential is reestablished.

The electrical activity about the heart creates an electrical field throughout the body. Because the salty body fluids provide an excellent conducting medium, the sequence of electrical events prior to and during each cardiac cycle can be picked up as voltage changes by electrodes placed on the skin's surface. The graphic record of the heart's electric activity is called the *electrocardiogram,* or simply *ECG.* A characteristic, normal electrocardiogram is presented in Figure 16-2.

The *P wave* represents the depolarization of the atria. It lasts about 0.15 second and heralds atrial contraction. The P wave is then followed by the relatively large *QRS complex.* This reflects the electric changes caused by the depolarization of the ventricles; at this point, the ventricles contract. Atrial repolarization following the P wave produces a wave so small that it is usually obscured by the large QRS complex. The *T wave* represents repolarization of the ventricles. This occurs during ventricular diastole.

Due to the heart's relatively long period of depolarization, approximately 0.20 to 0.30 second is required before it can receive another impulse and contract again. This "rest" or *refractory period* serves an important function because it provides sufficient time for ventricular filling between beats.

The electrocardiogram serves useful purposes for the cardiologist and exercise specialist. For one thing, it provides an effective means for monitoring heart rate objectively during exercise. Radio telemetry makes it possible to transmit the ECG while the subject is free to perform various types of exercise including football, weight lifting, basketball, ice hockey, and even swimming.

Electrocardiography also serves as an extremely valuable tool for uncovering abnormalities in heart function, especially those related to cardiac rhythm, electric conduction, myocardial oxygen supply, and actual tissue damage (see Chap. 29). Its application is especially valuable during exercise stress testing.

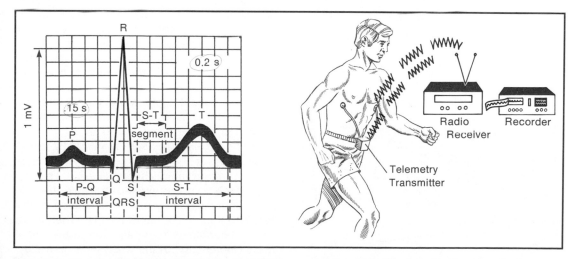

FIG. 16-2. *The normal electrocardiogram. At right is an example of bipolar chest leads and radio telemetry routinely used to obtain the exercise ECG.*

Extrinsic Regulation of Heart Rate

Neural influences are superimposed on the inherent rhythmicity and conductivity of the myocardium. These originate in the cardiovascular center in the medulla and are transmitted through the sympathetic and parasympathetic components of the autonomic nervous system. As shown in Figure 16-3, the atria are supplied with large numbers of both sympathetic and parasympathetic neurons, whereas the ventricles receive sympathetic fibers almost exclusively.

SYMPATHETIC INFLUENCE. Stimulation of the sympathetic cardioaccelerator nerves releases epinephrine and norepinephrine. Collectively, these neural hormones are called *catecholamines*. They act to accelerate the depolarization of the sinus node, which causes the heart to beat faster. This acceleration in heart rate is termed *tachycardia*. The catecholamines also significantly increase myocardial contractility. It has been estimated that maximum sympathetic stimulation nearly doubles the force of ventricular contraction. Epinephrine released from the medullary portion of the adrenal glands in response to a general sympathetic activation also produces a similar though slower acting effect on cardiac function.

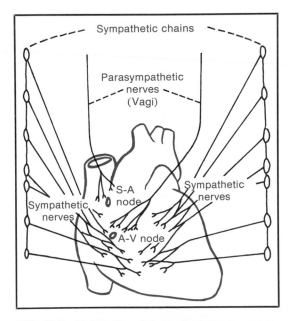

FIG. 16-3. *Distribution of sympathetic and parasympathetic nerves to the heart.*

PARASYMPATHETIC INFLUENCE. *Acetylcholine,* the hormone of the parasympathetic nervous system, retards the rate of sinus discharge and slows the heart. This slowing of heart rate is termed *bradycardia*. The effect is mediated through the action of the *vagus nerve* whose cell bodies originate in the cardioinhibitory center in the medulla. Vagal stimulation has essentially no effect on myocardial contractility.

TRAINING EFFECTS. It appears that physical training creates an imbalance between the tonic activity of the sympathetic accelerator and parasympathetic depressor neurons in favor of greater vagal dominance. This is probably mediated by an increase in parasympathetic activity and a concomitant decrease in sympathetic discharge. In addition, training may also decrease the intrinsic rate of firing of the S-A node.[2,8] These adaptations probably account for the significant bradycardia often observed in highly conditioned endurance athletes or in sedentary subjects following aerobic training.

PERIPHERAL INPUT. The cardiovascular center in the medulla receives sensory input from peripheral receptors in blood vessels, joints, and muscles. Stimuli from these receptors modify either vagal or sympathetic outflow to bring about the appropriate cardiac response. Receptors in the aortic arch and carotid sinus, for example, respond to changes in arterial blood pressure. As blood pressure increases, the stretch of the arterial vessels activates these *baroreceptors* to bring about a reflex slowing of the heart, as well as a compensatory dilation of the peripheral vasculature. This causes blood pressure to decrease toward more normal levels. To some degree, this particular feedback mechanism is overridden during exercise, since heart rate and blood pressure are both increased considerably. More than likely, the baroreceptors act as a brake to prevent abnormally high pressure levels in exercise.

Carotid artery palpation significantly slows the heart rate and occasionally produces electrocardiographic abnormalities.[10] This effect, which is demonstrated in Table 16-1, is probably mediated by direct stimulation of the baroreceptors in the carotid sinus. When heart rate is determined from palpation at the radial artery (thumb side of the wrist) or temporal artery (side of head at temple), no changes in heart rate or ECG are noted. This indicates that

TABLE 16-1. *Heart rate following palpation of the carotid, radial, and temporal arteries prior to, during, and immediately following exercise*[a]

	HEART RATE (beats · min⁻¹)		
	BEFORE PALPATION	DURING PALPATION	DIFFERENCE
Carotid artery			
Preexercise	79.1	68.1	−11.0[b]
Exercise	155.2	152.9	− 2.3
Postexercise	153.7	138.1	−15.6[b]
Radial artery			
Preexercise	78.8	79.9	+ 1.1
Exercise	156.6	156.0	− 0.6
Postexercise	154.6	155.1	+ 0.5
Temporal artery			
Preexercise	78.8	79.0	+ 0.2
Exercise	154.8	155.4	+ 0.6
Postexercise	153.6	154.0	+ 0.4

[a]Modified from White, J.R.: EKG changes using carotid artery for heart rate monitoring. *Med. Sci. Sports,* 9:88, 1977. Copyright 1977, the American College of Sports Medicine. Reprinted by Permission.
[b]Statistically significant.

these sites are preferable for obtaining a valid estimate of heart rate during exercise or in immediate recovery. An accurate measure of heart rate is especially important for training when specific "target" heart rates are assigned or modified to regulate training intensity (see Chap. 20) If the method used to monitor the pulse rate consistently gave low values (as could be the case with carotid palpation), the person would unwittingly be pushed to a higher work level. This would certainly be undesirable in exercise prescription for cardiac patients.

CORTICAL INPUT. Impulses from the cerebral cortex pass through the cardiovascular center in the medulla. Consequently, variations in one's emotional state significantly affect cardiovascular responses and make it difficult to obtain "true" values for resting heart rate or blood pressure. Cerebral impulses also cause the heart rate to rise rapidly and considerably in anticipation of exercise. This *anticipatory heart rate* is probably the result of both an increase in sympathetic discharge and reduction of vagal tone.

The extent of the anticipatory response is clearly demonstrated in Figure 16-4. The heart rate of trained sprint runners was telemetered at rest, at the starting commands, and during a 60-, 220-, and 440-yard race.[6] Heart rate averaged 148 beats per minute at the starting com-

mands in anticipation of the 60-yard sprint; this represented 74% of the total heart rate adjustment to the run! The magnitude of the anticipatory heart rate was greatest in the short sprint events and successively lower prior to the longer sprint distances.

As shown in Table 16-2, this pattern of anticipation was also demonstrated in events of longer duration. For example, the anticipatory heart rate of four athletes trained for the 880-yard run averaged 122 beats per minute, whereas heart rates during the starting commands of the 1-mile and 2-mile runs averaged only 118 and 108 beats, respectively. This represented only 33% of the total heart rate adjustment to the 2-mile run. As indicated in Table 16-2, untrained subjects also demonstrated an anticipatory increase in heart rate prior to the start of exercise. For these subjects, however, the pattern of anticipation in relation to the distance to be run was not as clear as in the runners trained for specific events. More than likely, the rather specific nature of the anticipatory heart rate with trained athletes reflects genetic differences between competitive runners and untrained subjects as well as specific long-term conditioning factors resulting from training. The initial neural outflow in anticipation of exercise would be desirable prior to intense activity of short duration (such as sprinting) to provide for the rapid mobilization of bod-

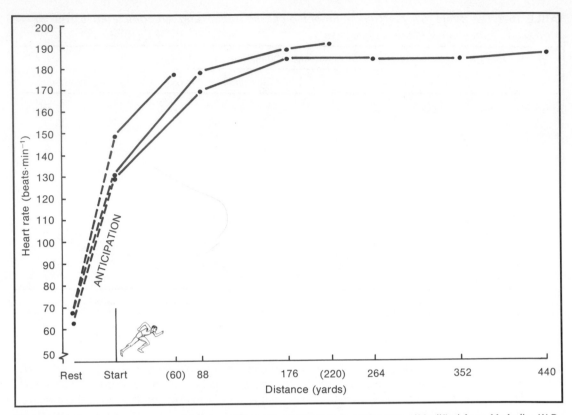

FIG. 16-4. *Heart rate response of runners trained to participate in sprint runs. (Modified from McArdle, W.D., Foglia, G.F., and Patti, A.V.: J. Appl. Physiol., 23:566, 1967.)*

✱ ily reserves. On the other hand, this mechanism for "reving the body's engine" might be wasteful in events of longer duration.

✱ It seems clear from the preceding observations that a large portion of the heart rate adjustment to exercise reflects cortical input that occurs during the initial stages of the activity.

More than likely, considerable accelerator input ✱ is also provided by the activation of receptors in joints and muscles as the exercise begins.[7] Even in the so called nonsprint events, heart rate is approximately 180 beats per minute within 30 seconds of 1- and 2-mile runs. Further increases in heart rate are gradual, with several ✱

TABLE 16-2. *Resting, anticipatory and maximum exercise heart rate in competitive runners and untrained subjects during all-out running*[a]

EVENT	N TRAINED	N UNTRAINED	REST TRAINED	REST UNTRAINED	ANTICIPATORY TRAINED	ANTICIPATORY UNTRAINED	EXERCISE TRAINED	EXERCISE UNTRAINED
60 yard	5	4	67	69	148	124	177	162
220 yard	5	4	67	67	130	115	191	186
440 yard	4	4	63	68	129	118	187	189
880 yard	4	4	62	70	122	129	186	194
1 mile	4	4	58	64	118	128	195	198
2 mile	4	4	59	74	108	109	206	199
Values are averages								

[a]From McArdle, W.D., Foglia, G.F., and Patti, A.V.: Telemetered cardiac response to selected running events. *J. Appl. Physiol., 23:566,* 1967. Values are averages.

plateaus being reached during the run. Almost identical results have been reported for telemetered heart rates during competitive swimming events; only the maximum exercise heart rates were lower in swimming.[5]

DISTRIBUTION OF BLOOD

Effect of Exercise

Increased energy expenditure usually requires rapid adjustments in blood flow that affect the entire cardiovascular system. For example, nerves and local metabolic conditions act on the smooth muscular bands of arteriole walls, causing them to alter their internal diameter almost instantaneously. In addition, stimulation of nerves to the venous capacitance vessels causes them to "stiffen." Such veno-constriction permits large quantities of blood to move from peripheral veins into the central circulation. It is this capability of large portions of the vasculature to either constrict or dilate that provides a rapid redistribution of blood to meet the tissue's metabolic requirements.

During exercise, the vascular portion of active muscles is considerably increased by the dilation of local arterioles. Concurrently, other vessels that can temporarily compromise their blood supply constrict or "shut down." Kidney function vividly illustrates this regulatory capacity for adjusting regional blood flow. Renal blood flow at rest is normally about 1100 ml per minute; this is about 20% of the cardiac output. In maximal exercise, however, renal blood flow may be reduced to only 250 ml per minute or about 1% of the exercise cardiac output.[4]

Regulation of Blood Flow

Blood flows through the vascular circuit in general accordance with the physical laws of hydrodynamics as applied to rigid, cylindric vessels. Because blood is not a homogeneous fluid and the blood vessels are not rigid tubes, these relationships are true mainly in a qualitative sense.

The volume of flow in any vessel is (1) directly proportional to the pressure gradient between the two ends of the vessel (P) and not to the absolute pressure within the vessel, and (2) in-

versely related to the resistance encountered to the flow (R). Resistance, which is the force impeding blood flow, is caused by friction between the blood and the internal vascular wall. This is determined by three factors: the thickness or *viscosity* of the blood, the *length* of the conducting tube, and, most important, the *diameter* of the blood vessel. The relationship between pressure, resistance, and flow can be expressed by an equation often referred to as *Poiseuille's law* where:

$$\text{Flow} = \frac{\text{Pressure gradient (P)} \times \text{Vessel radius}^4}{\text{Vessel length} \times \text{Viscosity}}$$

In the body, the viscosity of the blood and the length of the transport vessel remain relatively constant under most circumstances. Therefore, the most important factor affecting blood flow is the *diameter* of the conducting tube. In fact, the resistance to flow changes with the vessel diameter raised to the fourth power; if the diameter is reduced by one-half, flow through the vessel decreases 16 times! Conversely, doubling the vessel's diameter increases the volume 16-fold. If the pressure within the vascular circuit were to remain relatively constant, a considerable alteration in blood flow would be achieved with only a small change in vessel diameter. *In a physiologic sense, constriction and dilation provide the most important mechanisms for regulating regional blood flow.*

LOCAL FACTORS.   At rest, only 1 out of every 30 to 40 capillaries in muscle tissue is actually open.[11] The opening of dormant capillaries in exercise serves three important functions: (1) It provides for a significant increase in muscle blood flow. (2) Because more channels are now open, the increased blood volume can be delivered with only a minimal increase in the velocity of flow. (3) The enhanced vascularization increases the effective surface for exchange between the blood and the muscle cells.

Local factors related to the level of tissue metabolism act directly on the smooth muscle bands of the small arterioles and precapillary sphincters to cause vasodilatation. The response is almost instantaneous and finely adjusted to the tissue's metabolic needs.[3] In fact, in muscle, the local vascular dilatation is proportional to the force of a contraction.[1] Local regulation even provides for adequate regional blood flow in patients in whom the nerves to the blood vessels have been surgically removed.

A decrease in a tissue's oxygen supply produces a potent local stimulus for vasodilatation in skeletal and cardiac muscle. Furthermore, local increases in temperature, carbon dioxide, acidity, adenosine, and the ions of magnesium and potassium enhance regional blood flow. These autoregulatory mechanisms for blood flow make sense from a physiologic standpoint because they reflect elevated tissue metabolism and increased need for oxygen. The most effective immediate step for increasing a tissue's oxygen supply is rapid and local vasodilatation.

NEURAL FACTORS. Superimposed on the vasoregulation afforded by local factors is a central vascular control mediated by the sympathetic, and to a minor degree, the parasympathetic portions of the autonomic nervous system. For example, muscles contain small sensory nerve fibers that are highly sensitive to substances released in local tissue during exercise. When these fibers are stimulated, they provide input to the central nervous system to bring about an appropriate cardiovascular response. With central regulation, blood flow in one area cannot dominate when a concurrent oxygen need exists in other more "needy" tissues. In exercise, for example, blood flow through the skin and kidneys is temporarily reduced, whereas the vessels to the active muscles dilate. This vascular response occurs even in anticipation of exercise.

Figure 16-5 is a schematic view of the distribution of sympathetic outflow. These nerve fibers end in the muscular layers of small arteries, arterioles, and precapillary sphincters.

Norepinephrine acts as a general vasoconstrictor and is released at certain sympathetic nerve endings. These sympathetic constrictor fibers are called *adrenergic fibers*. Other sympathetic neurons, especially those in skeletal and heart muscle, release acetylcholine; these are the *cholinergic fibers* and their action is vasodilatation.

From the preceding discussion, it is clear that the sympathetic nervous system consists of *both* adrenergic constrictor and cholinergic dilator fibers. The constrictor nerves are constantly active so that certain blood vessels are always in a state of constriction. The relative degree of this constrictor activity is often referred to as *vasomotor tone*. Dilatation of blood vessels under the influence of adrenergic neurons is due more to a reduction in vasomotor tone than to an increase in the action of either sympathetic or parasympathetic dilator fibers.

HORMONAL FACTORS. Sympathetic nerves also terminate in the medullary portion of the adrenal glands. In response to sympathetic activation, this glandular tissue secretes large quantities of epinephrine and a smaller amount of norepinephrine into the blood. These hormones then act as chemical messengers to bring about a generalized constrictor response, except in the blood vessels of the heart and skeletal muscles. During exercise, the hormonal control of regional blood flow is relatively minor in comparison to the more local, rapid, and powerful sympathetic neural drive.

INTEGRATED RESPONSE IN EXERCISE

The chemical, neural, and hormonal adjustments prior to and during exercise are summarized in Table 16-3. At the onset of exercise

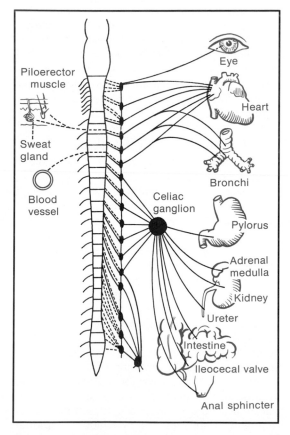

FIG. 16-5. *Schematic view of vascular regulation via sympathetic outflow.*

Piloerector muscle

Sweat gland

Blood vessel

Celiac ganglion

Eye

Heart

Bronchi

Pylorus

Adrenal medulla

Kidney

Ureter

Intestine

Ileocecal valve

Anal sphincter

TABLE 16-3. *Summary of integrated chemical, neural, and hormonal adjustments prior to and during exercise*

CONDITION	ACTIVATOR	RESPONSE
Preexercise "anticipatory" response	Activation of motor cortex and higher areas of brain causes increase in sympathetic outflow and reciprocal inhibition of parasympathetic activity.	Acceleration of heart rate; increased myocardial contractility; vasodilatation in skeletal and heart muscle (cholinergic fibers); vasoconstriction in other areas, especially skin, gut, spleen, liver, and kidneys (adrenergic fibers); increase in arterial blood pressure.
Exercise	Continued sympathetic cholinergic outflow; alterations in local metabolic conditions due to hypoxia, $\downarrow$pH, $\uparrow$PCO$_2$, $\uparrow$ADP, $\uparrow$Mg^{2+}, $\uparrow$Ca^{3+}, and $\uparrow$temperature.	Further dilation of muscle vasculature.
	Continued sympathetic adrenergic outflow in conjunction with epinephrine and norepinephrine from the adrenal medullae.	Concomitant constriction of vasculature in inactive tissues to maintain adequate perfusion pressure throughout arterial system. Venous vessels stiffen to reduce their capacity. This venoconstriction facilitates venous return and maintains the central blood volume.

(and even before exercise begins), cardiovascular changes are initiated from nerve centers above the medullary region. These adjustments provide for a significant increase in the rate and pumping strength of the heart, as well as predictable alterations in regional blood flow that are proportional to exercise severity. As exercise continues, sympathetic cholinergic outflow plus local metabolic factors, which act on chemosensitive nerves as well as directly on the blood vessels, cause dilatation of resistance vessels in active muscles. This reduced peripheral resistance permits the active areas to accommodate greater blood flow. As exercise continues, there are further constrictor adjustments in less active tissues; thus, an adequate perfusion pressure can be maintained even with the large dilatation of the muscle's vasculature. This constrictor action provides for the appropriate redistribution of blood to meet the metabolic requirements of working muscles.

Factors affecting venous return are equally as important as those regulating arterial blood flow. The action of the muscle and ventilatory pumps and the stiffening of the veins themselves (probably mediated by sympathetic activity) immediately increase the return of blood to the right ventricle. In fact, as cardiac output increases, venous tone also increases proportionally in both working and nonworking muscles.[9] With these adjustments, the balance between cardiac output and venous return is maintained. The factors affecting blood flow in the venous system are especially important in upright exercise where the force of gravity tends to counter the venous pressure in the extremities.

SUMMARY

1. The cardiovascular system provides for rapid regulation of heart rate as well as for effective distribution of blood in the vascular circuit in response to the body's metabolic and physiologic needs.

2. The cardiac rhythm is initiated at the S-A node. The impulse then travels across the atria to the A-V node where it is delayed and then

rapidly spreads across the large ventricular mass. With this normal conduction pattern, the atria and ventricles contract effectively to provide impetus for blood flow.

3. The electrocardiogram provides a record of the sequence of the heart's electric events during the cardiac cycle. Electrocardiography is important for detecting various abnormalities in heart function at rest and during exercise.

4. The sympathetic catecholamines, epinephrine and norepinephrine, act to accelerate heart rate and increase myocardial contractility. The parasympathetic neurotransmitter, acetylcholine, acts via the vagus nerve to slow the heart.

5. Neural and hormonal extrinsic factors

modify the heart's inherent rhythmicity, enabling it to speed up rapidly in anticipation of exercise and to increase to 200 beats per minute in maximum exercise.

6. A large part of the heart rate adjustment to exercise is probably due to cortical influence prior to and during the initial stages of the activity.

7. Nerves, hormones, and local metabolic factors act on the smooth muscle bands in various blood vessels. This causes them to alter their internal diameter to regulate blood flow. Adrenergic sympathetic fibers release norepinephrine, which causes vasoconstriction; cholinergic sympathetic neurons secrete acetylcholine, which brings about vasodilation.

References

1. Bevegård, B.S., and Shepherd, J.T.: Regulation of the circulation during exercise in man. Physiol. Rev., *47:*178, 1967.
2. Bolter, C. et al.: Intrinsic rate and cholinergic sensitivity of isolated atria from trained and sedentary rats. Proc. Soc. Exp. Biol. Med., *144:*364, 1973.
3. Corcondilas, A. et al.: Effect of a brief contraction of forearm muscles on forearm blood flow. J. Appl. Physiol., *19:*1942, 1964.
4. Grimby, G. et al.: Cardiac output during submaximal and maximal exercise in active middle-aged athletes. J. Appl. Physiol., *21:*1150, 1966.
5. Magel, J.R. et al.: Telemetered heart rate response to selected competitive swimming events. J. Appl. Physiol., *26:*764, 1969.
6. McArdle, W.D. et al.: Telemetered cardiac response to selected running events. J. Appl. Physiol., *23:*566, 1967.
7. Petro, J.K. et al.: Instantaneous cardiac acceleration in a man induced by voluntary muscle contractions. J. Appl. Physiol., *29:*794, 1970.
7a. Rowell, L.B.: Human cardiovascular adjustments to exercise and thermal stress. Physiol. Rev., *54:*75, 1974.
8. Scheuer, J. et al.: Experimental observations on the effects of physical training upon intrinsic cardiac physiology and biochemistry. Am. J. Cardiol., *33:*744, 1974.
9. Shepherd, J.T.: Behavior of resistance and capacity vessels in human limbs during exercise. Circ. Res., *20* (Suppl. 1):70, 1967.
10. White, J.R.: EKG changes using carotid artery for heart rate monitoring. Med. Sci. Sports, *9:*88, 1977.
11. Zweifach, B.J.: The microcirculation of the blood. Sci. Am., January, p. 54, 1959.

Functional Capacity of the Cardiovascular System

17

MEASUREMENT OF CARDIAC OUTPUT

Cardiac output is the primary indicator of the functional capacity of the circulation to meet the demands of physical activity. Output from the heart, as with any pump, is determined by its rate of pumping (*heart rate*) and by the quantity of blood ejected with each stroke (*stroke volume*). Thus, cardiac output is computed as:

Cardiac output = Heart rate × Stroke volume

The output from a hose, pump, or faucet can easily be determined. One need only open the valve, collect and measure the volume of fluid ejected, and record the time. This, however, is not the case with the measurement of cardiac output. Even if such a *direct* technique were applied, the disruption of the main output vessel in a closed circulatory system would in itself dramatically alter the output. With advances in biomedical engineering, however, electromagnetic and ultrasonic flowmeters can be surgically implanted around a main artery in the vascular circuit. For obvious reasons, this technique is usually limited to animal research and has little application for use in a typical exercise setting with healthy humans. The direct Fick, indicator dilution, and CO_2 rebreathing methods are commonly used in human measurement.

Direct Fick Method

Cardiac output can be easily computed if one knows a person's oxygen consumption during a minute and the average difference between the oxygen content of arterial and mixed venous blood (a-$\bar{v}$ O_2 difference). The question to be answered is: How much blood must have circulated during the minute to account for the observed oxygen consumption, given the observed a-$\bar{v}$ O_2 difference? The formula expressing the relationship between cardiac output, oxygen consumption, and a-$\bar{v}$ O_2 difference embodies the principle set forth by Fick in 1870 and is termed the *Fick equation*.

$$\begin{array}{c} \text{Cardiac} \\ \text{output} \\ (\text{ml} \cdot \text{min}^{-1}) \end{array} = \frac{\begin{array}{c}O_2 \text{ consumption} \\ (\text{ml} \cdot \text{min}^{-1})\end{array}}{\begin{array}{c}\text{a-}\bar{v}\ O_2 \text{ difference} \\ (\text{ml per 100 ml blood})\end{array}} \times 100$$

The Fick principle for determining cardiac output is illustrated in Figure 17-1. In this example, 250 ml of oxygen are consumed during a minute at rest, and the a-$\bar{v}$ O_2 difference during this time averages 5 ml of oxygen per 100 ml of blood. Substituting these values in the Fick equation,

$$\begin{array}{c} \text{Cardiac} \\ \text{output} \\ (\text{ml} \cdot \text{min}^{-1}) \end{array} = \frac{250 \text{ ml } O_2}{5 \text{ ml } O_2} \times 100 = \frac{5000 \text{ ml}}{\text{blood}}$$

Although the Fick principle is straightforward, the actual measurement of cardiac output by this technique is complex and is usually limited to a clinical setting where the benefits of measurement exceed any potential risk. The measurement of oxygen consumption involves the methods of open-circuit spirometry summarized in Chapter 8. A more difficult aspect is the sampling of arterial and mixed venous blood to obtain the a-$\bar{v}$ O_2 difference. A representative sample of arterial blood can be obtained from any convenient systemic artery such as the femoral, radial, or brachial artery. Although

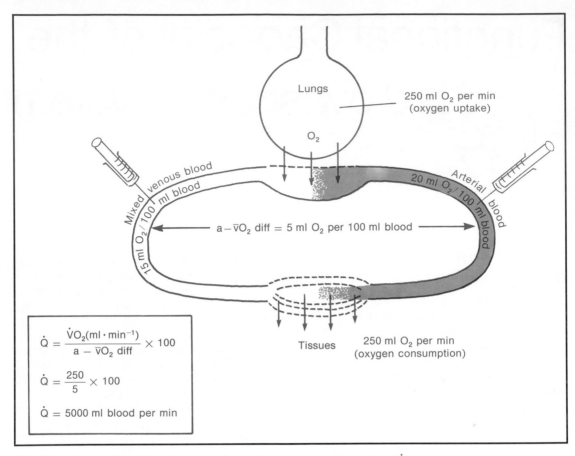

FIG. 17-1. *Application of the Fick principle for determining cardiac output ($\dot{Q}$).*

these arteries are easily located, the actual arterial puncture can be traumatic to the patient. Sampling of mixed venous blood presents additional difficulties because the blood in each vein only reflects the metabolic activity of the specific area it drains. To obtain an accurate estimate of the average oxygen content of venous blood, it is necessary to sample from an anatomic "mixing chamber" such as the right atrium, right ventricle, or even the pulmonary artery. This is achieved by threading a small flexible tube or catheter through the antecubital vein in the arm, up into the superior vena cava, and into the right heart. Arterial and mixed venous blood are then sampled during the same period that oxygen consumption is measured.

The direct Fick technique has been used in numerous studies of cardiovascular dynamics under a variety of experimental conditions. In fact, this method generally provides the criterion to validate other techniques for cardiac output measurement. The main criticism of the method is that by its very nature of being *inva-*

sive to the body, cardiovascular dynamics may be altered during the measurement period. Thus, although the obtained value for cardiac output may be accurate, it may not reflect the person's "normal" cardiovascular response in a particular situation.

Indicator Dilution Method

This technique involves venous and arterial punctures, but does not require cardiac catheterization. A known quantity of harmless dye such as idocyanine green or of a radioactive substance is injected into a large vein. The indicator material remains in the vascular stream and is usually bound to plasma proteins or red blood cells. It is then mixed as the blood travels to the lungs and back to the heart before being ejected into the systemic circuit. Arterial blood samples are continually measured with a radioactive counter or photosensitive device. The area under the dilution–concentration curve obtained by this repetitive sampling indicates the average concentration of indicator material as blood is pumped from the heart. From the dilution of a known quantity of dye in an unknown quantity of blood, the cardiac output is calculated as follows:

$$\text{Cardiac output} = \frac{\text{Quantity of dye injected}}{\text{Average conc. dye in blood for duration of curve} \times \text{Duration of curve}}$$

CO_2 Rebreathing Method

Cardiac output can be determined from values of carbon dioxide substituted in the Fick equation. By using a rapid carbon dioxide gas analyzer and making certain reasonable assumptions, it is possible to obtain valid estimates of venous and arterial carbon dioxide levels. The technique is noninvasive or "bloodless," and simply requires a breath-by-breath analysis of carbon dioxide.[16a]

Once venous and arterial carbon dioxide concentrations are estimated, cardiac output is calculated in accordance with the Fick principle as follows:

$$\text{Cardiac output} = \frac{\text{Carbon dioxide production}}{\bar{v}\text{-a } CO_2 \text{ difference}} \times 100$$

The advantages of the CO_2 rebreathing method over the direct Fick and indicator dilution techniques are obvious. The method is bloodless, involves minimal interference with the subject, and does not require close medical supervision. Because the method is noninvasive, it may provide more accurate estimates of the cardiovascular dynamics during exercise than would be obtained by more direct techniques.[10] One limitation of the method is that it requires the subject to exercise at a steady metabolic rate. This may place some restrictions on its use during maximal and "supermaximal" exercise or during the transition from rest to exercise.

CARDIAC OUTPUT AT REST

Cardiac output at rest is widely variable. It is affected by emotional conditions that alter cortical outflow to the cardioaccelerator nerves as well as to nerves that act on the resistance and capacitance vessels. On the average, however, the entire blood volume of approximately 5 liters is pumped from the left ventricle each min-

ute. This value is similar for both trained and untrained subjects. For the average person, a 5-liter cardiac output is usually sustained with a heart rate of about 70 beats per minute. Substituting this heart rate value in the cardiac output equation, the calculated stroke volume of the heart equals 71 ml per beat. Stroke volumes for females usually average 25% below values for men and are 50 to 70 ml per beat at rest. This "sex difference" is essentially due to the smaller body size of the average woman as compared to the average man.

Endurance training causes the sinus node of the heart to come under greater influence of acetylcholine, the parasympathetic hormone that has a slowing effect on heart rate.[29] This effect is probably accompanied by a concomitant reduction in resting sympathetic activity. This training adaptation partially explains the relatively low resting heart rates of many male and female endurance athletes. Their heart rates generally average about 50 beats per minute at rest, although heart rates below 40 beats per minute have been reported for apparently healthy endurance athletes. (Extreme bradycardia at rest is not necessarily a general phenomenon with well-trained athletes. For example, resting pulse rates of 64 to 76 beats per minute have been observed for Jim Ryun, former world-record-holder in the 1-mile run.[7]) Because the resting cardiac output of endurance athletes also averages 5 liters per minute, blood is circulated with the proportionately larger stroke volume of 100 ml per beat. Average values for cardiac output, heart rate, and stroke volume of trained and sedentary people at rest are summarized as follows:

Rest

$$\text{Cardiac output} = \text{Heart rate} \times \text{Stroke volume}$$

Sedentary: 5000 ml = 70 b · min⁻¹ × 71 ml
Trained: 5000 ml = 50 b · min⁻¹ × 100 ml

Although these calculations are straightforward, the underlying physiologic mechanisms are still poorly understood. It is not clear whether the bradycardia that occurs with endurance training "causes" a larger stroke volume or vice versa, because the myocardium itself is strengthened through aerobic exercise. Both factors are probably operative with training: (1) endurance training increases vagal tone that slows the heart, and (2) the heart muscle strengthened through training is capable of a more forceful stroke with each contraction.

CARDIAC OUTPUT
DURING EXERCISE

Blood flow increases in proportion to the severity of exercise. In progressing from rest to steady-rate exercise, cardiac output undergoes a rapid increase followed by a gradual rise until a plateau is reached. At this point, blood flow is presumably sufficient to meet the metabolic requirements of exercise.

In relatively sedentary, college-aged males, cardiac output during *strenuous* exercise increases by about four times the resting level to an average maximum of 20 to 22 liters of blood per minute. Maximum heart rate for these young adults usually averages about 195 beats per minute. Consequently, the stroke volume is generally 103 to 113 ml of blood per beat during maximal exercise. In contrast, world-class endurance athletes have maximum cardiac outputs of 35 to 40 liters per minute. This is even more impressive if one considers that the trained person may have a slightly lower maximum heart rate than the sedentary person of similar age.[17,20] Thus, *the endurance athlete achieves a large cardiac output compared with his or her sedentary counterpart due to a considerably larger stroke volume.* For example, the cardiac output of an Olympic medal winner in cross-country skiing increased almost 8 times above rest to 40 liters per minute in maximum work with an accompanying stroke volume of 210 ml per beat. This is nearly twice the volume of blood pumped per beat in comparison to the maximum stroke volume of healthy, sedentary people of similar age.

The functional capacity of the heart during maximal exercise in trained and untrained men is summarized as follows:

Maximum Exercise

$$\frac{\text{Cardiac}}{\text{output}} = \frac{\text{Heart}}{\text{rate}} \times \frac{\text{Stroke}}{\text{volume}}$$

Sedentary: 22,000 ml = 195 b · min⁻¹ × 113 ml
Trained: 35,000 ml = 195 b · min⁻¹ × 179 ml

Stroke Volume in Exercise:
Training Effects

Figure 17-2 illustrates the stroke volume response for two groups of men during upright exercise of increasing severity. One group consisted of six highly trained endurance athletes who had trained for several years; the other group was comprised of three sedentary col-

lege students. The students' exercise responses were evaluated before and after a 55-day training program designed to improve aerobic fitness.[28]

From these data, several important conclusions can be drawn: (1) The endurance athlete's heart has a considerably larger stroke volume during both rest and exercise than an untrained person of the same age. (2) For both trained and untrained individuals, the greatest increase in stroke volume in upright exercise occurs in the transition from rest to moderate exercise. As exercise becomes more intense, stroke volume increases are small. (3) Maximum stroke volume is reached at 40% to 50% of the maximal oxygen consumption; this usually represents a heart rate of 110 to 120 beats per minute. Stroke volume does not decrease at the more intense exercise levels. This suggests that even at rapid heart rates there is still adequate time for the ventricles to fill during diastole, so the stroke volume is not diminished. (4) For untrained individuals, there is only a small increase in stroke volume in the transition from rest to exercise. For these individuals, the major increase in cardiac output is brought about by an acceleration in heart rate. For the trained endurance athletes, *both* heart rate and stroke volume increase to augment cardiac output, with the increase in the athlete's stroke volume being generally 50% to 60% above resting values. For previously sed-

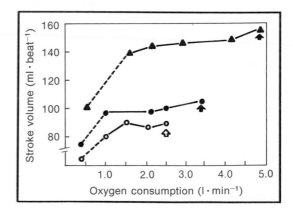

FIG. 17-2. *Stroke volume in relation to oxygen consumption during upright exercise in endurance athletes (▲) and sedentary college students prior to (0) and following (●) 55 days of aerobic training; (⬦, ♠ = maximal values). (From Saltin, B.: Physiological effects of physical conditioning. Med. Sci. Sports, 1:50, 1969. Copyright 1969, the American College of Sports Medicine. Reprinted by Permission.)*

entary subjects, 8 weeks of aerobic training substantially increases stroke volume, but these values are still well below values observed for elite athletes. The degree to which this difference reflects prolonged training, genetics, or a combination of both has yet to be determined.

The importance of stroke volume in differentiating people with very high and very low max $\dot{V}O_2$ is amplified in Table 17-1.

These data were obtained from three groups: athletes, healthy but sedentary men, and patients with mitral stenosis, a valvular disease of the heart that results in inadequate filling of the left ventricle. The differences in max $\dot{V}O_2$ between groups are closely related to differences in maximal stroke volume. Patients with mitral stenosis had an aerobic capacity and maximum stroke volume that was half that of the sedentary subject's. This relationship was also apparent in comparisons between healthy subjects. The maximal oxygen uptakes of the athletes averaged 62.5% larger than those of the sedentary group. This was paralleled by a 60% larger stroke volume. Since the maximal heart rates of both groups were similar, differences in cardiac output (and max $\dot{V}O_2$) were almost entirely due to differences in maximal stroke volume.

Stroke Volume: Systolic Emptying Versus Diastolic Filling

Essentially, two physiologic mechanisms regulate stroke volume. The first is intrinsic to the myocardium and requires enhanced cardiac filling that is followed by a more forceful contraction. The second mechanism is under neurohormonal influence. It involves normal ventricular filling that is accompanied by an increased stroke due to a forceful systolic ejection that brings about a greater cardiac emptying.

ENHANCED DIASTOLIC FILLING. Any factor that increases venous return or slows the heart causes greater ventricular filling during the diastolic phase of the cardiac cycle. This increase in *end-diastolic volume* stretches the myocardial fibers and causes a powerful ejection stroke as the heart contracts. As a result, the normal stroke volume is expelled plus the additional blood that entered the ventricles and stretched the myocardium.

The relationship between the force of contraction and the resting length of muscle fibers was described by two physiologists, Frank and Starling, in the early 1900s. The improved contractility probably results from a more optimum arrangement of myofilaments as the muscle stretches. This phenomenon as applied to the myocardium has been termed *Starling's law of the heart.*

For many years it was taught that the Frank-Starling mechanism provided the "modus operandi" for *all* increases in stroke volume during exercise. Physiologists believed that the enhanced venous return in exercise caused a greater cardiac filling, so that the ventricles were stretched in diastole and subsequently responded with a more forceful ejection. In all likelihood, this is the pattern of response for stroke volume as a person moves from the upright to the recumbent position. Enhanced diastolic filling probably also occurs in certain activities, such as swimming, in which the body's horizontal position optimizes the flow of blood into the heart.

From the data in Table 17-2, it is clear that body position has a significant effect on circulatory dynamics.[6] Cardiac output and stroke volume are highest and most stable in the horizontal position. In this position, the stroke volume is nearly maximum at rest and increases only slightly during exercise. In contrast, the

TABLE 17-1. *Maximal values of oxygen uptake, heart rate, stroke volume, and cardiac output in three groups having very low, normal, and high max $\dot{V}O_2$*[a]

GROUP	MAX $\dot{V}O_2$ (l · min^{-1})	MAX HEART RATE (beats · min^{-1})	MAX STROKE VOLUME (ml)	MAX CARDIAC OUTPUT (l · min^{-1})
Mitral stenosis	1.6	190	50	9.5
Sedentary	3.2	200	100	20.0
Athlete	5.2	190	160	30.4

[a] Modified from Rowell, L.B.: Circulation. *Med. Sci. Sports,* 1:15, 1969.[29] Copyright 1969, the American College of Sports Medicine. Reprinted by Permission.

TABLE 17-2. *The effect of body position on cardiac output, stroke volume, and heart rate at rest and during exercise (active subjects)*[a]

	REST		MODERATE EXERCISE		STRENUOUS EXERCISE	
	SUPINE	UPRIGHT	SUPINE	UPRIGHT	SUPINE	UPRIGHT
Cardiac output, $l \cdot min^{-1}$	9.2	6.6	19.0	16.9	26.3	24.5
Stroke volume, ml	141	103	163	149	164	155
Heart rate, beats $\cdot min^{-1}$	65	64	115	112	160	159
Oxygen consumption, $l \cdot min^{-1}$	345	384	1769	1864	3364	3387

[a] Data from Bevegård, S. et al.: Circulatory studies in well-trained athletes at rest and during heavy exercise, with special reference to stroke volume and the influence of body position. *Acta Physiol. Scand., 57:26,* 1963.

force of gravity in the upright position acts to counter the return flow of blood to the heart; this results in diminished stroke volume and cardiac output. This postural effect is especially apparent in comparing circulatory dynamics at rest in the upright and supine positions. As the intensity of upright exercise increases, however, stroke volume increases and more closely approaches the maximum stroke volume in the supine position.

GREATER SYSTOLIC EMPTYING. In most forms of upright exercise, the heart does not fill to an extent that would cause a significant increase in cardiac volume.[27] Actually, some reports even indicate a decrease in the diastolic size of the heart during such exercise.[26] It is now generally agreed that in upright exercise both the sedentary and trained heart increase stroke volume by means of a more complete emptying during systole.

A greater systolic ejection without an accompanying increase in end-diastolic volume is possible because the heart possesses a *functional residual volume.* At rest in the upright position, 40% to 50% of the total end-diastolic blood volume remains in the left ventricle after a contraction; this amounts to approximately 50 to 70 ml of blood. Myocardial strength is enhanced in exercise by the action of the sympathetic hormones epinephrine and norepinephrine, which produce augmented stroke power and greater systolic emptying of the heart. In addition, endurance training enhances the contractile state of the myocardium itself and improves its capability for achieving a large stroke volume.

Heart Rate During Exercise: Training Effects

The large stroke volume of topflight endurance athletes and the increases in stroke volume of sedentary subjects following aerobic training are usually accompanied by a proportionate heart rate reduction during submaximal exercise. The relationship between heart rate and oxygen consumption is shown in Figure 17-3.

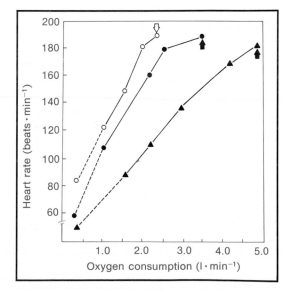

FIG. 17-3. *Heart rate in relation to oxygen consumption during upright exercise in endurance athletes (▲) and sedentary college students prior to (0) and following (●) 55 days of aerobic training; (⇧ = maximal values).* (From Saltin, B.: Physiological effects of physical conditioning. Med. Sci. Sports, *1:*50, 1969. Copyright 1969, the American College of Sports Medicine. Reprinted by Permission.)

As with the previous figure for stroke volume, comparisons are made between athletes and sedentary students before and after training.

The lines relating heart rate and oxygen consumption are essentially linear for both groups throughout the major portion of the work range. Whereas the untrained students' heart rates accelerated rapidly as exercise severity increased, the heart rates of the athletes accelerated to a much lesser extent; that is, the slope or rate of change of the lines differed considerably. Consequently, an athlete (or trained student) with good cardiovascular response to exercise will do more work and achieve a higher oxygen consumption before reaching a particular submaximal heart rate than a sedentary student. At an oxygen consumption of 2.0 liters per minute, for example, the heart rates of the athletes averaged 70 beats per minute lower than those of the sedentary students! Following 55 days of training, this difference in submaximal heart rate was reduced to about 40 beats per minute. In each instance, the cardiac output was approximately the same—*the difference was the stroke volume.*

DISTRIBUTION OF CARDIAC OUTPUT

The blood flow to specific tissues is generally proportional to their metabolic activity. However, blood flow to the kidneys, skin, and splanchnic areas can also vary with the physiologic function of these tissues in a specific circumstance.

Blood Flow at Rest

At rest in a comfortable environment, the five-liter cardiac output is distributed in roughly the proportions shown in Table 17-3. As can be seen, about one-fifth of the cardiac output is directed to muscle tissue whereas the major portion of blood flows to the digestive tract, liver, spleen, brain, and kidneys.

Blood Flow During Exercise

The percentage distribution of the cardiac output during light, moderate, and strenuous exercise is shown in Table 17-4. Although regional blood flow during physical activity varies considerably depending on environmental conditions, level of fatigue, and the type of exercise, *the major portion of the exercise cardiac output is diverted to the working muscles.* At rest, about 4 to 7 ml of blood are delivered each minute to every 100 g of muscle. This output increases steadily until at maximum exertion, muscle blood flow may be as high as 50 to 75 ml per 100 g of tissue. This represents about 85% of the total cardiac output.

The increase in muscle blood flow in exercise is due largely to increased cardiac output. However, muscle blood flow is disproportionately large in relation to blood flow in other tissues. Due to neural and hormonal vascular regulation and the local metabolic conditions of the muscles themselves, blood is redistributed and directed through working muscles from areas that can temporarily tolerate a reduction in normal blood flow. This *shunting* of blood from specific tissues occurs primarily during maximum exercise. Blood flow to the skin increases during light and moderate exercise so the metabolic heat generated in muscle can be dissipated at the skin's surface. During intense work of short duration, however, this tissue temporarily restricts its bloodflow, even if the exercise is performed in a hot environment.[25] In some instances, blood flow is reduced by as much as four-fifths of an organ's blood supply at rest! The kidneys and splanchnic tissues, for example, utilize only 10% to 25% of the oxygen available in their blood supply. Consequently, a considerable reduction in blood flow to these tissues can be tolerated before oxygen demand exceeds supply and function is compromised.[27] With reduced blood flow, the energy needs of the tissues are maintained by increased extraction of oxygen from the available blood supply. A substantial reduction in blood flow to the visceral organs can be sustained for more than an hour during heavy exercise. Redistribution of

TABLE 17-3. *Relative distribution of a five-liter cardiac output*

ORGAN	PERCENTAGE	VOLUME PER MINUTE (ml)
① Hepatic-splanchnic	27	1350
② Kidneys	22	1100
③ Muscles	20	1000
④ Brain	14	700
⑤ Skin	6	300
⑥ Heart	4	200
⑦ Other	7	350
TOTAL	100	5000

TABLE 17-4. *Distribution of cardiac output during light, moderate, and strenuous exercise, as well as the oxygen extraction in these various tissues at rest*[a]

TISSUE	RESTING a-v̄ O_2 DIFFERENCE (ml O_2 PER 100 ml BLOOD)	EXERCISE BLOOD FLOW, ml · min^{-1}		
		LIGHT	MODERATE	MAXIMUM
Splanchnic	4.1	1100 (12%)	600 (3%)	300 (1%)
Renal	1.3	900 (10%)	600 (3%)	250 (1%)
Cerebral	6.3	750 (8%)	750 (4%)	750 (3%)
Coronary	14.0	350 (4%)	750 (4%)	1000 (4%)
Muscle	8.4	4500 (47%)	12,500 (71%)	22,000 (88%)
Skin	1.0	1500 (15%)	1900 (12%)	600 (2%)
Other		400 (4%)	400 (3%)	100 (1%)
		9500	17,500	25,000

[a]Modified from Anderson, K.L.: The cardiovascular system in exercise. *In* Exercise Physiology, Edited by H.B. Falls. New York, Academic Press, 1968.

blood from these tissues occurs even without an increase in cardiac output; this "frees" as much as 600 ml of oxygen per minute for use by the working muscles.[24] However, prolonged reduction in blood flow to the liver and kidneys may have its consequences and may partially account for the fatigue eventually observed in continuous, submaximal exercise.

Blood Flow to the Heart

Some tissues cannot compromise their blood supply (Table 17-4). The myocardium normally uses about 75% of the oxygen in the blood flowing through the coronary circulation at rest. With this limited margin of safety, the increased myocardial oxygen needs in exercise can be met *only* by an increase in coronary blood flow. Thus, a four- to fivefold increase in cardiac output is accompanied by a similar increase in coronary circulation; in maximum exercise this amounts to about 1 liter of blood per minute.

CARDIAC OUTPUT AND OXYGEN TRANSPORT

Rest

Each 100 ml of arterial blood carries about 20 ml of oxygen or 200 ml of oxygen per liter of blood (see Chap. 13). The oxygen-carrying capacity of blood normally varies only slightly because the hemoglobin content of the blood fluctuates little with one's state of training. Because about 5 liters of blood are circulated each minute at rest, potentially 1000 ml of oxygen are available to the body (5 liters blood ×

200 ml O_2). Because the oxygen consumption at rest averages only 250 ml per minute, about 750 ml of oxygen return unused to the heart. This, however, is not an unnecessary waste of cardiac output. On the contrary, this extra oxygen above the resting needs represents oxygen in reserve—a margin of safety that can be released immediately should a tissue's metabolic needs suddenly increase.

Exercise

A person with a maximum heart rate of 200 beats per minute and a stroke volume of 80 ml per beat generates a maximum cardiac output of 16 liters (200 × 80 ml). Even during maximum exercise, the saturation of hemoglobin with oxygen is nearly complete, so each liter of blood carries about 200 ml of oxygen. Consequently, 3200 ml of oxygen are circulated each minute via a 16-liter cardiac output (16 liters × 200 ml O_2). If all the oxygen could be extracted from this 16-liter cardiac output as it traveled through the body, the greatest possible max $\dot{V}O_2$ would be 3200 ml. This is only theoretical, however, because the oxygen needs of certain tissues such as the brain do not increase greatly with exercise, yet these tissues require a constant supply of blood.

Any increase in the maximum cardiac output directly affects a person's capacity to circulate oxygen. Based on the preceding example, if the heart's stroke volume was increased from 80 to 200 ml per beat while the maximum heart rate remained unchanged at 200 beats per minute, maximum cardiac output would be dramatically increased to 40 liters of blood per minute. This means that the quantity of oxygen circulated in

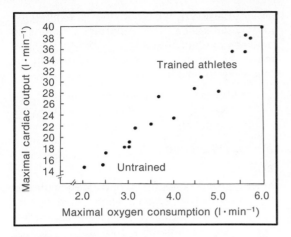

FIG. 17-4. *Relationship between maximal cardiac output and maximal aerobic power.*

maximum exercise each minute would have increased approximately $2\frac{1}{2}$ times from 3200 to 8000 ml. *An increase in maximum cardiac output clearly results in a proportionate increase in the potential for aerobic metabolism.*

The relationship between maximum cardiac output and the capacity for achieving a high level of aerobic metabolism is shown in Figure 17-4. Included are values for the sedentary and untrained as well as elite endurance athletes.

The relationship is unmistakable. A low aerobic capacity is clearly associated with a low maximum cardiac output, whereas the ability to generate a 5- or 6-liter max $\dot{V}O_2$ is always accompanied by a 30- to 40-liter cardiac output.

Figure 17-5 further amplifies the important role of cardiac output in sustaining aerobic metabolism. For both trained athletes and students, the cardiac output increases linearly with oxygen consumption throughout the major portion of the work range. Each one-liter increase in oxygen consumption is generally accompanied by a 6-liter increase in blood flow. The distinguishing feature for the endurance athletes is a high level of oxygen consumption *and* of cardiac output capacity. The 35% increase in max $\dot{V}O_2$ noted for the students after 55 days of training was accompanied by an almost proportionate increase in maximum cardiac output.

DIFFERENCES IN CARDIAC OUTPUT BETWEEN MEN AND WOMEN. The response pattern of cardiac output during exercise is similar between boys and girls and men and women. However, both teenage and adult females have a 5% to 10% *larger* cardiac output at any level of submaximal oxygen uptake than males. This apparent "sex difference" in cardiac output in submaximal

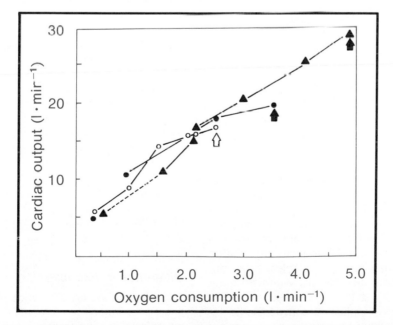

FIG. 17-5. *Cardiac output in relation to oxygen consumption during upright exercise in endurance athletes (▲) and sedentary college students prior to (0) and following (●) 55 days of aerobic training, (⇧, ♠ = maximal values).* (From Saltin, B.: Physiological effects of physical conditioning. Med. Sci. Sports, *1*:50, 1969. Copyright 1969, the American College of Sports Medicine. Reprinted by Permission.)

exercise may be due to the lower hemoglobin content of the blood of women, which is about 10% below the values for men.[2] Consequently, within limits, a small decrease in the blood's oxygen-carrying capacity due to lower hemoglobin is compensated for by a proportionate increase in cardiac output in submaximal exercise.

TRAINING AND SUBMAXIMAL CARDIAC OUTPUT. Several reports have demonstrated that training, although improving the maximal cardiac output, also tends to reduce the minute volume of the heart during moderate exercise in young adult and middle-aged subjects.[1,13] This apparent training adaptation has also been observed in comparisons of trained endurance athletes and sedentary subjects.[1,12,13,32] In one study, the average cardiac output of young men after 16 weeks of training was reduced by 1.5 and 1.1 liters per minute at a 1.0- and 2.0-liter submaximal oxygen uptake, respectively.[9] As expected, the maximal cardiac output for these men increased 8% from 22.4 to 24.2 liters per minute. With the reduction in submaximal cardiac output, the exercise oxygen requirement was met by a corresponding increase in a-$\bar{v}$ O$_2$ difference. This greater oxygen extraction was presumably the result of an enhanced ability of the trained muscles to generate ATP aerobically and function at a lower partial pressure of oxygen.

EXTRACTION OF OXYGEN: THE a-$\bar{v}$ O$_2$ DIFFERENCE

If blood flow were the only means for increasing a tissue's oxygen supply, then cardiac output would have to increase from 5 liters per minute at rest to 100 liters per minute in maximum exercise in order to achieve a 20-fold increase in oxygen consumption—an increase in oxygen consumption that is not uncommon among trained people. Fortunately, such a large cardiac output is unnecessary during exercise because hemoglobin releases a considerable ''extra'' quantity of oxygen from the blood that perfuses the active tissues. Consequently, two mechanisms are available to increase the capacity for oxygen consumption. The *first* is to speed up the rate of blood flow, that is, increase cardiac output; the *second* is to utilize the relatively large quantity of oxygen

already carried by the blood, that is, expand the a-$\bar{v}$ O$_2$ difference. The important relationship between cardiac output, a-$\bar{v}$ O$_2$ difference, and maximum aerobic power is summarized in the following equation:

$$\begin{array}{ccc} \text{Maximal} & \text{Maximal} & \text{Maximal} \\ \text{oxygen} & = \text{cardiac} \times & \text{a-}\bar{v}\text{ O}_2 \\ \text{consumption} & \text{output} & \text{difference} \end{array}$$

a-$\bar{v}$ O$_2$ Difference at Rest

At rest, an average of 5 ml of oxygen is utilized from the 20 ml of oxygen in each 100 ml of arterial blood as it passes through the capillaries. Thus, 75% of the blood's original oxygen load still remains bound to the hemoglobin.

a-$\bar{v}$ O$_2$ Difference in Exercise

Figure 17-6 is a comparison of the relationship between oxygen extraction (a-$\bar{v}$ O$_2$ difference) and exercise intensity for trained athletes and sedentary students. For the sedentary students, a-$\bar{v}$ O$_2$ difference increases steadily during light and moderate exercise and reaches a maximum value of about 15 ml of oxygen per 100 ml of blood. Following 55 days of training, the student's maximum capability for oxygen extraction increased about 11% to 17 ml of oxygen. This means that about 85% of the oxygen was extracted from arterial blood during heavy exercise. Actually, even more oxygen is released in the working muscles because the value for a-$\bar{v}$ O$_2$ difference reflects an *average* based on calculations from mixed venous blood. This contains blood returning from tissues whose oxygen utilization during exercise is not nearly as high as that of active muscle.

The post-training value for the maximal a-$\bar{v}$ O$_2$ difference for the students is identical to that achieved by the endurance athletes. Obviously, the rather large difference in max $\dot{V}O_2$ that still exists between the athletes and students is due to the lower cardiac output capacity of the students.

Factors Affecting a-$\bar{v}$ O$_2$ Difference in Exercise

The maximal a-$\bar{v}$ O$_2$ difference attained during exercise is influenced to some degree by one's capacity to divert a large portion of the cardiac output to working muscles. As mentioned previously, certain tissues can temporarily compromise their blood supply considerably during

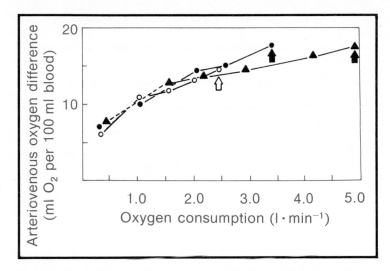

FIG. 17-6. *a-∇ O₂ difference in relation to oxygen consumption during upright exercise in endurance athletes (▲) and sedentary college students prior to (0) and following (●) 55 days of training; (⇧, ♠ = maximal values).* (From Saltin, B.: Physiological effects of physical conditioning. Med. Sci. Sports, *1*:50, 1969. Copyright 1969, the American College of Sports Medicine. Reprinted by Permission.)

exercise for purposes of shunting blood and increasing the quantity of oxygen available for muscle metabolism. This redirection of the central circulation is facilitated by exercise training.

At the local level, the microcirculation of skeletal muscle is also enhanced with aerobic training.[28a] Several studies with humans and animals have demonstrated a greater capillary density in specific muscles trained by endurance exercise. Muscle biopsies from the *quadriceps femoris* showed a significantly larger ratio of capillaries to muscle fibers in trained than in sedentary men.[14] Although the evidence for increased capillarization with training is far from conclusive, an increase in the capillary-to-fiber ratio would certainly appear to be a positive adaptation because it would provide for a greater interface for the exchange of nutrients and metabolic gases in exercise.

Another important factor determining the capacity for oxygen extraction is the ability of individual muscle cells to generate energy aerobically. Aerobic training improves the metabolic capacity of the specific cells trained by exercise. The mitochondria enlarge and even increase in number, whereas the quantity of enzymes for aerobic energy transfer also increases.[15] All of these local improvements within the muscle ultimately result in an enhanced capacity for the aerobic production of ATP.

CARDIAC HYPERTROPHY AND THE "ATHLETE'S HEART"

A *moderate* increase in heart size is a *normal* response to exercise training. This cardiac *hypertrophy* can be viewed as a fundamental biologic adaptation of muscle to an increased work load.[11,19] In such situations, a greater synthesis of cellular protein occurs with a concomitant reduction in protein breakdown. This accelerated protein synthesis is due largely to an increase in the muscle's content of RNA.[4] Individual myofibrils thicken; at the same time, the number of these contractile filaments within the muscle fiber increases.[22]

The heart volume, determined by x-ray examination of 30 young girl swimmers, was generally much larger than expected for their body size.[3] In terms of functional significance, the heart volume correlated well with the girls' maximal oxygen uptake. Additional evidence is presented in Table 17-5 to support the case that in healthy individuals, some cardiac hypertrophy results from training.

In sedentary men, the average heart volume was about 800 ml; this volume increased in athletes in relation to the aerobic nature of the sport, so that for endurance athletes the average heart volumes were about 25% larger than those of sedentary men. The degree to which

TABLE 17-5. *Heart volumes estimated from areas of heart shadow determined by x-ray examination*[a]

SPORTS CATEGORY	NUMBER OF SUBJECTS	MEAN VOLUME (ml)	RANGE
Normal	67	790	490–1080
Wrestlers and high jumpers	30	782	610–920
Swimmers, soccer players, and tennis players	86	876	605–1130
Skiers, long-distance runners, and swimmers	66	923	645–1180
Professional cyclists	18	1104	880–1460

[a] From Anderson, K.L.: The cardiovascular system in exercise. *In* Exercise Physiology. Edited by H.B. Falls. New York, Academic Press, 1968.

the relatively large heart volumes of some endurance athletes reflect genetic endowment or training adaptations, or both, has yet to be determined.

Cardiac hypertrophy is also seen in certain diseases. In chronic hypertension, for example, the heart must continually work against an excessive resistance to the flow of blood. As a result, the heart muscle stretches and, in accordance with the Frank-Starling mechanism, generates compensatory force to overcome the added vascular resistance. In addition to this ventricular stretching or dilation, the individual muscle cells hypertrophy to adjust to the increased myocardial work imposed by vascular disease. As the untreated hypertension progresses, the myocardial fibers are eventually stretched beyond their optimal length, and the dilated, hypertrophied heart weakens and eventually fails. To the pathologist, the "hypertrophied" heart of the cardiac patient is enlarged, flabby, and functionally inadequate to deliver even enough blood to meet the minimal resting requirements.

At times, the cardiac hypertrophy in response to chronic pathologic states has been confused with the moderate compensatory growth of the myocardium with endurance training. Although the stress of exercise requires that myocardial fibers generate increased tension, *a critical requirement for initiating compensatory hypertrophy,* the application of this overload differs considerably from that of the chronic resistance imposed by vascular disease. For one thing, during exercise training the myocardial overload is only temporary so a "recuperative" time is available during nonexercise periods. Also, if compensatory heart growth does occur with training, it is not accompanied by a dilation

and weakening of the ventricles, a frequent response to chronic hypertension. It is true that the hearts of elite, endurance-trained athletes are usually larger than the hearts of untrained counterparts—*but heart size is generally within the upper range of normal limits.*[21] *The "athlete's heart" is a muscular heart capable of generating a relatively large stroke volume. This enhanced stroke capacity is not the result of a greater filling and subsequent stretching of the myocardium in diastole, but rather of a more forceful systolic ejection and greater ventricular emptying.*

Specific Nature of Training Hypertrophy

The ultrasonic techniques of *echocardiography* have been used to evaluate the structural characteristics of the hearts of athletes and to determine if different patterns of cardiac hypertrophy and enlargement were associated with different types of physical conditioning.[18] Male competitive swimmers, long-distance runners, wrestlers, and shot putters were studied during their competitive seasons and compared to 16 untrained, healthy college men. The swimmers and runners were considered representative of athletes participating in "isotonic" or endurance events; the wrestlers and shot putters represented the "isometric" or resistance-trained athletes. It is clear from the results in Table 17-6 that the structural characteristics of the hearts of apparently healthy athletes differ considerably from those of normal individuals. Also, the pattern of these differences appears to depend on the nature of the exercise conditioning. For example, left ventricular volume and mass were 181 ml and 308 g, respectively for the swim-

TABLE 17-6. *Comparative average cardiac dimensions in college athletes, world-class athletes, and normal subjects*[a]

DIMENSION[b]	COLLEGE RUNNERS (N = 15)	COLLEGE SWIMMERS (N = 15)	WORLD-CLASS RUNNERS (N = 10)	COLLEGE WRESTLERS (N = 12)	WORLD-CLASS SHOT PUTTERS (N = 4)	NORMALS (N = 16)
LVID	54	57	48–59[c]	48	43–52[c]	46
LVV, ml	160	181	154	110	122	101
SV, ml	116	—[d]	113	75	68	—[d]
LV wall, mm	11.3	10.6	10.8	13.7	13.8	10.3
Septum, mm	10.9	10.7	10.9	13.0	13.5	10.3
LV mass, g	302	308	283	330	348	211

[a]From Morganroth, J. et al.: Comparative left ventricular dimensions in trained athletes. Ann. Intern. Med. 82:521, 1975.
[b]LVID, left ventricular internal dimension at end diastole; LVV, left ventricular volume; SV, stroke volume; LV wall, posterobasal left ventricular wall thickness; Septum, ventricular septal thickness; LV mass, left ventricular mass.
[c]Range.
[d]Values not reported.

mers, and 160 ml and 302 g for the runners; the nonathletic controls averaged 101 ml for ventricular volume and 211 g for ventricular mass. Ventricular wall thickness was normal for the endurance athletes. In contrast, the athletes involved in resistance exercises had normal left ventricular volumes but the largest ventricular wall thickness and ventricular mass.

These structural and dimensional differences may largely reflect specific training demands. For example, the training overload for endurance athletes often requires the maintenance of a relatively large cardiac output for many hours each week. As shown in Table 17-5, the myocardial adaptations to this training are certainly in keeping with the development of a large stroke volume. On the other hand, athletes who engage in straining-type, isometric exercise are not subjected to a volume overload, but rather to acute episodes of elevated arterial pressure caused by static muscular contractions. Consequently, this added workload of the left ventricle is compensated for by an increase in ventricular wall thickness. The implications of these apparent differences in training response to long-term cardiovascular health are unknown.

Other Training Adaptations

Although considerable debate in this area exists, endurance training may also improve the vascularization of the myocardium,[13a,30a] especially at the arteriole level.[8,31] In addition, several experimenters have reported an increase in mitochondrial mass and cellular concentra-

tion of respiratory enzymes in the hearts of animals trained by forced running or swimming.[29] In some instances, it appeared that new components were actually being added to the existing mitochondria.[16] Of what significance these vascular and cellular adaptations are to the functional capacity of the heart during exercise has yet to be determined because it is not believed that the healthy untrained heart suffers from an oxygen lack during maximum exercise. These training changes may, however, enable myocardial tissue to function at a lower percentage of its total oxidative capacity during exercise. In addition, they may provide *some* protection from the degenerative process of heart disease.

SUMMARY

1. Cardiac output reflects the functional capacity of the circulatory system. The two factors determining the heart's output capacity are heart rate and stroke volume. The relationship is:

Cardiac output = Heart rate × Stroke volume

2. Several invasive and noninvasive methods are available to measure cardiac output. Each has its specific advantages and disadvantages for use with humans, especially during exercise.

3. Cardiac output increases in proportion to the severity of exercise, from about 5 liters per minute at rest to a maximum of 20 to 25 liters per minute and 35 to 40 liters per minute in college-aged men and elite male endurance athletes, respectively. These differences in

maximum cardiac output are due entirely to the large stroke volumes of the athletes.

4. During upright exercise, stroke volume increases during the transition from rest to light exercise with maximum values reached at about 45% of max $\dot{V}O_2$. Thereafter, cardiac output is increased by increases in heart rate.

5. Increases in stroke volume in upright exercise are generally the result of a more complete systolic emptying rather than a greater filling of the ventricles during diastole. Systolic ejection is augmented by sympathetic hormones. Endurance training improves myocardial strength, which also greatly contributes to stroke power during systole.

6. Heart rate and oxygen consumption are linearly related for both trained and untrained individuals through the major portion of the work range. With endurance training, this line shifts significantly to the right due to improvements in the heart's stroke volume. Consequently, heart rate becomes significantly reduced at any submaximal work level.

7. Blood flow to specific tissues is gener-ally regulated in proportion to their metabolic activity. This causes the major portion of exercise cardiac output to be diverted to the working muscles. In addition, a significant quantity of blood is shunted to the muscles from the kidneys and splanchnic regions, which can temporarily compromise their blood supply.

8. The maximal oxygen uptake is determined by the maximum cardiac output and the maximum a-$\bar{v}O_2$ difference. Although large cardiac outputs clearly differentiate endurance athletes from untrained counterparts, the ability to generate a large a-$\bar{v}O_2$ difference is also enhanced with training.

9. Cardiac hypertrophy is a fundamental adaptation to the increased work load imposed by exercise training. It results in a stronger heart that can generate a relatively large stroke volume. There is no scientific evidence that a normal heart is harmed by exercise training.

10. The pattern of structural and dimensional changes in the left ventricle appears to vary with specific forms of exercise training.

References

1. Andrew, G.M. et al.: Effect of athletic training on exercise cardiac output. J. Appl. Physiol., *21:*603, 1966.
2. Åstrand, P.O. et al.: Cardiac output during submaximal and maximal work. J. Appl. Physiol., *19:*268, 1964.
3. Åstrand, P.O. et al.: Girl swimmers—with special references to respiratory and circulatory adaption and gynaecological and psychiatric aspects. *Acta Paediatr., (Suppl.) 147:*5, 1963.
4. Badeer, H.S.: The stimulus to hypertrophy of the myocardium. Circulation, *30:*128, 1964.
5. Bar-Or, O. et al.: Cardiac output of 10- to 13- year-old boys and girls during submaximal exercise. J. Appl. Physiol., *30:*219, 1971.
6. Bevegård, S. et al.: Circulatory studies in well-trained athletes at rest and during heavy exercise, with special reference to stroke volume and the influence of body position. Acta Physiol. Scand., *57:*26, 1963.
7. Daniels, J. T.: Running with Jim Ryun: a five-year study. Physician Sportsmed., *2:*62, 1974.
8. Eckstein, R.W.: Effect of exercise and coronary artery narrowing on coronary collateral circulation. Circ. Res., *5:*230, 1957.
9. Ekblom, B. et al.: Effect of training on circulatory response to exercise. J. Appl. Physiol., *24:*518, 1968.

10. Ferguson, R.J. et al.: Comparison of cardiac outputs determined by CO_2 rebreathing and dye dilution method. J. Appl. Physiol., 25:450, 1968.
11. Goldberg, A.L.: Mechanism of work-induced hypertrophy of skeletal muscle. Med. Sci. Sports, 7:185, 1975.
12. Hanson, J.S., and Tabakian, B.S.: Comparison of the circulatory response to upright exercise in 25 "normal" men and 9 distance runners. Br. Heart J., 27:211, 1965.
13. Hanson, J.S. et al.: Long-term physical training and cardiovascular dynamics in middle aged men. Circulation, 38:783, 1968.
13a. Heaton, W.H., et al.: Beneficial effect of physical training on blood flow to myocardium perfused by chronic collaterals in exercising dog. Circulation, 57:575, 1978.
14. Hermansen, L., and Wachtlova, M.: Capillary density of skeletal muscle in well trained and untrained men. J. Appl. Physiol., 30:860, 1971.
15. Holloszy, J.O., and Booth, F.W.: Biochemical adaptations to endurance exercise in muscle. Annu. Rev. Physiol., 38:273, 1976.
16. Laugens, R.P., and Gomez-Dumm, L.A.: Fine structure of myocardial mitochondria in rats after exercise for one-half to two hours. Circ. Res., 11:271, 1967.
16a. Magel, J.R., and Andersen, K.L.: Cardiac output in muscular exercise measured by the CO_2 rebreathing technique. In Ergometry in Cardiology. Edited by H. Denolin, et al. Boehringer Mannheim GmbH, 1968.
17. McArdle, W.D. et al.: Specificity of run training on VO_2 max and heart rate changes during running and swimming. Med. Sci. Sports, 10:16, 1978.
18. Morganroth, J. et al.: Comparative left ventricular dimensions in trained athletes. Ann. Intern. Med., 82:521, 1975.
19. Oscai, L. et al.: Cardiac growth and respiratory enzyme levels in male rats subjected to a running program. Am. J. Physiol., 220:1238, 1971.
20. Pechar, G.S. et al.: Specificity of cardio-respiratory adaptation to bicycle and treadmill training. J. Appl. Physiol., 36:753, 1974.
21. Pollack, M.L. et al.: Comprehensive analysis of world calibre distance runners. Track Field Quart. Rev., 77:6, 1977.
22. Richter, G.W., and Kellner, A.: Hypertrophy of the human heart at the level of fine structure: an analysis of two postulates. J. Cell Biol., 18:195, 1965.
23. Rowell, L.B.: Human cardiovascular adjustments to exercise and thermal stress. Physiol. Rev., 54:75, 1974.
24. Rowell, L.B.: Vascular blood flow and metabolism during exercise. In Frontiers of Fitness. Edited by R.J. Shephard. Springfield, Ill., C.C Thomas, 1971.
25. Rowell L.B. et al.: Reductions in cardiac output, central blood volume, and stroke volume with thermal stress in normal men during exercise. J. Clin Invest. 45:1801, 1966.
26. Rushmer, R.F.: Cardiovascular Dynamics. Philadelphia, W.B. Saunders Co., 1976.
27. Rushmer, R.F., and Smith, O.A.: Cardiac control. Physiol. Rev., 39:41, 1959.
28. Saltin, B.: Physiological effects of physical conditioning. Med. Sci. Sports, 1:50, 1969.
28a. Saltin, B., et al.: Fiber types and metabolic potentials of skeletal muscles in sedentary man and endurance runners. Ann. N.Y. Acad. Sci., 301:3, 1977.
29. Scheuer, J., and Tipton, C.M.: Cardiovascular adaptations to training. Ann. Rev. Physiol., 39:221, 1977.
30. Seely, J.E. et al.: Heart and lung function at rest and during exercise in adolescence. J. Appl. Physiol., 36:34, 1974.
30a. Spear, K.L., et al.: Coronary blood flow in physically trained rats. Circ. Res., 12:135, 1978.
31. Stevenson, J.A.F. et al.: Effect of exercise on coronary tree size in the rat. Circ. Res., 15:265, 1964.
32. Tabakian, B.S. et al.: Effect of physical training on the cardiovascular and respiratory response to graded upright exercise in distance runners. Br. Heart J., 27:205, 1965.

Skeletal Muscle:
Structure and Function

18

Human movement depends on transforming the chemical energy in ATP into mechanical energy. This specific energy transformation is achieved through the action of skeletal muscles. Muscular forces acting on the body's bony lever system cause one or more bones to move about their joint axis; this enables a person to propel an object, move the body itself, or do both simultaneously. In the sections that follow, we present the architectural organization of *skeletal muscle* and focus on its gross and microscopic structure. The discussion includes the sequence of chemical and mechanical events in muscular contraction and relaxation, as well as the differences in muscle characteristics between sedentary and highly trained people.

GROSS STRUCTURE OF SKELETAL MUSCLE

Each of the more than 430 voluntary muscles in the body contains various wrappings of fibrous connective tissue. Figure 18-1 shows the cross section of a muscle consisting of thousands of cylindric muscle cells called *fibers.* These long, slender multinucleated fibers (whose number is probably fixed by the second trimester of fetal development) lie parallel to each other, and the force of contraction is along the long axis of the fiber.

Each fiber is wrapped and separated from its neighboring fibers by a fine layer of connective tissue, the *endomysium.* Another layer of connective tissue, the *perimysium,* surrounds a bundle of up to 150 fibers called a *fasciculus.* Surrounding the entire muscle is a fascia of fibrous connective tissue known as the *epimysium.* This protective sheath is tapered at its dis-

tal ends as it blends into and joins the intramuscular tissue sheaths to form the dense, strong connective tissue of the *tendons.* The tendons connect both ends of the muscle to the outermost covering of the skeleton, the *periostium.* Thus, the force of muscular contraction is transmitted directly from the muscle's connective tissue harness to the tendons, which in turn pull on the bones at their points of attachment. The region where the tendon joins a relatively stable skeletal part is the *origin* of the muscle; the point of attachment to the moving bone is the *insertion.* The origin is generally at the proximal or fixed end of the lever system or nearest the body's midline, whereas the *insertion* is the distal or movable attachment.

Beneath the endomysium and surrounding each muscle fiber is the *sarcolemma.* This thin, elastic membrane encloses the fiber's cellular contents. The aqueous protoplasm or *sarcoplasm* of the cell contains the contractile proteins, enzymes, fat and glycogen particles, the nuclei, and various specialized cellular organelles. Embedded within the sarcoplasm is an extensive interconnecting network of tubular channels and vesicles known as the *sarcoplasmic reticulum.* This highly specialized system provides the cell with structural integrity and also serves important functions in muscular contraction.

Chemical Composition

Seventy-five percent of skeletal muscle is water, 20% is protein, and the remaining 5% is made up of inorganic salts and other sub-

234

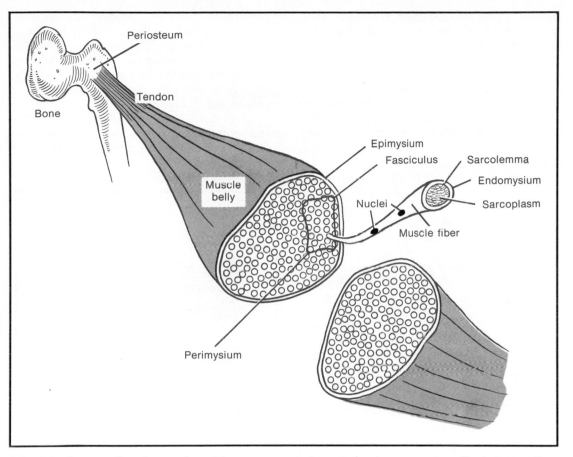

FIG. 18-1. *Cross section of a muscle and the arrangement of connective tissue wrappings. The individual fibers are covered by the endomysium. Groups of fibers called fasciculi are surrounded by the perimysium, and the entire muscle is wrapped in a fibrous sheath of connective tissue, the epimysium. The sarcolemma is a thin, elastic membrane that covers the surface of each muscle fiber.*

stances including high-energy phosphates, urea, lactic acid, the minerals calcium, magnesium, and phosphorous, various enzymes and pigments, ions of sodium, potassium, and chloride, and amino acids, fats, and carbohydrates.

The most abundant muscular proteins are *myosin, actin,* and *tropomyosin.* They comprise about 52%, 23%, and 15%, respectively, of the muscle's total protein content. Also, about 700 mg of the conjugated protein *myoglobin* is incorporated into each 100 g of muscle tissue. The specifics of myoglobin function were presented in Chapter 13.

Blood Supply

During exercise requiring an oxygen uptake of 4.0 liters per minute, the muscle's oxygen consumption increases nearly 70 times to about 11 ml per 100 g per minute or a total of about 3400 ml per minute. To accommodate this large oxygen requirement of exercising muscles, the local vascular bed must channel large quantities of blood through the active tissues. In rhythmic exercise such as running, swimming, or cycling, the blood flow fluctuates; it decreases during the muscle's contraction phase and increases during the relaxation period. This provides a "milking action" facilitating blood flow through the muscles and back to the heart. Complementing this pulsatile flow is the rapid dilatation of previously dormant capillaries so that in strenuous exercise, more than 4000 capillaries may be delivering blood to each square millimeter of muscle cross section.

Straining-type activities present a somewhat different picture. When a muscle contracts to about 60% of its force-generating capacity, blood flow to the muscle is occluded due to elevated intramuscular pressure. With a sustained static or isometric contraction, the compressive force of the contraction actually stops the flow of blood. Under such conditions, energy for continued muscular effort is generated mainly from the stored phosphogens and via the anaerobic reactions of glycolysis.

One factor often proposed for the improved exercise capacity with training is an *increase in capillary density of the trained muscles.* Aside from its role in delivering oxygen, nutrients, and hormones, the capillary circulation also provides the means for removing heat and metabolic by-products from the active tissues. All of these functions would be enhanced by a higher capillary density in muscle tissue.

Several investigations show favorable effects of endurance training on the capillarization of skeletal muscle. In one study using the electron microscope,[2] the number of capillaries per muscle (as well as the capillaries per square millimeter of muscle tissue) averaged about 40% greater in endurance athletes than in untrained counterparts. This was almost identical to the 41% difference in maximal oxygen uptake between the two groups. One research group cited unpublished observations that skeletal muscle capillaries "can be easily increased, and that the increase is closely related to the activity level of the muscle."[15] They also report a high positive relationship between maximal oxygen uptake and the average number of muscle capillaries for both men and women. The functional significance of this relationship is that increased capillarization enhances the oxygenation of the entire muscle cell. This would be especially beneficial during strenuous exercise requiring a high level of steady-rate aerobic metabolism. Further research is necessary to clarify the role of exercise in capillary development and to establish the precise physiologic role of these adaptations.

ULTRASTRUCTURE OF SKELETAL MUSCLE

The ultrastructure or microscopic anatomy of skeletal muscle has been revealed with the aid of electron microscopy, x-ray diffraction, and histochemical staining techniques. Figure 18-2 shows the different levels of subcellular organization within skeletal muscle fibers. Each muscle fiber is composed of smaller functional units that lie parallel to the long axis of the

fiber. These *fibrils* or *myofibrils* are approximately 1 micron (μm) in diameter (1 micron = 1/1000 mm) and are composed of even smaller subunits, the *filaments* or *myofilaments,* that also lie parallel to the long axis of the myofibril. The myofilaments are made up mainly of two proteins, *actin* and *myosin,* that account for about 84% of the myofibrillar complex. Six other proteins have also been identified that have either a structural function or a significant

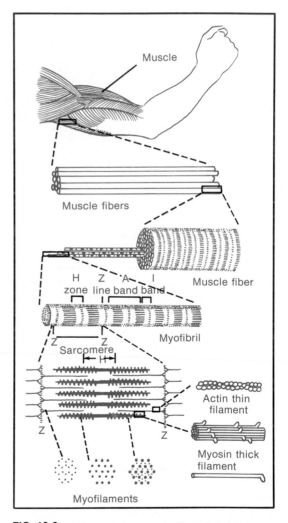

FIG. 18-2. *Microscopic organization of skeletal muscle. The whole muscle is composed of fibers; these in turn are made up of myofibrils, of which the actin and myosin protein filaments are a part. If viewed under a microscope, magnification would be approximately 205,000 x. (From Vander, A.J., Sherman, J.H., Luciano, D.S.: Human Physiology, 2nd Edition. New York, McGraw-Hill, © 1975. Used with permission of McGraw-Hill Book Company.)*

effect on the interaction of protein filaments during contraction. These are (1) *tropomyosin,* located along the actin filaments (5%); (2) *troponin,* also located in the actin filaments (3%); (3) *α-actinin,* distributed in the region of the Z band (7%); (4) *β-actinin,* found in the actin filaments (1%); (5) *M protein,* identified in the region of the M lines within the sarcomere (<1%); and (6) *C protein* (<1%), thought to maintain the structural integrity of the sarcomere.

The Sarcomere

At low magnification, the alternating light and dark bands along the length of the muscle fiber give it its characteristic *striated* appearance. Figure 18-3 illustrates the structural details of this cross-striation pattern within a myofibril. The lighter area is referred to as the I band, whereas the darker zone is known as the A band. The Z line bisects the I band and adheres to the sarcolemma to give stability to the entire structure.* The repeating unit between two Z lines is called the *sarcomere, which is the func-*

tional unit of the muscle cell. The actin and myosin filaments within the sarcomere are primarily involved in the mechanical process of muscular contraction.

The position of the thin actin and thicker myosin proteins in the sarcomere results in an overlap of the two filaments. The center of the A band contains the H zone, a region of lower optical density due to the absence of actin filaments in this area. The central portion of the H zone is bisected by the M line, which delineates the sarcomere's center. The M line consists of the protein structures that support the arrangement of the myosin filaments.

Actin-Myosin Orientation

The top portion of Figure 18-4 illustrates the actin-myosin orientation within a sarcomere at resting length. The bottom portion of the figure shows the hexagonal arrangement of actin and myosin filaments. A thick filament [150 angstroms (Å) in diameter and 1.5 microns (μm) long] is bordered by six thinner filaments, each about 50 Å in diameter and 1 μm long. Three thick filaments surround each thin filament. This muscular substructure is extremely impressive. For example, a myofibril 1 μm in diameter contains about 450 thick filaments in the center of the sarcomere and 900 thin filaments at each end of the sarcomere. A single muscle fiber 100 μm in diameter and 1 cm long contains about 8000 myofibrils, each myofibril consisting of 4500 sarcomeres. This results in a total of 16 billion thick and 64 billion thin filaments in a single fiber![17]

Figure 18-5 is a detailed illustration of the spatial orientation of the various proteins that comprise the contractile filaments. Projections or "cross-bridges" spiral about the myosin filament at the region where the filaments of actin and myosin overlap. These cross-bridges are repeated at intervals of about 450 Å along the filament. Their globular "lollipoplike" heads extend perpendicularly to interact with the thinner strands of actin; this is the structural and functional link between the myofilaments.

Tropomyosin and troponin are two other important constituents of the actin helix structure. These proteins appear to regulate the make-

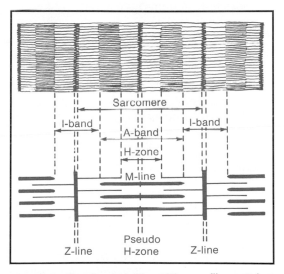

FIG. 18-3. *Structural position of the myofilaments in a sarcomere. A sarcomere is bounded at both ends by the Z line. In a single muscle fiber consisting of 4,500 sarcomeres, there are approximately 16 billion thick and 64 billion thin filaments. (From Huxley, H.E.: The Mechanism of Muscular Contraction. Copyright © 1965 by Scientific American, Inc. All rights reserved.)*

---

* The bands are named according to their optical properties. When a light passes through the I band, its velocity is the same in all directions (isotropic). Polarized light passing through the A band does not scatter equally (anisotropic). The letter Z is from the German *zwischen,* which means "between."

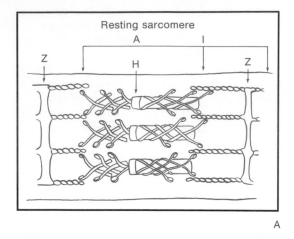

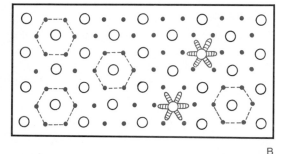

FIG. 18-4. *A, Ultrastructure of actin–myosin orientation within a resting sarcomere. B, Representation of electron micrograph through a cross section of myofibrils in a single muscle fiber. Note the hexagonal orientation of the smaller actin and larger myosin filaments, as well as an example of the cross-bridges that extend from a thick to the thin filament.*

and-break contacts between the myofilaments during contraction. Tropomyosin is distributed along the length of the actin filament in a groove formed by the double helix. It is believed to inhibit actin and myosin interaction or coupling and prevent a permanent bonding of these filaments. Troponin, which is embedded at fairly regular intervals along the actin strands, has a high affinity for calcium ions (Ca^{2+}). It is the action of Ca^{2+} and troponin that triggers the myofibrils to interact and slide past each other. When the fiber is stimulated, the troponin molecules appear to undergo a conformational change that in some way "tugs" on the tropomyosin protein strand. This moves the tropomyosin deeper into the groove between the two actin strands. This action "uncovers" the active sites of the actin and allows contraction to proceed.

The M line consists of transversely and longitudinally oriented proteins that serve to maintain the proper orientation of the thick filament within a sarcomere. As can be observed in Figure 18-5, the perpendicularly oriented M bridges connect with six adjacent thick (myosin) filaments in a hexagonal pattern.

Intracellular Tubule Systems

Figure 18-6 illustrates the tubule system within a muscle fiber. An extensive network of interconnecting tubular channels, the *sarcoplasmic reticulum,* lies parallel to the myofibrils. The lat-

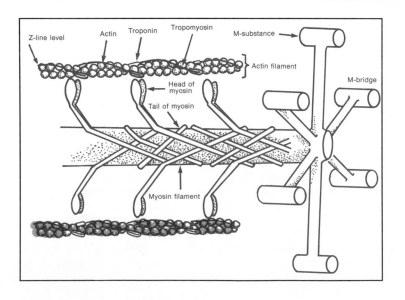

FIG. 18-5. *Details of the thick and thin protein filaments, including tropomyosin, troponin, and the M line. The myosin AT-Pase is located on the globular head of the myosin; this "active" head frees the energy from ATP to be used in muscle contraction. (From The Biology of Physical Activity by D.W. Edington and V.R. Edgerton. Copyright © 1976 by Houghton Mifflin Company. Reprinted by permission of the publisher.)*

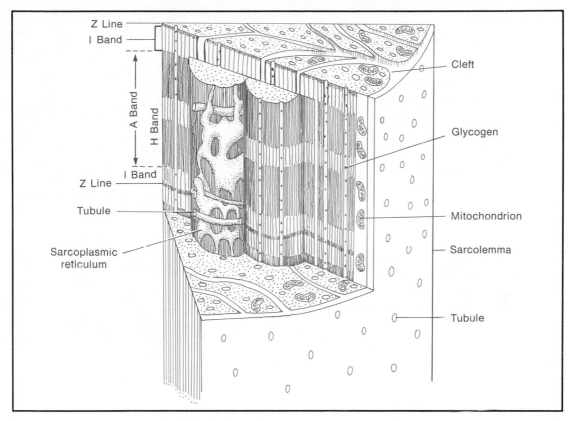

FIG. 18-6. *Three-dimensional view of sarcoplasmic reticulum and T-tubule system within the muscle fiber. (From Grahm, H.: How is muscle turned on and off? Sci. Am., 222:84, 1970.)*

oral end of each tubule terminates in a saclike vesicle that stores Ca^{2+}. Another network of tubules known as the transverse tubule system or *T-system* runs perpendicular to the myofibril. The T tubules are situated between the lateralmost portion of two sarcoplasmic channels with the vesicles of these structures abutting the T tubule. This repeating pattern of two vesicles and T tubules in the region of each Z line is known as a *triad*. There are two triads in each sarcomere, and the pattern is repeated regularly throughout the length of the myofibril.

The T tubules pass through the fiber and open externally from the inside of the muscle cell. *The triad and T-tubule system appear to function as a microtransportation or plumbing network for spreading the action potential (wave of depolarization) from the fiber's outer membrane inward to the deep regions of the cell.* During this depolarization process, calcium ions are released from the triad sacs and diffuse a short distance to the filaments, presumably to "activate" the actin filaments. Con-traction is initiated when the cross-bridges of the myosin filaments are attracted to the active sites on the actin filaments. When electric excitation ceases, there is a decrease in free calcium concentration in the cytoplasm; this is associated with the relaxation of the muscle.

CHEMICAL AND MECHANICAL EVENTS DURING CONTRACTION AND RELAXATION

The electron microscope has helped unravel many secrets of cellular structure that have led to the formulation of reasonable hypotheses concerning the chemical and mechanical events during muscular contraction and relaxation. Although many gaps remain, there is considerable evidence to support a "sliding-fila-ment theory" of muscle contraction that fits nicely with the detailed ultrastructure of muscle discussed previously.

Sliding-Filament Theory

The sliding-filament theory proposes that a muscle shortens or lengthens because the thick and thin myofilaments slide past each other without the filaments themselves changing length. This causes a major change in the relative size of the various zones and bands within a sarcomere. Figure 18-7 illustrates that the thin actin myofilaments slide past the myosin myofilaments and move into the region of the A band during contraction (and move out in relaxation). The major structural rearrangement during contraction, therefore, occurs in the region of the I band, which decreases markedly. The Z bands are essentially pulled toward the center of each sarcomere. There is no change in the width of the A band, although the H zone can disappear when the actin filaments are in contact at the center of the sarcomere. In an isometric muscular contraction, force is generated while the fiber's length remains relatively unchanged and the relative spacing of I and A bands stays constant; in this situation, the same molecular groups react with one another repeatedly. In an eccentric contraction where force is generated while the muscle lengthens, the A band becomes broader.

MECHANICAL ACTION OF THE CROSS-BRIDGES. The globular head of the myosin cross-bridge

provides the mechanical means for the actin and myosin filaments to slide past each other. Figure 18-8 shows schematically the oscillating to-and-fro nature of the cross-bridges, which move in a way somewhat similar to the action of oars in water. However, unlike oars, the cross-bridges do not all move in a synchronous manner. During contraction, each cross-bridge undergoes many repeated but independent cycles of movement. Thus, at any one time, only about 50% of the bridges are in contact with the thin actin filaments to form the protein complex *actomyosin,* which has contractile properties; the others are at some other position in their vibrating cycle.

As illustrated in the right side of Figure 18-8, each action of a cross-bridge contributes only a small longitudinal displacement in terms of the total sliding action of the filaments. This process has been likened to the action of a person climbing a rope. The arms and legs represent the cross-bridges. Climbing is accomplished by first reaching with the arms, then grabbing, pulling and breaking contact, and then repeating this process over and over throughout the climb.

LINK BETWEEN ACTIN, MYOSIN, AND ATP. The interaction and movement of the protein filaments during muscular contraction necessitate that the myosin cross-bridges continually undergo oscillatory movements by combining, detaching, and recombining to new sites along the actin strands.

The detachment of the myosin cross-bridges from the actin filament is brought about when an ATP molecule is joined to the actomyosin complex. This reaction enables the myosin cross-bridge to return to its original state so it is available to bind a new active site on the actin. The dissociation of actomyosin occurs in the following way:

Actomyosin + ATP $\longrightarrow$ Actin + Myosin – ATP

ATP also serves an important function in the contraction process. Energy is provided for cross-bridge movement when the terminal phosphate is split from ATP. One of the reacting sites on the globular head of the myosin cross-bridge binds to the reactive site on actin. The other myosin active site acts as the enzyme *myofibrilar adenosinetriphosphatase,* or more commonly, *myosin ATPase.* This enzyme splits ATP so that its energy can be used for muscle contraction. The rate of ATP splitting is relatively slow if myosin and actin remain apart;

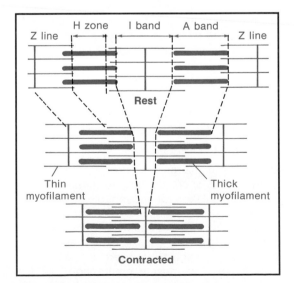

FIG. 18-7. *Structural rearrangement of actin and myosin filaments at rest and during contraction.*

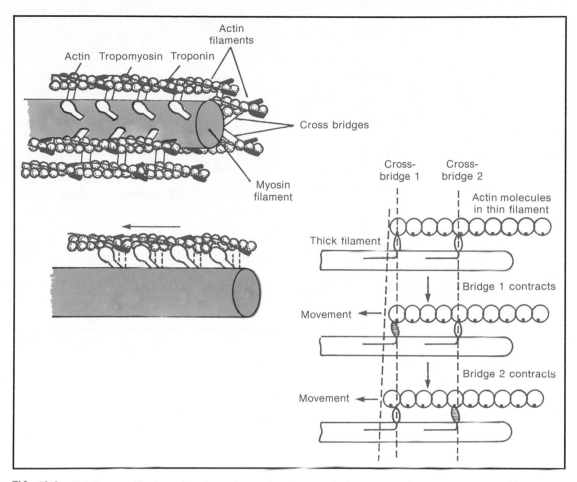

FIG. 18-8. *Relative positioning of actin and myosin filaments during the oscillating movement of the cross-bridges. The action of each bridge contributes a small displacement of movement. For clarity, one of the actin strands is omitted from the left-hand figure.*

when they join, however, the reactive rate of myosin ATPase increases considerably. It is believed that energy released from ATP splitting somehow activates the cross-bridges, causing them to oscillate. It is possible that this energy transfer process causes a conformational change in the shape of the globular head of the myosin cross-bridge so that it interacts with the appropriate actin molecule.

Fast-twitch muscle fibers with the ability for rapid and powerful contraction possess a relatively high activity level of myosin ATPase. It is tempting to speculate that specific forms of speed and power training modify enzymatic activity in a manner that facilitates the sequence of events in muscular contraction. More will be said concerning fiber types and training effects shortly.

Excitation–Contraction Coupling

Excitation–contraction is the physiologic mechanism whereby an electric discharge at the muscle initiates the chemical events that lead to contraction. We shall explore this process.

In the resting state, a muscle's Ca^{2+} concentration is relatively low. When a muscle fiber is stimulated to contract, there is an immediate increase in intracellular Ca^{2+}. This is brought about by the arrival of the action potential at the transverse tubules, which causes Ca^{2+} to be released from the lateral sacs of the sarcoplasmic reticulum. The inhibitory action of troponin that prevents actin-myosin interaction is released when Ca^{2+} ions bind rapidly with troponin in the actin filaments. In a sense, the muscle is now "turned on."

Actin + Myosin ATPase ⟶
Actomyosin ATPase

When the active sites on the actin and myosin are joined, myosin ATPase is activated, which in turn splits ATP. During this process, the transfer of energy causes movement of the myosin cross-bridges and the muscle generates tension.

Actomyosin ATPase ⟶ Actomyosin + ADP
+ P + Energy

The cross-bridges uncouple from actin when ATP *binds* to the myosin bridge. Coupling and uncoupling continues as long as the Ca^{2+} concentration remains at a sufficient level to inhibit the troponin–tropomyosin system. When the nerve stimulus to the muscle is removed, Ca^{2+} moves back into the lateral sacs of the sarcoplasmic reticulum. This restores the inhibitory action of the troponin–tropomyosin, and actin and myosin remain separated as long as ATP is present. (In *rigor mortis,* the muscles become stiff and rigid soon after death. This occurs because ATP is no longer available in the muscle cells. Without ATP, the myosin cross-bridges and actin remain attached and cannot be pulled apart.) Figure 18-9 illustrates the interaction between the actin and myosin filaments, Ca^{2+}, and ATP in a relaxed and contracted muscle.

Relaxation

When a muscle is no longer stimulated, the flow of Ca^{2+} ceases and troponin is free once again to inhibit actin-myosin interaction. During recovery, Ca^{2+} is actively pumped into the sarcoplasmic reticulum where it concentrates in the lateral vesicles. The retrieval of Ca^{2+} from the troponin–tropomyosin proteins "turns off" the active sites on the actin filament. This deactivation accomplishes two things; (1) It prevents any mechanical link between the myosin cross-bridges and the actin filaments. (2) It reduces the activity of myosin ATPase so there is no more ATP splitting. The muscle's relaxation is brought about by the return of the actin and myosin filaments to their original state.

Sequence of Events in Muscular Contraction

The following is a list of the main events in muscular contraction and relaxation. The sequence begins with the initiation of an action potential by the motor nerve. This impulse is then propagated over the entire surface of the muscle fiber as the cell membrane becomes depolarized: (1) The muscle action potential depolarizes the transverse tubules at the A-I junction of the sarcomere. (2) The depolarization of the transverse or T tubules causes Ca^{2+} to be released from the lateral sacs of the sarcoplasmic reticulum. (3) Ca^{2+} ions bind to troponin-tropomyosin in the actin filaments. This releases the inhibition that prevented actin from combining with myosin. (4) Actin combines with myosin-ATP. Actin also activates the myosin ATPase, which then splits ATP. The energy from this reaction is used to produce movement of the myosin cross-bridge, and tension is created. (5) ATP binds to the myosin bridge. This breaks the actin-myosin bond and allows the cross-bridge

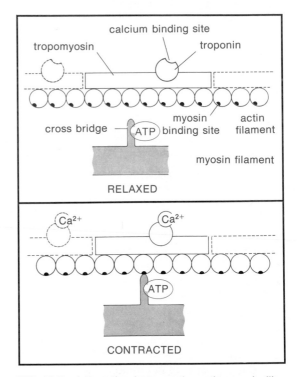

FIG. 18-9. *Interaction between the actin-myosin filaments, Ca^{2+}, and ATP in relaxed and contracted muscle. In the relaxed state, troponin and tropomyosin interact with actin, preventing the coupling of the myosin cross bridge to actin. During contraction, the cross bridge couples with actin due to the binding of Ca^{2+} with troponin-tropomyosin. (From Vander, A.J., et al.: Human Physiology, 2nd ed., New York, McGraw-Hill Book Company, 1975.)*

to dissociate from actin. This leads to a relative movement or sliding of the thick and thin filaments past each other and the muscle shortens. (6) Cross-bridge activation continues as long as the concentration of Ca^{2+} remains high enough (due to membrane depolarization) to inhibit the action of the troponin–tropomyosin system. (7) When the muscle is no longer stimulated, the concentration of Ca^{2+} ions rapidly decreases as they move back into the lateral sacs of the sarcoplasmic reticulum by an energy process that splits ATP. (8) The removal of Ca^{2+} ions restores the inhibitory action of troponin–tropomyosin. In the presence of ATP, actin and myosin remain in the dissociated, relaxed state.

MUSCLE FIBER TYPE

Skeletal muscle is not simply a homogeneous group of fibers with similar metabolic and functional properties. Although considerable confusion has existed concerning the method and terminology for classifying human skeletal muscle, distinct fiber types have been identified and classified by their *contractile* and *metabolic* characteristics.

Fast-twitch muscle fibers have a high activity level of myosin ATPase that relates to their ability to generate energy rapidly for quick, forceful contractions. It should be recalled that it is myosin ATPase that splits ATP to provide energy for muscle contraction. In fact, their speed of contraction is nearly twice as fast as that of fibers classified as slow-twitch fibers (next section). The fast-twitch fibers rely largely on a well-developed, short-term glycolytic system for energy transfer. They have been labeled *FG fibers* to signify their fast-glycolytic capabilities. *Fast-twitch fibers are generally activated in short-term, sprint activities that depend almost entirely on anaerobic metabolism for energy.*[8] The metabolic and contractile capacities of these fibers are also important in the stop-and-go or change-of-pace sports such as basketball or field hockey, which at times require rapid energy that only the anaerobic metabolic pathways supply.

Slow-twitch fibers generate energy for ATP resynthesis predominantly by means of the relatively long-term system of aerobic energy transfer. They are distinguished by a low activity level of myosin ATPase, a slow speed of

contraction, and a glycolytic capacity less well developed than that of their fast-twitch counterparts. However, the slow-twitch fibers contain relatively large and numerous mitochondria. Accompanying this enhanced metabolic machinery is a high concentration of mitochondrial enzymes required to sustain aerobic metabolism.[5,6,10] *Thus, slow-twitch fibers are well suited for prolonged aerobic exercise.* These fibers have been labeled *SO fibers* to describe their slow contraction speed and great reliance on oxidative metabolism. Unlike the FG fibers that fatigue readily, the SO fibers are adapted for prolonged work and are recruited for aerobic activities.[7,8]

Many researchers classify slow twitch (SO) fibers as *type I*, whereas the fast-twitch FG fibers (and proposed subdivisions) are categorized as *type II*. When a person is exercising at near maximum aerobic and anaerobic levels, as in middle-distance running or swimming, or in sports such as basketball, field hockey, or soccer, which require a blend of aerobic and anaerobic energy, both types of muscle fibers are activated.[8]

A subdivision of the fast-twitch fiber appears to be present in humans. This fiber is considered intermediate in that its fast contraction speed is combined with a moderately well developed capacity for both aerobic and anaerobic energy transfer. These are the fast-twitch, oxidative-glycolytic or *FOG fibers* (type IIA). Two other subdivisions of the type II fiber have also been proposed: the type IIB and type IIC fibers. In contrast to the type IIA fiber, the type IIB fiber possesses the greater anaerobic potential. The type IIC fiber is normally a rare and undifferentiated fiber that may be involved in re-innervation or motor unit transformation.[11a]

Effects of Training

Several interesting observations can be made concerning muscle fiber types and the possible influence of specific training on fiber composition and metabolic capacity. For one thing, sedentary men and women as well as young children[1] possess 45% to 55% slow-twitch fibers. Although there are no sex or age differences in fiber distribution, the individual variation is large, especially among men. In addition, for a particular person, the fiber type can vary considerably from muscle to muscle. Also, among those who achieve high levels of proficiency in various sports, certain patterns of fiber distribution are readily apparent. Those athletes who are highly successful in endurance activities generally demonstrate a predominance of slow-twitch fibers in the muscles activated in their sport. For successful sprint athletes, the fast-twitch muscle fiber predominates. This is shown in Figure 18-10 for top Scandinavian competitors representing different sports. Athletic groups with the highest aerobic and endurance capacities, such as distance runners and cross-country skiers, also have the highest relative number of slow-twitch fibers. Weight lifters, ice-hockey players, and sprinters, on the other hand, tend to have more fast-twitch fibers and a relatively lower max $\dot{V}O_2$.[1a] As might be expected, other studies show that men and women who perform in middle-distance events have an approximately equal percentage of the two types of muscle fibers.[15] This distribution is also often the case for certain power athletes such as throwers, jumpers, and high jumpers.[3] It should be noted that these relatively clear-cut distinctions between performance and muscle fiber composition are for *elite* athletes who have achieved highly in a specific sport category. However, a person's fiber composition is clearly not the sole determinant of performance as several researchers have shown that for a particular group, either trained or untrained, knowledge of a person's predominant fiber type is of limited value in predicting the outcome of specific exercise performances.[2a,11a] This is not surprising because performance capacity is the end result of the blending of many physiologic,

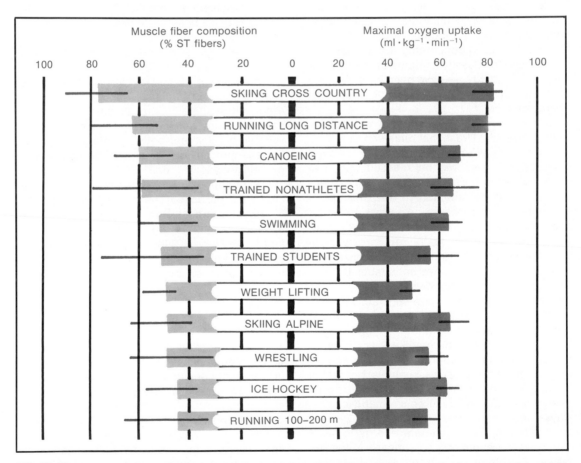

FIG. 18-10. *Muscle fiber composition (percent slow-twitch fibers) (left side) and maximal oxygen uptake (right side) in athletes representing different sports. The dark horizontal bar denotes the range. (From Bergh, U. et al.: Maximal oxygen uptake and muscle fiber types in trained and untrained humans. Med. Sci. Sports 10:151, 1978. Copyright 1978, the American College of Sports Medicine. Reprinted by permission.)*

biochemical, neurologic, and biomechanical components—and is not simply from a single factor such as muscle fiber type.

In terms of muscle size, endurance athletes exhibit slow-twitch fibers of relatively normal size.[8] Power athletes, on the other hand, show a definite enlargement, especially in the fast-twitch fibers.[16] These fibers may be 45% larger than those of endurance athletes or of sedentary people of the same age.[4] This is because power and strength training induce a definite enlargement of the fiber's contractile apparatus—specifically the actin and myosin filaments as well as its total glycogen content.[12,13] The basic distinction between the sexes is the generally larger muscle fibers of the male athletes.[3]

Can Fiber Type be Changed?

To determine whether the fiber composition characteristics of specific athletic groups are due to training or natural endowment (that is, can fiber composition be changed?), six men participated in a 5-month program of aerobic bicycle training.[6] Muscle biopsies from the lateral portion of the quadriceps before and after training indicated *no change* in fiber composition, although all men improved considerably in work capacity and aerobic power. Similar observations have been noted for the fiber composition of subjects after endurance or sprint training programs,[14] or after a period of weight training. These data support the argument that a fast-contracting fiber before training will still be a fast-contracting fiber after training with the same holding true for the slow-twitch fibers.

However, additional studies of 18 weeks of "aerobic" and 11 weeks of "anaerobic" training in four athletes suggest the possibility of a progressive fiber type transformation process with specific training.[10a] In these subjects, anaerobic training caused an *increase* in the percentage of type IIC fibers and a *decrease* in the percentage of type I fibers; the opposite was observed in the aerobic phase of the training sequence. These findings suggest that specific training (and perhaps inactivity) may induce an *actual conversion* of type I to type II fibers (or vice versa) and that the fiber of transformation may be the *type IIC fiber.* It is clear that more research needs to be done in this intriguing area before definitive statements can be made

concerning the fixed nature of a muscle's fiber composition.

In summary, considerable variation in fiber type distribution is noted from muscle to muscle and from person to person. These characteristics appear to be determined largely by genetic code[8,10] with the major direction of a muscle's fiber composition probably being fixed before birth or early in life. Whether this status can be modified with prolonged training is still open to question. It also seems likely that, at elite levels of certain sports performances, a particular fiber distribution is "required" for success. Although this suggests an obvious genetic predetermination, it is well documented that specific training significantly enhances aerobic and possibly anaerobic power of both fiber types.[7,10] In fact, enhancement of the oxidative capacity of fast-twitch fibers with high-intensity endurance training brings them to a level that markedly surpasses the aerobic capacity of the slow-twitch fibers of untrained subjects![5] This training adaptation in young and mature adults[8] is brought about by the well-documented increase in mitochondrial size and number and the accompanying enhancement in the activity level of enzymes relevant to Krebs cycle and electron transport function.[9]

The fact that *only* the specific muscles (more precisely, muscle fibers) used in training show adaptation to exercise certainly explains why highly trained athletes who switch to a sport requiring different muscle groups feel essentially untrained for the new activity. Within this framework, swimmers or canoeists will not necessarily transfer their upper body "fitness" to a running sport.

The changes occurring in skeletal muscle resulting from specific training are summarized in Table 18-1. It should be kept in mind that both fiber types are involved in most activities; it is just that certain activities require activation of a much greater proportion of one type over another.

Practical Implications

A scheme is proposed to summarize adaptive changes in active muscle accompanying changes in max $\dot{V}O_2$ with endurance training.[15] As shown in Figure 18-11, maximal oxygen uptake increases about 15% to 30% in the first 3 months of intensive training and may rise as much as 50% over a 2-year period. When train-

TABLE 18-1. *Effects of specific forms of training on skeletal muscle*[a]

MUSCLE FACTOR	SLOW-TWITCH FIBERS		FAST-TWITCH FIBERS	
	TYPE OF TRAINING			
	STRENGTH	ENDURANCE	STRENGTH	ENDURANCE
Percent composition	0	0	0	0
Size	+	0	+ +	0
Contractile property	0	0	0	0
Oxidative capacity	0	+ +	0	+
Anaerobic capacity	0 or ?	0	0 or ?	0
Glycogen content	0	+ +	0	+ +
Fat oxidation	0	+ +	0	+
Capillary density	?	? or +	?	? or +
Blood flow during work	?	?	?	?

0 = no change; ? = unknown; + = moderate increase; + + = large increase.

[a] Modified from Gollnick, P.D., and Sembrowich, W.L.: Adaptations in human skeletal muscle as a result of training. Reproduced with permission from Amsterdam, E.A., Wilmore, J.H., DeMaria, A.N. (Eds.): Exercise in Cardiovascular Health and Disease. New York, Yorke Medical Books, 1977. Copyright © 1977 by Yorke Medical Books, a division of Dun-Donnelley Publishing Corporation.

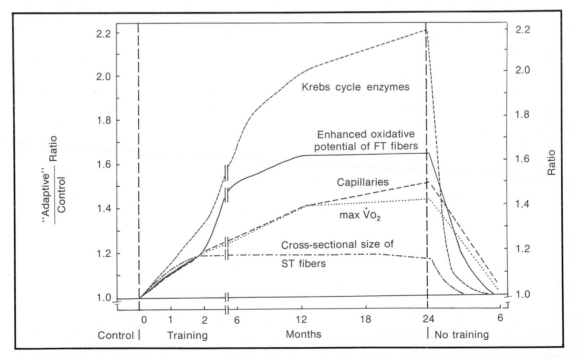

FIG. 18-11. *A schematic, and in part, hypothetical summary of some of the adaptations taking place in active muscle with endurance training. The graph is based on longitudinal and cross-sectional studies of humans. When there is a lack of data from humans (as in the case for capillarization after training), results from other species have been used. It should be pointed out that in endurance-trained muscles the ST fibers can be smaller than what is observed in the same muscle of sedentary people. (From Saltin, B. et al.: Fiber types and metabolic potentials of skeletal muscles in sedentary man and endurance runners. Ann. N.Y. Acad. Sci. 301:3, 1977.*

ing stops, the aerobic capacity slowly returns to the pretraining level. The picture for the aerobic enzymes of the Krebs cycle and electron transport system is even more impressive. These enzymes, which facilitate carbohydrate and fat breakdown, increase rapidly and substantially throughout the training period. Conversely, this metabolic adaptation is lost within a few weeks after training ceases. Although data on capillarization in humans are limited, it is hypothesized that the number of muscle capillaries continues to increase throughout training; this adaptation in blood supply is also probably lost at a relatively slow rate with detraining.

As illustrated in Figure 18-11, intensive training lasting longer than 6 months causes an increase in the oxidative capacity of the trained muscles. This "local" metabolic improvement greatly outstrips the body's ability to circulate, deliver, and use oxygen during intense exercise (as demonstrated by the increase in max $\dot{V}O_2$). In this phase of training, however, a muscle's lactate production may be much lower than that observed in submaximal exercise of similar relative intensity prior to training. *These cellular adjustments may account for a trained person being able to do prolonged steady-rate work at a larger percentage of max $\dot{V}O_2$.* In addition, the local metabolic and circulatory adaptations with long-term training may partially explain the lowered rate of glycogen utilization and concomitant increase in free fatty acid metabolism in exercise. This glycogen-sparing effect is of extreme importance in prolonged strenuous exercise.

SUMMARY

1. Skeletal muscle is encased in various wrappings of connective tissue. These eventually blend into and join the tendinous attachment to bone. This harness enables muscles to act on the bony levers to transform the chemical energy of ATP into mechanical energy and motion.

2. Seventy-five percent of skeletal muscle is water, 20% is protein, and the remainder consists of inorganic salts, enzymes, pigments, fats, and carbohydrates.

3. In vigorous exercise, the muscle's oxygen consumption increases nearly 70 times above the resting level. Supporting this metabolic requirement are immediate adjustments and longer term training adaptations in the local vascular bed.

4. The sarcomere is the functional unit of the muscle cell. It contains the contractile proteins actin and myosin. There are 4500 sarcomeres and a total of 16 billion thick (myosin) and 64 billion thin (actin) filaments in an average-sized fiber.

5. Projections or "cross-bridges" provide the structural link between the thin and thick contractile filaments. Tropomyosin and troponin, two proteins of the myofibrillar complex, regulate the make-and-break contacts between the filaments during contraction. Tropomyosin inhibits actin and myosin interaction; troponin with calcium triggers the myofibrils to interact and slide past each other.

6. The triad and T-tubule system serve as a microtransportation network for spreading the action potential from the fiber's outer membrane inward to deep regions of the cell. Contraction occurs when calcium activates actin, causing the myosin cross-bridges to attach to active sites on the actin filaments. Relaxation occurs when calcium concentration decreases.

7. The "sliding filament theory" proposes that a muscle shortens or lengthens because the protein filaments slide past each other without changing their length. Excitation–contraction coupling is the mechanism by which electrochemical and mechanical events are linked to achieve muscular contraction.

8. Two types of muscle fibers can be classified by their contractile and metabolic characteristics: (1) fast-twitch fibers, in which energy is generated anaerobically and rapidly for a quick, powerful contraction (these are labeled *FG* fibers to signify their fast speed of contraction and high glycolytic properties), and (2) slow-twitch fibers that contract relatively slowly and generate energy for ATP synthesis predominantly via aerobic metabolism. These are called *SO* fibers to denote their slow contraction speed and reliance on oxidative metabolism. There is some indication that an intermediate, fast-twitch, oxidative-glycolytic (FOG) fiber is also present.

9. Percentage distribution of fiber type differs significantly among people and between various muscle groups of a particular person. This distribution is probably determined by genetic code and cannot be changed to any large extent by physical training. However, both types of fibers can be markedly improved in metabolic capacity by specific endurance and power training.

References

1. Bell, R.D. et al.: Muscle fiber types and morphometric analysis of skeletal muscle in six-year-old children. Med. Sci. Sports, *12:*28, 1980.

1a. Bergh, U. et al.: Maximal oxygen uptake and muscle fiber types in trained and untrained humans. Med. Sci. Sports, *10:*151, 1978.

2. Brodal, P. et al.: Capillary supply of skeletal muscle fibers in untrained and endurance trained men. Acta Physiol. Scand. (Suppl.) *440,* 1976.

2a. Campbell, C.J. et al.: Muscle fiber composition and performance capacities of women. Med. Sci. Sports, *11:*260, 1979.

3. Costill, D.L. et al.: Skeletal muscle enzyme and fiber composition in male and female track athletes. J. Appl. Physiol., *40:*149, 1976.

4. Edström, L., and Ekblom, B.: Differences in sizes of red and white muscle fibers in vastus lateralis of musculus quadriceps of normal individuals and athletes; relation to physical performance. Scand. J. Clin. Lab. Invest., *30:*175, 1972.

5. Essén, B. et al.: Metabolic characteristics of fiber types in human skeletal muscles. Acta Physiol. Scand., *95:*153, 1975.

6. Gollnick, P.D.: Effects of training on enzyme activity and fiber composition of human skeletal muscle. J. Appl. Physiol., *34:*107, 1973.

7. Gollnick, P.D., and Hermansen, L.: Biochemical adaptations to exercise. Anaerobic metabolism. *In* Exercise and Sport Sciences Reviews. Edited by J.H. Wilmore. New York, Academic Press, 1973.

8. Gollnick, P.D., and Sembrowich, W.L.: Adaptations in human skeletal muscle as a result of training. *In* Exercise in Cardiovascular Health and Disease. Edited by E.A. Amsterdam et al. New York, Yorke Medical Books, 1977.

9. Holloszy, J.O.: Adaptation of skeletal muscle to endurance exercise. Med. Sci. Sports, *7:*155, 1975.

10. Jansson, E., and Kaijser, L.: Muscle adaptation to extreme endurance training in man. Acta Physiol. Scand., *100:*315, 1977.

10a. Jansson, E. et al.: Changes in muscle fibre type distribution in man after physical training. Acta Physiol. Scand. *104:*235, 1978.

11. Karlsson, J.B. et al.: LDH isozymes in skeletal muscles of endurance and strength trained athletes. Acta Physiol. Scand., *93:*150, 1975.

11a. Komi, P.V., and Karlsson, J.: Skeletal muscle fibre types, enzyme activities and physical performance in young males and females. Acta Physiol. Scand., *103:*210, 1978.

12. MacDougall, J.D. et al.: Biochemical adaptation of human skeletal muscle to heavy resistance training and immobilization. J. Appl. Physiol. *43:*700, 1977.

13. MacDougall, J.D. et al.: Mitochondrial volume density in human skeletal muscle following heavy resistance training. Med. Sci. Sports, *11:*164, 1979.

14. Saltin, B. et al.: The nature of the training response; peripheral and central adaptations to one-legged exercise. Acta Physiol., Scand., *96:*289, 1976.

15. Saltin, B. et al.: Fiber types and metabolic potentials of skeletal muscles in sedentary man and endurance runners. Ann. N.Y. Acad. Sci., *301:*3, 1977.

16. Thorstensson, A.: Muscle strength, fiber types and enzyme activities in man. Acta Physiol. Scand. (Suppl.) *443,* 1976.

17. Vander, A.J. et al.: Human Physiology: The Mechanisms of Body Function. New York, McGraw-Hill, 1976.

Neural Control of Human Movement

19

The correct application of force in relatively complex, learned movements like a tennis serve or the shot put depends on a series of coordinated neuromuscular patterns and not *just* on the strength of the muscle groups recruited for the activity. Such movements are regulated by neural control mechanisms linked together by pathways in the central nervous system. This neural circuitry in the brain and spinal cord is somewhat analogous to a modern computer system, although the integrative and organizational structure of the nervous system is far more highly advanced and specialized. In response to changing internal and external stimuli, bits of sensory input are automatically and rapidly transmitted for processing by the neural control mechanisms. The input is properly organized, routed, and retransmitted to the effector organs, the muscles.

In the sections that follow, we present a general outline describing the neural control of human movement. This includes (1) the structural organization for motor control, (2) neuromuscular transmission, (3) the motor unit—the functional unit of neuromuscular activity, and (4) sensory input for muscular activity. For a more thorough discussion of neuromotor regulation and skill acquisition, texts dealing with neuroanatomy, neurophysiology, and motor-skill learning should be consulted.

ORGANIZATION OF THE NEUROMOTOR SYSTEM

Central Organization

Figure 19-1 presents the general scheme for the various subdivisions of the nervous system that regulate and program the sequential patterns required for motor control. Each block represents a major neural subdivision. The arrows show the direction of nerve impulses along the motor (brown) or *efferent* and sensory (blue) or *afferent* pathways. The circular insert illustrates the basic control mechanism of the motor system. In this closed loop system, the afferent neurons transmit sensory impulses from muscle and also interface with motor neurons that send impulses to muscle.

Tracts of nerve tissue descending from the brain terminate at neurons in the spinal cord. Two major pathways serve this function, the *pyramidal* and *extrapyramidal* tracts. Nerves in the pyramidal or *corticospinal* tract transmit their impulses downward through the spinal cord. By means of direct routes and interconnecting neurons in the spinal cord, these nerves eventually excite alpha (α) *motoneurons* that control the various skeletal muscles. Each of the descending extrapyramidal nerve tracts is named for its area of origin and final connection. For example, nerves in the *vestibulospinal* tract originate in the vestibular nucleus of the cerebellum, whereas the *rubrospinal tract* nerves originate in the red nucleus of the midbrain, and the *reticulospinal tract* nerves have their origin in the reticular formation, a mass of nervous tissue that passes through the brain stem. The neurons of the extrapyramidal tract essentially control posture and provide a continual background level of neuromuscular tone. This is in contrast to the discrete movements stimulated by the nerves in the pyramidal tract.

The extrapyramidal nerves originate in the brain stem and connect at all levels of the spinal cord. The *reticular formation* provides impor-

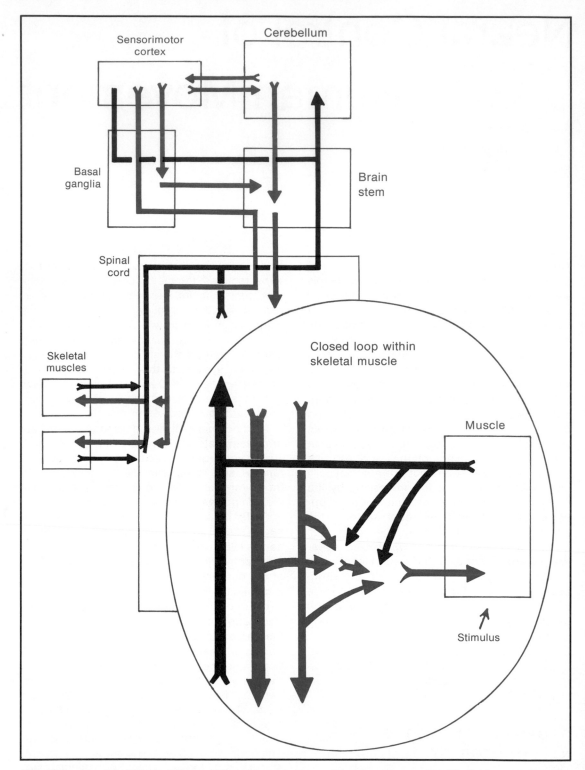

FIG. 19-1. *Simplified block diagram of the nervous system related to motor control. The interconnections between the various subdivisions are indicated by motor (brown) and sensory (blue) motoneurons. The circular insert represents the closed loop that links each muscle with the spinal cord. The arrows show the direction of the neural impulses between subdivisions.*

tant interconnections between the spinal cord, cerebral cortex, basal ganglia, and cerebellum. It integrates various input that flows through it. This input originates from the stretching of sensors in joints and muscles, or from pain receptors in the skin, visual signals from the eye, or auditory impulses from the ear. Once activated, the reticular system produces either an inhibitory or facilitory effect on other neurons.

The reticular inhibitory center transmits impulses that inhibit neurons to the antigravity muscles involved in postural control. Excitation of the facilitory sensory neurons arouses the reticular nerve cells. This causes excitation in the cerebral cortex, and signals are transmitted back to the reticular system to maintain an appropriate level of cortical arousal. Superimposed on this feedback system is another feedback network that transmits impulses through the spinal cord to the muscles. For example, if the neural outflow goes to the postural muscles, the tension of these muscles then becomes increased. This increased "neuromuscular tone" also stimulates the muscle's own set of sensory modulators, the spindles, to redirect excitatory impulses back to the central nervous system to maintain the excitatory level of the reticular formation. Such a system of multiple feedback control is one of the most complex aspects of the nervous system.

The *basal ganglia* are made up of masses of nerves that receive descending connections from the cortex and pass them through to the brain stem. Although the exact functions of the basal ganglia are unknown, it is believed that this nerve tissue is involved in the coordination of movement at both the volitional and subconscious levels.

The *cerebellum,* located behind the brain stem, functions by means of intricate feedback circuits to monitor and coordinate other areas of the brain involved in motor control. It receives signals concerning motor output from the cortex and sensory information from receptors in muscles, tendons, joints, and skin, as well as from visual, auditory, and vestibular end-organs. The cerebellum influences all motor centers from the cortex down to the spinal cord. It provides a special damping function for movement that would otherwise be jerky. *This specialized brain tissue is the major comparing, evaluating, and integrating center for postural adjustments, locomotion, maintenance of equilibrium, perceptions of speed of body movement, and many other reflex func-* *tions related to movement. In essence, it provides the "fine tuning" for muscular activity.*

The Reflex Arc

The diagram in Figure 19-2 shows a typical neural arrangement for a *reflex arc* in one of the 31 spinal cord segments. Sensory input is transmitted from the receptor by sensory (afferent) nerves that enter the spinal cord through the dorsal or sensory root. These nerves interconnect or synapse in the cord via *interneurons* that serve as relay stations to distribute information to various levels of the cord. The impulse is then passed over the *motor root pathway* via anterior motoneurons to the effector organ, the muscles.

The operation of the reflex arc is illustrated when one unknowingly touches a hot object. Pain receptors in the fingers are stimulated and send sensory information rapidly over afferent fibers to the spinal cord. Here, the efferent or motor fibers are activated to bring about the appropriate muscular response, and the hand is rapidly pulled away. Concurrently, the signal is transmitted up the cord to sensory areas in the brain where the sensation of pain is actually "felt." These various levels of operation for sensory input, processing, and motor output, including the reflex action just described, account for the fact that the hand is removed from the hot object before the pain is actually perceived. Many muscle functions are controlled by reflex actions in the spinal cord and other subconscious areas of the central nervous system.

NERVE SUPPLY TO MUSCLE

One nerve or its terminal branches innervates at least one of the approximately 250 million muscle fibers in the human body. Because there are only about 420,000 motor nerves, this means that a single nerve usually supplies many individual muscle fibers. *The ratio of muscle to nerve is generally related to a muscle's particular movement function.* The delicate and precise work of the eye muscles, for example, requires that a neuron control fewer than 10 muscle fibers. For less complex movements of the big muscles, a motoneuron may innervate

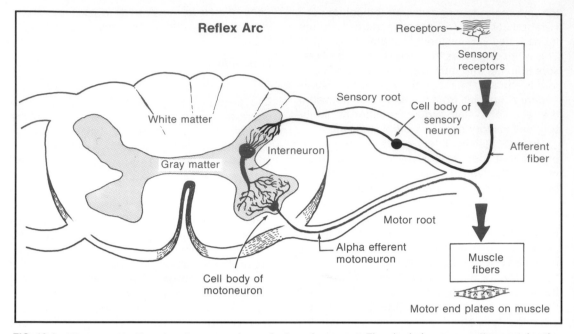

FIG. 19-2. *Afferent and efferent motoneurons in a spinal cord segment. The shaded or gray matter contains the neuron cell bodies; the white matter is made up of longitudinal columns of nerve fibers. Stimulation of a single alpha motoneuron could affect as many as 300 muscle fibers. The motoneuron and the fibers it innervates are collectively referred to as a motor unit. Only one side of the spinal–nerve complex is shown.*

as many as 2000 or 3000 fibers. In terms of muscular activity, the spinal cord is the major processing center for motor control. We will now take a closer look at how information processed in the central nervous system is delivered to the muscles to bring about an appropriate motor response.

The Anterior
Motoneuron

The anterior motoneuron illustrated in Figure 19-3 consists of a *cell body, axon,* and *dendrites.* Its unique design enables it to transmit an electrochemical nerve impulse from the spinal cord to the muscle. The cell body houses the control center—the structures involved with replication and transmission of the genetic code. This part of the motoneuron is located within the gray matter of the spinal cord. The axon extends from the cord to deliver the impulse to the muscle; the dendrites are the short neural branches that receive impulses through numerous connections and conduct them toward the cell body. Nerve cells conduct impulses in one direction—down the axon away from the point of stimulation.

The larger nerve fibers are encased in a *myelin sheath,* a lipid–protein membrane that wraps around the axon over most of its length. A specialized cell known as a *Schwann cell* encases the bare axon and then spirals around it, sometimes up to 100 times in the biggest fibers. Myelin forms a large part of this sheath and insulates the axon. A thinner membrane, the *neurolemma,* covers the myelin sheath. The Schwann cells and myelin are interrupted every one or two millimeters along the axon's length at the *nodes of Ranvier.* Whereas the myelin sheath insulates the axon to the flow of ions, the nodes of Ranvier permit depolarization of the axon to occur. This alternating sequence of myelin sheath and node of Ranvier permits impulses to ''jump'' from node to node as the electric current travels toward the terminal branches at the *motor end-plate.* This means of conduction is responsible for the higher transmission velocity in myelinated than in unmyelinated fibers. In fact, the speed of conduction in a nerve fiber is proportional to its diameter and to the thickness of the myelin sheath.

The anterior motoneurons are also known as *type A α nerve fibers.* Their diameter is large, ranging from about 8 to 20 μm. Other smaller type A fibers are known as gamma (γ) *efferent motoneurons*. They have a diameter no larger than about 10 μm and a conduction velocity about one-half that of the larger α fibers. As is discussed in the section on proprioception, the γ fibers connect with special stretch sensors in skeletal muscle that facilitate detecting minute changes in the length of muscle fibers.

Neuromuscular Junction (Motor End-plate)

The interface between the end of a myelinated motoneuron and a muscle fiber is known as the *neuromuscular junction* or *motor end-plate*. Its function is to transmit the nerve impulse to the muscle. For each skeletal muscle fiber, there is

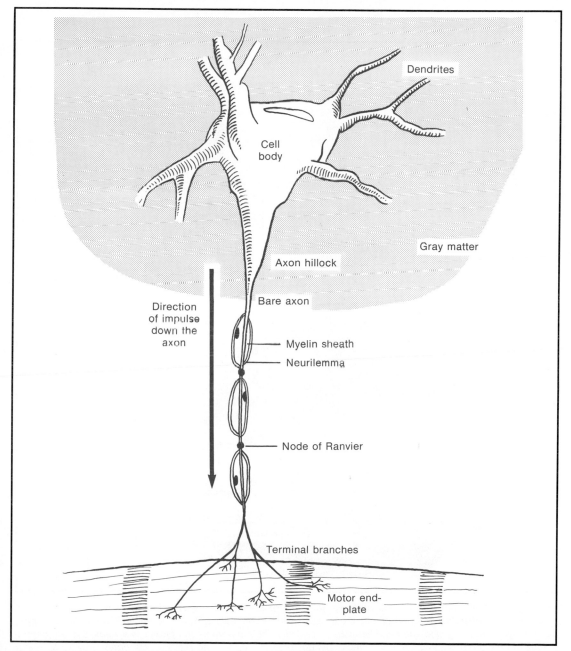

FIG. 19-3. *The anterior motoneuron.*

usually only one neuromuscular junction. Figure 19-4 illustrates the details of the neuromuscular junction based on electron-microscopic studies.

The terminal portion of the axon below the myelin sheath forms several smaller axon branches whose endings are the *presynaptic terminals.* They lie close to, but not in contact with, the sarcolemma of the muscle fiber. The invaginated region of the *postsynaptic mem-* *brane* or *synaptic gutter* has many infoldings that increase its surface area. The region between the synaptic gutter and presynaptic terminal of the axon is called the *synaptic cleft.* The transmission of the neural impulse takes place in this region.

The neurotransmitter responsible for changing a basically electric neural impulse into a chemical stimulus at the motor end-plate is *acetylcholine.* It is released from small, saclike

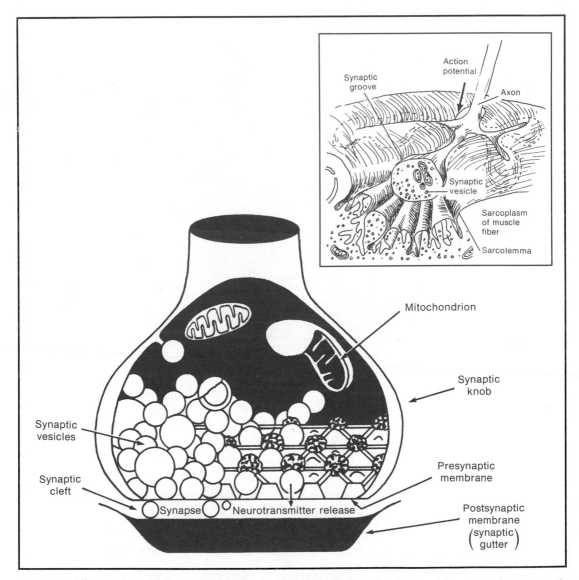

FIG. 19-4. *Microanatomy of the neuromuscular junction. Inset displays the details of the pre- and postsynaptic contact area between the motoneuron and the muscle fiber it innervates. (From K. Akert, K. Pfenninger, C. Sandri, and H. Moor. Freeze etching and cytochemistry of vesicles and membrane complexes in synapses of the central nervous system. In* Structures and Functions of Synapses *(G.D. Pappas and D.P. Purpua, eds.). New York: Raven Press, 1972.)*

vesicles within the terminal axons. When an impulse arrives at the neuromuscular junction, acetylcholine is released into the synaptic cleft and combines with a transmitter–receptor complex in the postsynaptic membrane. This complex increases the postsynaptic membrane's permeability to sodium and potassium ions that ultimately causes the membrane to become depolarized. The impulse then begins to spread over the entire muscle fiber.

Within about 5 milliseconds after acetylcholine is released from the synaptic vesicles, it is destroyed by the enzyme *cholinesterase,* which is concentrated at the borders of the synaptic cleft. The destruction of acetylcholine by cholinesterase allows the postsynaptic membrane to repolarize. Acetic acid and choline, the by-products of cholinesterase action, can be taken up by the axon and resynthesized to acetylcholine so the entire process can begin again with the arrival of another nerve impulse.

EXCITATION. Excitation occurs *only* at the neuromuscular junction. The change in the electric properties of the postsynaptic membrane elicits an *end-plate potential* that spreads from the motor end-plate to the extrajunctional sarcolemma. It then causes an *action potential* to travel the length of the fiber and down the T tubules. Once this occurs, the contractile machinery of the muscle fiber is primed for its major function—to contract.

Acetylcholine is probably one of the interneuronal excitatory transmitter substances. When it is released from the synaptic vesicles, it excites the postsynaptic membrane of its neighboring neuron. This changes the membrane permeability and permits sodium ions to diffuse rapidly to the inside of a neuron. An action potential is generated if the change in microvoltage is sufficient to reach the *threshold for excitation.* This change in membrane potential at the junction between two neurons (which increases the positive charges inside the cell) is referred to as the *excitatory postsynaptic potential* or *EPSP.* If the EPSP is subthreshold, the neuron does not discharge, but its resting membrane potential is lowered and its tendency to "fire" is temporarily increased. The neuron fires when many subthreshold excitatory impulses arrive in rapid succession. In terms of neural activity, this condition is known as *temporal summation. Spatial summation* occurs when different presynaptic terminals on the same neuron are stimulated at the same time. Their individual effects are "summed" and an action potential is initiated.

INHIBITION. Some presynaptic terminals set up inhibitory impulses. The inhibitory transmitter substance increases the permeability of the postsynaptic membrane to potassium and chloride ions. This produces an increase in the membrane's electric potential, creating an *inhibitory postsynaptic potential* or *IPSP.* The IPSP hyperpolarizes the neuron, making it more difficult to fire. No action potential is generated if a motoneuron is subjected to both excitatory and inhibitory influences and if the IPSP is large. The reflex to pull one's hand away when removing a splinter, for example, can usually be overridden (inhibited) so the hand can be steadied to expedite this rather painful task.

The exact neurochemical that provokes an IPSP is unknown, although gamma aminobutyric acid (GABA) and the protein glycine are thought to be involved in the inhibitory process. Neural inhibition serves protective functions and also reduces the input of "unwanted" stimuli so that smooth, purposeful responses can occur. Removing inhibitory influences is important under certain exercise conditions. In all-out strength and power activities, for example, the ability to "disinhibit" and maximally activate all motoneurons required for a movement may be crucial to topflight performance. Central nervous system excitation (neuronal facilitation) is perhaps the mechanism by which intense concentration or "psyching" enhances maximal performances. The "psychologic" influence on strength performance is discussed in Chapter 20.

Motor Units

Although each muscle fiber generally receives only one nerve fiber, a motor nerve may innervate many muscle fibers. This is because the terminal end of an axon forms numerous branches. *The anterior motoneuron and the specific muscle fibers it innervates are called a motor unit.* This is the functional unit of neuromuscular control; all fibers in the specific motor unit have similar metabolic and contractile properties. Some motor units contain up to two thousand muscle fibers whereas others contain relatively few. For example, the first dorsal interosseous muscle of the finger contains 120 motor units that control 41,000 fibers; the medial gastrocnemius muscle (calf) has 580 motor units and 1,030,000 muscle fibers. The ratio of muscle fibers per motor unit is therefore 340 for the finger muscle and 1900 for the gastrocnemius.[2]

ALL-OR-NONE PRINCIPLE. If the stimulus is strong enough to trigger an action potential in the motoneuron, *all* of the accompanying muscle fibers in the motor unit are stimulated to contract synchronously. There is no such thing as a strong or weak contraction from a motor unit—either the impulse is strong enough to elicit a contraction or it is not. Once the neuron is "fired" and the impulse reaches the neuromuscular junction, the muscle cells always contract. This is the principle of "all-or-none" in relation to the normal action of skeletal muscle.

How then is the force of contraction varied from slight to maximal? This occurs in two ways: (1) increasing the number of motor units recruited for the activity, and (2) increasing their frequency of discharge. Clearly, if all motor units are active, the force generated will be considerable compared to that generated by the activation of only a few. Also, if repetitive stimuli reach a muscle before it has relaxed, the total tension produced is increased. By blending these two factors, recruitment of motor units and the rate of their firing, optimal patterns of neural discharge permit a wide variety of graded contractions.

CHARACTERISTICS OF MOTOR UNITS. Motor units are comprised of fibers of one specific fiber type (or subdivision of a particular fiber type). Consequently, these units can be classified into one of three categories depending on their speed of contraction, the amount of force they generate, and the relative fatigability of the fibers. Figure 19-5 illustrates these characteristics for the three categories of motor units: (1) fast twitch, high force, and high fatigue; (2) fast twitch, moderate force, and fatigue resistant; (3) slow twitch, low tension, and fatigue resistant.

The fast-twitch fibers are innervated by relatively large motoneurons with fast conduction velocities. These units reach greater peak tension, and develop it nearly twice as fast as slow-twitch motor units. The slow-twitch motor units are innervated by small motoneurons with slow conduction velocities. These units are much more fatigue-resistant than fast-twitch

units. It should be recalled from our discussion of muscle fiber type, however, that the particular metabolic characteristics of *all* fibers can be modified by specific endurance training. *With prolonged training, some fast-twitch units can become almost as fatigue-resistant as the slow-twitch units.*

There is some evidence that the particular neurons themselves have a trophic or stimulating effect on the muscle fibers they innervate in a way that influences the fibers' growth and development.[4] Innervating fast-twitch fibers with the neuron from a slow-twitch motor unit, for example, eventually alters the twitch characteristics of the fast fibers. If this neurotrophic effect is as great as believed, then the myoneural junction takes on much greater significance than *only* being the site of muscle depolarization.

FIRING PATTERN. Not all of the motor units in a muscle fire at the same time. If they did, it would be virtually impossible to control the force of a contraction. This is easy to demonstrate if one considers the tremendous gradation of forces and speeds that muscles generate. For example, when lifting a barbell, specific muscles contract to move the limb and weight at some particular speed of movement under a given rate of tension development. If the weight is not too heavy, it can be lifted at a number of speeds. If a heavier weight is used, the speed options decrease accordingly. With a light object like a pencil, the proper force is generated by the muscles to lift the pencil, regardless of how fast or slow the arm is moved. *From the standpoint of neural control, the fast- and slow-twitch motor units are selectively recruited and modulated in their firing pattern to produce the desired response.* During sustained activities such as jogging or cycling on a level grade or during slow swimming, motor units of slow-twitch fibers are selectively recruited; for rapid, powerful movements the fast-twitch fibers take preference. More than likely, as a runner reaches a hill during a distance race some fast-twitch units are also activated so that a constant pace is maintained over varying terrain.

The differential control of the motor unit firing pattern is probably the major factor that distinguishes not only skilled from unskilled performances, but also specific athletic groups. For example, weight lifters generally demonstrate a synchronous pattern of motor-unit firing (i.e.,

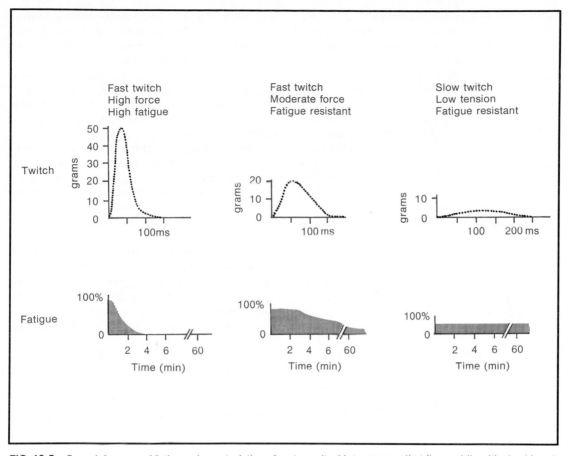

FIG. 19-5. *Speed, force, and fatigue characteristics of motor units. Motoneurons that fire rapidly with short bursts are termed phasic, those that fire slowly but continuously are tonic. (Modified from Edington, D.W., and Edgerton, V.R.: The Biology of Physical Activity. Boston: Houghton Mifflin Co., 1976.)*

many motor units recruited simultaneously during lifting), whereas the firing pattern of endurance athletes is asynchronous (i.e., some units fire while others recover).[6] As discussed previously, the compositional characteristics of a muscle in terms of its specific motor units (muscle fibers) largely determine the performance characteristics of various athletes.[1,3,5] In addition, the synchronous firing of a muscle's fast-twitch fibers certainly aids the weight lifter to generate force quickly for the desired lift. For the endurance athlete, on the other hand, the asynchronous firing of predominantly slow-twitch fatigue-resistant units provides a built-in recuperative period.

NEUROMUSCULAR FATIGUE. Muscular fatigue is the result of many factors, each related to the specific demands of the exercise that produces

it. As was shown in Chapter 1, a significant reduction in muscle glycogen is related to fatigue during prolonged submaximal exercise. This "nutrient fatigue" occurs even though sufficient oxygen is available to generate energy through aerobic pathways. Muscle fatigue in short-term maximal exercise is associated with oxygen lack and an increased level of blood and muscle lactic acid. This anaerobic condition may cause drastic intracellular changes within the active muscles. These could include a depletion of stored high-energy phosphates, a disturbance in the tubular system for transmitting the impulse throughout the cell, and ionic imbalances. Certainly a change in Ca^{2+} distribution could alter the activity of the myofilaments and impair muscular performance. This would cause fatigue even though nerve impulses continue to bombard the muscle fiber.

Fatigue can also be demonstrated at the neuromuscular junction when an action potential fails to cross from the motoneuron to the muscle fiber. The precise mechanism for this aspect of neural fatigue is unknown.

As muscle function becomes impaired during prolonged submaximal exercise, additional motor-unit recruitment takes place to maintain the required force output for the particular activity. In all-out exercise, when all motor units are presumably maximally activated, fatigue is accompanied by a decrease in neural activity (as measured by the electromyogram). The fact that neural activity decreases supports the argument that this form of fatigue is partially caused by a failure in neural or myoneural transmission.

RECEPTORS IN MUSCLES, JOINTS, AND TENDONS: THE PROPRIOCEPTORS

Specialized sensory receptors in the muscles, joints, and ligaments are sensitive to stretch, tension, and pressure. These end-organs, known as *proprioceptors,* rapidly relay information concerning muscular dynamics and limb movement to conscious and unconscious portions of the central nervous system for processing. Thus, the progress of any movement or sequence of movements is continually charted to provide the basis for modifying subsequent motor behavior.

Muscle Spindles

The *muscle spindles* provide sensory information concerning changes in the length and tension of muscle fibers. Their main function is to respond to stretch on a muscle and, through reflex action, to initiate a stronger contraction to reduce this stretch.

STRUCTURAL ORGANIZATION. As shown in Figure 19-6, the spindle is fusiform in shape and is attached in parallel to the regular or *extrafusal fibers* of the muscle. Consequently, when the muscle is stretched so is the spindle. The number of spindles contained per gram of muscle varies widely depending on the muscle group. On a relative basis, there are more spindles in muscles requiring complex movements than in those requiring gross movements. The spindle is covered by a sheath of connective tissue. Within the spindle, there are two types of specialized muscle fibers called *intrafusal fibers.* One type, known as *nuclear bag fibers,* is fairly large and has numerous nuclei centrally packed throughout its diameter. There are usually two bag fibers per spindle. The other type of intrafusal fiber contains many nuclei along its length. These are the *nuclear chain fibers* attached to the surface of the longer nuclear bag fibers. There are usually four to five chain fibers in each spindle. The ends of the intrafusal fibers are striated (they contain actin and myosin) and are capable of contracting.

Three different nerve fibers service the spindles; two are afferent or sensory, one is efferent or motor. A primary afferent nerve fiber is entwined about the midregion of the bag fiber. This is the *annulospiral* nerve fiber that responds directly to the stretch of the spindle; its frequency of firing is proportional to the degree of stretch. A second group of smaller sensory nerve fibers, known as *flower-spray endings,* make connections mainly on the chain fibers, although there are also attachments to the bag fibers. These endings are less sensitive to stretch than the annulospiral fibers are. Activation of the annulospiral and flower-spray sensors relays impulses through sensory roots into the cord to cause a reflex activation of the motoneurons to the muscle. This causes the muscle to contract more forcefully and to shorten; this in turn causes the stretch stimulus to be removed from the spindles.

The third type of spindle nerve fiber has a motor function. These are the thin *gamma efferent* fibers that innervate the contractile, striated ends of the intrafusal fibers. These fibers, activated by higher centers in the brain, provide the mechanism for maintaining the spindle at peak operation at all muscle lengths. Stimulation of the gamma efferents causes the ends of the spindles to contract, thereby regulating their length and sensitivity independent of the overall length of the muscle itself. This activation mechanism prepares the spindle for other lengthening reactions that are about to occur, even though the muscle may already be shortened to a new length. These adjustments enable the spindle to monitor continuously the length of the muscles in which they are located.

THE STRETCH REFLEX. The functional significance of the muscle spindle is its ability to detect, respond to, and control changes in the

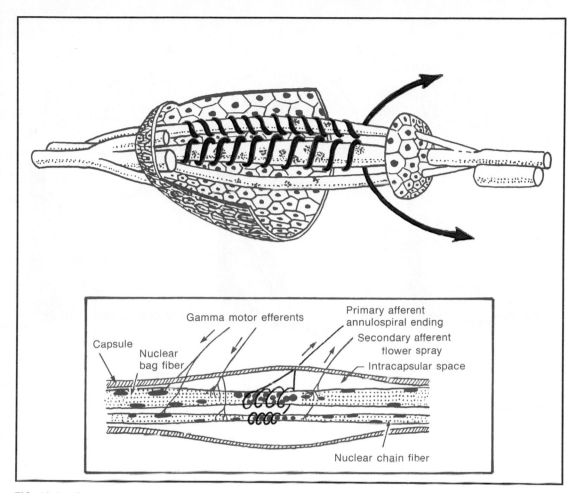

FIG. 19-6. *Structural organization of the muscle spindle. The insert shows an enlarged view of the equatorial region of the spindle. (Modified from Schade, J.P., and Ford, D.H.: Basic Neurology; 2nd ed. Amsterdam: Elsevier/North-Holland Biomedical Press, 1973.)*

length of extrafusal muscle fibers. This is of tremendous importance in the regulation of movement and maintenance of posture. Postural muscles are continuously bombarded by neural input; they must maintain their readiness to respond to voluntary movements or to maintain some degree of constant activity to counter the pull of gravity for upright posture. The stretch reflex is fundamental to achieving this end.

There are three main components to the stretch reflex: (1) the muscle spindle, the sensory receptor within the muscle that responds to stretch, (2) an afferent nerve fiber that carries the sensory impulse from the spindle to the spinal cord, and (3) an efferent motor neuron in the spinal cord that signals the muscle to contract.

Figure 19-7 illustrates schematically the neural pathways involved in this basic reflex. In part A, the bicep muscle is contracted to maintain the bony lever at a 90° angle while holding a 5-kg block. If the block is suddenly increased twofold in weight (part B), the muscle is stretched. This causes the spindles' sensory endings to direct impulses through the dorsal root into the spinal cord where they directly activate the motoneuron. The returning motor impulses (part C) cause the muscle to contract more forcefully to return the limb to its original position. During this reflex process, interneurons in the cord are also activated to facilitate the appropriate movement response. Excitatory impulses are conveyed to muscles that support the desired movement (*synergistic* muscles),

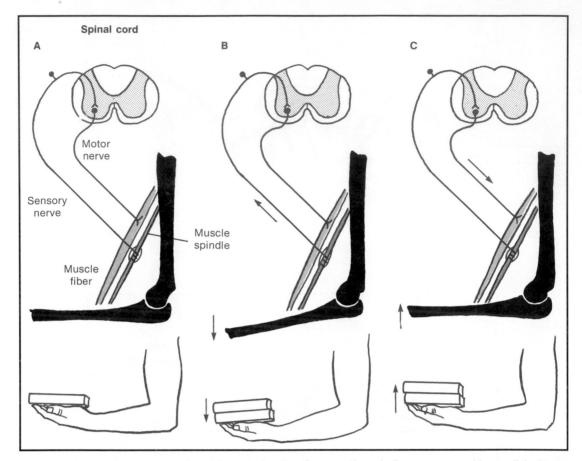

FIG. 19-7. *Schematic representation of the stretch reflex. Because the spindles are arranged in parallel with the extrafusal fibers, they become stretched when these fibers are stretched. This causes a stretch of intrafusal fibers, causing the spindle sensory receptors to fire. This discharge reflexly stimulates the alpha motoneurons to cause the extrafusal fibers to contract. This takes the stretch off of the intrafusal fibers and silences the spindle afferents. In the diagram, the stretch reflex acts as a self-regulating mechanism to maintain the relative constancy of limb position. (From Merton, P.O.: How we control the action of our muscles. Sci. Am., 226: 30, 1972.)*

whereas inhibitory impulses flow to the neurons of muscles that are *antagonists* of the movement. In this way, the stretch reflex acts as a self-regulating or compensating mechanism; it enables the muscle to adjust automatically to differences in load (and length) without immediately processing information through higher centers.

Golgi Tendon Organs

Unlike the muscle spindles that lie parallel to the extrafusal muscle fibers, the *Golgi tendon organs* are connected in series to as many as 25 extrafusal fibers. These sensory receptors are also located in the ligaments of joints and are mainly responsible for detecting differences in muscle tension rather than length. As shown in Figure 19-8, the Golgi tendon organs respond as a feedback monitor to discharge impulses under one of two conditions: (1) in response to tension created in the muscle when it shortens, and (2) in response to tension when the muscle is passively stretched.

When stimulated by excessive tension or stretch, the Golgi receptors conduct their signals rapidly to bring about a *reflex inhibition* of the muscles they supply. This occurs because of the overriding influence of the inhibitory spinal interneuron on the motoneurons supplying the muscle. Thus, the Golgi tendon organ functions as a protective sensory mechanism. If the change in tension or stretch is too great, the sensor's discharge increases; this further depresses the activity of the motoneurons and reduces the tension generated in the muscle fibers. If the muscle contraction produces little tension, Golgi receptors are only weakly activated and exert little influence. *The ultimate function of the Golgi tendon organs is to protect the muscle and its connective tissue harness from injury due to an excessive load.*

Pacinian
Corpuscles

Pacinian corpuscles are small elipsoidal bodies located close to the Golgi tendon organs. These small, onionlike sensory receptors that are sensitive to quick movement and deep pressure are embedded in a single, nonmyelinated nerve fiber. Deformation or compression of the capsule by a mechanical stimulus transmits pressure to the sensory nerve endings within its core. This produces a change in the electric potential of the nerve ending. If this *generator potential* is of sufficient magnitude, a sensory signal is established and propagated down the myelinated axon leaving the corpuscle.

Pacinian corpuscles are "fast-adapting" mechanical sensors because they discharge a few impulses at the onset of a steady stimulus and then remain electrically silent or may discharge a second volley of impulses when the stimulus is removed. Consequently, they detect changes in movement or pressure, rather than how much movement occurred or how much pressure was applied.

SUMMARY

1. Human movement is finely regulated by neural control mechanisms located in the central nervous system. In response to internal and external stimuli, bits of sensory input are automatically and rapidly routed, organized, and transmitted to the effector organs, the muscles.

2. Tracts of nerve tissue descend from the brain to influence neurons in the spinal cord. Neurons in the extrapyramidal tract control posture and provide a continual background level of neuromuscular tone; the pyramidal tract neurons provide for discrete muscular movement.

3. The cerebellum is the major comparing, evaluating, and integrating center that provides the "fine tuning" for muscular activity.

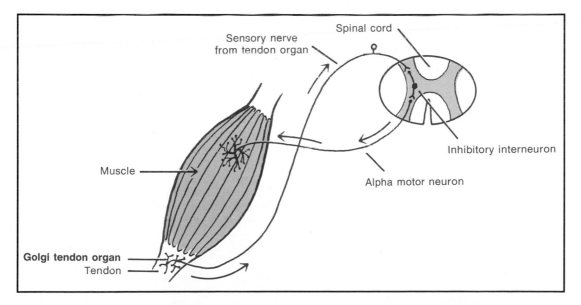

FIG. 19-8. *The Golgi tendon organ. Excessive tension or stretch on a muscle activates the Golgi receptors, which rapidly brings about a reflex inhibition of the muscles they supply. In this way, the Golgi tendon organs function as a protective sensory mechanism.*

4. Many muscular functions are controlled in the spinal cord and other subconscious areas of the central nervous system. The reflex arc is the basic mechanism for processing these automatic muscular movements.

5. The number of muscle fibers in a motor unit depends on the muscle's movement function. Intricate movement patterns require a small fiber-to-neuron ratio whereas for gross movements, a single neuron may innervate several thousand muscle fibers.

6. The anterior motoneuron (cell body, axon, and dendrites) transmits the electrochemical nerve impulse from the spinal cord to the muscle. The dendrites receive impulses and conduct them toward the cell body, whereas the axon transmits the impulse in one direction only—down the axon to the muscle.

7. The neuromuscular junction is the interface between the motoneuron and the muscle fiber. Acelytcholine is released here to provide the chemical stimulus that activates muscles.

8. Both excitatory and inhibitory impulses continually bombard the synaptic junctions between neurons. These alter a neuron's threshold for excitation by either increasing or decreasing its tendency to "fire." In all-out power exercise, a high degree of disinhibition is beneficial because it enables maximal activation of a muscle's motor units.

9. There are three types of motor units depending on speed of contraction, force generated, and fatigability: (1) fast twitch, high force high fatigue, (2) fast twitch, moderate force, fatigue resistant and (3) slow twitch, low tension fatigue resistant.

10. Special sensory receptors in muscles tendons, and joints relay information concerning muscular dynamics and limb movement to specific portions of the central nervous system This provides important sensory feedback during physical activity.

References

1. Costill, D.L. et al.: Skeletal muscle enzyme and fiber composition in male and female track athletes. J. Appl. Physiol., *40:*149, 1976.
2. Feinstein, B. et al.: Morphologic studies of motor units in normal human muscle. *Acta Anat.* (Basel), *23:*127, 1955.
3. Gollnick, P.D., and Sembrowich, W.L.: Adaptations in human skeletal muscle as a result of training. *In* Exercise in Cardiovascular Health and Disease. Edited by E.A. Amsterdam, et al. New York, Yorke Medical Books, 1977.
4. Gutman E.: Neurotrophic relations. Annu. Rev. Physiol., *38:*177, 1976.
5. Saltin, B. et al.: Fiber types and metabolic potentials of skeletal muscles in sedentary man and endurance runners. Ann. N.Y. Acad. Sci., *301:*3, 1977.
6. Stepanov, A.S. and Burlakov, M.L.: Electrophysiological investigation of fatigue in muscular activity. Sechenov Physiol. J. USSR, *47:*43, 1961.

Applied
And
Exercise
Physiology

SECTION IV
Enhancement of Energy Capacity

In many cases, exercise training is more an art than a science. The success of different conditioning programs is usually evaluated by individual achievements or won–loss records rather than by scientific inquiry and discovery. Too often, coaches of sports such as basketball or soccer place considerable importance on the development of cardiovascular or aerobic capacity and devote little time to various phases of vigorous anaerobic conditioning. It is true that these sports require a relatively steady release of aerobic energy. However, in those crucial situations that demand all-out effort, if the relative capacity of the athlete's anaerobic energy transfer system is poor, the player is unable to perform at full potential. Training the anaerobic capacity of endurance athletes, on the other hand, would be wasteful because the contribution of anaerobic energy to successful performance is minimal. Rather, these activities demand a well-conditioned heart and vascular system capable of circulating large quantities of blood as well as a high capacity of muscle cells to generate ATP aerobically. At the other extreme, one's capacity for aerobic metabolism contributes little to overall success in sprint activities and sports such as football. Here, performance is largely dependent on muscular strength and power where energy is generated primarily from reactions that do not utilize oxygen.

With a clear understanding of energy transfer and the effects of specific training on the systems of energy delivery and utilization, it should be possible to construct a sound training program to achieve optimum performance. In Chapters 20 and 21 we discuss the basis of training for muscular strength and aerobic and anaerobic power, the physiologic consequences of such training, and the important factors affecting training success. In Chapter 22, we take a closer look at factors purported to increase human exercise performance.

Training for Anaerobic and Aerobic Power

20

Throughout this book we have stressed that different activities, depending on their duration and intensity, require the activation of specific energy systems. This is shown in Figure 20-1 in which exercise is broadly classified in terms of duration and predominant energy pathways.

We realize that it is difficult to place certain activities in one category. For example, as a person increases aerobic fitness, an activity previously classified as anaerobic might be reclassified as aerobic. In many cases, all three energy transfer systems, the ATP-CP system, the glycolytic or lactic acid system, and the aerobic system, operate at different times during exercise. Their relative contributions to the energy continuum, however, are directly related to the length of time and intensity (power output) the specific activity is performed.

Brief power activities lasting about 6 seconds rely almost exclusively on "immediate" energy generated from the breakdown of the stored intramuscular phosphates, ATP and CP. Consequently, power athletes like sprinters must gear training to improve the capacity of this energy transfer system. As all-out exercise progresses up to 60 seconds and power output becomes somewhat reduced, the major portion of energy is still generated via anaerobic pathways. These metabolic reactions involve the short-term energy system of glycolysis and subsequent lactic acid formation. As exercise intensity diminishes somewhat and duration extends to 2 to 4 minutes, reliance on energy from phosphate stores and anaerobic glycolysis decreases, whereas the aerobic production of ATP becomes increasingly more important. Prolonged exercise progresses on a "pay-as-you-go" basis with more than 99% of the en-

ergy requirement being generated by aerobic reactions. Clearly, an efficient training program is one that allocates a proportionate commitment to training the specific energy systems involved in the activity. In the sections that follow, we discuss anaerobic and aerobic conditioning with special emphasis on principles, methods, and short- and long-term adaptations. The approach to physiologic conditioning is basically the same for men and women; both respond and adapt to training in essentially the same manner.[4,12]

PRINCIPLES OF TRAINING

The major objective in training is to cause biologic adaptations in order to improve performance in a specific task. This requires adherence to carefully planned and executed activities. Attention is focused on factors such as frequency and length of workouts, type of training, speed, intensity, duration, and repetition of the activity, and appropriate competition. Although these factors vary depending on the performance goal, it is possible to identify several principles of physiologic conditioning common to the performance classifications shown in Figure 20-1.

Overload Principle

To enhance physiologic improvement effectively and to bring about a training change, a specific exercise overload must be applied. By

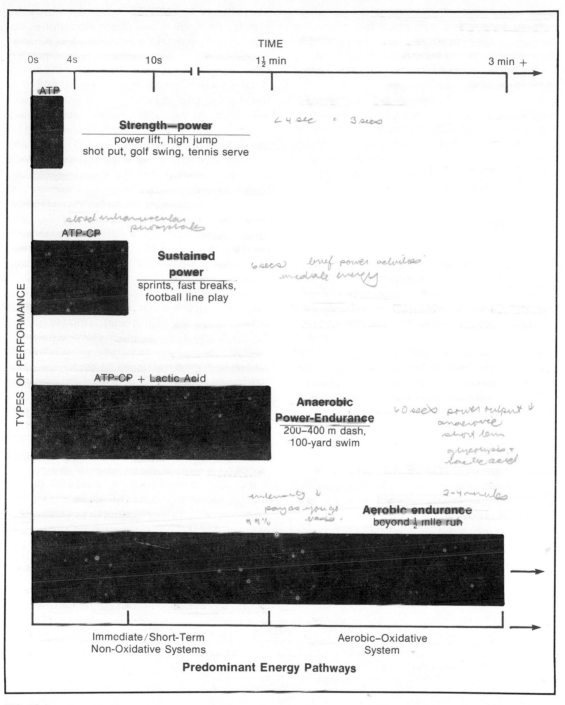

FIG. 20-1. *Classification of activities based on duration of performance and the predominant intracellular energy pathways.*

exercising at a level above normal, a variety of training adaptations take place that cause the body to function more efficiently. The appropriate overload for each person can be achieved by manipulating combinations of training *frequency, intensity,* and *duration.*

This concept of individualized and progressive overload applies to the athlete, the sedentary person, and even the cardiac patient. In fact, an increasing number in this latter group use an appropriately formulated exercise rehabilitation program to walk, jog, and eventually run and complete marathons![27a]

Specificity Principle

The important principle of specificity has been mentioned in numerous sections of this text. When applied to training, specificity refers to adaptations in the *metabolic* and *physiologic* systems depending on the type of overload imposed. It is known that a specific exercise stress such as strength–power training induces specific strength–power adaptations, and that specific aerobic or cardiovascular exercise elicits specific endurance-training adaptations.[24,51,52] The specificity principle, however, goes beyond this because development of aerobic fitness for swimming,[31] bicycling,[39,53] or running[33] is most effectively achieved when the exerciser trains the specific muscles involved in the desired performance. Truly, *specific exercise elicits specific adaptations creating specific training effects.*

SPECIFICITY OF MAX $\dot{V}O_2$. Table 20-1 shows the results of a study in one of our laboratories designed to investigate specificity of endurance swim training on improvements in maximal aerobic power.[31] Fifteen men trained 1 hour a day, 3 days a week, for 10 weeks. Before and after the training, the max $\dot{V}O_2$ of all subjects was measured during both treadmill running and swimming. A complete specificity was noted for the 11% improvement in max $\dot{V}O_2$ with swim training. Because a vigorous training exercise such as swimming provides a general overload to the central circulation, we had expected at least some improvement or "transfer" in aerobic power from swimming to running. This was not the case, however. In fact, if only treadmill running had been used to evaluate swim training effects, we would have mistakenly concluded "No effect"!

Based on available research,[32,33,39] it is reasonable to advise that in training for specific aerobic activities like cycling, swimming, rowing, or running, the overload must engage the appropriate muscles required by the activity as well as provide an exercise stress for the cardiovascular system. There is little improvement noted when aerobic capacity is measured by a dissimilar exercise, yet there are significant improvements when the test exercise is the same exercise used in training. Thus, one can appreciate how difficult it is to be in "good shape" for diverse forms of aerobic exercise.

It is also noteworthy from Table 20-1 that although swimming max $\dot{V}O_2$ improved 11% with swim training, the maximum work time in-

TABLE 20-1. *Effects of 10 weeks of interval swim training on changes in max $\dot{V}O_2$ and endurance performance as measured during running and swimming[a]*

SUBJECTS	MEASURE	RUNNING TEST			SWIMMING TEST		
		PRE-TRAINING	POST-TRAINING	% CHANGE	PRE-TRAINING	POST-TRAINING	% CHANGE
Swim training	Max $\dot{V}O_2$						
	$l \cdot min^{-1}$	4.05	4.11	+1.5	3.44	3.82	+11.0
N = 15	$ml \cdot kg^{-1} \cdot min^{-1}$	54.9	55.7	+1.5	46.6	51.8	+11.0
	Max work time, min	19.6	20.5	+4.6	11.9	15.9	+34.0
Nontraining Controls	Max $\dot{V}O_2$						
	$l \cdot min^{-1}$	4.12	4.18	+1.5	3.51	3.40	3.1
N = 15	$ml \cdot kg^{-1} \cdot min^{-1}$	55.1	55.5	+0.7	46.8	45.0	−3.8
	Max work time, min	20.7	19.7	−4.8	11.5	11.5	0

[a]From Magel, J.R. et al.: Specificity of swim training on maximum oxygen uptake. *J. Appl. Physiol.* 38:151, 1975.

creased 34% during the swim test. Max $\dot{V}O_2$ improvements probably reach a peak in training, and, thereafter, improvements in performance are supported by other mechanisms only partly related to the oxygen transport system. The partial independence of performance measures from physiologic measures may explain why max $\dot{V}O_2$ values of certain endurance athletes of the 1930s and 1940s were similar to those of present-day athletes, even though the performances of contemporary athletes substantially exceed those of athletes from that time. This illustrates the necessity for clearly distinguishing between *physiologic* and *performance* changes with training.

SPECIFICITY OF LOCAL CHANGES. In endurance training, the overload of specific muscle groups enhances work performance and aerobic power by facilitating both oxygen transport and utilization at the local level.[24] The oxidative capacity of the vastus lateralis muscle, for example, is greater in well-trained cyclists than in endurance runners,[18] and is improved significantly following training on a bicycle ergometer.[19] Such adaptations would certainly increase the capacity of the trained muscles to generate ATP aerobically. The specificity of aerobic improvement may also result from greater regional blood flow in active tissues due either to increased microcirculation or to more effective distribution of cardiac output, or both. Regardless of the mechanism, such adapta-

tions would occur *only* in the specifically trained muscles and would only be seen when these muscles were activated.

Individual Differences Principle

Many factors contribute to individual variation in training response. Of considerable importance is the person's relative fitness level at the start of training. It is unrealistic to expect different people to be in the same "state" of training at the same time. Consequently, it is counterproductive to insist that all performers of the same team (or even the same event) train the same way or at the same relative or absolute work rate. It is also unrealistic to expect all individuals to respond to a given training dosage in precisely the same manner. *Training benefits are optimized when programs are planned to meet the individual needs and capacities of the participants.*

Reversibility Principle

Detraining occurs rapidly when a person stops exercising. After only 2 weeks of detraining, significant reductions in working capacity can be measured, and almost all of the training improvements are lost within several months. Table 20-2 shows the physiologic and metabolic consequences of various durations of

TABLE 20-2. Changes in physiologic and metabolic values resulting from various durations of detraining

STUDY[a]	N	SEX	DURATION (DAYS)	VARIABLE	PRE-DETRAINING AVERAGE	POST-DETRAINING AVERAGE	PERCENT CHANGE
(45)	5	M	20 (bedrest)	Max $\dot{V}O_2$, $l \cdot min^{-1}$	3.3	2.4	−27
				Stroke volume, ml	116	88	−24
				Cardiac output, $l \cdot min^{-1}$	20	14.8	−26
(10)	7	F	84	Max $\dot{V}O_2$, $ml \cdot kg^{-1} \cdot min^{-1}$	47.8	40.4	−15.5
				Ve max, $l \cdot min^{-1}$	77.5	69.5	−10.3
				O_2 pulse, $ml \cdot beat^{-1}$	12.7	10.9	−14.2
(34)	17	M	70	Sum of 3-min recovery heart rate	190	237	−24.7
(30)	9	M	35	CP, $mmols \cdot g$ wet wt^{-1}	17.9	13.0	−27.4
				ATP, $mmols \cdot g$ wet wt^{-1}	5.97	5.08	−14.9
				Glycogen, $mmols \cdot g$ wet wt^{-1}	113.9	57.4	−49.6
				Elbow extension strength, ft, lb	39.0	25.5	−34.6

[a]Number in parenthesis refers to study in reference list.

detraining as evaluated in several studies. The research of one group of workers is especially interesting.[45] For five subjects confined to bed for 20 consecutive days, there was a 25% decrease in max $\dot{V}O_2$ accompanied by a similar decrement in maximal stroke volume and cardiac output. This corresponded approximately to a 1% decrease in physiologic function each day.

The important point is that the beneficial effects of exercise training are *transient* and *reversible*. For this reason, most athletes begin a reconditioning program several months prior to the start of the competitive season. Many ex-athletes are in poorer physiologic condition several years after they retire from active participation than is the 50-year-old business executive who plays racquetball on a regular basis.

PHYSIOLOGIC CONSEQUENCES OF TRAINING

Many of the biologic changes that accompany training have been presented in appropriate sections throughout this book. We will now summarize the various training adaptations outlined in Table 20-3.

Anaerobic System Changes

Figure 20-2 summarizes the metabolic adaptations in *anaerobic function* accompanying strenuous physical training.

In keeping with the concept of specificity of training, activities that demand a high level of anaerobic metabolism bring about specific

TABLE 20-3. *Typical metabolic and physiologic values for trained and untrained men*[a]

VARIABLE	UNTRAINED	TRAINED	PERCENT DIFFERENCE[b]
Glycogen, mmol · g wet muscle⁻¹	85.0	120	41
Number of mitochondria, mmol³	0.59	1.20	103
Mitochondrial volume, % muscle cell	2.15	8.00	272
Resting ATP, mmol · g wet muscle⁻¹	3.0	6.0	100
Resting CP, mmol · g wet muscle⁻¹	11.0	18.0	64
Resting creatine, mmol · g wet muscle⁻¹	10.7	14.5	35
Glycolytic enzymes			
Phosphofructokinase, mmol · g wet muscle⁻¹	50.0	50.0	0
Phosphorylase, mmol · g wet muscle⁻¹	4–6	6–9	60
Aerobic enzymes			
Succinate dehydrogenase, mmol · kg wet muscle⁻¹	5–10	15–20	133
Max lactic acid, mmol · kg wet muscle⁻¹	110	150	36
Muscle fibers			
Fast twitch, %	50	20–30	−50
Slow twitch, %	50	60	20
Max stroke volume, ml · beat⁻¹	120	180	50
Max cardiac output, l · min⁻¹	20	30–40	75
Resting heart rate, beats · min⁻¹	70	40	−43
Max heart rate, beats · min⁻¹	190	180	−5
Max (a-v̄) O₂ diff, ml · 100 ml⁻¹	14.5	16.0	10
Max V̇O₂, ml · kg⁻¹ · min⁻¹	30–40	65–80	107
Heart volume, l	7.5	9.5	27
Blood volume, l	4.7	6.0	28
Hemoglobin, g · kg⁻¹	11.6	13.7	18
Ve max, l · min⁻¹	110	190	73
Percent body fat	15	11	−27

[a] In some cases, approximate values are used. In *all* cases, the trained values represent data from endurance athletes. Caution is advised in assuming that the percent differences between trained and untrained are necessarily the result of training, because genetic differences between individuals probably exert a strong influence on many of these factors.

[b] Computed as the percent that the trained differs from the corresponding value for the untrained.

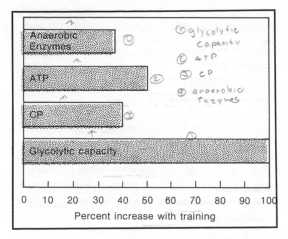

FIG. 20-2. *Changes in the anaerobic potential of skeletal muscle as a result of heavy physical training.*

changes in the immediate and short-term energy systems. Specifically, the metabolic changes that occur with power-type training include:

1. *Increases in resting levels of anaerobic substrates.*[25,27,30] As shown in Table 20-4, these changes were determined from muscle biopsies taken before and after resistance weight training. A 28% improvement in strength was accompanied by significant increases in the muscle's resting levels of ATP, CP, free creatine, and glycogen.

2. *Increases in the quantity and activity of key enzymes controlling the anaerobic phase of glucose breakdown.* These changes are not of the magnitude observed for oxidative enzymes with aerobic training. The most dramatic alterations in anaerobic enzyme function and increase in fiber size occur in the fast-twitch muscle fibers.[19,52]

3. *Increases in capacity for levels of blood lactic acid during all-out exercise following anaerobic training.* This is probably due to enhanced glycolytic enzyme activity as well as to improved motivation and "pain" tolerance to fatiguing exercise. Concurrent with metabolic adaptations, increased anaerobic exercise capacity is also observed.[8,25,30]

Aerobic System Changes

Aerobic overload training significantly improves a variety of functional capacities related to oxygen transport and utilization. The most notable adaptations accompanying aerobic training include the following:

1. *Mitochondria from trained skeletal muscle have a greatly increased capacity to generate ATP aerobically by oxidative phosphorylation.*[3]

2. *Associated with the increased capacity for mitochondrial oxygen uptake is an increase in both the size and number of mitochondria and a potential twofold increase in the activity level of aerobic system enzymes.*[3,28] These changes may be of extreme importance in sustaining a high percentage of aerobic capacity during prolonged exercise.

3. *Skeletal muscle myoglobin content increases* by as much as 80%.[38] As a result, the quantity of oxygen within the cell at any one time is increased, which probably facilitates oxygen diffusion to the mitochondria.

4. *There is an increase in the trained muscle's capacity to mobilize and oxidize fat.*[36] This increase is brought about by an increase in the activity of fat-mobilizing and fat-metabolizing enzymes. Thus, at any submaximal work rate, a trained person uses more free fatty acids for

TABLE 20-4. *Changes in resting concentrations of CP, creatine, ATP, and glycogen following 5 months of heavy-resistance weight training in nine male subjects*[a]

VARIABLE[b]	CONTROL	POST-TRAINING	PERCENT DIFFERENCE[c]
CP	17.07	17.94	+5.1
Creatine	10.74	14.52	+35.2
ATP	5.07	5.97	+17.8
Glycogen	86.28	113.90	+32.0

[a] From MacDougall, J.D. et al.: Biochemical adaptation of human skeletal muscle to heavy resistance training and immobilization. *J. Appl. Physiol., 43:* 700, 1977.
[b] All values are expressed in mmol per gram of wet muscle tissue.
[c] All percent differences are statistically significant.

energy than an untrained counterpart does. This is beneficial to endurance athletes because it conserves the carbohydrate stores so important in prolonged exercise.

5. *Trained muscle also exhibits a greater capability to oxidize carbohydrate.*[7] Consequently, large quantities of pyruvic acid move through the aerobic energy pathways. This is consistent with the increased oxidative potential of the mitochondria, as well as with increased glycogen storage within the trained muscles.

6. *Aerobic training produces metabolic adaptations in the different types of muscle fibers.* It is generally believed that the basic fiber type does not "change,"[18,51,52] but instead, all fibers develop their already existing aerobic potential.[18]

7. *There may also be selective hypertrophy of different muscle fibers to specific overload training.*[18,52] Highly trained endurance athletes show larger slow-twitch fibers than fast-twitch fibers in the same muscle. Conversely, for athletes trained in predominantly anaerobic activities, the fast-twitch fibers occupy a greater cross-sectional area.

Related Cardiovascular and Respiratory Changes

Because the cardiovascular and respiratory systems are intimately linked with aerobic processes, related changes occur that are both functional and dimensional.

HEART SIZE. The weight and volume of the heart generally increase with aerobic training.[37] This cardiac hypertrophy is a normal training adaptation characterized by an increase in the size of the left ventricular cavity as well as by a thickening of its walls.

BLOOD VOLUME. Blood volume and total hemoglobin tend to increase with endurance training.[29] This adaptation may enhance circulatory dynamics to facilitate one's oxygen delivery capacity during exercise.

HEART RATE. Resting and submaximal exercise heart rate decrease during an aerobic training program. This is especially true for previously sedentary individuals. Consequently, heart rate changes provide a convenient index to measure training improvement.

STROKE VOLUME. The heart's stroke volume increases significantly at rest and during exercise as a result of aerobic training. Large stroke volumes are particularly evident among endurance athletes and generally result from a large ventricular volume accompanied by enhanced myocardial contractility.

CARDIAC OUTPUT. The most significant change in cardiovascular function with aerobic training is the increase in maximum cardiac output. Because the maximal heart rate may even decrease slightly, the heart's increased outflow capacity with training results directly from improved stroke volume. A large cardiac output is a major factor that distinguishes champion endurance athletes from well-trained and untrained individuals.

OXYGEN EXTRACTION. Training produces significant increases in the amount of oxygen extracted from the circulating blood.[32,44] An increase in the arteriovenous oxygen difference is the result of a more effective distribution of the cardiac output to working muscles as well as of enhanced capacity of the trained muscle cells to extract and utilize oxygen.

BLOOD FLOW AND DISTRIBUTION. There is some indication that trained individuals perform submaximal exercise with a relatively lower cardiac output than untrained counterparts. This is probably the result of specific biochemical cellular changes with training. As the cell's ability to extract and utilize oxygen increases, less regional blood flow is required to meet the muscle's oxygen needs. This decrease in muscle blood flow would "free" blood that could now be delivered to nonworking but important tissues such as the skin, liver, and kidneys. This could be of considerable benefit in sustaining prolonged submaximal exercise.

Of course, training causes large increases in total muscle blood flow during maximal exercise due to: (1) improvements in maximal cardiac output, and (2) redistribution of blood from nonworking areas that temporarily compromise their blood flow in response to all-out effort.[45]

BLOOD PRESSURE. Regular aerobic training reduces both systolic and diastolic blood pressure during rest and submaximal exercise. The largest decreases occur in systolic pressure and are especially apparent in hypertensive subjects.

↑ed breathing vol   higher max vent   ↑initial vol +breathing freq
In submax - ventilates less   - ↑ventilatory efficiency → more O₂ to working mm

RESPIRATORY FUNCTION.

Increased breathing volumes accompany improvements in max $\dot{V}O_2$. Higher maximum ventilation is due to increases in both tidal volume and breathing frequency. In submaximal exercise, however, the trained person ventilates less than he or she did before training. This adaptation may be helpful in prolonged exercise because increased ventilatory efficiency means more oxygen available to the working muscles.

Other Training-Induced Changes

↑ ex performance

PERFORMANCE CHANGES.

Enhanced exercise performance usually accompanies the physiologic adjustments with training. For example, a training study consisted of long-distance cycling for 40 to 60 minutes, 4 days per week for 10 weeks at an intensity of 85% of max $\dot{V}O_2$. The performance test consisted of trying to maintain a constant work rate of 1620 kg-m per minute for 8 minutes. As shown in Figure 20-3, there was significantly less drop-off from the prescribed initial pace following training.

BODY COMPOSITION CHANGES.

For obese and borderline obese people, regular endurance exercise causes a reduction in body weight accompanied by a decrease in body fat. Increases in lean body weight often accompany

↓in body wgt   ↓ in body fat
↗ in lean body wgt (strength training)

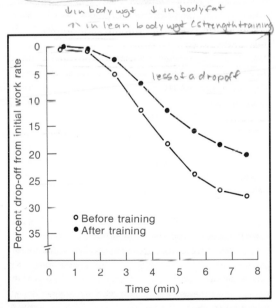

less of a dropoff

○ Before training
● After training

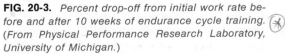

FIG. 20-3. *Percent drop-off from initial work rate before and after 10 weeks of endurance cycle training. (From Physical Performance Research Laboratory, University of Michigan.)*

strength training programs. If weight loss is attempted by diet *alone,* a significant reduction in lean body tissue also accompanies fat loss. When diet is combined with exercise, however, more of the weight lost is fat because exercise appears to have a conserving effect on the body's lean tissues.[55]

diet → ↓lean body tissue   ↓fat loss
diet + ex → more wgt lost is fat
ex → conserving effect on lean tissue

BODY HEAT TRANSFER.

Trained individuals exercise more comfortably in hot environments because of a more responsive heat regulatory mechanism. Trained individuals dissipate heat faster and more economically and thereby cool the body more effectively. This means that the metabolic heat generated by exercise causes less heat strain and thus prolongs one's exercise tolerance.

body heat transfer better
& ex more comfortably in hot
- more responsive heat regulatory mech

- dissipate heat faster + more economically cool more effectively
→ metabolic heat during ex → less heat strain + prolongs ex tolerance

FACTORS AFFECTING TRAINING

An appropriate exercise prescription must consider the major factors related to training improvement: (1) initial fitness level, (2) frequency of training, (3) intensity of exercise, (4) duration of exercise, and (5) type of exercise.

Initial Fitness Level

less fit → more room for improvement
more fit → less room for improvement
→ 5 - 25% improvement

The amount of training improvement depends on one's initial fitness level.[46,47] If someone rates low at the start, there is room for considerable improvement. If capacity is already high, then naturally there will be relatively little improvement. In studies of sedentary, middle-aged men with heart disease, maximal aerobic power improved by 50%, whereas for the same type of training in normally active, healthy adults only a 10% to 15% improvement occurs.[41] Of course, a 5% improvement in physiologic function for an elite athlete is just as important as a 40% increase for a sedentary person. As a general guideline, however, aerobic fitness improvements of 5% to 25% can be expected from systematic endurance training.

Exercise Intensity

↑ on intensity of overload
- reflects calorie cost of work + specific energy system activated
- absolute or relative basis

Training-induced physiologic changes depend *primarily* on the intensity of the overload. Exercise intensity reflects both the caloric cost of

minimal stimulus ↑ heart rate 70% of max or 50-55% OK may VO₂

ceiling for intensity 55% max VO₂ 90% max heart rate

the work and the specific energy systems activated, and intensity can be applied either on an absolute or relative basis.

An example of an absolute training intensity would be to have *all* individuals do the *same* work at the same rate, such as 1200 kg-m per minute on the bicycle ergometer or expend 300 kcal in a 30-minute exercise session. With everyone doing the same amount of work, however, a considerable exercise stress for one person might be below the training threshold intensity for another more highly conditioned person. For this reason, training is usually assigned based on the relative stress placed on a person's physiologic systems. Relative intensity is usually assigned as some percentage of maximum function, for example, max $\dot{V}O_2$, maximum heart rate, or maximum work capacity. The general practice for establishing aerobic training intensity is to either directly measure or estimate the person's max $\dot{V}O_2$ or maximum heart rate, and then assign a work schedule that corresponds to some percentage of these maximums.

Although establishing training intensity from measures of oxygen consumption is highly accurate, it is impractical without sophisticated equipment. An effective alternative is to use heart rate to classify exercise in terms of relative intensity and to establish a training protocol. This practice is based on the fact that the percent of one's max $\dot{V}O_2$ and percent of maximum heart rate (HR max) are related in a predictable way regardless of sex or age. Selected values for percent max $\dot{V}O_2$ and corresponding percentages of HR max obtained from several sources are presented in Table 20-5.[2,50] The error in estimating percent max $\dot{V}O_2$ from percent HR max, or vice versa, is about ± 8%. Because of this intrinsic relationship, it is only necessary to monitor heart rate in order to estimate percent max $\dot{V}O_2$.

TABLE 20-5. *Relation between percent max $\dot{V}O_2$ and percent max heart rate*

PERCENT MAX HR	PERCENT MAX $\dot{V}O_2$
50	28
60	42
70	56
80	70
90	83
100	100

TRAINING AT A PERCENTAGE OF MAXIMUM HEART RATE. *As a general rule, aerobic capacity will improve if exercise is of sufficient intensity to increase heart rate to about 70% of maximum.* This is equivalent to about 50% to 55% of the maximum aerobic capacity or, for college-aged men and women, to a heart rate of 130 to 140 beats per minute. This intensity appears to be the *minimal* stimulus required to provide training improvements.

[An alternate and equally effective method of establishing the training threshold is to exercise at a heart rate about 60% of the distance between resting and maximal.[26] This is calculated as:

$$HR_{threshold} = HR_{rest} + 0.60 \, (HR_{max} - HR_{rest})]$$

Clearly, exercise need not be strenuous in order to obtain positive results. An exercise heart rate of 70% maximum represents moderate exercise that can be continued for a long time with little or no discomfort. This training level is frequently referred to as "conversational exercise" in that it is sufficiently intense to stimulate a training effect yet not so strenuous that it limits a person from talking during the workout. It is unnecessary to exercise above this heart rate in order to improve physiologic capacity. Figure 20-4 shows that as cardiovascular fitness improves and the person starts to become "trained," the exercise heart rate is gradually reduced. It is common for submaximal heart rate to be lowered by 10 to 20 beats per minute during an aerobic conditioning program. To keep pace, the work rate must be increased periodically to achieve the threshold heart rate or whatever target rate has been established. A person who began training by walking will now have to walk more briskly; this will gradually be replaced by jogging for periods of the workout, and, eventually, continuous running will be required to achieve the same relative strenuousness at the desired target heart rate.

IS STRENUOUS TRAINING MORE EFFECTIVE? Generally, the greater the relative training intensity above threshold, the greater is the training improvement.[40,47] However, this is only true within certain limits. Although there may be a minimal threshold intensity below which a training effect will not occur, there may also be a ceiling "threshold" above which there are no further gains.[5] The lower and upper limits may depend

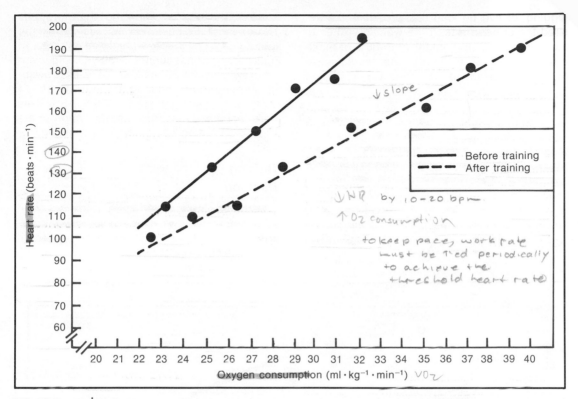

FIG. 20-4. *HR-$\dot{V}O_2$ line for a 20-year-old woman before and after a 10-week aerobic conditioning program.*

[handwritten] relatively poor condition   training threshold 60% HR max — 45% max $\dot{V}O_2$
[handwritten] higher fitness level → higher threshold

[handwritten annotations on figure: ↓ slope; ↓ HR by 10-20 bpm; ↑ O_2 consumption; to keep pace, work rate must be ↑ed periodically to achieve the threshold heart rate]

on the participant's initial capacity and state of training. For people in relatively poor condition, the training threshold may be closer to 60% of HR max that corresponds to about 45% max $\dot{V}O_2$; persons at higher fitness levels generally have a higher threshold level. The ceiling for training intensity is unknown, although 85% max $\dot{V}O_2$ (corresponding to 90% HR max) is thought to be the upper limit—however, no definitive research is available to either prove or disprove this notion.

THE "TRAINING-SENSITIVE ZONE." Maximum heart rate for a specific activity can usually be determined immediately after 2 to 4 minutes of all-out exercise in that form of work. This level of exercise, however, requires considerable motivation and certainly is not advisable for adults without medical clearance or those predisposed to coronary heart disease. Consequently, people should consider themselves "average" and use the age-adjusted maximum heart rates presented in Figure 20-5. Although all people of a particular age do not possess the same maximum heart rate, the loss in accuracy due to individual variation (usually ± 10 beats per minute at any age-predicted heart rate) is of small significance in establishing an effective training program. As a convenient "rule of thumb," maximum heart rate is established as 220 minus the person's age. Figure 20-5 also shows the "training-sensitive zone" in relation to age. Conditioning of the aerobic systems occurs as long as the exercise heart rate is maintained within this zone.

If a 40-year-old woman wishes to train at moderate intensity, yet still be at or above the threshold level, a training heart rate would be selected that is equal to 70% of the age-predicted maximum heart rate, i.e., a target exercise heart rate of 126 beats per minute (0.70 × 180). Then, by trial and error (using progressive increments in light to moderate exercise), the woman can arrive at a walking,

[handwritten left margin: max heartrate – after 2-4 min of all-out ex → considerable motivation not advisible for adults b out medical clearance → use age adjusted max heartrate]

[handwritten right margin: training sensitive zone conditioning as long as heart rate maintained within zone]

[handwritten bottom right: of same age all people do not possess same max hr → ±10 b/m → small sign max heart rate = 220 – age]

cling load that produces the de-
:eart rate. If the woman wishes to
:raining intensity to 85% of maxi-
:ercise heart rate would have
:sed to 153 beats per minute

RUNNING VERSUS SWIMMING. If swimming is
used for training, an adjustment should be
made in estimating maximum heart rate. *Maxi-*
mum heart rate swimming averages about 13
beats per minute lower than running in both
trained and untrained subjects.[31,33] This difference is probably due to the horizontal body
position during swimming and the cooling effect of the water. To establish the appropriate

exercise intensity for swimming, therefore, this
difference of 13 beats per minute should be
subtracted from the age-predicted HR max in
Figure 20-5. Consequently, a 30-year-old wishing to swim at 70% HR max would select a swimming speed that produced a heart rate of 124
beats per minute $[(0.70) \times (190 - 13)]$. This
more accurately represents the appropriate
threshold training heart rate for swimming.

Training Duration

A threshold duration per workout has *not* been
identified for optimal cardiovascular improvement. Such a threshold is probably dependent

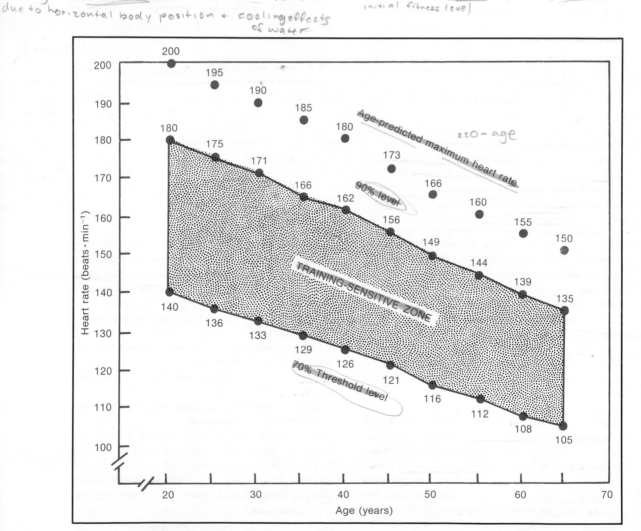

FIG. 20-5. *Maximal heart rates and training-sensitive zones for use in aerobic training programs for people of different ages. (From Nutrition, Weight Control, and Exercise by Frank I. Katch and William D. McArdle. Copyright © 1977 by Houghton Mifflin Company. Reprinted by permission of the publisher.)*

on many factors including the total work done, exercise intensity, training frequency, and initial fitness level. Activity of lower intensity generally requires a relatively longer exercise duration. Whereas 3- to 5-minute periods of daily exercise will produce training effects in some poorly conditioned people, 20 to 30 minutes of exercise per session is more optimal (yet still practical in terms of time), if the intensity is at 70% HR max. With high-intensity training, significant improvements will occur with 10- to 15-minute exercise periods per workout.

How long before improvements are noted? This, of course, depends on the specific systems affected. It is likely that adaptations in cardiovascular fitness and aerobic capacity occur rapidly, and significant improvements are often noted within 1 or 2 weeks.[11,22] Figure 20-6 shows absolute and percentage improvements in max $\dot{V}O_2$ for subjects who trained 6 days a week for 10 weeks. Training consisted of 30 minutes of bicycling 3 days a week combined with running for up to 40 minutes on alternate days. As illustrated, there was continuous week-by-week improvement in aerobic capacity. This suggests that for relatively sedentary people, training improvements occur rapidly and continue in a relatively steady fashion. Of course, these adaptive responses eventually begin to level off as the person approaches his or her "genetically determined" maximum. The exact duration until this leveling-off occurs is unknown, especially for individuals undergoing high-intensity training. It no doubt varies depending on the particular physiologic and metabolic systems affected.

Training Frequency

Is it better to work out 2 days or 5 days a week if the duration and intensity of each training session are the same? Unfortunately, a precise answer is unavailable. Although some investigators report that training frequency is an important factor in causing cardiovascular improvements,[16,43] others maintain that this factor is considerably less important than either the intensity or duration of exercise.[9,40,47] Several studies using interval training showed that 2 days-per-week training resulted in changes in max $\dot{V}O_2$ similar to those observed with 5-days-per week training.[13,14] In other studies where total work was held constant,[21,49] there were no differences in max $\dot{V}O_2$ improvements when training was 2 versus 4, or 3 versus 5 days a week.

It seems that an extra investment of time may not be that profitable in terms of producing changes in physiologic function. On the other hand, if exercise is used as a means for weight control, strong consideration should be given to exercising 5 or 6 days a week, because this frequency of exercise represents a considerable caloric expenditure when compared with training only 2 days a week. To bring about weight loss through exercise, it is recommended that each exercise session last at least 20 to 30 minutes and be of sufficient intensity to expend about 300 kcal. Training fewer than 2 days a week does not produce adequate changes in either anaerobic or aerobic capacity or body composition.[1]

Typical training programs are conducted 3 days a week with a rest day spaced between two workout days. A meaningful question, however, is whether training could occur on con-

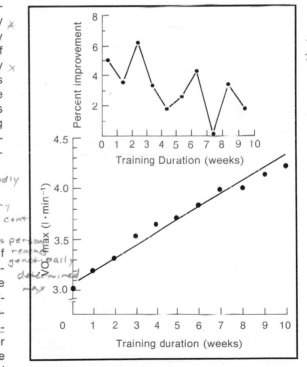

FIG. 20-6. *Improvements in $\dot{V}O_2$ max over 8 weeks of high-intensity endurance training. The upper graph shows the week-by-week percent improvement. (From Hixson, R.C. et al.: Linear increases in aerobic power induced by a program of endurance exercise. J. Appl. Physiol., 42:373, 1977.)*

secutive days and still produce equally effective results? In an experiment concerned with this exact question, improvements in max $\dot{V}O_2$ were nearly *identical* regardless of the sequence of the 3-day-a-week training schedule.[35] This result suggests that perhaps the stimulus for aerobic training is closely tied to the *intensity* and *total work accomplished* and *not to the sequence of training.*

Exercise Mode

If intensity, duration, and frequency are held constant, training improvements will be similar, regardless of training mode—as long as the exercise involves large muscle groups activated in a rhythmic, aerobic nature. Bicycling, walking, running, swimming, and rope skipping are all excellent exercises to stress the aerobic systems.[43,54] Of course, based on the specificity concept, the magnitude of training changes may vary considerably depending on the *mode of testing.* Individuals trained on a bicycle show greater improvements when tested on the bicycle than on the treadmill.[39,53] Likewise, those trained by running show the greatest improvements when measured with an exercise involving the leg muscles rather than muscles of the upper body.[33]

METHODS OF TRAINING

Each year improvements in performance are noted in almost all athletic activities. These advances are generally attributed to increased opportunities for participation, so that those individuals with "natural endowment" are more likely to be exposed to particular sports. Also contributing to superior performances are improved nutrition and health care, better athletic equipment, and a more systematic and scientific approach to athletic training and conditioning. In the following sections, general guidelines for both anaerobic and aerobic training are presented with particular emphasis on three general training classifications: (1) *interval training*, (2) *continuous training*, and (3) *fartlek training*.

Anaerobic Training

We showed in Figure 20-1 that the capacity to perform and persist in all-out exercise for brief periods of time up to 60 seconds is largely dependent on ATP generated by the immediate and short-term anaerobic energy systems.

THE PHOSPHATE POOL. Sports such as football, weightlifting, and various other brief sprint activities rely almost exclusively on energy derived from the muscle's phosphate pool. Developing the capacity of the ATP-CP energy system to the fullest is of paramount importance.

The phosphate pool can be overloaded by engaging specific muscles in repeated *maximum* bursts of effort for 5 to 10 seconds. Because the high-energy phosphates supply energy for intense, intermittent exercise, only small amounts of lactic acid are produced and recovery is rapid. Thus, a subsequent exercise bout can begin after a 30- to 60-second rest period. This use of brief all-out work periods interspersed with recovery represents a specific application of *interval training* especially useful for anaerobic training.

In training to enhance the ATP-CP energy capacity of specific muscles, the activities selected must engage the muscles at the appropriate speed of movement for which the athlete desires improved anaerobic power. Not only does this enhance the anaerobic metabolic capacity of the specific trained muscle fibers, but it also facilitates the recruitment of the appropriate motor units used in the actual movement.

LACTIC ACID. As the duration of all-out effort extends beyond 10 seconds, dependence on anaerobic energy from the phosphates decreases while the quantity of anaerobic energy generated in glycolysis increases. To improve capability for anaerobic energy release via the short-term lactic acid energy system, the physiologic conditioning program must overload this aspect of energy metabolism.

Heavy anaerobic training is psychologically taxing and requires considerable motivation. Repeat bouts of up to 1 minute of maximum running, swimming, or cycling, stopped about 30 seconds before subjective feelings of exhaustion, cause lactic acid to increase to near maximum levels. Each exercise bout should be repeated after 3 to 5 minutes of recovery. Several repeats cause a "lactate stacking" that results in higher levels of lactic acid than just one bout of all-out effort to the point of voluntary exhaustion.[20] Of course, it is critical to use the specific muscle groups that require this enhanced anaerobic capacity. A backstroke swimmer should train by swimming backstroke, a cyclist must bicycle, and the basketball, hockey, or soccer player should rapidly perform various movements and direction changes similar to those required by the demands of the sport.

When exercise involves a significant anaerobic component, the time necessary for recovery can be considerable. For this reason, anaerobic power training should occur at the end of the conditioning session. Otherwise, fatigue would carry over and perhaps hinder the efficiency of subsequent aerobic training.

Aerobic Training

Figure 20-7 indicates the two important factors in formulating an aerobic training program. For one thing, the training must be geared to provide a sufficient cardiovascular overload to stimulate increases in stroke volume and cardiac output. This central overload should be accomplished with the appropriate muscle groups so as to concurrently enhance the local circulation and "metabolic machinery" within the specific muscles. This essentially embodies the specificity principle as applied to aerobic training. Simply stated, runners should run, cyclists should bicycle, and swimmers should swim.

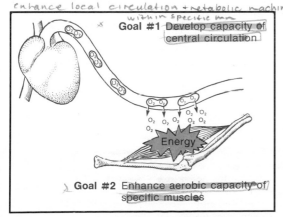

Goal #1 Develop capacity of central circulation

Energy

Goal #2 Enhance aerobic capacity of specific muscles

FIG. 20-7. *The two major goals of aerobic conditioning. (From Nutrition, Weight Control, and Exercise by Frank I. Katch and William D. McArdle. Copyright © 1977 by Houghton Mifflin Company. Reprinted by permission of the publisher.)*

Brief bouts of repeated exercise (interval training) as well as continuous, long-duration work (continuous training) enhance aerobic capacity, provided the exercise is sufficiently intense to overload the aerobic systems. Interval training, continuous training, and fartlek training are three common methods to improve aerobic fitness.

INTERVAL TRAINING. Many elite athletes attribute their success to interval training.[15] With the correct spacing of exercise and rest periods, a tremendous amount of work can be accomplished that would not normally be completed in a workout in which the exercise was performed continuously. Repeated exercise bouts (with rest periods or *relief intervals*) can vary from a few seconds to several minutes or more depending on the desired outcome. The interval training prescription can be modified in terms of intensity and duration of the exercise interval, the length and type of relief interval, the number of work intervals (repetitions), and the number of repetition blocks or sets per workout. Adjustment of any or all of these can easily be made to meet the specific requirements for different performances. This offers flexible options for developing the anaerobic and aerobic energy transfer systems. A longer work interval engages the aerobic systems, whereas shorter exercise intervals place greater overload on the anaerobic energy systems.

One value of interval training is that it permits high-intensity, intermittent exercise for a relatively long period. For example, few people can maintain a "4-minute mile" pace for longer than a minute, let alone complete a mile within 4 minutes. However, if running intervals were limited to only 15 seconds followed by 30 seconds of recovery, it would not be exceedingly difficult to maintain these exercise–rest intervals and complete the mile in 4 minutes of actual running! Although this does not suggest a world-class performance, the point is that a significant quantity of normally exhausting work can be achieved with the proper spacing of rest and work intervals.

In the example of a continuous run at a 4-minute mile pace, a major portion of energy would be supplied through anaerobic glycolysis. Within a minute or two, lactic acid levels would rise precipitously and the runner would become exhausted. With interval training, repeated work bouts of about 15 seconds would permit a severe load to be imposed on the aerobic energy system of specific muscles without an appreciable buildup of lactic acid. Fatigue incurred during the work interval would be minor and recovery could take place quickly. The work interval could then begin after only a brief rest period, and a high level of aerobic metabolism would be sustained (see "Intermittent Exercise," Chap. 7).

A practical system for determining interval training work rates is presented in Table 20-6.

1. *Exercise interval*: Generally 1.5 to 5.0 seconds are added to the exerciser's "best time" for training distances between 55 and 220 yards for running and 15 to 55 yards for swimming.[15,54] If a person can run 60 yards from a running start in 8 seconds, the training time for each repeat would therefore be 8 + 1.5 or 9.5 seconds. For interval training distances of 110 and 220 yards, 3 and 5 seconds are added, respectively, to the best running times. This particular application of interval training is suited for anaerobic power training, especially the immediate energy system.

For training distances of 440 yards running or 110 yards swimming, the work rate is determined by *subtracting* 1 to 4 seconds from the best 440-yard part of a mile run or 110-yard part of a 440-yard swim. If a person runs a 7-minute mile averaging 105 seconds per 440 yards, the interval time for each 440-yard repeat would be between 104 seconds (105 − 1) and 101 seconds (105 − 4). For training intervals beyond 440 yards, 3 to 4 seconds are added for each 440-yard portion of the interval distance. In running an interval of 880 yards, the 7-minute miler would thus run each interval at about 216 seconds [(105 + 3) × (2) = 216].

2. *Relief interval*: The relief interval can be either passive (rest-relief) or active (work-relief). The recommended duration of relief is usually expressed as a ratio of work duration to recovery duration. The ratio of 1 to 3 is generally recommended for training the immediate energy systems. Thus, for a sprinter who runs 10-second intervals, the relief interval is usually about 30 seconds. For training the short-term glycolytic energy system, the relief interval is twice as long as the work interval or a ratio of 1 to 2. These specific ratios of work-to-relief for anaerobic training supposedly ensure sufficient restoration of the phosphagen pools or lactic acid removal so that the next work bout can proceed without undue fatigue.

For training the long-term aerobic energy system, the work–recovery interval ratio is usually 1 to 1 or 1 to 1.5. During a 60- to 90-second exercise interval, for example, oxygen consumption does not have enough time to meet the energy requirements of the exercise. The recommended recovery interval enables the succeeding exercise interval to begin before recovery is complete. This ensures that the cir-

TABLE 20-6. *Guidelines for determining interval-training work rate for running and swimming different distances*[a]

INTERVAL TRAINING DISTANCES (YARDS)		WORK RATE FOR EACH EXERCISE INTERVAL OR REPEAT
Run	Swim	
55	15	1.5 seconds *slower* than best
110	25	3 times from running
220	55	5 (or swimming) start for each distance
440	110	1 to 4 seconds *faster* than the averge 440-yard run or 110-yard swim times recorded during a mile run or 440-yard swim
660–1320	165–320	3 to 4 seconds *slower* than the average 440-yard run or 100-yard swim times recorded during a mile run or 440-yard swim

[a] From Fox, E.L., and Mathers, D.K.: Interval Training. Philadelphia, W.B. Saunders Co., 1974.

culatory and aerobic metabolic stress will reach near peak levels even though the exercise intervals are relatively short. With longer periods of intermittent exercise there is sufficient time for metabolic and circulatory adjustments; thus, the duration of the rest interval is not as crucial.

CONTINUOUS TRAINING. Continuous training involves steady-paced exercise performed at either moderate or high intensity for a sustained duration. The exact pace can vary, but it must be of sufficient threshold intensity to ensure physiologic adaptation. The method to establish this threshold so that the person might exercise in the "training-sensitive zone" was outlined previously (see page 275). Continuous training is popular among joggers and other fitness enthusiasts as well as competitive endurance athletes. It is not uncommon for distance runners to run between 100 and 150 miles each week. In one report,[7] a man training for the 52.5 mile "ultramarathon" ran twice a day, 20 miles each morning and 13 miles each evening, interspersed with an occasional 30- to 60-mile nonstop run at a 7- to 8-minute per mile pace. With this schedule, he ran more than 800 miles each month and totaled 9,600 miles per year! The precise effects and benefits of such considerable training are unknown.

By its nature, continuous exercise training is submaximum and, therefore, can be engaged in for considerable time in relative comfort. Because of the potential hazards of high-intensity interval training for coronary-prone individuals (as well as an almost total dedication required by such strenuous exercise), continuous training is particularly suitable for those just beginning an exercise program. When applied in athletic training, continuous training is really "over-distance" training, with most athletes covering between two to five times the actual distance of their racing event. It is believed that over-distance training produces the largest aerobic adaptations. Overload is generally accomplished by increasing exercise duration, although the work rate increases progressively as training improvements are achieved.

One of the advantages of continuous training is that it permits training at nearly the same intensity as actual competition. Because the recruitment of appropriate motor units is dependent on work rate, continuous training may be best suited for the endurance athlete. This is in contrast to interval training, which may place a disproportionate stress on the fast-twitch mus-

cle fibers; these are *not* the fibers predominantly recruited in endurance competition!

FARTLEK TRAINING. Fartlek is a Swedish word meaning "speed play." This training method is a relatively "unscientific" adaptation of interval training that is well suited for exercising out-of-doors over natural terrain. With this system, alternate running is done at both fast and slow speeds.

In contrast to the precise exercise prescription in interval training, fartlek training does not require systematic manipulation of the work and relief bouts. Instead, the performer determines the training scheme based on "how it feels" at the time. If done properly, this system will develop one or all of the energy systems. An added advantage is the flexibility it affords in determining the extent of training. Although lacking the systematic and quantified base of interval and continuous training, fartlek training is ideally suited for general conditioning or off-season training and for maintaining a certain "freedom" and variety in workouts.

At present, there is insufficient evidence for the superiority of any specific training method for improving aerobic capacity. *Each* training procedure results in success; they probably can be used interchangeably and certainly should be used to modify training and achieve a more pleasing psychologic set.

INITIATING A TRAINING PROGRAM

Although few studies have compared the "trainability" of men and women, it appears that the amount of improvement in aerobic capacity with training is similar for both sexes.[4,12] In addition, other observations show little difference in training response between older and younger, middle-aged groups (49 to 65 years).[42]

Aims and Objectives

The most important aspect in formulating a training program is to identify specific aims and achievement objectives. This is equally important for both the Olympic decathlon hopeful and the person simply wishing to "get-in-shape." Whether the goal is a 4-minute mile, a sub-3-hour marathon, or a nonstop jog or run for 20 minutes, motivation, willingness, and dedication during training are enhanced if individuals know their performance goals and the specific directions to meet their training objectives.

Specific goals are usually expressed in performance terms, such as being able to complete a marathon. It is also possible to state goals in physiologic terms, for example, achieving a certain increase in max $\dot{V}O_2$ or a decrease in heart rate on a step test.

Assessment of Individual Status

Measuring initial status prior to a conditioning program depends on available facilities and technical expertise, as well as the exerciser's training goals. For competitive athletes, a complete assessment is provided with the help of films, coaches' expert opinion, and field and laboratory tests.[49] For others, adequate fitness assessment may consist of simple tests easily administered at home.[48] Regardless of the method or extent of assessment, we believe it is prudent for previously sedentary individuals to have medical clearance for exercise. For some over the age of 35, this may involve a supervised exercise stress test (Chap. 29, Page 435). As a minimum for adults considering an exercise program, we advise a physical examination that includes assessment of the cardiovascular system, blood pressure and blood chemistry, muscles, and joints. The assessment of fitness status involves four major areas: (1) muscular strength, (2) joint flexibility, (3) body composition (percent fat, lean body weight, and desirable body weight), and (4) cardiovascular–respiratory functional capacity.

The Program

Training should begin at a relatively moderate intensity and gradually lead up to the target level. *The quickest way to extinguish enthusiasm for exercise is to prescribe too much too soon!* Several minutes of mild calisthenics or jogging in place generally provide a sufficient warm-up so that the heart and circulation are not suddenly taxed.[3a] A 5-minute "cool-down" consisting of exercise of gradually lessening intensity is generally advocated before exercise is stopped. This makes sense because it re-duces the chances of abrupt physiologic alterations, especially those involving cardiovascular dynamics, which are more likely with the sudden cessation of strenuous exercise.

Provision should be made for progressive improvements, adequate use of facilities, variety, some competition, and periodic evaluation. It is desirable to sketch out the whole program at the beginning, with full realization that changes and modifications will be necessary to meet individual needs and rates of change. With a well-planned yet flexible program, both the exercise specialist and participant will know exactly what to expect and in what fitness areas to concentrate. This does not mean the program must be complex or excessively time-consuming. In fact, in one school district, simply adding between 5 and 14 minutes of jogging to the daily physical education program significantly improved the students' running endurance by 18% at the end of the semester.[6]

Leadership

We maintain that individuals trained in the science of exercise are most qualified to establish, lead, and direct individual and community fitness and training programs. Although it is often argued that practical experience is the best teacher, it is our belief that knowing the *why* of training and exercise is fundamental. It is no longer sufficient to have been a "letter winner" or former athlete to qualify for a job in the "fitness marketplace." Programs of certification as exercise leaders and program directors, laboratory stress-test coordinators or exercise technicians, athletic trainers, physical educators, and coaches are being established. Such certification programs demand knowing both the hows and the whys of exercise and training.

SUMMARY

1. It is possible to classify activities in terms of their predominant activation of a specific system of energy transfer. An effective training program is one that allocates a proportionate time commitment to training the specific energy system(s) involved in the activity.

2. Proper physical conditioning is based on sound principles that produce optimum improvements. Of crucial importance are *the overload principle, the specificity of exercise*

principle, the individual difference principle, and *the reversibility principle.*

3. Exercise training brings about specific metabolic and physiologic adaptations that involve subtle cellular as well as gross physiologic changes. Anaerobic training increases resting levels of anaerobic substrates and key glycolytic enzymes. This is usually accompanied by concomitant increases in all-out exercise performance. Aerobic training changes include increases in mitochondrial size and number as well as the activity of aerobic enzymes, increased myoglobin, and enhanced oxidation of fat and carbohydrate. These adaptations are geared to a greater aerobic production of ATP.

4. Aerobic training brings about both functional and dimensional changes in the cardiovascular system. These include decreases in resting and submaximal exercise heart rate, enhanced stroke volume and cardiac output, and an expanded a-$\bar{v}$ O_2 difference.

5. The major factors affecting training are initial fitness level, frequency of training, exercise intensity, duration of exercise, and type (mode) of training.

6. Training intensity can be applied either on an absolute basis in terms of exercise load, or relative to an individual's physiologic response. It is practical and effective to set exercise intensity to a percent of a person's maxi-

mum heart rate response. Training levels corresponding to 70% to 90% of maximum heart rate are most desirable for inducing aerobic fitness changes.

7. Training duration and intensity are intimately related. Nevertheless, 20 to 30 minutes per session seems to be optimum in terms of exercise duration.

8. Frequency for optimum aerobic training appears to be a minimum of 3 days per week. Maximum frequency levels have not been established.

9. If intensity, duration, and frequency are held constant, training improvements are similar regardless of training mode, as long as large muscle groups are exercised.

10. Methods of training differ markedly. Interval, continuous, and fartlek training can be used effectively for conditioning the different energy systems. The merits of interval training for both anaerobic and aerobic system changes have recently been stressed.

11. Aerobic training must be geared to enhance *both* circulatory function and the metabolic capacity of the specific muscles.

12. When initiating a training program, care must be given to establishment of individual aims and objectives, assessment of performance and physiologic status, design of the program, and appropriate leadership.

References

1. American College of Sports Medicine. Position Statement on "The Recommended Quantity and Quality of Exercise for Developing and Maintaining Fitness in Healthy Adults." Sports Med. Bull., *13:*1, 1978.
2. Åstrand, P.O., and Rodahl, K.: Textbook of Work Physiology. New York, McGraw-Hill Co., 1977.
3. Barnard, R.J. et al.: Effects of exercise on skeletal muscle: I. Biochemical and histochemical properties. J. Appl. Physiol., *28:*762, 1970.
3a. Barnard, R.J. et al.: Ischemic response to sudden strenuous exercise in healthy men. Circulation, *48:*936, 1973.
4. Burke, E. J.: Physiological effects of similar training programs in males and females. Res. Quart., *48:*510, 1977.
5. Burke, E. J., and Franks, B. D.: Changes in $\dot{V}O_2$ max resulting from bicycle training at different intensities holding total mechanical work constant. Res. Quart., *46:*31, 1975.
6. Cooper, K. H. et al.: An aerobics conditioning program for Fort Worth, Texas school district. Res. Quart., *46:*345, 1975.

7. Costill, D., and Fox, E.: The ultra-marathoner. Distance Running News, *3:* 4, 1968.
8. Cunningham, D. A., and Faulkner, J. A.: The effect of training on aerobic and anaerobic metabolism during a short exhaustive run. Med. Sci. Sports, *1:* 65, 1969.
9. Davies, C.T.M., and Knibbs, A.V.: The training stimulus: The effects of intensity, duration and frequency of effort on maximum aerobic power output. Int. Z. Angew. Physiol., *29:* 299, 1971.
10. Drinkwater, B., and Horvath, S.: Detraining effects on young women. Med. Sci. Sports, *4:* 91, 1972.
11. Durnin, J.V.G.A. et al.: Effects of a short period of training of varying severity on some measurement of physical fitness. J. Appl. Physiol., *15:* 161, 1960.
12. Eddy, D. O. et al.: The effects of continuous and interval training in women and men. Eur. J. Appl. Physiol., *37:* 83, 1977.
13. Fox, E.L., and Mathews, D. K.: *Interval Training: Conditioning for Sports and General Fitness.* Philadelphia, W. B. Saunders Co., 1974.
14. Fox, E. et al.: Intensity and distance of interval training programs and changes in aerobic power. Med. Sci. Sports, *5:* 18, 1973.
15. Fox, E. et al.: Frequency and duration of interval training programs and changes in aerobic power. J. Appl. Physiol., *38:* 481, 1975.
16. Gettman, L. R. et al.: Physiological responses of men to 1, 3, and 5 day per week programs. Res. Quart., *47:* 638, 1976.
17. Gollnick, P., and Hermansen, L.: Biochemical adaptation to exercise: Anaerobic metabolism. *In* Exercise and Sport Sciences Reviews, Vol. 1, Edited by J. Wilmore. New York, Academic Press, 1973.
18. Gollnick, P. et al.: Enzyme activity and fiber composition in skeletal muscle of untrained men. J. Appl. Physiol., *33:* 312, 1972.
19. Gollnick, P. et al.: Effects of training on enzyme activity and fiber composition of human skeletal muscle. J. Appl. Physiol., *34:* 107, 1973.
20. Hermansen, L.: Lactate production during exercise. *In* Muscle Metabolism During Exercise. Edited by B. Pernow and B. Saltin. New York, Plenum Press, 1971.
21. Hill, J. S.: The effects of frequency of exercise of cardiorespiratory fitness of adult men. Unpublished M.S. Thesis, University of Western Ontario, London, Ontario, 1969.
22. Hixson, R.C. et al.: Linear increases in aerobic power induced by a strenuous program of endurance exercise. J. Appl. Physiol., *42:* 373, 1977.
23. Holloszy, J. O.: Effects of exercise on mitochondrial oxygen uptake and respiratory enzyme activity in skeletal muscle. J. Biol. Chem., *242:* 2278, 1967.
24. Holloszy, J. O.: Adaptation of skeletal muscle to endurance exercise. Med. Sci. Sports, *7:* 155, 1975.
25. Houston, M.E., and Thomson, J. A.: The response of endurance adapted adults to intense anaerobic training. Eur. J. Appl. Physiol., *36:* 207–213, 1977.
26. Karvonen, M. J. et al.: The effects of training on heart rate. A longitudinal study. Ann. Med. Exp. Biol. Fenn., *35:* 305, 1957.
27. Karlsson, J. et al.: Muscle lactate, ATP, and CP levels during exercise after physical training in man. J. Appl. Physiol., *33:* 199, 1972.
27a. Kavanagh, T. et al.: Characteristics of postcoronary marathon runners. Ann. N.Y. Acad. Sci., *301:*455, 1977.
28. Kiessling, K.: Effects of physical training on ultrastructural features in human skeletal muscle. *In* Muscle Metabolism During Exercise. Edited by B. Pernow, and B. Saltin. New York, Plenum Press, 1971.
29. Kjellberg, S. et al.: Increase of the amount of hemoglobin and blood volume in connection with physical training. Acta Physiol. Scand., *19:* 146, 1949.
30. MacDougall, J. D. et al.: Biochemical adaptation of human skeletal muscle to heavy resistance training and immobilization. J. Appl. Physiol., *43:* 700, 1977.
31. Magel, J. R. et al.: Specificity of swim training on maximum oxygen uptake. J. Appl. Physiol., *38:* 151, 1975.

32. Magel, J. R. et al.: Metabolic and cardiovascular adjustment to arm training. J. Appl. Physiol.: Respiration., Environmental and Exercise Physiology, *45:* 75, 1978.
33. McArdle, W. D. et al.: Specificity of run training on $\dot{V}O_2$ max and heart rate changes during running and swimming. Med. Sci. Sports, *10:* 16, 1978.
34. Michael, E. et al.: Physiological changes of teenage girls during five months of detraining. Med. Sci. Sports, *4:* 214, 1972.
35. Moffatt, R.: Placement of tri-weekly training sessions: Importance regarding enhancement of aerobic capacity. Res. Quart., *48:* 583, 1977.
36. Molé, P. et al.: Adaptation of muscle to exercise. Increase in levels of palmityl Co A synthetase, carnitine palmityltransferase, and palmityl Co A dehydrogenase, and in the capacity to oxidize fatty acids. J. Clin. Invest., *50:* 2, 323, 1971.
37. Morganroth, J. et al.: Comparative left ventricular dimensions in trained athletes. Ann. Intern. Med., *82:* 521, 1975.
38. Pattengale, P. K., and Holloszy, J. O.: Augmentation of skeletal muscle myoglobin by programs of treadmill running. Am. J. Physiol., *213:* 783, 1967.
39. Pechar, G. S. et al.: Specificity of cardiorespiratory adaptation to bicycle and treadmill training. J. Appl. Physiol., *36:* 753, 1974.
40. Pollock, M.: The quantification of endurance training programs. *In* Exercise and Sport Sciences Reviews, Vol. 1. Edited by J. Wilmore. New York, Academic Press, 1973.
41. Pollock, M. et al.: Effects of mode of training on cardiovascular function and body composition of adult men. Med. Sci. Sports, *7:*139, 1975.
42. Pollock, M.L. et al.: Physiologic response of men 49 to 65 years of age to endurance training. J. Am. Geriatr. Soc., *XXIV:*97, 1976.
43. Pollock, M.L. et al.: Effects of frequency and duration of training on attrition and incidence of injury. Med. Sci. Sports, *9:*31, 1977.
44. Rowell, L.: Human cardiovascular adjustments to exercise and thermal stress. Physiol. Rev., *54:*75, 1974.
45. Saltin, B. et al.: Response to exercise after bed rest and after training. Circulation, *38:* Suppl. 7, 1968.
46. Sharkey, B. J.: Intensity and duration of training and the development of cardiorespiratory endurance. Med. Sci. Sports, *2:* 197, 1970.
47. Shephard, R. J.: Intensity, duration, and frequency of exercise as determinants of the response to a training regime. Int. Z. Angew. Physiol., *26:* 272, 1968.
48. Shephard, R. J. et al.: Development of the Canadian home fitness test. Can. Med. Assoc., *114:* 675, 1976.
49. Sidney, K. H. et al.: *In* Training: Scientific Basis and Application Edited by, A. W. Taylor. Springfield, Ill.: Charles C Thomas, 1972.
50. Taylor, H. L. et al.: Exercise Tests: A summary of procedures and concepts of stress testing for cardiovascular diagnosis and function evaluation. *In* Measurement in Exercise Electrocardiography, Edited by H. Blackburn. Springfield, Ill.: Charles C Thomas, 1969.
51. Thorstensson, A. et al.: Enzyme activities and muscle strength after sprint training in man. Acta Physiol. Scand., *94:* 313, 1975.
52. Thorstensson A. et al.: Effect of strength training on enzyme activities and fiber characteristics in human skeletal muscle. Acta Physiol. Scand., *96:* 392, 1976.
53. Wilmore, J. et al.: Physiological alterations consequent to 20-week conditioning programs of bicycling, tennis, and jogging. Med. Sci. Sports., *12:*1, 1980.
54. Wilt, F.: Training for competitive running. *In* Exercise Physiology. Edited by H. Falls. New York, Academic Press, 1968.
55. Zuti, W.B., and Golding, L.A.: Comparing diet and exercise as weight reduction tools. Physician Sportsmed., *4:*49, 1976.

Muscular Strength: Training Muscles to Become Stronger

21

PART 1
Measuring and Improving Muscular Strength

Years ago, specific strength or "weight lifting" exercises were used predominantly by body builders, competitive weight lifters, and some wrestlers. Most other athletes refrained from weight lifting for fear that such exercises would slow them down and increase muscle size to the point where they would lose joint flexibility. In other words, they would become *muscle-bound!* This myth was essentially dispelled by subsequent research in the 1950s and 1960s that showed that exercises that strengthen muscles do not reduce movement speed or flexibility. In fact, the opposite was usually the case because elite weight lifters and body builders demonstrated exceptional joint flexibility and were certainly not limited in general movement speed. In longitudinal experiments with untrained healthy subjects, heavy-resistance exercises have increased both speed and power of muscular effort. Certainly, these effects would not be detrimental to sports performance.

In the sections that follow, we explore the underlying rationale, the process, and the physiologic adjustments that occur as muscles are trained to become stronger. Discussion centers on the various ways muscular strength is measured, strength differences between men and women, and the various training programs designed to increase muscular strength.

MEASUREMENT OF MUSCULAR STRENGTH

Muscular strength, or more precisely, *the maximum force or tension generated by a muscle* (or muscle groups), is generally measured by one of four methods: (1) tensiometry, (2) dynamometry, (3) one-repetition maximum or 1-RM, and the newest approach, (4) computer-assisted force and work output determinations.

Cable Tensiometry

Figure 21-1 shows a cable tensiometer and its use for measuring muscular force during knee extension. As the force on the cable increases, the riser over which the cable passes is depressed. This deflects the pointer and indicates the subject's strength score. This instrument measures the pulling force of a muscle during a static or isometric contraction where there is

286

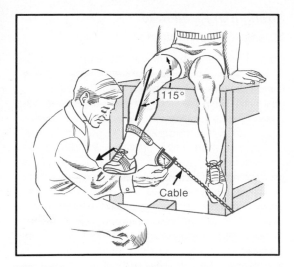

FIG. 21-1. *Measurement of knee extension static force using the cable tensiometer.*

essentially no change in the muscle's external length. This application of the tensiometer is considerably different from its original use for measuring the tension of the steel cables linking various parts of an airplane.

The tensiometer is lightweight, portable, durable, easy to use, and has the advantage of versatility for recording force measurements at virtually all angles in the range of motion of a specific joint. Cable tension strength-test batteries have been developed to measure the static force of muscles activating the fingers, thumb, wrist, forearm, elbow, shoulder, trunk, neck, hip, knee, and ankle.[3,4,6,8] These tests are excellent for isolating and evaluating stength impairment in specific muscles weakened as a result of disease or injury. The muscle can be isolated and evaluated at a specific joint angle. This can then be objectively reproduced on repeated measurement to determine the status of specific muscle groups at the beginning of a therapeutic exercise program and during rehabilitation. In addition, since more than one muscle group is usually activated in a particular movement, the tensiometer can be applied in many phases of the movement. This may give a clearer picture of "strength" (or weakness) than standard weight-lifting tests do.

Dynamometry

Hand-grip and back-lift dynamometers used for strength measurement are shown in Figure

21-2. Both devices operate on the principle of compression. When an external force is applied to the dynamometer, a steel spring is compressed and moves a pointer. By knowing how much force is required to move the pointer a particular distance, it is then a simple matter to determine exactly how much external "static" force has been applied to the dynamometer.

One-Repetition Maximum (1-RM)

A dynamic method of measuring muscular strength makes use of the one-repetition maximum or 1-RM method. This refers to the maximum amount of weight lifted *one time* during the performance of a standard weight-lifting exercise. To test 1-RM for any particular muscle group or groups such as forearm flexors, leg extensors, or shoulders, a suitable starting weight is selected close to but below the subject's maximum lifting capacity. If one repetition is completed, weight is added to the exercise device until maximum lift capacity is achieved. The weight increments are usually 5, 2 and 1 kg during the period of measurement. The 1-RM

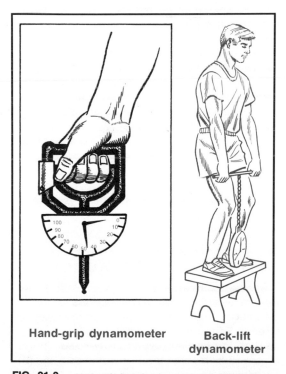

Hand-grip dynamometer   **Back-lift dynamometer**

FIG. 21-2. *Use of hand-grip and back-lift dynamometers.*

technique is usually used with barbells and dumbells but can also be applied with most commercial exercise machines.

Computer-Assisted, Electromechanical, and Isokinetic Methods

The emergence of microprocessor technology has made possible a rapid way to quantify accurately muscular forces generated during a variety of movements. Sensitive instruments are currently available to measure force, acceleration, and velocity of body segments in various movement patterns.

Force platforms can be used to measure the external application of muscular force by a limb such as in jumping. Other electromechanical devices measure the force generated during all phases of an exercise movement such as cycling or during a supine bench press or leg press.

An *isokinetic dynamometer* is an electromechanical instrument containing a speed-controlling mechanism that accelerates to a preset speed when any force is applied. Once this constant speed is attained, the isokinetic loading mechanism accommodates automatically to provide a counterforce equal to the force generated by the muscle. *Thus, maximum force (or any percentage of maximum effort) can be applied during all phases of the movement at a constant velocity.* A load cell inside the dynamometer continuously monitors the immediate level of applied force (and matching resistance) and feeds this information into an appropriate recorder. An electronic integrator placed in series with the recorder provides a readout of the average force generated for a given time. The voltage output from the integrator can be interfaced directly with a computer to provide almost instantaneous readouts of average force and total work.[26]

STRENGTH DIFFERENCES BETWEEN MEN AND WOMEN

Three basic approaches have been used to determine whether true "sex differences" exist between men and women in terms of muscular strength. Strength has been evaluated (1) in relation to muscle cross-sectional area, (2) on an *absolute* basis as total force exerted, and (3) as *relative* strength, that is, strength in relation to body weight or lean body weight.

Strength in Relation to Muscle Cross Section

Human skeletal muscle can generate approximately 3 to 4 kg of force per cm^2 of muscle cross section regardless of sex. In the body, however, this force-output capacity varies depending on the arrangement of the bony levers. Figure 21-3 is a comparison of the arm flexor strength of men and women in relation to the cross-sectional area of muscle. Clearly, the greatest force is exerted by individuals with the largest muscle cross section. However, the linear relationship between strength and muscle size indicates little difference in arm flexor strength for the same size muscle in men and women. This is further demonstrated in the insert graph when the strength of males and females is expressed per unit area of muscle cross section.[24]

Absolute Muscular Strength

When strength is compared on an *absolute* score basis (that is, *total* force in pounds or kilograms), men are usually stronger than women for all muscle groups tested. This is true regardless of the device used to measure strength. The exceptions occur for strength-trained female track and field athletes who significantly increase the strength of specific muscle groups by resistance exercises designed to enhance the muscle's force-generating capacity.

ISOMETRIC MEASUREMENTS. In a review of seven studies comparing the isometric strengths of men and women,[27] the *absolute* strength of the upper extremities measured in 11 different positions in women was about 56% less than that of their male counterparts; for five other tests of leg strength, the women's strength scores averaged about 72% of the maximum values recorded by men.

DYNAMIC MEASUREMENTS. The tallest portion of the vertical bars in Figure 21-4 compare the *absolute* weight-lifting and dynamometric strength of men and women. Strength differences are expressed as the ratio of the absolute strength of men divided by the absolute strength of women. Grip and leg static strengths were measured with dynamometers: two-arm curl and bench-press dynamic strengths were assessed by the 1-RM method. The results were clear—the absolute strength for the men was about one-third greater than that for women for each measurement. Similar findings have been reported by others[33,34] and indicate that the dynamic strength of women averaged about 70% that of men, with a range of 59% to 84% depending on the muscle groups tested.

Strength in Relation to Body Weight and Lean Body Weight

The two smaller portions of the vertical bars in Figure 21-4 illustrate the differences between men and women when strength is expressed in relation to body weight and lean body weight, that is, body weight minus body fat. When body size and composition are considered, the large strength differences between men and women are reduced considerably. In fact, leg-press strength per kilogram of lean body weight for females was below 1.0. In this case, the women could be considered "stronger" than the men when their scores are computed in a way that more precisely considers a person's quantity of muscle mass.

These observations provide a strong argument that few sex differences exist in muscle quality, at least as reflected by force output capacity. From a practical standpoint, however, because men generally develop a larger muscle

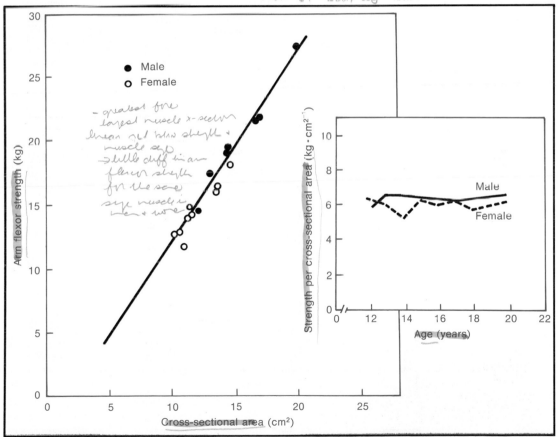

FIG. 21-3. *Arm flexor strength of men and women plotted as a function of muscle cross-sectional area. The insert displays strength per unit cross-sectional area of muscle in males and females 12 to 20 years of age. (From Ikai, M., and Fukunaga, T.: Calculation of muscle strength per unit cross-sectional area of human muscle by means of ultrasonic measurements. Arbeitsphysiologie, 26:26, 1968.)*

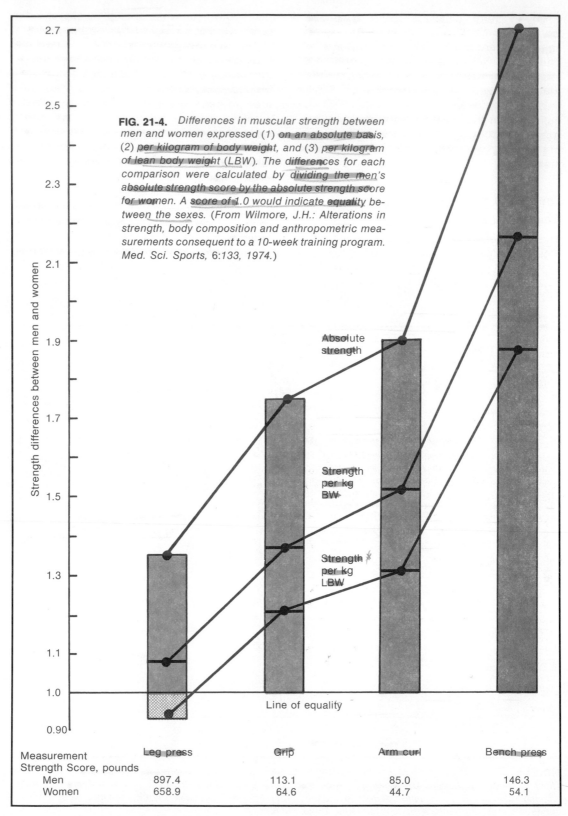

FIG. 21-4. *Differences in muscular strength between men and women expressed (1) on an absolute basis, (2) per kilogram of body weight, and (3) per kilogram of lean body weight (LBW). The differences for each comparison were calculated by dividing the men's absolute strength score by the absolute strength score for women. A score of 1.0 would indicate equality between the sexes. (From Wilmore, J.H.: Alterations in strength, body composition and anthropometric measurements consequent to a 10-week training program. Med. Sci. Sports, 6:133, 1974.)*

Measurement Strength Score, pounds	Leg press	Grip	Arm curl	Bench press
Men	897.4	113.1	85.0	146.3
Women	658.9	64.6	44.7	54.1

mass than women, their absolute strength is
proportionately greater. Also, because women
usually have more body fat than men, they are,
in a sense, loaded down with more "dead
weight" than male counterparts of the same
body weight. Consequently, their strength per
unit of body weight is also usually lower.

TRAINING MUSCLES TO BECOME STRONGER

As a general rule, a muscle worked close to its
force-generating capacity will increase in
strength. The overload can be applied with
standard weight-lifting equipment, pulleys or
springs, immovable bars, or a variety of isokinetic devices. The important point is that
strength improvements are generally governed
by the *intensity of overload* and not by the specific method. It is just that certain methods lend
themselves to a precise and systematic overload application. *Progressive resistance weight
training, isometric training,* and *isokinetic training* are three common exercise systems used
for training muscles to become stronger. These
systems rely, to varying degrees, upon the three
types of muscular contractions illustrated in
Figure 21-5A-C. With a *concentric* muscular
contraction (Fig. 21-5A), the muscle shortens
as it develops tension and overcomes the resistance. This type of contraction is common to
weight lifting as well as to most other sports
activities. When a muscle contracts *eccentrically* (Fig. 21-5B), the external resistance overcomes the active muscle and the muscle
lengthens while developing tension. This usually occurs as a muscle acts to oppose the
force of gravity. In weight lifting, muscles frequently contract eccentrically as the exerciser
slowly returns the weight to the starting position
to begin again the next concentric contraction.
These combinations of concentric and eccentric contractions in weight lifting have frequently, but imprecisely, been termed *isotonic
exercise* (from the Greek *iso,* the same or
equal; *tonos,* tension or strain). Although the
absolute weight lifted in a specific exercise
remains constant, the bony lever system pre-

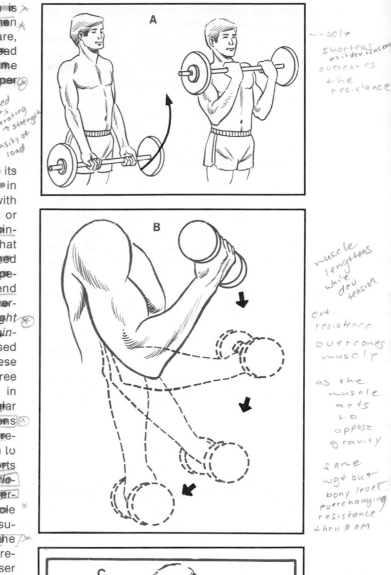

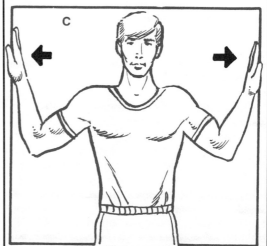

FIG. 21-5. *A, Concentric contraction; B, Eccentric
contraction; C, Isometric contraction. (From Nutrition,
Weight Control, and Exercise by Frank I. Katch and
William D. McArdle. Copyright © 1977 by Houghton
Mifflin Company. Reprinted by permission of the
publisher.)*

sents the muscle with an ever-changing resistance through the full range of motion.

In Figure 21-5C, the object is too heavy to move and the muscle contracts *isometrically*. Considerable force may be generated with no noticeable shortening of the muscle fibers.

Progressive Resistance Weight Training

Probably the most popular form of strength training involves weight lifting. With this method, exercises are designed to strengthen specific muscles by causing them to overcome a fixed resistance, usually in the form of a barbell or dumbbell.

PROGRESSIVE RESISTANCE EXERCISE (PRE). Working in a rehabilitation setting following World War II, researchers devised a method of weight training to improve the strength capacity of previously injured limbs.[10,11] Their method involved three sets of exercises—each set consisting of ten repetitions done consecutively without resting. The first set was done with one-half of the maximum weight that could be lifted 10 times or 1/2 10-RM; the second set was done with 3/4 10-RM, whereas the final 10-RM set was done with maximum weight. As patients trained, the exercised limbs became stronger, and it was necessary to increase periodically the 10-RM resistance so that continued strength improvements would occur. Even when the progression of exercise intensity was reversed so that the 10-RM was performed first, similar improvements were observed.

This technique of *progressive resistance exercise* or *PRE* is a practical application of the overload principle and forms the basis of most weight training programs.

VARIATIONS OF PRE. Variations of PRE for weight training have been studied to determine the optimal number of sets and repetitions, and the frequency and relative intensity of training required to improve muscular strength.[7] The findings can be summarized as follows: (1) Performing an exercise between 3-RM and 9-RM is the most effective number of repetitions for increasing muscular strength. (2) PRE training once weekly with 1-RM for one set increases strength significantly after the first week of training and each week up to at least the sixth week. (3) No particular sequence of PRE training with different percentages of 10-RM is more effective for strength improvement, as long as one set of 10-RM is performed each training session. (4) Performing one set of an exercise is less effective for increasing strength than performing two or three sets, and there is some indication that three sets are more effective than two sets. (5) The optimum number of training days per week with PRE for improving muscular strength is unknown. Significant increases have occurred training 1 day weekly to 5 days per week for beginners. (6) When PRE training uses several different exercises, training 4 or 5 days a week may be less effective for increasing dynamic strength than training 2 or 3 times per week. The more frequent strength training may prevent sufficient recuperation between training sessions. This possibly could retard progress in neuromuscular adaptation and strength development.

PRACTICAL RECOMMENDATIONS FOR INITIATING A WEIGHT TRAINING PROGRAM. In the beginning stages of a program, maximum lifts should be avoided. Excessive weight contributes little to strength development and greatly increases the chances for muscle or joint injury. In fact, a load that is equal to 60% to 80% of a muscle's force-generating capacity is sufficient to increase strength. This generally permits the completion of about ten repetitions of a particular exercise. Using a lighter weight (and thus more repetitions) may be more effective when starting a weight training program. Experience has shown that beginners should initially attempt to complete 12 to 15 repetitions. This will not place an excessive strain on the muscles during the beginning phase of the muscular conditioning program. A heavier weight should be used if the weight selected for the 12 repetitions feels too easy. The weight is too heavy if the exerciser cannot do 12 repetitions. This is a trial-and-error process and may take several exercise sessions before a proper starting weight is selected. After a week or two of training, when the muscles have adapted and the correct movements are learned, the number of repetitions can be reduced to six to eight. Each time this new target number of repetitions is reached, more weight is added. This is progressive resistance training—as the muscles become stronger, the weight is adjusted and a heavier load is attempted.

THE LOWER BACK. Many orthopedists consider muscular weakness, especially in the abdominal region, and poor joint flexibility in the back and legs, prime factors related to the *low back pain syndrome*. Both strengthening and flexibility exercises are commonly prescribed for the prevention and rehabilitation of chronic low back strain.

The proper application of strength training provides an excellent means for strengthening the abdomen and muscles of the lower back, which provide the necessary support and protection for the spine. If done improperly, however, with heavy weight and hips thrust forward and back arched, weight lifting can impose a considerable strain on the lower spine. Pressing and curling exercises, if performed with excessive hyperextension or arch to the back may also create tremendous shearing stresses on the lumbar vertebrae. This spinal pressure can trigger low back pain. Proper execution should not be sacrificed in order to lift a heavier load or "squeeze out" an additional repetition. The extra weight lifted through improper technique will not facilitate strengthening the desired muscle groups and may precipitate an injury.

Isometric Strength Training

Research in Germany[22] showed that a weekly increase in isometric strength of about 5% of the initial strength level could be achieved by performing a daily single, maximum isometric contraction of only 1 second duration or a 6-second contraction at two-thirds maximum. Repeating this contraction 5 to 10 times daily produced greater increases in isometric strength. These results have been observed for subjects who differed in initial strength[30] and age.[9,32]

Although isometric exercise is effective in providing muscular overload and improving strength, its use may be limited for sports training. For one thing, it is difficult to evaluate progress in training. Because there is no movement, it is impractical to measure force output or whether a person's strength is actually improving. Also, the development of isometric strength is highly *specific*. Thus, a muscle trained isometrically demonstrates improved strength mainly when the muscle contracts isometrically, especially at the joint angle and body position at which the strength was developed.

If isometric training is used to develop "strengths" in a particular movement, it is probably necessary to train isometrically at several points through the range of motion. This can become time-consuming, especially if conventional weight training and, more recently, isokinetic methods are available. The isometric method, however, does seem to be especially beneficial in muscle testing and rehabilitation. With isometric techniques,[5,7,8] specific muscle weakness can be detected and strengthening exercises performed at the appropriate joint angle.

Which Is Better, Isometrics or Isotonics?

Although it is generally true that both isometric and isotonic training methods produce significant increases in muscular strength,[3] no one system can really be considered "superior" to the other. The crucial consideration is the intended purpose for the newly acquired strength. The strength training method selected must be determined by the individual's specific needs. The isometrically trained muscle is stronger when measured isometrically; the weight-trained muscle is stronger when evaluated during weight lifting. This *specificity of strength training* is probably explained by the fact that all voluntary movements depend on a finely regulated series of neuromuscular patterns and not merely on the strength of the muscles used in the movement. Likewise, all-out muscular effort is dependent not only on local factors such as muscle fiber type and cross section, but also on neural factors that determine effective recruitment and firing of the appropriate motor units.

The complex interaction between the nervous and muscular systems provides some explanation for the observation that the leg muscles, when strengthened in an activity like squats or deep knee bends, do not usually show improved force capability when used in another leg movement such as jumping. Also, a muscle group strengthened with weights does not generate an equal improvement in force when measured isometrically. Consequently, strengthening muscles for use in a specific activity such as golf, rowing, swimming, or football requires more than just identifying and overloading muscles involved in the movement. It requires that training be specific with regard to the exact movements involved. Training the muscles of the arms to become stronger by weight lifting does not necessarily mean that the performance of *all* subsequent arm movements will be improved. There is little transfer of newly acquired strength to other types of movements, even though the *same* muscles are involved. *To improve a specific performance by the strengthened musculature, the muscles must be trained with movements as close as possible to the desired movement or actual skill.*

Within this framework of training specificity, isokinetic methods appear to show great promise for effective strength improvement at various speeds of movement.

Isokinetic Strength Training

Isokinetic strength training combines the best features of both isometrics and weight training to provide muscular overload at a preset speed while the muscle mobilizes its maximum force-generating capacity through the full range of movement. Any effort encounters an equal and opposing force; this is an *accommodating resistance exercise* accomplished with the aid of a mechanical device. Isokinetic training makes it possible to activate the largest number of motor units and consistently overload muscles to achieve their maximum tension-developing or force output capacity at every point in the range of motion, even at the relatively "weaker" joint angles.

ISOKINETICS VERSUS STANDARD WEIGHT LIFTING. An important distinction can be made between a muscle overloaded isokinetically and one overloaded with a standard weight-lifting exercise. When strength training with weights, the resistance is usually fixed at the greatest load that allows completion of the movement. Consequently, the resistance can be no greater than the maximum strength of the weakest muscle (or joint position) in the range of motion. Otherwise, the movement would not be completed. Weight lifters frequently refer to this point in a range of motion as the "sticking point." A main limitation of weight-lifting exercise is that the force generated by the muscles during a contraction is not maximum through-

out *all* phases of the movement. This is not the case in an isokinetically loaded muscle. The desired speed of movement occurs almost instantaneously, and the muscle is able to generate peak power output at a specific, but controlled speed of contraction.

EXPERIMENTS WITH ISOKINETIC EXERCISE AND TRAINING. Experiments using isokinetic exercise have been designed to explore the force–velocity relationships in various exercises and to relate this to the muscle's fiber composition.[36] Figure 21-6 displays the progressive decline in peak torque output in relation to increasing angular velocity of the knee extensor muscles in two groups of subjects who differed in sports training and muscle fiber composition. In the experiments that involved movement at 180 degrees per second, the power athletes, elite Swedish track and field sprinters and jumpers (closed circles), produced significantly higher torque values than the other group of athletes, which included downhill skiers, competition walkers, and cross-country runners. At this angular velocity, the decrement in maximal

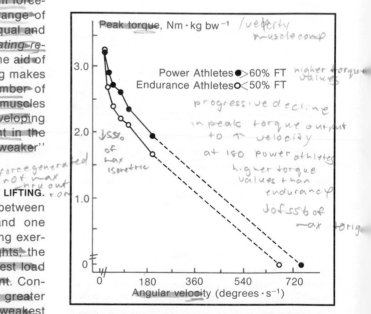

FIG. 21-6. *Peak torque output expressed as a function of increasing angular velocity in two groups of athletes with different muscle fiber composition. The torque–velocity curves were extrapolated to the approximated values for maximal velocity of knee extension. (From Thorstensson, A.: Muscle strength, fiber types and enzyme activities in man. Acta Physiol. Scand. (Suppl.) 443, 1976.)*

torque was equal to about 55% of the maximal isometric torque.

The two curves in Figure 21-6 can also be distinguished in terms of peak torque depending on the group's muscle fiber composition. At zero velocity (isometric contraction), peak force was the same for athletes with relatively high or low percentages of fast-twitch fibers; this indicated that both fast- and slow-twitch motor units were activated in maximal isometric knee extension. *As movement velocity increased, however, greater torque was achieved by individuals with a higher percentage of fast-twitch fibers.* This suggests that a high percentage of fast-twitch fibers is desirable for power activities where success is largely influenced by one's ability to generate large muscular torque in rapid velocities of movement.

SUMMARY

1. The most common methods for measuring muscular strength are (1) tensiometry, (2) dynamometry, (3) 1-RM testing with weights, and (4) computer-assisted force and work-output determinations including isokinetic measurements of muscle force.

2. Human skeletal muscle can generate about 3 to 4 kg of force per square centimeter

of muscle cross section, regardless of sex. On an absolute basis, men are usually stronger than women. An exception to this is strength-trained female track athletes who demonstrate high levels of muscular strength, especially in the legs. When body size and body composition are considered, the large strength differences between men and women are reduced considerably, and in some cases women score higher than men.

3. Muscles become stronger in response to overload training. Overload is created by either increasing the load, increasing the speed of muscular contraction, or by a combination of the above.

4. A load that represents 60% to 80% of a muscle's force-generating capacity is usually sufficient overload to produce strength gains.

5. The three major systems for developing strength are progressive resistance weight training (PRE), isometrics, and isokinetic training. Each system results in strength gains that are highly specific to the type of training. Isokinetic training, because of the possibility for generating maximum force throughout the full range of motion, appears to offer a superior method for strength training. For all strength training, appropriate attention must be given to proper technique and safety.

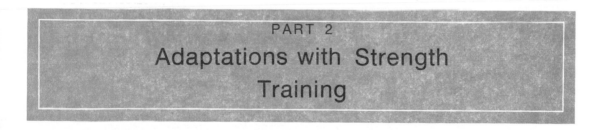

PART 2

Adaptations with Strength Training

FACTORS MODIFYING THE EXPRESSION OF HUMAN STRENGTH

A variety of factors, broadly categorized as psychologic and muscular, influence the expression of human strength. Many are readily modified by a program of systematic strength training, whereas others appear to be training-resistant; these are probably determined by natural endowment or are fixed early in life.

Psychologic Factors

In a series of unique experiments conducted at George Williams College,[25] a group of college men and women was subjected to various treatments designed to evaluate "psychologic" influences on human stength. Arm strength was measured under normal conditions, immediately after a loud noise or while the subject screamed loudly at the time of exertion, under the influence of alcohol and amphetamines or "pep pills," and under hypnosis in which they were told they would be considerably stronger than usual and should have no fear of injury. Each of these factors generally increased strength above normal levels. In fact, the greatest increments were observed under hypnosis, the most "mental" of all treatments!

The investigators speculated that strength improvements under the various experimental treatments were due to a temporary modification in central nervous system function. It was argued that most people normally operate at a level of neural inhibition that prevents them from expressing their true strength capacity. This capacity is largely established by the cross section and fiber type of the muscle and by the mechanical arrangement of bone and muscle. Neuromuscular inhibition could be the result of unpleasant past experiences with exercise, an overly protective home environment, or a fear of injury. Regardless of the reason, the person is usually unable to express his or her maximum strength capability. However, during the excitement of intense competition, or under the influence of disinhibitory drugs or hypnotic suggestion, inhibition is removed, motoneurons are optimally recruited, and an apparent supermaximal performance is attained.

An enhanced arousal level and accompanying disinhibition (or neural facilitation) may explain the so-called unexplainable feats of strength of men and women in emergency situations. In all likelihood, under such circumstances, the person is now able to achieve maximum strength. In fact, drugs, loud noises, and hypnotic suggestion are not the only factors that might improve a strength performance. Highly trained athletes in many sports create an almost self-hypnotic state by intensely concentrating or "psyching" prior to competition. Changes in neural facilitation probably also occur in the early stages of strength training and may largely account for the rapid improvement ratio in the early phase of the program.

Muscular Factors

Although psychologic inhibition and learning factors greatly modify one's ability to express muscular strength, the ultimate limit for strength is determined by anatomic and physiologic factors within the muscle. These factors are not immutable and can be modified with appropriate training procedures. The changes in strength-trained muscles are generally limited to adaptations in the contractile mechanisms and are usually accompanied by substantial increases in ability to exert force through a given range of movement.

MUSCULAR HYPERTROPHY. Increases in skeletal muscle size with strength training can be viewed as a fundamental biologic adaptation to an increased work load. This compensatory adjustment ultimately leads to an increase in the muscle's capacity to generate tension.

Muscular growth in response to overload training occurs primarily from an enlargement or *hypertrophy* of individual muscle fibers. The fast-twitch muscle fibers of weight lifters, for example, were 45% larger than those of healthy sedentary people and endurance athletes.[16] The process of hypertrophy is directly related to the synthesis of cellular material, particularly the protein that constitutes the contractile elements. Within the cell, myofibrils thicken and increase in number as protein synthesis is accelerated, and protein breakdown correspondingly decreases.[17] It appears that the primary requirement for initiating muscular hypertrophy is an increase in the tension or force the muscle must generate. In fact, an increased tension-output by the muscle stimulates hypertrophy independent of a variety of hormonal influences.

The increase in total contractile protein with heavy resistance training appears to occur without a parallel increase in the total volume of mitochondria within the muscle cell.[28] Thus, the ratio of mitochondrial volume to myofibrillar (contractile protein) volume is reduced in strength-trained muscle. Although this training adaptation is apparently beneficial to strength and power athletes, it may actually be detrimental to endurance performance by decreasing the fiber's aerobic potential per unit of muscle mass.

Aside from enlarging existing muscle fibers, tension overload may also stimulate a proliferation of connective tissue and satellite cells that surround the individual muscle fibers.[17] This thickens and strengthens the muscle's connective tissue harness.[15] Muscular overload also improves the structural and functional integrity of both tendons and ligaments.[37] These adaptations may provide some protection from joint and muscle injury; this supports the use of resistance exercise in preventive and rehabilitative strength programs for athletes.

Figure 21-7 shows the changes in muscle fiber size that accompany exercise-induced hypertrophy. The top figure compares the exercised and unexercised *soleus* muscle of a rat. The hypertrophied muscle is on the right. The bottom figures are typical cross sections of untrained and hypertrophied muscles. Not only was the average diameter of the hypertrophied muscle larger by about 30%, but there was also a 46% increase in the number of nuclei present within the cells. These compensatory changes with intense muscular overload are related to a marked increase in DNA synthesis as well as to a proliferation of small, mononucleated satellite cells located under the basement membrane adjacent to the muscle fibers.[17]

ARE NEW MUSCLE FIBERS MADE? Whether the actual number of muscle cells increases with training is a question that is frequently raised. If this does take place, to what extent does it contribute to muscular hypertrophy in humans? Researchers have reported that some muscle fibers from trained animals undergo a process of *longitudinal splitting*.[19,20] In such cases, the split fibers become two individual daughter cells through a process of lateral budding.

One of the problems often encountered with animal research is generalizing the findings to humans. For example, most animals do not undergo the massive hypertrophy observed in humans with strength training. Thus, for various animal species, fiber splitting may be an important compensatory adjustment to overload. Whether this takes place in humans has yet to be shown. Even if these findings are replicated in well-controlled human studies (and even if the response is a positive adjustment), *the greatest contribution to muscular hypertrophy with overload training is made by the increase in size of existing individual muscle cells.*

A

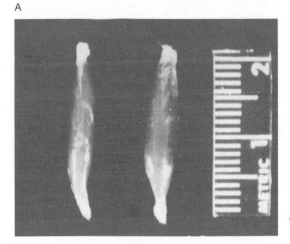

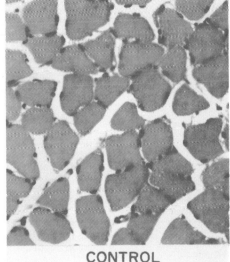

B

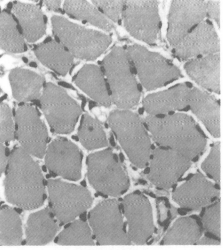

CONTROL   HYPERTROPHY

FIG. 21-7. *A, Control and hypertrophied rat soleus muscle. B, Cross sections of control and hypertrophied muscles shown in A. The average diameter for 50 fibers of the hypertrophied muscle was 24% to 34% greater than in controls; the average number of nuclei in the hypertrophied muscle was 40% to 52% greater than in the control. (From Goldberg, A. L. et al.: Mechanism of work-induced hypertrophy of skeletal muscle. Med. Sci. Sports, 3: 185, 1975.)*

CHANGES IN MUSCLE FIBER COMPOSITION. The effects of 8 weeks of progressive resistance exercise on muscle fiber size and composition were evaluated for the leg extensor muscles of 14 men who performed three sets of 6-RM leg squats 3 times a week.[36] Muscle biopsies were taken from the *vastus lateralis* before and after training. The results for muscle fiber type were clear; there was *no change* with strength training in the percentage distribution of fast- and slow-twitch muscle fibers as indicated by the activity level of myofibrillar ATPase. This was consistent with previous studies using both strength[21] and endurance-type training[18] and strongly suggests that relatively short-term strength training in adults does not alter the basic fiber composition of skeletal muscle. It is still open to question whether specific training early in life or for the prolonged time periods engaged in by Olympic-caliber athletes can cause a change in the inherent twitch (speed of shortening) characteristics of muscle fibers. Although research indicates a possible potential for progressive fiber type transformation with prolonged, specific training (see Chap. 18), the position presently taken is that the predominant muscle fiber distribution is established early in life and is largely determined by genetic factors.[16,18]

Although one's basic fiber type probably does not change dramatically during life,[19a] other characteristics of specific fibers undergo change with training. In the strength training experiment just described, there were significant increases in the volume of fast-twitch fibers in the leg extensor muscles. This is clearly shown in Figure 21-8, where the relative areas of the fast- and slow-twitch fibers are presented for each subject before and after strength training. Progressive resistance training produces a significant and selective hypertrophy of the fast-twitch fibers.[31,36] This makes sense within the framework of exercise specificity, because the fast-twitch motor units are predominantly recruited in near-maximal exercise involving powerful contractions that require anaerobic energy transfer.

COMPARATIVE RESPONSES OF MEN AND WOMEN TO STRENGTH TRAINING

In today's society, women are successfully participating in just about all sports and physical activities. One area that women have generally shied away from, however, is strength training. Many women fear that these exercises will develop overly enlarged muscles similar to those observed for men engaged in heavy weight-lifting programs. This is unfortunate because both men and women often lack sufficient strength to successfully perform activities such as tennis, golf, skiing, dance, and gymnastics. Appropriate forms of muscular overload rapidly improve strength to levels required to learn basic sport skills. A proper program of strength training improves muscular strength and may have a favorable effect on body composition.

Muscular Strength Increases

Table 21-1 summarizes the results of an experiment designed to evaluate the strength "trainability" of 26 previously untrained college-aged men and 47 untrained women of similar age.[38] Strength was measured before and after 10 weeks of a standard weight-training program conducted 2 days a week for 40 minutes. At the start of training, the men were significantly stronger than the women in all muscle groups tested, averaging 28% and 26% greater strength in muscles of the upper and lower body, respectively. However, when leg strength was expressed in relation to body weight—as

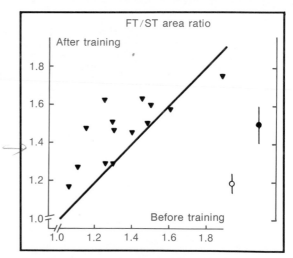

FIG. 21-8. *Individual changes for 14 male subjects in the ratio of the area of fast- to slow-twitch fibers following 8 weeks of PRE strength training. Open circle on right indicates average pretraining FT/ST area ratio while dark circle is the post-training average. (From Thorstensson, A.: Muscle strength, fiber types, and enzyme activities in man. Acta Physiol. (Suppl.) 443: 1976.)*

TABLE 21-1. *Strength changes in men and women as a result of a 10-week weight-training program*[a]

EXERCISE	WOMEN			MEN		
	BEFORE	AFTER	IMPROVEMENT, %	BEFORE	AFTER	IMPROVEMENT, %
Leg press, pounds	659	853	29.5	897	1130	26.0
Arm curls, pounds	45	50	10.6	85	101	18.9
Bench press, pounds	54	70	28.6	146	170	16.5
Grip strength, pounds	65	73	12.8	113	119	5.0

[a] From Wilmore, J.H.: Alterations in strength, body composition and anthropometric measurement consequent to a 10-week weight training program. Med. Sci. Sports, 6:133, 1974.

strength per pound of body weight—this strength difference between the sexes was eliminated. This indicated that the greater absolute leg strength of the men was due primarily to their larger body size (and accompanying muscle mass), and not to some inherent sex difference in a muscle's capability to generate force per unit area of muscle. This was further substantiated when strength improvement was evaluated. Although strength gains as large as 30% were noted, the improvement was *equal* for both sexes. This brought the leg strength of the trained women to a level that was about the same as that of the men prior to training. Relating upper body strength to body weight reduced the differences between the sexes, but the men still remained stronger in these strength measures.

Hypertrophy

The basic sex difference in response to strength training appeared to be the degree of muscle hypertrophy. Despite similar strength improvements, the increase in muscle girth was substantially less for the women. The researchers speculated that this was due to differences in hormonal levels between the sexes, especially the male hormone *testosterone*, which exerts a strong anabolic or tissue-building effect. More research is needed before definitive statements can be made concerning similarities and differences in the strength training responses of men and women. The limited data from relatively short-term studies do suggest that women can utilize conventional weight-lifting exercise without developing overly large muscles.

METABOLIC STRESS OF STRENGTH TRAINING

Although the various strength training methods are effective in enhancing a muscle's force-generating capacity, these exercises provide only minimal stimulus to improve aerobic capacity and reduce body fat. For example, data obtained during standard isometric and weight-lifting exercises with young adult men indicated that such exercise would be classified as light to moderate in terms of heart rate (generally <130 beats per minute) and oxygen consumption (about 3 to 4 times rest).[29] In all instances, resting levels were reached within 1 or 2 minutes of recovery.

Undoubtedly, the stress on specific muscles is considerable in strength training. However, due to the brief activation period and the relatively small muscle mass used, the cardiovascular and aerobic metabolic demands are small compared to those of vigorous walking or running, swimming, and cycling, or any other activity utilizing large muscles. Although a person may spend an hour or more completing a weight-training workout, the total time spent in actual exercise is relatively small, usually no more than 6 or 7 minutes per hour. Clearly, traditional strength training exercise should not make up the major portion of a program designed for cardiovascular overload and weight control.

By modifying the standard approach to strength training it is possible to increase the caloric cost of exercise and bring about improvements in more than one aspect of fitness.[38a, 38b] This approach, called circuit weight training, deemphasizes the heavy local muscle overload of standard strength training in order to provide for a more general conditioning to improve body composition, muscular strength, and endurance, and some cardiovascular fitness. With this approach, a person lifts a weight that is 40% to 55% of his or her maximum (I-RM) strength. The weight is then lifted as many times as possible for 30 seconds. After a 15-second rest the participant moves to the next weight lifting station and so on until the circuit is completed. Between 8 to 15 exercise stations are usually used. The circuit is repeated several times to allow for 20 to 30 minutes of continuous exercise. As strength increases, the weight lifted at each station also increases. This modification of standard weight lifting is an attractive alternative for those fitness enthusiasts desiring a generalized conditioning program. It may also be a good supplemental off-season conditioning for athletes involved in sports requiring a high level of strength, power, and muscular endurance.

MUSCLE SORENESS AND STIFFNESS

Following an extended layoff from exercise, most of us have experienced soreness and stiffness in the exercised muscles and joints. A temporary soreness may persist for several hours immediately after exercise, whereas a residual soreness may appear later and last for 3 to 4 days. Any one of at least four factors may be the causative agent: (1) minute tears in the muscle tissue itself, (2) osmotic pressure changes causing retention of fluids in the surrounding tissues, (3) muscle spasms, and (4) overstretching and perhaps tearing of portions of the muscle's connective tissue harness.

Although the precise cause of muscle soreness remains unknown, the degree of discomfort depends to a large extent on the type of exercise performed. Figure 21-9 shows that muscle soreness as rated by subjects immediately after exercise, and after 24, 48, and 72 hours postexercise, was greater when the exercise involved repeated eccentric contractions than when it involved concentric and isometric contractions.[35]

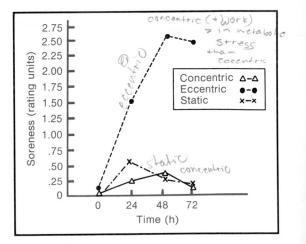

FIG. 21-9. Muscular soreness determined by a rating scale of eccentric, concentric, and static contractions. (From Talag, T. S.: Residual muscular soreness as influenced by concentric, eccentric, and static contractions. Res. Quart., 44: 458, 1973.)

When the subjects were tested for elbow flexion strength at the same time that soreness ratings were made, strength was significantly depressed in conjunction with the residual soreness from eccentric contractions. There was no decrement in stength after concentric and static muscular exercise.

The *tear theory* of muscle soreness proposes that minute tears or ruptures of individual fibers cause the soreness.[23] This is essentially speculation, because experimental verification of actual tissue damage with exercise has yet to be presented. A competing *excess metabolite theory* proposes that prolonged exercise following a layoff causes an accumulation of metabolites in the muscle. This accumulation causes osmotic changes in the cellular environment and fluid is retained. The edema caused by increased osmotic pressure excites sensory nerve endings, causing pain. This explanation is also inadequate.[2] It should be recalled from Figure 21-9 that muscle soreness was much greater following eccentric exercise than following static or concentric contractions. The metabolic stress of concentric (positive) work, however, is usually about five to seven times greater than that of eccentric work. Consequently, one would expect the metabolite buildup and accompanying soreness to be greater in the concentric exercise, not in the eccentric exercise, as is generally reported.

Tonic muscular spasms may also cause the temporary and residual soreness following exercise. It is argued that exercise above some minimal level produces a diminished oxygen supply due to inadequate blood flow in the active muscles. This ischemia can produce pain and initiate a reflex contraction of the muscle. This situation further prolongs the ischemia and sets up repeated cycles of pain, ischemia, and spasm. *Static stretching* is recommended to alleviate muscle soreness. With this form of stretching, a body position is held that stabilizes the joint in a position that places the sore muscle at the greatest possible length. The recommended duration of the stretch is 2 minutes, followed by a 1-minute rest and then another 2 minutes of stretching. The static stretch results in the least possible reflex stimulation (and thus contraction) to the particular muscle via the stretch reflex. A *bouncing stretch* may have an undesirable effect because the sore and rapidly stretched muscle would be stimulated to contract, and the spasms, pain, and soreness would be prolonged.[14]

Experimental Studies

THE SPASM HYPOTHESIS. Several experiments provide evidence to support the spasm hypothesis of muscle soreness. In one study,[12] soreness was produced in both arms by repeated wrist hyperextensions against a 4.3-kg resistance. The muscles of the nondominant arm were stretched by the static technique. This was beneficial because significantly greater levels of soreness occurred 24 and 48 hours after exercise in the dominant arm, which was not stretched. In another study,[13] the resting electrical (electromyographic, EMG) activity of the anterior lower leg muscles was evaluated as a consequence of static stretching procedures in subjects with shin splints, a musculoskeletal disorder involving severe pain in the anterior portion of the lower leg. Static stretching procedures brought about marked reductions in EMG activity. Symptomatic relief with stetching was also accompanied by a decrease in the amplitude of the EMG tracings.

CONNECTIVE TISSUE DAMAGE. In other studies,[1] muscle soreness was induced by repeated bouts of arm-curl weight-lifting exercise and by bench stepping. Several measures were employed to evaluate the degree of soreness and to shed light on possible causative mechanisms. Surface electrodes recorded the electric activity of the muscles for durations of up to 48 hours. Urine samples were obtained at selected intervals to detect postexercise *myoglobinuria*, because the presence of myoglobin in the urine is an accurate indicator of trauma to muscle fibers. To evaluate connective tissue damage, urinary levels of *hydroxyproline* were measured. This assay is useful for determining specific breakdown products of connective tissue and for evaluating collagen metabolism. Subjects also rated the degree of muscle soreness by a subjective rating scale. Analysis of these results showed *no* relationship between muscle pain and EMG activity in the sore muscles. When static stretching procedures were used to alleviate the soreness, there was *no* change in EMG activity, although pain was reduced somewhat for 1 to 2 minutes. In fact, slowly flexing and extending the arm relieved the pain to the same extent as the static stretching procedures!

The results for postexercise myoglobinuria showed that myoglobin release was unrelated to the development of muscle soreness. Elevated myoglobin levels were found in the urine of 7 of 8 subjects in the arm-soreness experiments and also after cycling, even though no soreness occurred following cycling at heavy loads. The presence of myoglobinuria, therefore, must have been a normal consequence of the exercise and was not necessarily due to the soreness per se.

Interesting results were observed for the hydroxyproline excretion rates in relation to muscle soreness produced by bench stepping. As a result of stepping, all subjects reported soreness in both the concentric (quadriceps) and eccentric (gastrocnemius) working muscles. There were statistically significant increases in the 48-hour postexercise hydroxyproline levels and in the total 4-day mean excretion levels for the exercise as compared to the nonexercise condition. The significant increase in hydroxyproline 48 hours after exercise, coupled with the fact that subjects complained of pain in the tendons of the eccentrically exercised muscles, suggests that *connective tissue damage in and around the muscles or an imbalance of collagen metabolism (a degradation process), is somehow involved in exercise-induced muscle soreness.*

SUMMARY

1. Our capacity for muscular strength is largely determined by physiologic factors such as size and type of muscle fibers, as well as by the anatomic-lever arrangement of bone and muscle. This strength capacity is probably greatly affected by neural influence from the central nervous system.

2. As muscles are overloaded and become stronger, they normally hypertrophy or grow larger. This process involves increased protein synthesis with resulting myofibril thickening, proliferation of connective tissue cells, and an increase in the number of satellite cells that surround each fiber.

3. Muscular hypertrophy generally involves structural changes within the contractile mechanism of individual fibers, especially that of the fast-twitch fibers. If new muscle fibers actually develop, their contribution to muscular enlargement is minimal.

4. In short-term training studies, women make strength improvements similar to those of men without accompanying muscular hypertrophy. This is probably due to hormonal differences between men and women.

5. Conventional weight-training exercises per se contribute little to cardiovascular–aerobic fitness and would not be effective major activities in weight-reducing programs.

6. There are several possible explanations for the muscle soreness and stiffness that accompany strength training: (1) minute tears in the muscle tissue, (2) osmotic pressure changes and water retention, (3) muscle spasms, and (4) overstretching and perhaps connective tissue tears. There is some experimental evidence supporting the argument for connective tissue damage.

References

1. Abraham, W. M.: Factors in delayed muscle soreness. Med. Sci. Sports, *9:*11, 1977.
2. Assmussen, E.: Observations on experimental muscle soreness. Acta Rheumatol. Scand. *1:*109, 1956.
3. Clarke, D. H.: Adaptations in strength and muscular endurance resulting from exercise. *In* Exercise and Sport Science Reviews. Edited by J. H. Wilmore, New York, Academic Press, 1973.
4. Clarke, D. H., and Clarke, H. H.: Research Processes in Physical Education, Recreation, and Health. Englewood Cliffs, N. J., Prentice-Hall, 1970.
5. Clarke, H. H.: Objective strength test of affected muscle groups in orthopedic disabilities. Res. Quart., *19:*118, 1948.
6. Clarke, H. H.: Improvements of objective strength tests of muscle groups by cable tension methods. Res. Quart., *21:*399, 1950.

7. Clarke, H. H.: Development of muscular strength and endurance. Phys. Fitness Res. Dig., President's Council on Physical Fitness in Sports. Washington, D. C., U.S. Government Printing Office, January, 1974.

8. Clarke, H. H. et al.: New objective strength tests of muscle groups by cable tension methods. Res. Quart., *23:*136, 1952.

9. Cotten, D.: Relationship of the duration of sustained voluntary isometric contraction to changes in endurance and strength. Res. Quart., *33:*366, 1967.

10. DeLorme, T. L., and Watkins, A. L.: Techniques of progressive resistance exercise. Arch. Phys. Med., *29:*263, 1948.

11. DeLorme, T. L., and Watkins, A. L.: Progressive Resistance Exercise. New York, Appleton-Century-Crofts, 1951.

12. DeVries, H. A.: Electromyographic observations of the effects of static stretching upon muscular distress. Res. Quart., *32:*468, 1961.

13. DeVries, H. A.: Prevention of muscular distress after exercise. Res. Quart., *32:*177, 1961.

14. DeVries, H. A.: Evaluation of static stretching procedures for improvement of flexibility. Res. Quart., *33:*222, 1961.

15. Edgerton, V. R.: Exercise and the growth and development of muscle tissue. *In* Physical Activity; Human Growth and Development. Edited by G. L. Rarick, New York, Academic Press, 1973.

16. Edstrom, L., and Ekblom, B.: Differences in sizes of red and white muscle fibers in vastus lateralis of musculus quadriceps femoris of normal individuals and athletes. Scand. J. Clin. Lab. Invest., *30:*175, 1972.

17. Goldberg, A. L. et al.: Mechanism of work-induced hypertrophy of skeletal muscle. Med. Sci. Sports, *7:*185, 1975.

18. Gollnick, P. D. et al.: Effect of training on enzyme activity and fiber composition of human skeletal muscle. J. Appl. Physiol., *34:*107, 1973.

19. Gonyea, W. J. et al.: Skeletal muscle fiber splitting induced by weight lifting exercise in cats. Acta Physiol. Scand., *99:*105, 1977.

19a. Grimby, G. et al.: Muscle morphology and function in 67- to 81 year-old men and women. Med. Sci. Sports., *12:* (abstract) 96, 1980.

20. Hall-Craggs, E. C. B.: The significance of longitudinal fiber division in skeletal muscle. J. Neurol. Sci., *15:*27, 1972.

21. Karlsson, J. B. et al.: LDH isozymes in skeletal muscles of endurance and strength trained athletes. Acta Physiol. Scand., *93:*150, 1975.

22. Hettinger, T. L., and Muller, E. A.: Muskelleistung und Muskeltraining. Int. Z. Angew. Physiol., *15:*111, 1953.

23. Hough, T.: Ergographic studies in muscular soreness. Am. J. Physiol., *7:*76, 1902.

24. Ikai, M., and Fukunaga, T.: Calculation of muscle strength per unit cross-sectional area of a human muscle by means of ultrasonic measurements. Int. Z. Angew. Physiol., *26:*26, 1968.

25. Ikai, M., and Steinhaus, A. H.: Some factors modifying the expression of human strength. J. Appl. Physiol., *16:*157, 1961.

26. Katch, F. I., and McArdle, W. D.: Nutrition, Weight Control, and Exercise. Boston, Houghton Mifflin, 1977.

27. Laubach, L. L.: Comparative muscular strength of men and women: a review of the literature. Aviation, Space, Environ. Med., *47:*534, 1976.

28. MacDougall, J. D.: Mitochondrial volume density in human skeletal muscle following heavy resistance training. Med. Sci. Sports, *11:*164–166, 1979.

29. McArdle, W. D., and Foglia, G. F.: Energy cost and cardiorespiratory stress of isometric and weight training exercises. J. Sports Med. Phys. Fitness, *9:*23, 1969.

30. Morehouse, C. A.: Development and maintenance of isometric strength of subjects with diverse initial strengths. Res. Quart., *38:*449, 1967.

31. Prince, F. P. et al.: Human muscle fiber types in power lifters, distance runners and untrained subject. Pflugers Arch., *363:*19, 1976.

32. Rarick, G. L., and Larsen, L. A.: Observations on frequency and intensity of isometric muscular effort in developing static muscular strength in prepubescent males. Res. Quart., *29:*333, 1958.

33. Snook, S. H. et al.: Maximum weights and work loads acceptable to male industrial workers. Am. Ind. Hyg. Assoc. J. *31:*579–586, 1970.

34. Snook, S. H., and Ciriello, V. M.: Maximum weights and work loads acceptable to female workers. J. Occup. Med., *16:*527, 1974.

35. Talag, T. S.: Residual muscular soreness influenced by concentric, eccentric, and static contractions. Res. Quart., *44:*458, 1973.

36. Thorstensson, A.: Muscle strength, fiber types and enzyme activities in man. Acta Physiol. Scand., Suppl. 443, 1976.

37. Tipton, C. M. et al.: The influence of physical activity on ligaments and tendons. Med. Sci. Sports, *7:*165, 1975.

38. Wilmore, J. H.: Alterations in strength, body composition and anthropometric measurements consequent to a 10-week weight training program. Med. Sci. Sports, *6:*133, 1974.

38a. Wilmore, J. H. et al.: Energy cost of circuit weight training. Med. Sci. Sports, *10:*75, 1978.

38b. Wilmore, J. H. et al.: Physiological alterations consequent to circuit weight training. Med. Sci. Sports, *10:*79, 1978.

39. Zinovieff, A. N.: Heavy resistance exercises: The Oxford Technique. Br. J. Phys. Med. *14:*129, 1951.

Special Aids
to Performance
and Conditioning

$\boxed{22}$

Coaches and athletes are continually searching for ways to gain the competitive "edge" and improve athletic performance. It is not surprising, therefore, that a variety of ergogenic* substances and procedures are used routinely at almost all competitive levels. Drugs are used most often by college and professional athletes, whereas nutrition supplementation and warm-up procedures are common to individuals who train for fitness and sports activities.

Considerable literature exists on the topic of ergogenic aids and athletic performance.[16,26,32,33] It includes studies of the potential performance benefits of alcohol, amphetamines, epinephrine, aspartates, red cell reinfusion, caffeine, steroids, protein, phosphates, oxygen-rich breathing mixtures, gelatin, lecithin, wheat-germ oil, vitamins, sugar, ionized air, music, hypnosis, and even cocaine! However, only a few of these aids are used routinely by athletes and only a few cause real controversy. Of specific interest is the use of anabolic steroids and amphetamines and the unique procedure of "blood doping." Because warm-up, oxygen administration, and nutritional supplementation are in common use, we also include these in our discussion of the practical implications of ergogenic aids for human exercise performance.

PHARMACOLOGIC AGENTS

It is well known that many male and female athletes use a variety of pharmacologic agents in the belief that a specific drug will have a positive influence on skill, strength, or endurance. In our drug-oriented, competitive culture, it is not surprising to find drug use for ergogenic purposes on the upswing among high school and even junior high school athletes. When winning becomes all important, there is little one can do to prevent the use and abuse of drugs by athletes, even if there is little "hard" scientific evidence of a direct relationship between drug use and improved athletic performance. It seems ironic that athletes go to great lengths to promote all aspects of their health; they train hard, they eat well-balanced meals, they seek and receive medical advice for various injuries (no matter how minor), yet they ingest synthetic agents, many of which can precipitate side effects ranging from nausea, hair loss, itching, and nervous irritability, to severe consequences such as sterility, liver disease, and drug addiction, and even death caused by liver and blood cancer.

We will now take a closer look at two categories of drugs often used by athletes—anabolic steroids and amphetamines.

---

* An ergogenic procedure or aid is supposed to improve physical work capacity or athletic performance.

305

Anabolic
Steroids

An anabolic steroid is a drug that functions in a manner similar to that of the male hormone testosterone. It is this hormone that greatly contributes to the male secondary sex characteristics and to the sex differences in muscle mass and strength that begin to develop at the onset of puberty. The hormone's androgenic or masculinizing effects can be minimized by synthetically manipulating the chemical structure of the steroid so that the anabolic tissue-building, nitrogen-retaining process is emphasized for purposes of promoting increased muscular growth (Dianabol, Nilevar). Nevertheless, the masculinizing effect is still noticeable, especially when the drug is used by females. Athletes who take the drug usually do so for several months (often much longer) in conjunction with a strength development program and augmented protein intake. Their aim is to improve performance in sports requiring strength, speed, and power. Steroids are taken by a wide variety of athletes including weight lifters, wrestlers, shot putters, discus and hammer throwers, football, basketball and baseball players, decathletes, cyclists, sprinters, rowers, boxers, and skiers.

The use of anabolic steroids by *men and women* in sports has generated considerable controversy because of the moral and ethical issues involved and the conflicting scientific data as to whether they even exert a positive influence on growth and performance in normal, healthy athletes.

Much of the confusion as to the ergogenic effectiveness of anabolic steroids has been due to variations in experimental design, poor controls, and differences in specific drugs, dosages, treatment duration, training intensity, measurement techniques, previous experience as subjects, and nutritional supplementation.[12a,19a,28b] There is also speculation that the relatively small residual androgenic action of the anabolic steroid may facilitate improvements by making the athlete more *aggressive* and *competitive* so that he or she trains harder for a longer period of time.[6a]

Recent research with animals suggests that treatment with anabolic steroids, when combined with exercise and adequate protein intake, may stimulate the complex process of protein synthesis and increase the content of skeletal muscle protein (myosin, myofibrillar,

and sarcoplasmic factors).[28a] Whether this occurs in humans is still to be determined. However, the distinct possibility of harmful side effects greatly outweighs any potential and, as yet, unproved performance benefits to be gained from steroid treatment. As part of a long-range educational program, the American College of Sports Medicine (ACSM) has taken a stand on the use and abuse of anabolic-androgenic steroids in sports.[1] We endorse their position paper which appears below.

ACSM POSITION STATEMENT ON ANABOLIC STEROIDS. The research background and specific references for this position statement are included in the original article.[1] Based on a comprehensive survey of the world literature and a careful analysis of the claims made for and against the efficacy of anabolic–androgenic steroids in improving human physical performance, it is the position of the American College of Sports Medicine that:

1) The administration of anabolic–androgenic steroids to healthy humans below age 50 in medically approved therapeutic doses often does not of itself bring about any significant improvements in strength, aerobic endurance, lean body mass, or body weight.

2) There is no conclusive scientific evidence that extremely large doses of anabolic–androgenic steroids either aid or hinder athletic performance.

3) The prolonged use of oral anabolic–androgenic steroids (C_{17}-alkylated derivatives of testosterone) has resulted in liver disorders in some persons. Some of these disorders are apparently reversible with the cessation of drug usage, but others are not.

4) The administration of anabolic-androgenic steroids to male humans may result in a decrease in testicular size and function and a decrease in sperm production. Although these effects appear to be reversible when small doses of steroids are used for short periods of time, the reversibility of the effects of large doses over extended periods of time is unclear.

5) Serious and continuing efforts should be made to educate male and female athletes, coaches, physical educators, physicians, trainers, and the general public regarding the inconsistent effects of anabolic-androgenic steroids on improvement of human physical performance and the potential dangers of taking certain forms of these substances,

especially in large doses, for prolonged periods.

STEROID USE AND LIFE-THREATENING DISEASE. In the ACSM position statement, evidence was presented concerning a possible link between anabolic steroid use and alterations in normal liver function. Table 22-1 amplifies the observations for liver disease.[19] We present these data not as a scare tactic, but to emphasize the potentially serious side effects, even when the drug is authorized by a physician in the recommended dosage. It should be noted that although the duration of drug treatment is greater than usually recommended for athletes, some athletes take steroids on and off for a period of years, with the dosage often greatly exceeding that prescribed for therapeutic purposes (50–200 mg per day versus the usual dosage of 5–20 mg). We believe that any potential gain in exercise performance from anabolic steroids is simply outweighed by the chances of developing severe and harmful side effects. Hopefully, the development of foolproof but simple drug detection techniques will discourage the continued widespread use of such drugs.

STEROID USE BY FEMALES. There is little information on the use of anabolic agents by female athletes but hearsay reports and "off-the-record" statements by coaches, physicians, and the athletes themselves give every reason to conclude that this form of drug abuse is on the upswing. In addition to the broad range of side effects discussed previously, women, especially those who have not fully matured, are susceptible to specific dangers. These include "masculinization, disruption of normal growth pattern, voice changes, acne, hirsutism, and enlargement of the clitoris. The long-term effects on reproductive function are unknown, but anabolic steroids may be harmful in this area. Their ability to interfere with the menstrual cycle has been well documented."[1]

Amphetamines

Amphetamines or "pep pills" are a group of pharmacologic compounds that exert a powerful stimulating effect on central nervous system function. Amphetamine (Benzedrine) and dextroamphetamine sulfate (Dexedrine) are the compounds used most frequently. Amphetamines are sympathomimetic in that their action mimics that of the sympathetic hormones epinephrine and norepinephrine. Consequently, they cause a rise in blood pressure, pulse rate, cardiac output, breathing rate, metabolism, and blood sugar level. Five to 20 mg of amphetamine usually exerts its effect for 30 to 90 minutes after ingestion. Aside from bringing about

TABLE 22-1. *Oral androgenic–anabolic steroids associated with detrimental side effects*[a]

CHEMICAL NAME	TRADE NAME	DAILY DOSAGE (mg)	DURATION IN AFFECTED PATIENTS (MONTHS)	COMPLICATIONS
Oxymetholone	Ora-Testryl Adroyd Anapolon Anadrol 50	10–250	10–51	Peliosis hepatis[b]
Methyltestosterone	Oreton Methyl Metandren Android	20–50	1–165	Hepatoma[c]
Stanazolol	Winstrol	15	18	Hepatoma[c]
Methandrostenolone	Dianabol	10–15	12–18	Hepatoma[c]
Fluoxymesterone	Halotestin	15–80	4–16	Peliosis hepatis[b]
Norethandrolone	Nilevar	20–30	1.5–9	Peliosis Hepatis[b]

[a] Data from Johnson, F.L.: The association of oral androgenic-anabolic steroids and life threatening disease. Med. Sci. Sports, 7:284, 1975. Copyright 1975, the American College of Sports Medicine. Reprinted by permission.
[b] Severe liver malfunction
[c] Liver cancer

an aroused level of sympathetic function, amphetamines are supposed to increase alertness and wakefulness as well as the capacity to perform increased amounts of work; this is achieved by depressing the sensation of muscle fatigue.[6b] It is not surprising, therefore, that athletes frequently use amphetamines with the hope of gaining an ergogenic edge.

DANGERS OF AMPHETAMINES. The use of amphetamines in athletics is ill-advised for the following medical reasons:

1. *Continual use* can lead to either physiologic or emotional drug dependency. This often brings about a cyclical dependency on "uppers" (amphetamines) or "downers" (barbiturates)—the barbiturates are taken to reduce or tranquilize the "hyper" state brought on by amphetamines.

2. *General side effects* of amphetamines are headaches, dizziness, and confusion—all of which can have a negative effect on sports performance requiring reaction, judgment, and a high level of mental concentration.

3. *Larger doses are* eventually required to achieve the same effect because individual tolerances to the drug increase with prolonged use; this may aggravate and even precipitate certain cardiovascular disorders.

4. Agents that inhibit or suppress the body's normal mechanisms for perceiving and responding to pain, fatigue, or heat stress can severely jeopardize the health and safety of the athlete.

5. The effects of prolonged intake of high doses of amphetamines are unknown.

AMPHETAMINE USE AND ATHLETIC PERFORMANCE. Table 22-2 summarizes the results of seven experiments that dealt with the effects of amphetamines on athletic performance. In almost all instances, amphetamines had little or no affect on exercise performances or on simple psychomotor skills.

The major reason athletes take amphetamines is to get "up" for the event *and* to keep up and be psychologically ready to compete. However, the day or evening before a contest, competitors are often nervous and irritable and have difficulty relaxing. Under these circumstances, a barbiturate is used to induce sleep. The athlete then regains the "hyper" condition by popping a "pep pill." Not only is this cycle of

depressant-to-stimulant undesirable and potentially dangerous, but the stimulant does not act in its normal manner after a barbiturate.

The moral, ethical, and legal considerations of drug use by athletes are beyond the scope of this chapter. From a physiologic point of view, however, most team physicians, trainers, and sports-controlling bodies consider the use of amphetamines undesirable and potentially harmful. Knowledgeable and prudent people urge that amphetamines be banned from sport competition. The International Olympic Committee, the American Medical Association, and most athletic governing groups have rules to disqualify athletes using amphetamines. Ironically, the majority of research has indicated that amphetamines do *not* enhance physical performance.[16] Perhaps their greatest influence is in the psychologic realm, where athletes are easily convinced that any supplement will bring on a superior performance. A placebo containing an inert substance often produces identical results!

CAFFEINE AND ENDURANCE. A possible exception to the general rule against stimulants is caffeine. It has been shown that consuming the amount of caffeine commonly found in 2.5 cups of regularly percolated coffee (330 mg) 60 minutes before exercising significantly extended endurance in moderately strenuous exercise.[7] With caffeine, subjects were able to perform an average of 90.2 minutes of exercise compared to 75.5 minutes during a decaffeinated exercise treatment. Even though values for heart rate and oxygen consumption during the two trials were similar, the caffeine also made the work feel easier. During exercise prior to which caffeine had been ingested, the plasma glycerol and free fatty acid levels and the respiratory exchange ratio (R) indicated a high level of fat metabolism and a corresponding reduced rate of carbohydrate oxidation. It is likely that this ergogenic effect of caffeine is due to the facilitated use of fat as a fuel for exercise, thus sparing the body's limited carbohydrate reserves. This would be of considerable benefit in prolonged exercise where glycogen depletion is intimately related to diminished work capacity. It is likely that a lessening of the subjective ratings of effort was due to the effect of caffeine on neuronal excitability, possibly via a lowering of the threshold for motor-unit recruitment and nerve transmission.[7]

RED BLOOD CELL REINFUSION— BLOOD DOPING

Red blood cell reinfusion or "blood doping" came into public prominence as a possible ergogenic technique during the 1976 Montreal Olympics when a champion endurance athlete was alleged to have used this in preparation for his eventual gold medal endurance run. With this procedure, 300 to 600 ml of a person's blood is withdrawn and stored for several weeks. During this time, the person reestablishes the normal red blood cell level. The stored red blood cells are then reinfused a day or two before an endurance event. It is theorized that the added blood volume contributes to a larger maximal cardiac output and that the red blood cell packing increases the blood's oxygen-carrying capacity and thus the quantity of oxygen available to the working muscles. An infusion of 500 ml of whole blood or its equivalent of 275 ml of packed red cells theoretically adds about 100 ml of oxygen to the total oxygen-carrying capacity of the blood. (This is because each 100 ml of whole blood carries about 20 ml of oxygen.) Because an athlete's total blood volume circulates five or six times

TABLE 22-2. *Summary of results on the use of amphetamines and athletic performance*

STUDY[a]	DOSE (mg)	TYPE OF EXPERIMENT	EFFECT OF AMPHETAMINES
(21)	10–20	2 exhaustive treadmill runs with 10 min rest between runs	None
		Consecutive 100 yd swims with 10 min rest intervals	None
		220–440 yd swims	None
		220 yd track runs for time	None
		100 yd to 2 mile track runs	None
(13)	10	Bench stepping to fatigue carrying weights equal to $\frac{1}{3}$ body weight, 3 times with 3 min rest intervals	None
(17)	5	100 yd swim for speed	None
(15)	15	All-out treadmill runs	None
(37)	10	Stationary cycling at work rates of 275–2215 kgm·min^{-1} for 25–35 min followed by treadmill run to exhaustion	None on submaximal or maximal oxygen consumption, heart rate, ventilation volume, or blood lactic acid; work time on the bicycle and treadmill increased significantly
(28)	20	Reaction and movement time to a visual stimulus	None; subjective feelings of alertness or lethargy unrelated to reaction or movement time
(25)	5	Psychomotor performance during a simulated airplane flight	Enhanced performance and lessened fatigue, but if preceded by secobarbital (barbiturate), decreased performance

[a] The number in parentheses refers to the specific reference listed at the end of the chapter.

each minute in all-out exercise, the potential "extra" oxygen available to the tissues from red cell reinfusion is about 0.5 liters. This would certainly be a considerable asset in endurance exercise that requires a high and sustained level of aerobic metabolism, especially if one's capacity for aerobic metabolism is limited by physiologic factors such as oxygen transport by the central circulation.

It is also possible that blood doping could have effects opposite to those intended. A large infusion of red blood cells (and resulting increase in cellular concentration) could increase blood viscosity and bring about a *decrease* in cardiac output, a *decrease* in blood flow velocity, and a *reduction* in peripheral oxygen content—all of which would *reduce* aerobic capacity.

Although a theoretical basis for blood doping exists, there is limited and conflicting experimental evidence to justify this procedure. Some researchers report significant and rapid increases in max $\dot{V}O_2$ following the infusion of whole blood.[10] Other well-controlled experiments, however, show no improvement in a maximal endurance treadmill run after red cell reinfusion.[34] In commenting on the reported 23% overnight increase in performance and 9% increase in maximal oxygen uptake after blood doping,[12] as well as the favorable results of other studies, researchers point out that control groups were not used, both subjects and investigators generally had knowledge of the specific conditions under which performance measures were made, and that subsequent work tests performed after blood withdrawal may have biased the results due to a training effect.[34]

In another experiment,[35] an attempt was made to control for or eliminate many confounding variables in order to more closely evaluate the effect of blood reinfusion on endurance capacity. Sixteen experienced distance runners ran four times to exhaustion. After the first all-out treadmill run (T_1), the men were matched on performance times and assigned to either a control or experimental group. Then, 460 ml of blood was withdrawn from each runner; 2 weeks later all subjects again ran to exhaustion (T_2). This represented the postwithdrawal test. One week later, the experimental group was infused with 460 ml of their own blood, whereas the controls received the same volume of saline solution. Neither group knew which of the solutions they re-

ceived. Two hours after infusion, a third all-out run was undertaken (T_3) followed by a fourth run one week later (T_4). During each run, subjects rated their perception of the exercise stress (*perceived exertion*) in terms of local stress on the legs, cardiorespiratory system, and general overall stress.

As shown in Table 22-3, the runs at T_3 and T_4 were significantly better than at the first trial. This more than likely reflects a training or learning effect or perhaps the psychologic effect of both groups believing they received the blood infusion and "should" perform better as a result of this treatment. Without the control group, however, one might falsely conclude that it was the blood infusion that increased performance. This was not the case, because no significant differences in running performance improvement or maximum heart rate were observed *between* groups—even though the blood hemoglobin was higher at T_3 and T_4 for the group receiving the blood infusion. In fact, after infusion at T_3, the experimental group had about 1.5 g of hemoglobin per 100 ml of blood more than the group receiving saline solution. In addition, subjects did not perceive the work as being any easier following blood infusion. Clearly, more research is needed concerning the precise physiologic and performance consequences of blood doping.

WARM-UP (PRELIMINARY EXERCISE)

Engaging in some type of physical activity or warm-up prior to vigorous exercise is generally accepted as a valid procedure by coaches, trainers, and athletes at all levels of competition. The underlying belief is that this preliminary exercise aids the performer in preparing either physiologically or psychologically for an event and may reduce the chances of joint and muscle injury. The warm-up is generally classified under one of two categories, although overlap often exists. These are (1) *general warm-up,* involving calisthenics, stretching, and general body movements or "loosening-up" exercises generally unrelated to the specific neuromuscular action of the anticipated performance, and (2) *specific warm-up,* which provides a skill rehearsal in the actual activity for which the participant is preparing. Swinging a golf club, throwing a baseball or football, ten-

TABLE 22-3. *Effects of blood cell infusion on endurance performance, heart rate, and hematology*[a]

VARIABLE	EXPERIMENTAL GROUP				CONTROL GROUP			
	T_1[b]	T_2	T_3	T_4	T_1	T_2	T_3	T_4
Run time to exhaustion (s)	2547	2595	2676	2656	2466	2561	2514	2550
Maximal heart rate (b·min^{-1})	189	188	190	189	191	189	189	190
Hemoglobin (g)	15.1	14.7	15.5	15.6	14.8	13.9	14.0	14.4
Hematocrit (%)	42.5	43.0	44.8	44.4	41.6	40.4	41.1	41.0
Red blood cells (10^6)	4.84	4.68	4.85	4.89	4.85	4.54	4.60	4.63

[a] From Williams, M.H. et al.: The effect of blood infusion upon endurance capacity and ratings of perceived exertion. Med. Sci. Sports, *10:*113, 1978.
[b] T_1, Prewithdrawal; T_2, 2 weeks postwithdrawal; T_3, 2 hours postinfusion; T_4, 1 week postinfusion.

nis practice, and preliminary lead-up in the high jump or pole vault are examples of specific warm-up.

Psychologic Considerations

Competitors at all levels often consider that some prior activity prepares them mentally for their event, so that their concentration and "psyche" become clearly focused on the upcoming performance. Some evidence supports the contention that a specific warm-up related to the activity itself improves the necessary skill and coordination. Consequently, sports requiring accuracy, timing, and precise movements generally benefit from some type of specific or "formal" preliminary practice.

There is also the notion that prior exercise, especially before a strenuous effort, gradually prepares a person to go "all out" without fear of injury. A good example is the ritual warm-up of baseball pitchers. Is it conceivable that a pitcher would ever enter a game, throwing at competitive speeds, without previously warming up? Would any athlete begin competition without first engaging in a particular form, intensity, or duration of warm-up? Although in most instances the answer is a definite "no," it would be nearly impossible to design an experiment with topflight athletes to resolve whether warm-up is really necessary and, in fact, whether it improves subsequent performance.

In certain situations, peak performance is expected as soon as play begins, and there is little time for warming up. For example, when a reserve player goes into the last few minutes of a game there is no time for stretching, vigorous calisthenics, or taking practice shots; the player is expected to go all out with no warm-up, except that done before the game or at intermission. Are more injuries recorded in such cases? Is physical performance such as shooting, rebounding, or basketball defense, for example, poorer during the first few minutes of this "unwarmed" condition than it is following a performance preceded by a warm-up?

Psychologic factors such as an athlete's ingrained belief in the importance of warming up establish a definite bias in comparing performance in the "no warm-up" condition.[22] It is difficult to obtain maximum effort with no warm-up if a subject believes warm-up is important. In this regard, some researchers have hypnotized their subjects to neutralize preconceived notions about warm-up. Even if verbal encouragement, money, grades, or other incentives are given to encourage maximum performance under all conditions, it is difficult to "prove" that the incentives were effective. This is often confounded in that "good" subjects may try to help the researcher prove what they perceive he or she believes, whereas "bad" subjects may try to prevent such results. In either case, the true effects are masked. It is noteworthy that no well-controlled research supports the belief that warm-up prevents injury or reduces its severity.[14]

Physiologic Considerations

On purely physiologic grounds, there are six possible mechanisms by which warm-up *should* improve performance due to subsequent increases in blood flow and muscle and core temperature:[9] (1) increased speed of contraction and relaxation of muscles; (2) greater mechanical efficiency because of lowered viscous resistance within the muscles; (3) facilitated oxygen utilization by the muscles because hemoglobin releases oxygen more readily at higher temperatures; (4) temperature effect of myoglobin similar to that of hemoglobin, (5) facilitated nerve transmission and muscle metabolism at higher temperatures; a specific warm-up may also facilitate the recruitment of motor units required in a subsequent all-out activity; and (6) increased blood flow through active tissues as the local vascular bed dilates with higher muscle temperatures.

Effects on Performance

There is little concrete evidence that warm-up per se directly affects subsequent exercise performance. That is not to say that warm-up is unimportant for such purposes. Rather, there is simply little justification from laboratory studies to support such practices. However, because of the strong psychologic component and possible physical benefits of warming up, whether it be passive (massage, heat applications, diathermy), general (calisthenics, jogging), or specific (practice of the actual movements), we recommend that such procedures be continued. Until there is substantial evidence justifying its elimination, a brief warm-up is certainly a comfortable way to lead up to more vigorous exercise. *The warm-up should be gradual and sufficient to increase muscle and core temperature without causing fatigue or reducing energy stores.* This consideration is highly individualized; adequate warm-up in terms of intensity and duration for an Olympic swimmer would totally exhaust the average recreational swimmer. To reap the possible benefits from increased body temperature, the actual event or activity should begin within several minutes from the end of the warm-up. In warming up, the specific muscles should be used in a way that mimics the anticipated activity and brings about a full range of joint motion. It should be kept in mind, however, that a healthy person in peak physical condition who has been competing on a regular basis would probably *not* be at a performance disadvantage without a warm-up, nor is injury more likely to occur from direct participation without some prior exercise.

Sudden Strenuous Exercise

Several studies have been done to evaluate the effects of preliminary exercise on cardiovascular response to sudden, strenuous exercise. The findings provide an essentially different physiologic framework for justifying warm-up that is of extreme importance to those involved in adult fitness and cardiac rehabilitation, as well as in occupations and sports requiring a sudden burst of high-intensity exercise.

In one study, 44 men, free from overt symptoms of coronary heart disease, ran on a treadmill at an intense workload for 10 to 15 seconds without prior warm-up.[3] Evaluation of the post-exercise ECG revealed that 70% of the subjects displayed abnormal electrocardiographic changes that could be attributed to inadequate oxygen supply to the heart muscle [ischemic S-T segment depression (N=19); T-wave flattening or inversion (N=5); minor S-T segment changes (N=6); and multiple premature ventricular contractions (N=2)]. These changes were not related to a man's age or fitness level. To evaluate the effect of a warm-up, 22 of the men jogged in place at moderate intensity (heart rate about 145 beats per min) for 2 minutes prior to the treadmill run. With warm-up, 10 men who had previously shown abnormal ECG responses to the treadmill run now had normal tracings and 10 men had improved their ST segment changes, whereas only two subjects still showed significant ST changes. The blood pressure response also improved with warm-up. For seven subjects with no warm-up, systolic blood pressure averaged 168 mm Hg immediately after the treadmill run. This was reduced to 140 mm Hg with the 2-minute jog-in-place warm-up.

In an extension of this research,[4] the same pattern of blood pressure and ECG response was obtained with regard to the beneficial warm-up effects on sudden strenuous exercise; warm-up exercise that preceded sudden exertion either eliminated or reduced the ischemic response of the myocardium. These observations indicate that the adaptation of coronary blood flow to a sudden and vigorous cardiac work load is not instantaneous and that transient myocardial ischemia may occur in apparently healthy and fit individuals. The effect of prior warm-up (at least 2 minutes of easy jogging) on the electrocardiogram and blood pressure appears to be significant in establishing a more favorable relationship between myocardial oxygen supply and demand.

Although warm-up preceding strenuous exercise is probably a prudent practice for all people, it is most important for those with cardiovascular problems that limit the heart's oxygen supply. Brief, prior exercise probably provides for more optimal blood pressure and hormonal adjustment at the onset of subsequent strenuous exercise. This warm-up would serve two purposes: (1) reduce the myocardial work load and thus the myocardial oxygen requirement, and (2) provide adequate coronary blood flow in sudden, high-intensity exercise.

OXYGEN INHALATION

It is common to observe athletes breathing oxygen-enriched gas mixtures during times out, at half-time, or following strenuous exercise. The belief is that this procedure enhances the blood's oxygen-carrying capacity and thus facilitates oxygen transport to the exercising muscles. If this were the case, oxygen breathing would certainly improve aerobic exercise capacity and possibly speed up recovery. The fact is, however, that when healthy people breathe ambient air at sea level, the hemoglobin in arterial blood leaving the lungs is about 95% to 98% saturated with oxygen. Thus, breathing high concentrations of oxygen could increase oxygen transport by hemoglobin to only a small extent, i.e., about 1 ml of extra oxygen for every 100 ml of whole blood. The oxygen dissolved in plasma when breathing a hyperoxic mixture would also increase slightly from its normal quantity of 0.2 ml to about 0.6 ml per 100 ml of blood. Thus, the blood's oxygen-carrying capacity under hyperoxic conditions would be increased potentially by about 1.4 ml of oxygen to every 100 ml of blood—1.0 extra ml attached to hemoglobin and 0.4 extra ml dissolved in plasma.

Preexercise Oxygen Breathing

A 70-kg person has about 5000 ml of blood. A hyperoxic breathing mixture could therefore potentially add or "store" about 70 ml of oxygen in the total blood volume (5000 ml blood $\times$ 1.4 ml "extra" O_2 per 100 ml blood or 1.4 ml $O_2 \times 50$). Thus, despite the potential psychologic benefit of the athlete believing that

preexercise oxygen breathing helps performance, this procedure might confer only a slight performance advantage due to the oxygen per se. However, this could occur only if the subsequent exercise took place almost immediately after oxygen administration and if ambient air was not breathed in the interval between hyperoxic breathing and exercise. The halfback who breathes oxygen on the sideline before returning to the game or the swimmer who takes a few breaths of oxygen before moving to the blocks for the starting instructions does not really gain the competitive edge due to physiologic benefits. This is especially ironic in football, because the energy to power each play is generated almost totally by metabolic reactions that do not utilize oxygen! The positive psychologic influence of oxygen breathing should not be discounted, however, for it may provide a useful rationale for continuing this practice.

Oxygen Breathing During Exercise

There is considerable evidence that breathing hyperoxic gas during submaximal and maximal aerobic exercise enhances physical performance.[8,18,20,24,29,36] Oxygen breathing during exercise has resulted in reduced blood lactic acid levels, lower submaximal heart rates and ventilation volumes, and a significant increase in maximal oxygen consumption.[11]

In one well-controlled study,[31] subjects performed a 6.5-minute enduranoe ride on a bicycle ergometer at a work level equivalent to 115% of max $\dot{V}O_2$ while breathing either room air or 100% oxygen. To mask a subject's knowledge of the breathing mixture, both air and oxygen were supplied from tanks of compressed gas. Figure 22-1A gives the details of the endurance ride showing there was superiority in endurance (with less drop-off in pedal revolutions) while breathing pure oxygen. Figure 22-1B shows the oxygen uptake curves during the endurance ride breathing oxygen and room air. The results were clear. Oxygen uptake was higher in the 100% oxygen condition with a correspondingly faster rate of oxygen uptake in the early stages of work. These differences can be explained by the fact that even a small increase in hemoglobin saturation during hyperoxia, as well as additional oxygen dissolved in the plasma, significantly increases total oxygen availability during strenuous exercise where the total blood volume is circulated 4 to 7 times

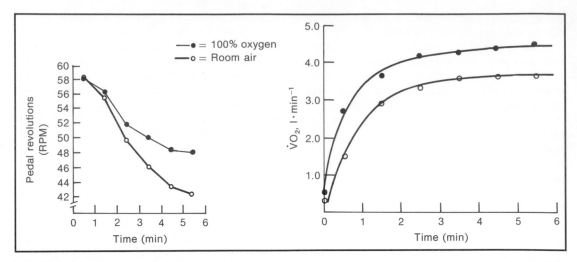

FIG. 22-1. *A, Superiority of endurance (measured by pedal revolutions each minute) breathing pure oxygen versus room air. B, Oxygen uptake curves during the endurance rides. (Data from Weltman, A. et al.: Effects of increasing oxygen availability on bicycle ergometer endurance performance. Ergonomics, 21:427, 1978.)*

each minute. The increase in partial pressure of oxygen in solution also facilitates its diffusion across the tissue-capillary membrane to the mitochondria. This may account for its more rapid rate of utilization in the beginning phase of exercise.

Although breathing hyperoxic mixtures appears to offer positive ergogenic benefits during endurance performance, its practical application in sports seems limited. Even if an appropriate breathing system could be devised, its "legality" in actual competition is unlikely.

Oxygen Breathing During Recovery

A study at the University of Michigan illustrates the effects of breathing hyperoxic gas during recovery from strenuous exercise on subsequent exercise performance.[30] Following one minute of all-out exercise on a bicycle ergometer, subjects recovered passively (quiet sitting) or actively (light pedaling) while breathing room air or 100% oxygen for either 10 or 20 minutes. They then repeated the all-out bicycle ride. Figure 22-2 shows that there were no significant differences in the 6-second revolutions and cumulative revolutions (note the insert graph) for the 1-minute ride after breathing room air or pure oxygen during recovery from previous all-out exercise. There were also no significant differences when comparing blood lactic acid measurements during the 10- and 20-minute

recovery periods breathing room air or oxygen. This indicated that oxygen inhalation did not preferentially alter lactate removal. These data, in conjunction with results from other stud-

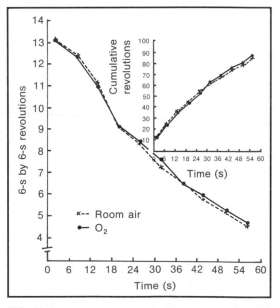

FIG. 22-2. *Absolute and cumulative (insert) endurance scores for 1 minute of all-out exercise following oxygen or room air inhalation during recovery from a previous all-out work bout. (From Weltman, A. et al.: Exercise recovery, lactate removal, and subsequent high intensity exercise performance. Res. Quart. 48:786, 1977.)*

ies,[6,20] do not support the use of hyperoxic breathing mixtures as an ergogenic aid during recovery, nor as an adjuvant to improved performance *following* different durations of recovery from previous exercise.

MODIFICATION OF CARBOHYDRATE INTAKE

Various nutritional aids and supplements are consumed during training and prior to competition in the belief that they confer a specific advantage compared to "normal" dietary practices. The ergogenic role of vitamin and mineral supplementation and the concept of optimal nutrition were presented in Chapters 2 and 3, respectively. The present discussion focuses on *carbohydrate loading,* one of the more popular methods of nutritional modification used by endurance athletes to improve performance. Although the judicious adherence to this dietary technique can significantly improve specific performances, there are also some negative aspects that could prove detrimental.

In the early stages of moderate exercise, about 40% to 50% of the energy requirements is supplied by the glycogen stored in the liver and the exercising muscles. If steady-rate exercise continues and the body's glycogen reserves become reduced, a progressively greater percentage of the energy for exercise must be supplied through the metabolism of fat. This food nutrient is mobilized from storage sites such as the adipose tissue and the liver and is delivered via the circulation to the working muscles. However, if exercise is performed to the point where muscle glycogen becomes severely lowered, fatigue can easily occur, even though sufficient oxygen is available to the muscles and the potential energy from stored fat remains almost unlimited. This is because the glycogen stored in the muscles becomes depleted. If a solution of glucose and water is ingested at the point of fatigue, exercise can be prolonged for an additional period of time, but for all practical purposes the muscles' "fuel tank" will read empty and continued energy production is severely limited.

In the late 1930s, scientists observed that endurance activities could be markedly improved by consuming a carbohydrate-rich diet. Conversely, if the diet consisted predominantly of fat, endurance capacity was drastically reduced. Because of this important relationship between diet and physical performance, researchers have evaluated several possible ways of increasing the body's glycogen reserves. In one series of experiments, subjects consumed three different diets.[5] One diet maintained the normal caloric intake but supplied the major quantity of calories in the form of fat. The second diet was normal and contained the recommended daily percentages of carbohydrates, fats, and proteins. The third diet provided 82% of the calories in the form of carbohydrates. The results showed that the glycogen content sampled from the leg muscles of subjects fed the high fat diet, the normal diet, and the high carbohydrate diet averaged 0.6, 1.75, and 3.75 g of glycogen per 100 g of muscle, respectively. (Similar observations have also been made for liver glycogen.) In addition, the endurance capacity of the subjects varied considerably depending on the diet each consumed in the days prior to the endurance test. As illustrated in Figure 22-3, the endurance capacity of the subjects fed the high-carbohydrate diet was more than three times greater than the endurance capacity of these same subjects on the high-fat diet. Clearly, a simple modification of the diet greatly altered the body's stores of carbohydrates, as well as affected subsequent performance in prolonged submaximal exercise. These observations are especially important not only for the endurance athlete but also for people who have modified their diets so that the normal, recommended percentage of carbohydrates is reduced. In fad diets such as the Atkins Diet,[2] a high fat intake is advocated with the corresponding elimination or severe restriction of carbohydrates. Similarly, high-protein diets are generally accompanied by a reduced intake of sugars and starches. Such diets would rapidly result in a drastic depletion of glycogen from the muscles and liver and make it extremely difficult to participate in vigorous physical activities or training.

Glycogen Supercompensation

Research has also shown that a particular combination of diet and exercise results in a significant "packing" of muscle glycogen. This procedure is termed *carbohydrate loading* or *glycogen supercompensation* and is commonly "in vogue" among endurance athletes, especially marathon runners. The end result of this

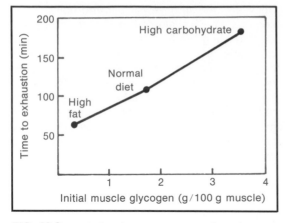

FIG. 22-3. *Relation between preexercise glycogen content of leg muscle and endurance performance in submaximal exercise. (Adapted from Bergstrom, J. et al.: Diet, muscle glycogen and physical performance. Acta Physiol. Scand., 71:140, 1967.)*

specific dietary modification is an even greater increase in muscle glycogen than that which occurs with the high-carbohydrate diet discussed previously. In fact, as many as 4 or 5 g of glycogen are "packed" into each 100 g of muscle.[23]

The basic procedure for achieving the supercompensation effect outlined in Table 22-4 is to reduce the muscle's glycogen content with prolonged steady-rate exercise about 6 days prior to competition. Because glycogen supercompensation occurs *only* in those specific muscles exercised, the athlete should be sure to engage the muscles involved in his or her sport. In preparation for a marathon, a 15- or 20-mile run is usually necessary, whereas for swimming and bicycling, moderately intense submaximal exercise, also for 90 minutes, is required. Then the athlete maintains a low-carbohydrate diet (about 60 to 100 g per day) for several days to further deplete glycogen stores.* During this time moderate training is continued. Then, at least 2 days before the competition, the athlete switches to a high-carbohydrate diet and maintains it up to and including the pre-event meal. The 2- to 3-day requirement for a high-carbohydrate intake is important because it generally takes this long for full restoration of muscle glycogen following severe depletion.[27] Of course, adequate daily protein, minerals and vitamins, and abundant water must also be part of the daily glycogen diet.

The reader should keep in mind that the po-

tential benefits from carbohydrate loading apply to aerobic activities of a prolonged nature. In most instances of sports competition and intense training, a daily diet containing about 50% to 60% of its calories as carbohydrate provides adequate muscle and liver glycogen reserves. Because most competitive endurance athletes normally maintain this carbohydrate intake, their levels of muscle glycogen are usually about twice those of untrained counterparts. For them, the supercompensation effect would be relatively small.

It is not necessary to supercompensate fully for all competitions. For activities of relatively short duration, it probably would be beneficial to increase the carbohydrate percentage in the diet for 1 or 2 days before the event. This ensures that glycogen stores are not low enough to limit performance. For events lasting 30 to 60 minutes, moderate supercompensation would suffice. This could be achieved by a 10-mile run 48 hours before competition, followed by a high-carbohydrate diet and rest. For competitions of longer duration, moderate supercompensation would certainly be beneficial, but utilization of the full protocol would produce better results.

---

*Although the precise mechanism is poorly understood, this glycogen depletion causes an increased level of the glycogen-storing enzyme *glycogen synthetase* in the muscle cell. A carbohydrate-rich diet without prior glycogen depletion increases glycogen storage but does *not* produce a supercompensation effect.

TABLE 22-4. *Two-stage dietary plan for increasing muscle glycogen storage*

Stage 1—Depletion
Day 1: Exhausting exercise performed to deplete muscle glycogen in specific muscles
Days 2, 3, 4: Low carbohydrate food intake (high percentage of protein and fat in the daily diet)
Stage 2—Carbohydrate Loading
Days 5, 6, 7: High carbohydrate food intake (normal percentage of protein and fat in the daily diet)
Competition Day
Follow high-carbohydrate pre-event meal outlined in Chapter 3.

TABLE 22-5. *Sample meal plan for carbohydrate depletion and carbohydrate loading diets preciding the endurance event*[a]

MEAL	STAGE 1 DEPLETION	STAGE 2 CARBOHYDRATE LOADING
Breakfast:	$\frac{1}{2}$ cup fruit juice 2 eggs 1 slice whole-wheat toast 1 glass whole milk	1 cup fruit juice hot or cold cereal 1 to 2 muffins 1 tbsp. butter coffee (cream/sugar)
Lunch:	6-oz hamburger 2 slices bread salad 1 tbsp. mayonnaise & salad dressing 1 glass whole milk	2–3-oz hamburger with bun 1 cup juice 1 orange 1 tbsp. mayonnaise pie or cake
Snack:	1 cup yogurt	1 cup yogurt, fruit or cookies

Dinner:	2 to 3 pieces chicken, fried
	1 baked potato with sour
	  cream
	$\frac{1}{2}$ cup vegetable
	iced tea (no sugar)
	2 tbsp. butter
		1–1$\frac{1}{2}$ pieces chicken, baked
		1 baked potato with sour
		  cream
		1 cup vegctable
		$\frac{1}{2}$ cup sweetened pineapple
		iced tea (sugar)
		1 tbsp. butter

Snack:	I glass whole milk	1 glass chocolate milk with 4 cookies

[a]During stage 1, the intake of carbohydrate is approximately 100 grams or 400 calories; in stage 2, the carbohydrate intake is increased to 400 to 625 grams or about 1600 to 2500 calories.

If, after weighing all the pros and cons, an athlete decides to supercompensate, It should be tried in stages during training. For example, the athlete should start with a long run followed by a high-carbohydrate diet. A detailed log should be kept of what is done and what happens. Subjective feelings should be noted during both exercise depletion and supercompensation phases. If the feelings are positive, then the athlete should try the entire series of depletion, low-carbohydrate diet, and high-carbohydrate diet—but stay on the low-carbohydrate diet for only one day. If there are no adverse effects, then the low carbohydrate diet should be gradually extended to a maximum of 3-4 days.

Sample Diets for Achieving the Supercompensation Effect

Table 22-5 provides an example of meal plans that can be used during carbohydrate depletion (stage 1) and carbohydrate loading (stage 2) preceding the endurance event.

Negative Aspects

The additional 2 7 g of water stored with each gram of muscle glycogen makes this a heavy fuel compared to an equal quantity of calories stored as fat. Body weight is increased and may make the athlete feel "too heavy" and uncomfortable; any extra weight load also directly adds to the energy cost of activities such as running. Extra weight may actually negate the potential benefits to be derived from the extra glycogen storage. On the positive side, the water liberated during glycogen breakdown is available for temperature regulation during exercise in the heat.

Supercompensation may be potentially hazardous to individuals with predispositions to specific health problems. A severe and chronic carbohydrate overload interspersed with periods of high fat or high protein intake could pose problems for individuals susceptible to adult diabetes and heart disease, or for those with certain muscle enzyme deficiencies or kidney disease. Although minor dietary alterations probably have little effect on overall health, there is no research on the long-term effects of repeated supercompensation or a prolonged carbohydrate overload in individuals unaccustomed to such a diet. Failure to eat a balanced diet may lead to deficiencies of some minerals and vitamins, particularly water-soluble vitamins; this may require some dietary supplementation. While in the glycogen-depleted state, a generally weakened condition may make the individual more susceptible to infection and injury and certainly reduces one's capability to engage in hard training. Athletes should become well informed about carbohydrate loading before trying to manipulate their dietary and exercise habits to achieve glycogen loading.

SUMMARY

1.   Ergogenic aids are substances or procedures that are thought to *improve* physical work capacity or athletic performance.

2.   The most common pharmacologic agents used as ergogenic aids are anabolic steroids and amphetamines. An anabolic steroid is a drug that functions in a manner similar to the hormone testosterone. There are no consistent findings to support the beneficial effects of steroids on muscular strength and power. The potential side effects of these drugs greatly outweigh any possible exercise benefits.

3.   There is little evidence that amphetamines or "pep pills" aid exercise performance or psychomotor skills, other than what can be derived from a simple placebo effect. The side effects of amphetamines include drug dependency, headache, dizziness, confusion, and upset stomach.

4.   Red blood cell reinfusion or "blood doping" involves the drawing, storage, and reinfusion several weeks later of 300 to 600 ml of blood. It is believed that the added blood volume contributes to a larger maximum cardiac output and an increase in the blood's oxygen-carrying capacity and hence max $\dot{V}O_2$. There is evidence both pro and con concerning blood doping. More research is needed in this area.

5.   There is a physiologic argument that warm-up enhances exercise performance. This includes the possible ergogenic effects of warm-up on muscular speed and efficiency, enhanced oxygen delivery and utilization, and facilitated transmission of nerve impulses. However, research to support the benefits of warm-up beyond a strong psychologic component is of limited quality. Likewise, there is no evidence justifying its elimination if the performer feels that warm-up is important.

6.   There is evidence to support the usefulness of a moderate warm-up prior to sudden strenuous exercise. It reduces cardiac work load and may provide for adequate coronary blood flow. In this instance, warm-up may prevent transient myocardial ischemia and potentially dangerous side effects.

7.   The inhalation of oxygen-rich breathing mixtures prior to, during, and following vigorous exercise is common practice in many sports. Breathing 100% oxygen *during* performance extends endurance by increasing oxygen uptake, reducing blood lactic acid production, and lowering the ventilation rate. Breathing hyperoxic mixtures prior to or following exercise is of no ergogenic benefit.

8.   Techniques for carbohydrate loading are generally effective for augmenting endurance in prolonged submaximal exercise. Athletes should become well informed about these nutritional modifications before trying to manipulate their diets to achieve glycogen loading.

References

1. American College of Sports Medicine. The use and abuse of anabolic–androgenic steroids in sports. Med. Sci. Sports, *9:*xi, 1977.
2. American Medical Association Council on Food and Nutrition. *Journal of the American Medical Association. 224:*1418, 1973.
3. Barnard, R.J. et al.. Cardiovascular responses to sudden strenuous exercise-heart rate, blood pressure, and ECG. J. Appl. Physiol., *34:*833, 1973.
4. Barnard, R.J. et al.: Ischemic response to sudden strenuous exercise in healthy men. Circulation, *48:*936, 1973.
5. Bergstrom, J. et al.: Diet, muscle glycogen and physical performance. Acta Physiol. Scand., *71:*140, 1967.
6. Bjorgum, R.K., and Sharkey, B.J.: Inhalation of oxygen as an aid to recovery after exertion. Res. Quart., *37:*472, 1966.
6a. Brooks, R.V.: Anabolic steroids and athletes. Physician Sportsmed., *8:*161, 1980.
6b. Chandler, J.V., and Blair, S.N.: The effct of amphetamines on selected physiological components related to athletic success. Med. Sci. Sports, *12:*65, 1980.
7. Costill, D.L. et al.: Effects of caffeine ingestion on metabolism and exercise performance. Med. Sci. Sports, *10:*155, 1978.
8. Davies, C.T.M., and Sargeant, A.J.: Physiological responses to one-and-two leg exercise breathing air and 45% oxygen. J. Appl. Physiol., *36:*142, 1974.
9. DeVries, H.A.: Physiology of Exercise for Physical Education and Athletics. DuBuque, Iowa, W.C. Brown, 1974.
10. Ekblom, B.: Response to exercise after blood loss and reinfusion. J. Appl. Physiol., *33.*175, 1972.
11. Ekblom, B. et al.: Effect of changes in actual oxygen content on circulation and physical performance. J. Appl. Physiol., *39:*71, 1975.
12. Ekblom, B. et al.: Central circulation during exercise after venesection and reinfusion of red blood cells. J. Appl. Physiol., *40:*379, 1976.
12a. Fahey, T.D., and Brown, C.H.: The effects of anabolic steroids on the strength, body composition and endurance of college males when accompanied by a weight training program. Med. Sci. Sports, *5:*272, 1973.
13. Foltz, E.E. et al.: The influence of amphetamine (Benzedrine) sulfate and caffeine on the performance of rapidly exhausting work by untrained subjects. J. Lab. Clin. Med., *28:*601, 1943.
14. Franks, B.D.: Physical warm-up. *In* Ergogenic Aids and Muscular Performance. Edited by W.P. Morgan. Academic Press, New York, 1972.
15. Golding, L.A., and Barnard, R.J.: The effects of d-amphetamine sulfate on physical performance. J. Sports Med. Phys. Fitness, *3:*221, 1963.
16. Golding, L.A.: Drugs and hormones. *In* Ergogenic Aids and Muscular Performance. Edited by W.P. Morgan. Academic Press, New York, 1972.
17. Haldi, J., and Wynn, W.: Action of drugs on efficiency of swimmers. Res. Quart., *17:*96, 1959.
18. Hughes, R.L. et al.: Effects of inspired O_2 on cardiopulmonary and metabolic responses in man. J. Appl. Physiol., *24:*336, 1968.
19. Johnson, F.L.: The association of oral androgenic-anabolic steroids and life-threatening disease. Med. Sci. Sports, *7:*284, 1975.

19a. Johnson, L.C., et al.: Anabolic steroids: Effects on strength, body weight, oxygen uptake, and spermatogenesis upon mature males. Med. Sci. Sports, *4:*43, 1972.

20. Karpovich, P.V.: Effects of oxygen inhalation on swimming performance. Res. Quart. *5:*24, 1934.

21. Karpovich, P.V.: Effect of amphetamine sulfate on athletic performance. J.A.M.A., *170:*558, 1959.

22. Karpovich, P.V.: Encyclopedia of Sport Sciences and Medicine. Macmillan, New York, 1971.

23. Londeree, B.: To Supercompensate or not? Runners World, *9:*26, 1974.

24. Margaria, R. et al.: Maximum exercise in oxygen. Int. Z. Angew. Physiol. *18:*465, 1961.

25. McKenzie, R.E., and Elliot, L.L.: Effects of secobarbital and D-amphetamine on performance during a simulated air mission. Aerosp. Med., *36:*774, 1965.

26. Morgan, W.P.: Ergogenic Aids and Muscular Performance. Academic Press, New York, 1972.

27. Piehl, K.: Time course for refilling of glycogen stores in human muscle fibers following exercise-induced glycogen depletion. Acta Physiol. Scand., *90:*297, 1974.

28. Pierson, W.R., Rasch, P.J., and Brubaker, M.L.: Some psychological effects of the administration of amphetamine sulfate and meprobamate on speed of movement and reaction time. Med. Sci. Sports, *1:*61, 1961.

28a. Rogozkin, V.: Metabolic effects of anabolic steroids on skeletal muscle. Med. Sci. Sports, *11:*160, 1979.

28b. Stamford, B., and Moffatt, R.: Anabolic steroids: Effectiveness as an ergogenic aid to experienced weight trainers. J. Sports Med., *14:*191, 1974.

29. Taunton, J.E. et al.: Physical work capacity in hyperbaric environments and conditions of hyperoxia. J. Appl. Physiol., *28:*421, 1970.

30. Weltman, A.L. et al.: Exercise recovery, lactate removal, and subsequent high intensity exercise performance. Res. Quart., *48:*786, 1977.

31. Weltman, A.L. et al.: Effects of increasing oxygen availability on bicycle ergometer endurance performance. Ergonomics *21:*427, 1978.

32. Williams, M.H.: Drugs and Athletic Performance. Springfield, Ill., Charles C Thomas, 1974.

33. Williams, M.H.: Nutritional Aspects of Human Physical and Athletic Performance. Springfield, Ill. Charles C Thomas, 1976.

34. Williams, M.H. et al.: Effect of blood reinjection upon endurance capacity and heart rate. Med. Sci. Sports, *5:*181, 1973.

35. Williams, M.H. et al.: The effect of blood infusion upon endurance capacity and ratings of perceived exertion. Med. Sci. Sports, *10:*13, 1978.

36. Wilson, B.A. et al.: Effects of hyperoxic gas mixtures on energy metabolism during prolonged work. J. Appl. Physiol., *30:*267, 1975.

37. Wyndham, C.H. et al.: Physiological effects of the amphetamines during exercise. S. Afr. Med. J., *45:*247, 1971.

SECTION V

Work Performance and Environmental Stress

Our main concern so far has been to focus on the physiologic and metabolic adjustments that enable humans to generate energy for exercise in "normal" environments. In this context, the stress on the organism is largely that imposed by the specific form of work, such as walking or running, bicycling, or swimming in relatively warm water. In many instances, however, the environment compounds the stress of exercise. Sport activities are often held at altitudes that impair the normal oxygenation of blood flowing through the lungs. Above a certain elevation, the capacity to generate aerobic energy for exercise is severely limited. At the other extreme, to explore beneath the water's surface poses a different challenge. In this case, we must bring our sea level environment with us. This usually takes the form of air compressed in a *scuba* tank carried on the diver's back. For some sports enthusiasts, however, no external assistance is provided, and the length of an underwater excursion is generally limited by the quantity of air inhaled into the lungs just prior to the dive. In both breathhold diving and diving with scuba, unique challenges and dangers are provided by the environment. These are often independent of the stress of exercise.

Exercising in a hot, humid environment or under conditions of extreme cold can also impose severe thermal stress. The total effect of each environmental stressor is clearly determined by the degree to which it deviates from neutral conditions as well as by the duration of the exposure. In addition, several environmental stressors operating at the same time (for example, extreme cold exposure at high altitude) may exceed and override the simple additive effects of each stressor were it imposed by itself.

In the three chapters that follow, we explore the specific problems encountered at altitude and during exercise in hot and cold environments. We also discuss the immediate physiologic adjustments and long-term adaptations by which the body strives to maintain internal consistency despite an environmental challenge. In the chapter on sport diving, the unique problems associated with this increasingly popular form of sport and recreation are explored.

Exercise at Medium
and High Altitude

23

More than 40 million people live, work, and recreate at terrestrial elevations between 3048 meters (m) (10,000 ft) to 5486 m (18,000 ft) above sea level. In terms of the earth's topography, these elevations encompass the range of what is generally considered *high altitude*. Although high-altitude natives are self-sustaining, some of them living in permanent settlements as high as 5486 m in the Andes and Himalaya mountains, prolonged exposure of an unacclimatized person to such an altitude may cause death from hypoxia, even if the person remains inactive. The physiologic challenge of even moderately high or *medium altitude* becomes readily apparent during physical activity. This is especially true for newcomers who have not had time to acclimatize to the decreased partial pressure of oxygen at high elevations.

THE STRESS
OF ALTITUDE

The challenge of altitude is essentially the decreased partial pressure of ambient oxygen (Po_2) and *not* the reduced total barometric pressure per se or the relative concentrations of the inspired gases. Figure 23-1 illustrates the barometric pressure, the pressures of the respired gases, and the percent saturation of hemoglobin at various terrestrial elevations.[8,31]

The density of air decreases progressively as one ascends above sea level. For example, the barometric pressure at sea level averages 760 mm Hg whereas at 3048 m the barometer reads 510 mm Hg, and at an elevation of 5486 m, the pressure of a column of air at the earth's surface is about half its pressure at sea level. Although dry ambient air at sea level and altitude contains 20.9% oxygen, the Po_2 or density of oxygen molecules is lowered in direct proportion to the fall in barometric pressure upon ascending to higher elevations (Po_2 = .209 × barometric pressure). Thus, ambient Po_2 at sea level averages about 150 mm Hg, but it is only 107 mm Hg at 3048 m. *It is this reduction in Po_2 (and accompanying arterial hypoxia) that precipitates the immediate physiologic adjustments to altitude as well as the long-term process of acclimatization.*

Oxygen Loading at
Altitude

Due to the s-shaped nature of the oxyhemoglobin dissociation curve (Chap. 13, Fig. 13-3), little change in the percent saturation of hemoglobin is observed with decreasing Po_2 until an altitude of about 3048 m. At 1981 meters (6500 ft), for example, the alveolar oxygen partial pressure is reduced from its sea level value of 100 mm Hg to 78 mm Hg, yet hemoglobin is still about 90% saturated with oxygen. Although this relatively small decrease in the amount of oxygen carried by the blood may have little effect on an individual at rest or even during mild exercise, vigorous aerobic activities are altitude sensitive. In fact, the relatively poor performances of men and women in middle and distance running and swimming during the 1968 Olympics in Mexico City (altitude 2300 m; 7546 feet) were attributed to the small reduction in oxygen transport at this altitude.[10,15] No world records were established in events lasting longer than 2.5 minutes.

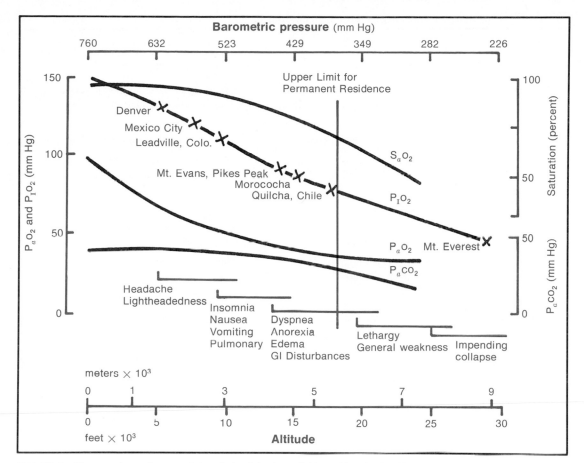

FIG. 23-1. *Changes in environmental and physiologic variables with altitude. (P_aO_2 = Partial pressure of arterial oxygen; P_aCO_2 = partial pressure of arterial carbon dioxide; P_IO_2 — partial pressure of oxygen in inspired air; S_aO_2 = oxygen saturation of hemoglobin) (From Kollias, J., and Buskirk, E.: Exercise and altitude. In Science and Medicine of Exercise and Sport. Edited by W. Johnson and C. Buskirk. New York, Harper and Row, 1974.)*

At higher elevations like the Andes and Himalayas, the reduced loading of hemoglobin with oxygen is readily apparent, and sustained physical activity is difficult. At altitudes above 5182 m (17,000 ft), permanent living is nearly impossible, and mountain climbing at these high elevations is usually done with the aid of oxygen equipment. At 5486 m[34] for example, arterial Po_2 is about 38 mm Hg, and hemoglobin is 73% saturated. Because this oxygen partial pressure is on the steep portion of the oxyhemoglobin dissociation curve, any further increase in altitude brings about a relatively large decrease in hemoglobin saturation and oxygen transport capacity. There are reports of acclimatized mountaineers who lived for weeks at 6706 m (28,000 ft) breathing only ambient air.[24] In fact, members of two Swiss expeditions to Mt. Everest remained at the summit (8848 m; 29,028 ft)

for 2 hours without using oxygen equipment![33] Although such performances are clearly the exception and not the rule, they do demonstrate the enormous adaptative capability of humans to work and survive without external support at extreme altitudes.

Acclimatization

During the many years that mountaineers have attempted to climb the world's highest peaks, it has been well known that weeks are required for sea-level residents to adjust to successively higher elevations. The adaptative responses that improve one's tolerance to altitude hypoxia are broadly termed *acclimatization. Each adjustment to a higher altitude is progressive, and full acclimatization requires time. Successful*

TABLE 23-1. *Immediate and longer term adjustments to altitude hypoxia*

SYSTEM	IMMEDIATE	LONGER TERM
Pulmonary	Hyperventilation	Hyperventilation
Acid–Base	Body fluids become more alkaline due to reduction in CO_2 with hyperventilation	Excretion of base via the kidneys and concomitant reduction in alkaline reserve
Cardiovascular	Increase in submaximal heart rate	Submaximal heart rate remains elevated
	Increase in submaximal cardiac output	Submaximal cardiac output falls to or below sea-level values
	Stroke volume remains the same or is slightly lowered	Stroke volume is lowered
	Maximum heart rate remains the same or is slightly lowered	Maximum heart rate is lowered
	Maximum cardiac output remains the same or is slightly lowered	Maximum cardiac output is lowered
Hematologic	—	Decrease in plasma volume
		Increased hematocrit
		Increased hemoglobin concentration
		Increase in total number of red blood cells
Local	—	Possible increased capillarization of skeletal muscle
		Increased red-blood-cell 2,3-DPG
		Increased mitochondria
		Increased aerobic enzymes

adjustment to medium altitude represents only partial adjustment to a higher elevation.

As summarized in Table 23-1, certain compensatory responses to altitude occur almost immediately whereas other physiologic and metabolic adaptations take weeks or even months. Although the intensity of the response is largely altitude-dependent, considerable *individual variability* exists for both the rate and success of an individual's acclimatization.

Immediate Responses to Altitude

Upon arrival at elevations of about 2300 m and higher, rapid physiologic adjustments occur to compensate for the thinner air and accompanying reduced alveolar oxygen pressure. The most important of these responses are (1) an

increase in the respiratory drive, which results in hyperventilation, and (2) an increase in blood flow at rest and during submaximal exercise.

HYPERVENTILATION. Probably the most important and clear-cut immediate response of the native lowlander to altitude exposure is hyperventilation brought on by the reduced arterial Po_2.[12] Once initiated, this "hypoxic drive" increases during the first few weeks and may remain elevated for a year or longer during prolonged altitude residence.[30,41]

It should be recalled from Chapter 14 that special receptors sensitive to reduced oxygen pressure are located in the aortic arch and at the branching of the carotid arteries in the neck. Any significant reduction in arterial Po_2 (e.g., which occurs at an altitude above 2000 m) progressively stimulates these chemoreceptors. This, in turn, modifies inspiratory activity to increase alveolar ventilation, which causes alveolar oxygen concentration to increase toward the level in ambient air—the greater the hyperventilation, the more closely alveolar air resembles inspired air. The increase in alveolar P_{O_2} with hyperventilation facilitates oxygen loading in the lungs and provides the rapid first line of defense against the stress of reduced ambient P_{O_2}.

INCREASED CARDIOVASCULAR RESPONSE. In the early stages of altitude adaptation, submaximal heart rate and cardiac output may increase 50% above sea level values,[27,43] whereas the heart's stroke volume remains essentially unchanged. Because the oxygen cost of work at altitude is essentially no different than it is at sea level,[27,35] this increase in submaximal blood flow partially compensates for the reduced oxygen in arterial blood. For example, a 10% increase in cardiac output at rest or in moderate exercise offsets a 10% reduction in arterial oxygen saturation, at least in terms of total oxygen circulated through the body.

The effects of *acute* altitude exposure on the metabolic and cardiorespiratory response to submaximal and all-out bicycle exercise in young men are shown in Table 23-2. Physio-logic measures were obtained at sea level and during a brief exposure to a simulated altitude of 4000 m (13,124 ft).[42] Even with the increase in pulmonary ventilation during submaximal exercise at "altitude" as compared to sea level, arterial oxygen saturation was reduced from 96% to about 70% at all work levels. However, in submaximal exercise, the blood's reduced oxygen content was *entirely* compensated for by an increase in cardiac output. This increased blood flow was due to an elevated heart rate because the heart's stroke volume remained unchanged during altitude exposure. With this circulatory adjustment, oxygen consumption was nearly identical in submaximal work at sea level and at altitude. The greatest effect of altitude on aerobic metabolism was observed during maximal exercise when the max $\dot{V}O_2$ was reduced to 72% of sea level values. At this exercise intensity, the ventilatory and circulatory adjustments to acute altitude exposure cannot compensate for the lower oxygen content of arterial blood.

ACUTE MOUNTAIN SICKNESS. Despite the body's rapid defense against the stress of altitude, many people experience acute discomfort termed *mountain sickness* during the first few

TABLE 23-2. *Cardiorespiratory and metabolic response during submaximal and maximal exercise at sea level and simulated altitude of 4,000 m (13,115 ft) in six young men*[a]

WORK LEVEL	$\dot{V}O_2$ (l·min^{-1})		$\dot{V}_E$ (l·min^{-1} BTPS)		ARTERIAL SATURATION (%)	
ALTITUDE, m	0	4000	0	4000	0	4000
600 kg. min^{-1}	1.50	1.56	39.6	53.7	96	71
900 kg. min^{-1}	2.17	2.23	59.0	93.7	95	69
Maximum	3.46	2.50	123.5	118.0	94	70

WORK LEVEL	$\dot{Q}$ (l·min^{-1})		H R (b·min^{-1})		S V (ml)		A-$\bar{V}O_2$ DIFF (ml O_2·100 ml^{-1})	
ALTITUDE, m	0	4000	0	4000	0	4000	0	4000
600 kg. min^{-1}	13.9	16.7	115	148	122	113	10.8	9.4
900 kg. min^{-1}	19.2	21.6	154	176	125	123	11.4	10.4
Maximum	23.7	23.2	186	184	127	126	14.6	10.8

[a]From Stenberg, J. et al.: Hemodynamic response to work at simulated altitude, 4000 m. J. Appl. Physiol. *21*:1589, 1966.

days at altitudes of about 3048 m or higher. These symptoms usually include headache (most frequent symptom), dizziness, nausea, vomiting, dimness of vision, insomnia, and generalized weakness.[25] Appetite suppression can be severe during the early stages of high altitude stay. This may result in an average reduction in energy intake of about 40% and an accompanying loss of body weight. Diets high in carbohydrates appear to be well tolerated by subjects during the early stay at high altitude and ameliorate the ill effects of altitude exposure. For one thing, the energy liberated per unit of oxygen consumed is greater in carbohydrate breakdown than in fat breakdown (5.0 kcal vs. 4.7 kcal per liter O_2). Also, high levels of circulating fats following a high-fat meal may reduce arterial oxygen saturation. In short-term hypoxia experiments, high-carbohydrate diets have the opposite effect. This improvement in arterial oxygen transport with a high-carbohydrate diet tends to (1) enhance altitude tolerance, (2) reduce the severity of mountain sickness, and (3) lessen the physical performance decrements during the early stages of altitude exposure. For people suffering the effects of mountain sickness, even moderate exercise can be intolerable. In the days and weeks that follow, as acclimatization progresses, symptoms subside and many disappear. Concurrently, a person's ability to exercise improves and considerably more work can be accomplished.

For unknown reasons, some people are unable to adjust to high altitude or, after a prolonged period at altitude, lose their acquired acclimatization. As a result, their general tolerance to hypoxia is lessened and the symptoms of mountain sickness return. To prevent severe disability or even death, these people must relocate at a lower altitude.

FLUID LOSS AT ALTITUDE. Because the air in mountainous regions is usually cool and dry, considerable body water can be lost through evaporation as air is warmed and moistened in the respiratory passages. This often leads to moderate dehydration and accompanying symptoms of dryness of the lips, mouth, and throat. This is especially true for active people for whom the daily total sweat loss and pulmonary ventilation (and hence water loss) are large. For these active people, body weight should be checked frequently and easy access to water provided at all times.

Longer Term Adjustments to Altitude

Hyperventilation and increased submaximal cardiac output provide a rapid and relatively effective counter to the challenge of altitude. Concurrently, other slower acting physiologic and metabolic adjustments occur during a prolonged altitude stay. The most important of these involve (1) maintenance of the acid–base balance of body fluids altered by hyperventilation, (2) increased formation of hemoglobin and red blood cells, and (3) changes in local circulation and cellular function. *All of these adaptations* generally reduce distress and improve tolerance to the relative hypoxia of medium and high altitudes.

ACID–BASE READJUSTMENT. Although hyperventilation at altitude favorably increases alveolar oxygen concentration, it has the opposite effect on carbon dioxide. Because ambient air contains essentially no carbon dioxide, the increased breathing at altitude tends to "wash out" or dilute this gas in the alveoli. This creates a larger-than-normal gradient for the diffusion of carbon dioxide from the blood to the lungs, and arterial carbon dioxide is reduced considerably. Upon exposure to an altitude of 3048 m, for example, alveolar P_{CO_2} falls to approximately 24 mm Hg. This is in contrast to the P_{CO_2} of 40 mm Hg usually maintained at sea level. During a prolonged stay at higher altitudes, the pressure of alveolar carbon dioxide falls as low as 10 mm Hg.

The loss of carbon dioxide from the body's fluids in hypoxic environments causes a physiologic disequilibrium. It should be recalled from our discussion of acid–base balance in Chapter 13 that the largest quantity of carbon dioxide is normally carried as carbonic acid. This relatively weak acid readily ionizes to H^+ and HCO_3^-, which are then transported to the lungs by the venous circulation. In the pulmonary capillaries, carbon dioxide and water re-form, and carbon dioxide diffuses into the alveoli. A decrease in carbon dioxide, as would occur in hyperventilation, causes the pH to rise and the blood becomes more alkaline.

Because hyperventilation is a normal response to altitude, adjustments must be made during acclimatization to minimize the accompanying "side effects" that disrupt acid–base balance. This control of respiratory alkalosis is accomplished slowly by the kidneys, which excrete base (HCO^-_3) through the renal tubules. In turn, the restoration of a normal pH increases the responsiveness of the respiratory center, and ventilation increases further to adjust to altitude hypoxia.

The establishment of acid–base equilibrium with acclimatization occurs at the expense of a loss of *alkaline reserve*. Thus, although the pathways of anaerobic metabolism are unaffected at altitude, the blood's buffering capacity for acids is gradually decreased, and the critical limit for the accumulation of acid metabolites is lowered.[26,30] A general depression in maximum lactate concentration is especially apparent in all-out exercise at altitudes above 4000 m.[36]

HEMATOLOGIC CHANGES. *The most important long-term adaptation to altitude is an increase in the blood's oxygen-carrying capacity.* Two factors are responsible: (1) an initial decrease in plasma volume, which is then followed by (2) a rapid formation of erythrocytes and hemoglobin.

1. *Decrease in plasma volume:* During the first few days at altitude, the red blood cells become more concentrated because of a decrease in plasma volume.[3,7,21] After a week at 2300 m, for example, the plasma volume decreases by about 8% whereas the concentrations of red blood cells (*hematocrit*) and hemoglobin increase 4% and 10%, respectively. A week at 4300 m (14,108 ft) causes a 16% to 25% decrease in plasma volume, whereas hematocrit rises about 6% and hemoglobin increases 20%.[7,21] This rather rapid adjustment in plasma volume and accompanying hemo-concentration causes the oxygen content of arterial blood to increase significantly above values observed immediately on ascent to altitude.

2. *Increase in red cell mass:* The reduced arterial oxygen pressure also stimulates an increase in the total number of red blood cells, a process termed *polycythemia.* This response is mediated by an erythrocyte-stimulating factor, *hemopoietin,* released from the kidneys and other tissues within 15 hours after altitude ascent.[1] In the weeks that follow, the production of erythrocytes in the marrow of the long bones increases considerably and remains elevated during residence at altitude.[17,39] A typical miner in the Andes, for example, has 38% more circulating red blood cells than his low-altitude counterpart. In some apparently healthy high-altitude natives, the red cell count may be more

than 50% greater than normal—8 million cells per cubic millimeter compared to 5.3 million for the native lowlander! In fact, during the 1973 Italian Mount Everest Expedition, a 40% increase in blood hemoglobin concentration and a 66% increase in hematocrit were noted for members acclimatized at 6500 m.[9] This probably approaches the limit of a beneficial rise in red blood cell concentration. Any further erythrocyte packing would increase the blood's viscosity and probably restrict oxygen diffusion and blood flow through the body.

In effect, polycythemia directly translates into a large increase in the blood's capacity to transport oxygen. The oxygen-carrying capacity of blood for high-altitude residents of Peru is 28% above sea level averages.[25] For well-acclimatized mountaineers, the oxygen-carrying capacity is 25 to 31 ml of oxygen per 100 ml of blood compared to about 19.7 ml for lowland residents.[34,45] Thus, even with the reduced saturation of hemoglobin at altitude, the actual *quantity* of oxygen in arterial blood closely approaches or even equals sea level values.

The general trend for increases in hemoglobin and hematocrit during altitude acclimatization is illustrated in Figure 23-2A. These data were obtained for eight young women at the University of Missouri (altitude 213 m) who lived and worked for 10 weeks at the 4267-m summit of Pikes Peak.[21] Because previous work of the researchers showed markedly fewer hematologic changes during acclimatization in women than in men, possibly due to inadequate iron intake, each woman received iron supplementation prior to, during, and on return from altitude.

Upon reaching Pikes Peak, red blood cell concentration increased rapidly. This was caused by a reduction in plasma volume during the first 24 hours at altitude. In the month that followed, hemoglobin concentration and hematocrit continued to increase and then stabilized for the remainder of the stay. Prealtitude values were established 2 weeks after the women returned to Missouri.

As shown in Figure 23-2B, iron supplementation increased the prealtitude values for hematocrit and hemoglobin. This is not surprising. As pointed out in Chapter 2, young women frequently suffer from mild iron deficiency. When the acclimatization curves for the iron-supplemented women were compared with those of another group of women not given additional iron, there was a greater hematocrit increase in

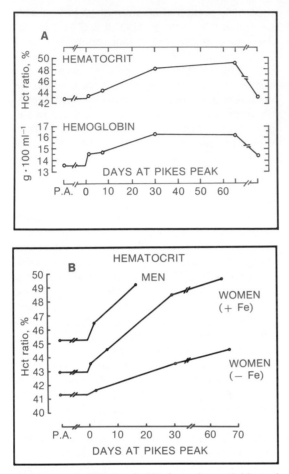

FIG. 23-2. *A, Effects of altitude on hemoglobin and hematocrit levels of 8 young women prior to, during, and 2 weeks after exposure to altitude of 4267 m. (From Hannon, J.P. et al.: Effects of altitude acclimatization on blood composition of women. J. Appl. Physiol., 26:540, 1968.) B, Hematocrit response of young women receiving supplemental iron (+ Fe) prior to and during altitude exposure compared to groups of male and female subjects receiving no supplemental iron (− Fe). P.A. = prealtitude values. (Courtesy of Dr. J.P. Hannon.)*

the group given supplements. Thus, at least in women, iron supplementation enhances the rate of hematocrit increase at altitude. The changes in these women were similar to hematologic observations for men at the same location.

CELLULAR ADAPTATIONS. Several local circulatory and cellular adaptations take place during long-term residence at high altitude that facili-

tate oxygen delivery and utilization.[13] For example, capillaries are more concentrated in the skeletal muscle of animals born and raised at high altitude than in those of animals of the same species born and raised at sea level.[44] This modification in local circulation reduces the distance for oxygen diffusion between the blood and tissues. Also, muscle biopsies from humans living at altitude indicate an increase in myoglobin by as much as 16% after acclimatization. This is complemented by an increase in the number of mitochondria and in the concentration of enzymes required for aerobic energy transfer.[38] Such adaptations increase the "storage" of oxygen in specific muscles and facilitate intracellular oxygen delivery and utilization, especially at low tissue P_{O_2}.

High-altitude natives also benefit from a slight shift to the right of the oxyhemoglobin dissociation curve. A decrease in the oxygen affinity of hemoglobin at altitude favors the release of available oxygen to the tissues for a given drop in P_{O_2}. This adaptation is probably due to an increase in the concentration of 2,3-diphosphoglycerate in red blood cells (see Chap. 13, "Red Blood Cell 2, 3-DPG") during long-term altitude residence.[14,32] An increase in 2,3-DPG coupled with an increased quantity of circulating hemoglobin places the altitude resident in a more favorable physiologic position for supplying oxygen to active tissue during strenuous exercise.

TIME REQUIRED FOR ACCLIMATIZATION

In general, the length of the acclimatization period is dependent on the altitude. Acclimation at one altitude ensures only partial adjustment to a higher elevation. As a broad guideline, about 2 weeks are required to adapt to altitudes up to 2300 m. Thereafter, for each 610-m increase in altitude, an additional week is required for full adaption up to an altitude of 4572 m.

For athletes desiring to compete at altitude, intense training should commence as soon as possible during the acclimatization period. This is necessary to minimize any detraining effects, especially since it is difficult to engage in hard training in the early days of one's altitude stay.[31] The benefits of acclimatization are probably lost *within 2 or 3 weeks* after returning to sea level.

METABOLIC, PHYSIOLOGIC, AND EXERCISE CAPACITIES AT ALTITUDE

The stress of high altitude imposes significant restrictions on work capacity and physiologic function. Even at lower altitudes, the body's adjustments do not fully compensate for the reduced oxygen pressure, and both physiologic function and exercise performance are compromised. In fact, certain circulatory parameters, especially stroke volume and maximum heart rate, are altered in a direction that contributes to a reduced capacity for oxygen transport.

Maximum Aerobic Capacity

Aerobic capacity shows a progressive and somewhat linear decrease with increases in altitude.[37] One can generally expect a 1.5 to 3.5% reduction in max $\dot{V}O_2$ for every 305 m (1000 ft) above 1524 m (5000 ft) altitude.[7,16,37] At 6248 m (20,500 ft), the max $\dot{V}O_2$ is approximately half the value at sea level whereas the maximum aerobic power of a relatively fit man atop Mount Everest would be about 960 ml of oxygen per minute.[33] This value corresponds to a work rate of only about 300 kg-m per minute on a bicycle ergometer.

The degree of physical conditioning prior to altitude exposure offers little protection, since the percentage reduction in max $\dot{V}O_2$ is equal in both trained and untrained individuals. For well-conditioned individuals, however, a particular work task at altitude still provides relatively less stress because it can be performed at a lower percentage of the trained person's maximum aerobic capacity.

Circulatory Factors

Even after several months of acclimatization, maximum aerobic power still remains significantly below sea level values.[16,19,30] This is partly due to the fact that the benefits of acclimatization are offset by a reduction in circulatory efficiency in moderate and strenuous exercise.[3,20,29]

SUBMAXIMAL EXERCISE. Although the immediate altitude response involves an increase in submaximal cardiac output (Table 23-2), the exercise cardiac output in the days and weeks of acclimatization that follow is significantly reduced and may even fall below sea level values.[3,27] This is due mainly to a *decrease in stroke volume* as the altitude stay progresses. With reduced cardiac output, oxygen consumption is maintained by an expanded a-$\bar{v}$ O_2 difference.

MAXIMAL EXERCISE. A reduction in maximum cardiac output also occurs after about a week at altitudes above 3048 m.[18,37,40,43] This reduction in blood flow during all-out exercise, which persists through one's altitude stay, is generally the combined effect of a decrease in maximum heart rate[30,40] and stroke volume.[20,27-29,37,40] The mechanism of diminished circulatory capacity is unclear, since myocardial hypoxia has not been demonstrated with ECG measurements,[22,40] or with coronary blood flow during vigorous exercise at high altitudes. The reduction in maximum heart rate at altitude may be influenced by enhanced parasympathetic tone induced by prolonged altitude exposure.[23]

Performance Measures

In order to perform aerobic exercise at the same relative intensity at altitude as at sea level, the pace must be slowed. If it is not, a larger portion of the energy for exercise is provided by anaerobic metabolism and fatigue develops. For example, a 2% to 13% decrement in performance is observed for fit subjects in the 1- and 3-mile runs at the medium altitude of 2300 meters.[16] This agrees with the 7.2% increase in 2-mile run times reported for highly trained middle-distance runners at the same altitude.[2] Even after 29 days of acclimatization, significant decrements in 3-mile running performance at high altitude are noted as compared to run times near sea level.[36]

ALTITUDE TRAINING AND SEA LEVEL PERFORMANCE

It is clear that altitude acclimatization improves one's capacity to work at altitude, especially at high altitude. What is not clear, however, is the effect of prior altitude exposure and altitude training on aerobic power and endurance performance immediately on return to sea level. Certainly, adaptations in local circulation and cellular function as well as the compensatory increase in ventilation and the blood's oxygen-carrying capacity should facilitate sea-level performance. Also, if tissue hypoxia is an important training stimulus, altitude *and* training should act synergistically so that the total effect exceeds that of similar training at sea level. Unfortunately, much of the previous altitude research has not been designed to evaluate adequately this possibility. Often, the activity level of the subjects is poorly controlled, so it is difficult to ascertain whether an improved max $\dot{V}O_2$ or performance score on return from altitude represents a training effect, an altitude effect, or synergism between altitude and training.[7,16]

Max $\dot{V}O_2$ on Return to Sea Level

When max VO_2 is used as the criterion, sea level performance is not significantly improved after living at altitude.[4,6,16] For example, a 14% decrement in aerobic capacity was noted in five runners when they arrived at an altitude of 2300 m. No significant improvement was observed during the next 6 weeks. When the athletes returned to sea level, max $\dot{V}O_2$ was no different than it had been before they left. Other researchers have also observed no significant change in the original 25% reduction in maximal aerobic power in young runners during 18 days at 3100 m.[19] On return to sea level, the max $\dot{V}O_2$ was about the same as the prealtitude measures. These findings have been duplicated at even higher altitudes.[6] Highly trained varsity trackmen from Pennsylvania State University were flown to Nunoa, Peru, altitude 4000 m (13,000 ft). They continued to train and acclimatize for 40 to 57 days. After the initial 3 days at altitude, max $\dot{V}O_2$ was reduced 29% below sea-level values; after 48 days, it was still

26% lower. Running performance after acclimatization was measured in the 440-yard, 880-yard, and 1- and 2-mile runs during a "track meet" with the altitude natives. Run times were still considerably slower than prealtitude times, especially in the longer runs. Furthermore, when the athletes returned to sea level, max $\dot{V}O_2$ and running performance were generally no different than they had been previously. On no occasion did a runner improve his previous prealtitude run time! In fact, running times in the longer events remained about 5% *below* prealtitude trials.

Even in those studies showing a small improvement in max $\dot{V}O_2$ at altitude and upon return to sea level,[13,15,28] the change is generally attributed to an increase in physical activity (that is, training and/or repeated testing) during the altitude exposure.

Some of the physiologic changes that occur during prolonged altitude exposure may actually negate adaptations that possibly could improve exercise performance upon return to sea level. The residual effects of a reduced maximum heart rate and stroke volume frequently observed at altitude certainly would not enhance sea-level performance. Any reduction in maximum cardiac output would offset the benefits derived from the blood's greater oxygen-carrying capacity. Although circulatory function does return to normal after a few weeks at sea level, so also do the potentially positive hematologic changes.[21]

Can Training Be Maintained at Altitude?

Exposure to altitudes of 2300 m and higher makes it nearly impossible for athletes to train at the same intensity as that engaged in at sea level. Table 23-3 shows this reduction in training intensity in relation to sea-level standards for six competitive college athletes.[31]

TABLE 23-3. *Effect of altitude on training intensity of six collegiate athletes*[a]

	ALTITUDE (M)			
	300	2300	3100	4000
Intensity of Workout (% of max $\dot{V}O_2$ at 200 m)	78	60	56	39

[a] From Kollias, J., and Buskirk, E.R.: Exercise and altitude. *In* Johnson, W.R., and Buskirk, E.R. (Eds.) Science and Medicine of Exercise and Sports, 2nd ed. New York, Harper and Row, 1974.

At successively higher elevations, the absolute training intensity was progressively below what was possible at a lower altitude. At 4000 m, for example, the runners were only able to train at 39% of the intensity of their sea-level workouts. This reduction in training intensity is possibly of such magnitude that an athlete may be unable to maintain peak condition for sea-level competition. Elite athletes might benefit by periodically returning from altitude to sea level for intensive training. This would help offset any "detraining" that takes place during a prolonged altitude stay. Such a procedure would not interfere with acclimatization and might even be beneficial to altitude performance.[11] If this approach is impractical, athletes should be sure to include speed work in their altitude training program to maintain muscle power.[5]

Is Altitude Training More Effective Than Sea-Level Training?

Equivalent groups were used to determine whether altitude training is more effective than sea-level training. Six highly trained middle-distance runners were trained at sea level for 3 weeks at 75% of sea level max $\dot{V}O_2$, whereas another group of six runners trained an equivalent distance at the same percentage of the max $\dot{V}O_2$ at 2300 m. The groups then exchanged training sites and continued training for 3 weeks at an intensity similar to that of the preceding group. Initially, 2-mile run times were 7.2% slower at altitude than at sea level. This improved about 2.0% for both groups after altitude training, but postaltitude performance at sea level was unchanged when compared to prealtitude sea-level runs. As shown in Figure 23-3, max $\dot{V}O_2$ for both groups at altitude was reduced initially by about 17.4%. This improved only slightly after 20 days of altitude training. When the runners were then measured at sea level, aerobic power was 2.8% *below* prealtitude sea level values! Clearly, for these well-conditioned middle-distance runners, there was no synergistic effect of hard aerobic training at medium altitude over equivalently severe training at sea level.

SUMMARY

1. The progressive reduction in ambient P_{O_2} upon ascent to altitude eventually leads to inad-

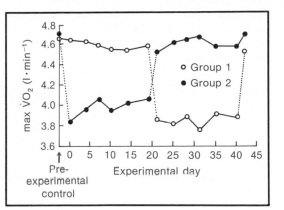

FIG. 23-3. *Maximal oxygen uptakes of two equivalent groups during training for 3 weeks at altitude and 3 weeks at sea level. Group 1 trained first at sea level and then continued training for 3 weeks at altitude. For group 2, the procedure was reversed as they trained first at altitude and then at sea level. (From Adams, W. C. et al.: Effects of equivalent sea-level and altitude training on $\dot{V}O_2$ max and running performance. J. Appl. Physiol., 39:262, 1975.)*

equate oxygenation of hemoglobin. This produces noticeable performance decrements in aerobic activities at altitudes of 2000 m and higher. Short-term anaerobic performances are not adversely affected at altitude, and certain activities may even show slight improvement.

2. The reduced P_{O_2} and accompanying hypoxia at altitude stimulate physiologic responses and adjustments that improve one's altitude tolerance during rest and exercise. The primary immediate responses are relative hyperventilation and increased submaximal cardiac output.

3. The longer term acclimatization process involves physiologic and metabolic adjustments that greatly improve tolerance to altitude hypoxia. The main adjustments involve (1) reestablishing the acid–base balance of the body fluids, (2) increased formation of hemoglobin and red blood cells, and (3) changes in local circulation and cellular function. Adjustments (2) and (3) significantly facilitate oxygen transport and utilization.

4. The rate of altitude acclimatization depends on the altitude. Noticeable improvements are generally observed within several days, and the major adjustments require about 2 weeks, although 4 to 6 weeks may be required to acclimatize to relatively high altitudes.

5. Acclimatization does not fully compensate for the stress of altitude. Even after accli-

matization, the max $\dot{V}O_2$ is decreased about 2% for every 300 m above 1500 m. This is paralleled by a drop in performance in endurance-related activities.

6. The inability to achieve sea level max $\dot{V}O_2$ values at altitude is partially explained by the fact that the beneficial effects of acclimatization are somewhat offset by altitude-related decrements in physiologic function. The latter involve mainly a reduction in maximum heart rate and stroke volume.

7. Although acclimatization to altitude would certainly seem to enhance aerobic power and endurance performance upon return to sea level, research results generally do not support this contention.

References

1. Abbrecht, P.H., and Littell, J.K.: Plasma erythropoietin in men and mice during acclimatization to different altitudes. J. Appl. Physiol., 32:54, 1972.
2. Adams, W.C. et al.: Effects of equivalent sea-level and altitude training on $\dot{V}O_2$ max and running performance. J. Appl. Physiol., 39:262, 1975.
3. Alexander, J.K. et al.: Reduction of stroke volume during exercise in man following ascent to 3,100 m altitude. J. Appl. Physiol. 23:849, 1967.
4. Balke, B. et al.: Effects of altitude acclimatization on work capacity. Fed. Proc., 15:7, 1966.
5. Balke, B. et al.: Variation in altitude and its effects on exercise performance. In Exercise Physiology. Edited by H.B. Falls. New York, Academic Press, 1968.
6. Buskirk, E.R. et al.: Maximal performance at altitude and on return from altitude in conditioned runners. J. Appl. Physiol., 23:259, 1967.
7. Buskirk, E.R. et al.: Physiology and performance of track athletes at various altitudes in the United States and Peru. In The International Symposium on the Effects of Altitude on Physical Performance. Edited by R.F. Goddard. Chicago, The Athletic Institute, 1967.
8. Buskirk, E.R.: Work and fatigue in high altitude. In Physiology of Work Capacity and Fatigue. Edited by E. Simonsen Springfield, Ill., Charles C Thomas, 1971.
9. Cerretelli, P.: Limiting factors to oxygen transport on Mount Everest. J. Appl. Physiol., 40:658, 1976.
10. Craig, A.B., Jr.: Olympics 1968: A post-mortum. Med. Sci. Sports, 1:177, 1969.
11. Daniels, J., and Oldridge N.: The effects of alternate exposure to altitude and sea level on world-class middle-distance runners. Med. Sci. Sports, 2:107, 1970.
12. Dempsey, J.A.: Effects of acute through life-long hypoxic exposure on exercise pulmonary gas exchange. Resp. Physiol. 13:62, 1971.
13. Gold, A.J. et al.: Effects of altitude stress on mitochondrial function. Am. J. Physiol. 224:946, 1973.
14. Eaton, J.W. et al.: Role of red cell 2, 3-diphosphoglycerate (DPG) in adaptation of men to altitude. J. Lab. Clin. Med. 73:603, 1969.
15. Faulkner, J.A. et al.: Effects of training at moderate altitude on physical performance capacity. J. Appl. Physiol. 23:85, 1967.
16. Faulkner, J.A. et al.: Maximum aerobic capacity and running performance at altitude. J. Appl. Physiol. 24:685, 1968.
17. Gordon, A.S. Hemopoietin. Physiol. Rev. 39:1, 1959.
18. Grover, R.F. et al.: Decreased stroke volume during maximum exercise in man at high altitude. Fed. Proc. 26:655, 1967.
19. Grover, R.F., and Reeves, J.T.: Exercise performance of athletes at sea level and 3,100 meters altitude. In The Effects of Altitude on Physical Performance. Edited by R.F. Goddard. Chicago, Ill., The Athletic Institute, 1967.

20. Grover, R.F. et al.: Alterations in coronary circulation of man following ascent to 3,100 m altitude. J. Appl. Physiol. *41:*832, 1976.
21. Hannon, J.P. et al.: Effects of altitude acclimatization on blood composition of women. J. Appl. Physiol., *26:*540, 1969.
22. Harris, C.W., and Hansen, J.E.: Electrocardiographic changes during exposure to high altitude. Am. J. Cardiol., *18:*183, 1966.
23. Hartley, L.H. et al.: Reduction of maximal exercise heart rate at altitude and its reversal with atropine. J. Appl. Physiol., *36:*362, 1976.
24. Hunt, J., and Hillary, E.: The Conquest of Everest. New York, E.P. Dutton Co., 1954.
25. Hurtado, A.: Animals in high altitudes: resident man. *In* Handbook of Physiology. Edited by D.B. Dill, E.F. Adolph, and C.G. Wilber. Baltimore, The Williams and Wilkins Co., 1964.
26. Hurtado, A. et al.: Mechanisms of natural acclimatization. Studies on the native resident of Morococha, Peru, at an altitude of 14,900 ft. Technical Documentary Report No. SAM-TDR-56-1, Washington, D.C., 1956, USAF School of Aerospace Medicine.
27. Klausen, K.: Cardiac output in man in rest and work during and after acclimatization to 3800 m. J. Appl. Physiol., *21:*609, 1966.
28. Klausen, K. et al.: Effect of high altitude on maximal working capacity. J. Appl. Physiol., *21:*1191, 1966.
29. Klausen K.: Exercise under hypoxic conditions. Med. Sci. Sports, *1:*43, 1969.
30. Klausen, K. et al.: Exercise at ambient and high oxygen pressure at high altitude and at sea level. J. Appl. Physiol., *29:*456, 1970.
31. Kollias, J., and Buskirk, E.R.: Exercise at altitude. *In* Science and Medicine of Exercise and Sports. Edited by W.R. Johnson and E.R. Buskirk. New York, Harper and Row, 1974.
32. Lenfant, C.P. et al.: Effect of chronic hypoxic hypoxia on the O_2-Hb dissociation curve and respiratory gas transport in man. Resp. Physiol., *7:*7, 1969.
33. Pugh, L.C.G.E.: Muscular exercise on Mount Everest. J. Physiol., *141:*233, 1958.
34. Pugh, L.C.G.E.: Physiological and medical aspects of the Himalayan Scientific and Mountaineering Expedition, 1960–61. Brit. Med. J. *2:*621, 1962.
35. Pugh, L.C.G.E.: Muscular exercise at great altitudes. J. Appl. Physiol., *19:*431, 1964.
36. Pugh, L.C.G.E.: Athletes at altitude. J. Physiol., *192:*619, 1967.
37. Pugh, L.C.G.E.: Animals in high altitudes: Man above 5000 meters—mountain exploration. *In* Handbook of Physiology. Edited by D.B. Dill, E.F. Adolph, and C.G. Wilber. Baltimore, The Williams and Wilkins Co., 1964.
38. Reynafarje, C.: Myoglobin content and enzymatic activity of muscle and alti-adaptation. J. Appl. Physiol., *17:*301, 1962.
39. Reynafarje, C.: Hematologic changes during rest and physical activity in man at high altitude. *In* The Physiological Effects of High Altitude. Edited by W.H. Weihe. New York, The Macmillan Co., 1964.
40. Saltin, B. et al.: Maximal oxygen uptake and cardiac output after 2 weeks at 4300 m. J. Appl. Physiol., *25:*400, 1968.
41. Sorensen, S.C., and Severinghaus, J.: Respiratory sensitivity to acute hypoxia in man born at sea level living at high altitude. J. Appl. Physiol., *25:*211, 1968.
42. Stenberg, J. et al.: Hemodynamic response to work at simulated altitude, 4,000 m. J. Appl. Physiol., *21:*1589, 1966.
43. Vogel, J.A. et al.: Cardiovascular responses in man during exhaustive work at sea level and high altitude. J. Appl. Physiol., *23:*531, 1967.
44. Valdivia, E.: Total capillary bed in striated muscle of guinea pigs native to Peruvian mountains. Am. J. Physiol., *194:*585, 1958.
45. West, J.B. et al.: Arterial oxygen saturation during exercise at high altitude. J. Appl. Physiol., *17:*617, 1962.

Exercise and Thermal Stress

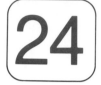
24

The requirements for *thermoregulation* can be considerable; the price for failure is death. Only a drop in deep body temperature of 10°C and an increase of 5°C can be tolerated. This has been vividly illustrated by the relatively large number of unnecessary deaths of football players that were the direct result of excessive heat stress during practice. Such tragedies can be minimized if not totally avoided with the proper understanding of thermoregulation and the best ways to support these mechanisms. A large part of this responsibility rests with the people who organize and guide sport and physical activity programs.

PART 1

Mechanisms of Thermoregulation

THERMAL BALANCE

As shown in Figure 24-1, body temperature or, more specifically, the temperature of the deeper tissues or *core,* is in dynamic equilibrium as a result of a balance between factors that add and subtract body heat. This balance is maintained by the integration of mechanisms that alter heat transfer to the periphery or *shell,* regulate evaporative cooling, and vary the body's rate of heat production. If heat gain outstrips heat loss, as can readily occur in vigorous exercise in a warm environment, core temperature rises; in the cold, on the other hand, heat loss often exceeds heat production and core temperature falls.

Heat is gained directly from the reactions of energy metabolism. When muscles become active, their heat contribution is tremendous.

From shivering alone, the total metabolic rate can increase three to fivefold.[35] During vigorous exercise, the metabolic rate increases to 20 to 25 times above the basal level, which theoretically can increase core temperature by about 1°C every 5 minutes! Heat is also absorbed from the environment by solar radiation and from objects that are warmer than the body. Heat is lost by the physical mechanisms of radiation, conduction, and convection, and the vaporization of water from the skin and respiratory passages.

Circulatory adjustments provide the "fine tuning" for temperature regulation. Heat is conserved by rapidly shunting blood deep to the cranial, thoracic, and abdominal cavities and portions of the muscle mass. This optimizes the insulation from subcutaneous fat and other portions of the body's shell. Conversely, when internal heat becomes excessive, peripheral

334

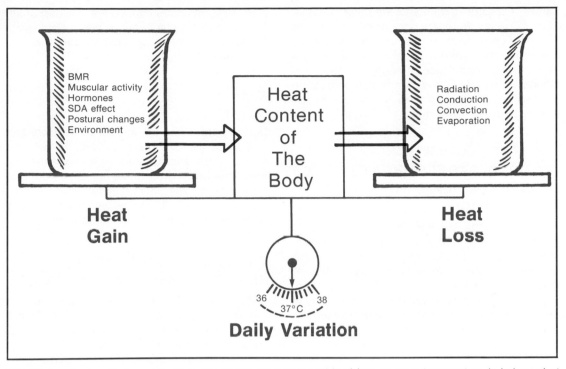

FIG. 24-1. *Factors that contribute to the body's heat gain and heat loss so core temperature is balanced at approximately 37°C.*

vessels dilate and warm blood is channeled to the cooler periphery. The drive for thermal balance is so strong that it may elicit a sweat rate of 3.5 liters per hour in exercise in the heat or an oxygen consumption of 1000 ml per minute brought on by shivering in severe cold.

HYPOTHALAMIC REGULATION OF TEMPERATURE

The *hypothalamus* contains the coordinating center for the various processes of temperature regulation. This group of specialized neurons at the floor of the brain acts as a "thermostat" (usually set and carefully regulated at 37°C±1°C) that makes thermoregulatory adjustments to deviations from a temperature norm. Unlike our home thermostat, however, the hypothalamus cannot "turn off" the heat; it can only initiate responses to protect the body from a buildup or loss of heat.

Heat-regulating mechanisms are activated in two ways: (1) by thermal receptors in the skin

that provide input to the central control center, and (2) by direct stimulation of the hypothalamus through changes in blood temperature perfusing these areas.

Peripheral thermal receptors, or sensors responsive to rapid changes in heat and cold, are distributed predominantly as free nerve endings in the skin. The cutaneous cold receptors are generally toward the skin surface and are more abundant than the deeper warmth receptors. They play an important role in initiating the regulatory response to a cold environment. The cutaneous thermal receptors act as an "early warning system" that relays sensory information to the hypothalamus and cortex to bring about appropriate heat-conserving or heat-dissipating adjustments and to cause the individual consciously to seek relief from the thermal challenge.

A central regulatory center plays an important role in maintaining thermal balance. In addition to peripheral input, cells in the anterior portion of the hypothalamus are themselves capable of detecting changes in blood temperature. These cells then activate other hypothalamic regions to initiate coordinated responses for heat conservation (posterior hypothalamus) or heat loss (anterior hypothalamus). In contrast to the importance of peripheral receptors in detecting cold, *body warmth is monitored mainly by the temperature of the blood perfusing the hypothalamus.*

THERMOREGULATION IN COLD STRESS: HEAT CONSERVATION AND HEAT PRODUCTION

Normally, the gradient for heat transfer is from the body to the environment, and core temperature is maintained without excessive physiologic strain. In extreme cold, however, excessive heat loss can occur. In this situation, heat production is increased and heat loss is retarded as adjustments are made to prevent a fall in internal temperature.

Vascular Adjustments

Stimulation of cutaneous cold receptors causes constriction of peripheral blood vessels, which immediately reduces the flow of warm blood to the body's cooler surface and redirects it to the warmer core. Consequently, skin temperature falls toward the ambient temperature, and the insulatory benefits of skin and subcutaneous fat are used to their maximal advantage. A fat person, therefore, can derive great benefits from this heat-conserving mechanism when exposed to cold stress.[43,46,48,51]

Muscular Activity

Although significant metabolic heat is generated through shivering, the greatest contribution of muscle to defense against cold occurs during physical activity. Exercise energy metabolism can sustain a constant core temperature in air temperature as low as $-30°C$ ($-22°$ F) without the need for heavy, restrictive clothing. It should be noted, however, that the thermoregulatory defense against cold is mediated by internal temperature and *not* by the heat production in the body per se.[47] Thus, shivering is observed even during exercise if the core temperature is low. As a result, exer-

cise oxygen consumption is proportionally higher (due directly to shivering) in cold stress than it is during the same exercise in a warmer environment.[20,43,48]

Hormonal Output

During cold exposure, increased heat production is due partially to the action of the two hormones of the adrenal medulla: epinephrine and norepinephrine. It is also possible that prolonged cold stress increases the release of the thyroid hormone, thyroxine, which leads to sustained elevation in resting metabolism.

THERMOREGULATION IN HEAT STRESS: HEAT LOSS

The mechanisms for thermoregulation are geared to protect against overheating. This is particularly important during exercise in hot weather when significant heat must be dissipated to the environment.[32] Body heat may be lost by *radiation, conduction, convection,* and *evaporation.*

Heat Loss by Radiation

Objects are continually emitting electromagnetic heat waves. Because our bodies are usually warmer than the environment, the net exchange of radiant heat energy is through the air to the solid, cooler objects in the environment. This form of heat transfer does not require molecular contact with the warmer object and is essentially the means by which the sun's rays warm the earth. A person can remain warm by absorbing radiant heat energy from direct sunlight (or reflected from the snow, sand, or water), even in subfreezing temperatures. When the temperature of objects in the environment exceeds skin temperature, radiant heat energy is absorbed from the surroundings. Under these conditions, the only avenue for heat loss is from evaporative cooling (see below).

Heat Loss by Conduction

This process of heat exchange involves the direct transfer of heat through a liquid, solid, or gas from one molecule to another. Although most of the body heat is transported to the shell by the circulation, a small amount continually moves by conduction directly through the deep tissues to the cooler surface. Here, heat loss by conduction involves the warming of air molecules and cooler surfaces in contact with the skin.

The rate of conductive heat loss depends on the temperature gradient between the skin and surrounding surfaces and their thermal qualities. For example, heat loss in water can be considerable.[20] This fact is clearly illustrated by placing one hand in water at room temperature. The hand in water feels much colder than the hand in air—even though the water is the *same* temperature as the air. This occurs because water can absorb several thousand times more heat than air and conduct it away from the warm body. For this reason, sitting in an indoor swimming pool is much more uncomfortable than sitting on the pool deck, even though the air and water are the *same* temperature.

Heat Loss by Convection

The effectiveness of heat loss by conduction depends on how rapidly the air (or water) adjacent to the body is exchanged once it becomes warmed. If air movement or *convection* is slow, the air next to the skin is warmed and acts as a zone of insulation. This minimizes further conductive heat loss. Conversely, if the warmer air surrounding the body is continually replaced by cooler air (as occurs on a breezy day or in a room with a fan or during running), heat loss increases as convective currents carry the heat away. Air currents at 4 miles per hour are about twice as effective for cooling as air currents at 1 mile per hour. This is the basis of the *wind chill index,* which gives the equivalent still air temperature for a particular ambient temperature at different wind velocities. In water, convection is also an important factor because heat is lost more rapidly while swimming than while lying motionless in the water.[48]

Heat Loss by Evaporation

Evaporation provides the major physiologic defense against overheating. Heat is continually transferred to the environment as water is vaporized from the respiratory passages and skin surface. For each liter of water that vaporizes, 580 kcal are extracted from the body and transferred to the environment.

Approximately 3 million sweat glands are distributed throughout the surface of the body. In response to heat stress, these glands secrete large quantities of weak saline solution (hypotonic—0.2%–0.4% NaCl). When sweat comes in contact with the skin, a cooling effect occurs as sweat evaporates. The cooled skin in turn serves to cool the blood that has been shunted from the interior to the surface. In addition to heat loss via sweating, about 500 ml of water seep through the skin each day and evaporate to the environment. Also, about 300 ml of water vaporize from the moist mucous membranes of the respiratory passages. This is seen as "foggy breath" in very cold weather.

HEAT LOSS AT HIGH AMBIENT TEMPERATURES. As ambient temperature increases, the effectiveness of heat loss by conduction, convection, and radiation decreases. When ambient temperature exceeds body temperature, heat is actually *gained* by these mechanisms of thermal transfer. In such environments (or when conduction, convection, and radiation are inadequate to dissipate a large metabolic heat load), the *only* means for heat dissipation is by sweat evaporation and the small contribution to cooling provided by the vaporization of water from the respiratory tract. In fact, the rate of sweating increases directly with the ambient temperature.[50]

HEAT LOSS IN HIGH HUMIDITY. The total sweat vaporized from the skin depends on three factors: (1) the surface exposed to the environment, (2) the temperature and humidity of the ambient air, and (3) the convective air currents about the body. *By far, relative humidity is the most important factor determining the effectiveness of evaporative heat loss.* Relative humidity is defined as the ratio of water in ambient air to the total quantity of moisture that can be carried in air at a particular ambient temperature, expressed as a percentage. For example, 40% relative humidity means that ambient air contains only 40% of the air's moisture-carrying capacity at the specific temperature. When humidity is high, the ambient vapor pressure approaches that of the moist skin (about 40 mm Hg) and evaporation is greatly reduced, Thus, this avenue for heat loss is essentially closed, even though large quantities of sweat bead on the skin and eventually roll off. This form of sweating represents a *useless* water loss that can lead to a dangerous state of dehydration and overheating.

Evaporative cooling is also thwarted by continually drying the skin with a towel before sweat has a chance to evaporate. *Sweat per se does not cool the skin; evaporation cools the skin.* As long as the humidity is low, relatively high environmental temperatures are tolerated. For this reason, hot–dry desert climates are more comfortable than cooler but more humid tropical climates.

Integration of Heat-Dissipating Mechanisms

The mechanisms for heat loss are the same whether the heat load is imposed internally (metabolic heat) or externally (environmental heat).

CIRCULATION. The circulatory system serves as the "workhorse" in maintaining thermal homeostasis. Superficial venous and arterial blood vessels dilate to divert warm blood to the body shell. This is seen as a flushed or reddened face on a hot day or during vigorous exercise. With extreme heat stress, 15% to 25% of the cardiac output passes through the skin. This greatly increases the thermal conductance of peripheral tissues and favors radiative heat loss to the environment, especially from the hands, forehead, forearms, ears, and tibial areas.

EVAPORATION. Sweating begins within 1.5 seconds after the start of vigorous exercise,[8] and, after about 30 minutes, reaches an equilibrium that is in direct relation to the work load.[32] An effective heat defense is established when evaporative cooling is combined with a large cutaneous blood flow. The cooled peripheral blood then returns to the deeper tissues to pick up additional heat.

HORMONAL ADJUSTMENTS. Because both water and electrolytes are lost through sweating, certain hormonal adjustments are initiated in heat stress as the body attempts to conserve salts and fluid. The pituitary gland releases *antidiuretic hormone* (ADH) to increase water reab-

sorption from the kidneys. This causes the urine to become more concentrated during heat stress. Concurrently, during repeated days of exercise in the heat,[62] or with just a single bout of exercise,[19] the sodium-conserving hormone *aldosterone* is released from the *adrenal cortex*. This hormone acts on the renal tubules to increase the reabsorption of sodium. Through as yet undefined mechanisms, the sodium concentration in sweat is also decreased during repeated heat exposure to aid in conserving electrolytes.[62]

EFFECTS OF CLOTHING ON THERMOREGULATION

Clothing insulates the body from its surroundings. It may reduce radiant heat gain in a hot environment or retard conductive and convective heat loss in the cold.

Cold-Weather Clothing

In providing insulation from the cold, the mesh of the cloth fibers traps air that then becomes warm. Because both cloth and air are poor heat conductors, a barrier to heat loss is established; the thicker the zone of trapped air next to the skin, the more effective is the insulation. For this reason, several layers of light clothing, or garments lined with animal fur, feathers, or synthetic fabrics (with numerous layers of trapped air), provide much greater insulation than a single bulky layer of winter clothing. When clothing becomes wet, through either external moisture or condensation from sweating, it loses its insulating properties and actually facilitates heat transfer *from* the body, because water conducts heat much faster than air.

When working in the cold, the problem is usually not one of adequate insulation but rather the dissipation of metabolic heat through a thick air–clothing barrier.[10] Cross-country skiers alleviate this problem by removing layers of clothing as the body becomes warm. In this way, core temperature is maintained without reliance on evaporative cooling. The ideal winter garment in dry weather is impermeable to air movement but permits the escape of water vapor from the skin through the clothing if sweating should occur.

Warm-Weather Clothing

Dry clothing, no matter how light, retards heat exchange compared to the same clothing soaking wet. The practice of switching to a dry tennis, basketball, or football uniform in hot weather makes little sense from the standpoint of temperature regulation. *Evaporative heat loss occurs only when the clothing becomes wet throughout.* A dry uniform simply prolongs the time lag between sweating and cooling.

Different materials absorb water at different rates. Cottons and linens absorb moisture readily. On the other hand, heavy "sweat shirts" and clothing made of rubber or plastic produce high relative humidity close to the skin and retard the vaporization of moisture from the skin surface; this significantly inhibits or even prevents evaporative cooling. Warm-weather clothing should be loose fitting to permit the free circulation of air between the skin and environment to promote water movement away from the skin. Color is also important because dark colors absorb light and add to the radiant heat gain whereas light colors reflect heat rays.

Football Uniforms

Of all athletic uniforms and equipment, those used in *football* present the most significant barrier to heat dissipation[30,42] Even with loose-fitting porous jerseys, the wrappings, the padding (with its plastic covering), the helmet, and other objects of "armour" effectively seal off 50% of the body surface from the benefits of evaporative cooling. To this is added the metabolic cost of carrying the 6 or 7 kg of equipment, frequently over a relatively hot artificial playing surface.

The metabolic and thermal stress provided by the football uniform is shown in Figure 24-2. In this experiment, nine men were tested at 25.6°C (78°F) and 35% relative humidity while running for 30 minutes.

In one test, the men wore only shorts; in another, they wore the complete football uniform including helmet and plastic padding. In a third series of measures, they wore shorts and carried a backpack containing 6.2 kg, exactly the weight of the uniform.

The effects of the uniform on heat dissipation are clear. Rectal temperature and skin temperature were significantly higher in both exercise and recovery than either of the other exercise conditions. The temperature directly beneath the padding averaged only 1°C less than rectal temperature. This meant that subcutaneous blood in these areas was cooled only about one-fifth as much as skin surface exposed to the environment. Because rectal temperature remained elevated in recovery with uniforms, it appears that a "rest" period is of limited value in normalizing thermal regulation unless the uniform is removed.

As shown by the dashed line, a large portion of the heat load was provided simply by the weight of the uniform. However, skin temperatures were much cooler and sweat rates less when the uniform was not worn. Without the uniform, evaporation from the skin was relatively free, whereas the uniform insulated the athlete and reduced the evaporative surface.

SUMMARY

1. Humans tolerate only relatively small variations in internal temperature. Consequently, exposure to heat or cold stress initiates thermoregulatory mechanisms that generate and conserve heat at low ambient temperatures and dissipate heat at high temperatures.

2. The "thermostat" for temperature regulation is located in the hypothalamus. This coordinating center initiates adjustments in response to input from thermal receptors in the skin as well as changes in the temperature of blood perfusing hypothalamic regions.

3. Heat conservation in cold stress is achieved by vascular adjustments that shunt blood from the cooler periphery to the warmer deep tissues of the body's core. If this is ineffective, shivering is initiated to provide a significant input of metabolic heat. Hormones that cause a sustained elevation in resting metabolism are also released.

4. In response to heat stress, warm blood is diverted from the body's core to the shell. Body heat is lost by radiation, conduction, convection, and evaporation. At high ambient temperatures and during exercise, evaporation provides the major physiologic defense against overheating.

5. In warm, humid environments, the effectiveness of evaporative heat loss is dramatically reduced. This makes one especially susceptible to a dangerous state of dehydration and spiraling core temperature.

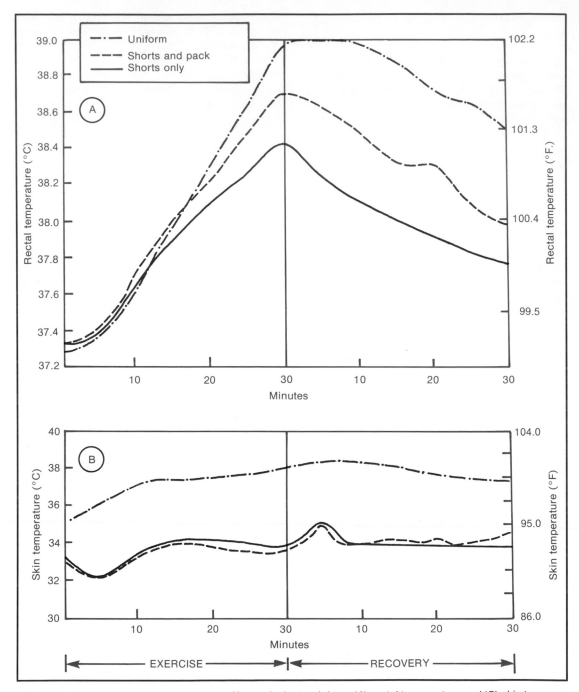

FIG. 24-2. *Effects of full football uniform and its equivalent weight on (A) rectal temperature and (B) skin temperature during exercise. Subjects ran at 9.6 km·h⁻¹ for 30 minutes at 26.5°C and 35% relative humidity. Due to its effect in retarding evaporative cooling, the uniform caused the largest heat stress as indicated by significant elevations in rectal and skin temperatures. (From Mathews, D.K. et al.: Physiological responses during exercise and recovery in a football uniform. J. Appl. Physiol., 26:611, 1969.)*

6. Several layers of light clothing provide a relatively thick zone of trapped air against the skin. This gives more effective insulation from the cold than a single thick layer of winter clothing. When clothing becomes wet, insulation is lost and heat flow from a body is greatly facilitated.

7. The metabolic heat generated during vigorous exercise generally maintains body temperature in cold environments, even if the person wears only little clothing.

8. The ideal warm-weather clothing is lightweight, loose-fitting, and light in color. Even wearing this clothing, heat loss is retarded until the clothing becomes wet and evaporative cooling can proceed.

9. Football uniforms impose a significant barrier to heat dissipation because they effectively seal off about 50% of the body's surface from the benefits of evaporative cooling.

PART 2

Thermoregulation During Exercise in the Heat

When exercising in the heat, the body is faced with two competitive demands: (1) the muscles require oxygen to sustain energy metabolism and, equally important, (2) metabolic heat must be transported by the blood from the deep tissues to the periphery. This blood cannot deliver its oxygen to the working muscles.

In addition to vascular adjustments, the dissipation of metabolic heat during exercise in hot weather is almost totally dependent on the refrigeration mechanism of evaporative cooling. A price is paid, however, as demands are placed on the body's fluid reserves, and a relative state of dehydration frequently occurs. Excessive sweating leads to more serious fluid loss and an accompanying reduction in blood volume. This can cause circulatory failure, and core temperature may rise to lethal levels.

CIRCULATORY ADJUSTMENTS

For reasons not fully understood, the stroke volume of the heart is usually lower during exercise in the heat,[56,68] This is compensated for, however, by a proportionate increase in heart rate at all levels of submaximal exercise. Consequently, cardiac outputs in submaximal exercise are similar in hot and cool environments.[59,60]

In the heat, adequate cutaneous and muscle blood flow are achieved at the expense of tissues that can temporarily compromise their blood supply.[57,68] For example, vasodilatation of the subcutaneous vessels is rapidly countered by compensatory constriction of the splanchnic vascular bed and renal tissues. Aside from redirecting blood to areas in great need, vasoconstriction in the viscera serves to increase total vascular resistance. In this way, arterial blood pressure is maintained during work in the heat.

Even when submaximal exercise is well tolerated in the heat, the work is generally accomplished with a greater dependence on anaerobic metabolism than in cooler conditions. This results in the early accumulation of lactic acid[11,29] and encroachment on glycogen stores[29] during submaximal exercise. An increased lactic acid level is probably due to (1) decreased lactate uptake by the liver, because significant reductions in hepatic blood flow occur during exercise in the heat,[59] and (2) reduced muscle circulation, because large quantities of blood are shunted to the periphery for heat dissipation. Both of these factors may be responsible for early fatigue during only moderate exercise in the heat.

CORE TEMPERATURE DURING EXERCISE

The heat generated in exercising muscles can raise body temperature to fever levels that would incapacitate a person if caused by external heat stress alone.[3] During 10 minutes of moderate bicycle exercise, for example, the temperature of the thigh muscles increases to about 38.8°C (102°F) whereas skin temperature remains relatively unchanged. In fact, champion distance runners show no ill effects from rectal temperatures as high as 41°C (105.8°F) recorded at the end of a 3-mile race.[54]

Within limits, the increase in core temperature in exercise does not reflect a failure of the heat-dissipating mechanisms. On the contrary it is a well-regulated response that even occurs during exercise in the cold.[52] Figure 24-3A illustrates the relationship between esophageal temperature and oxygen consumption for four men and two women of varying fitness levels during exercise of increasing severity.[61]

For all subjects, body temperature increases to a higher level as the exercise becomes more intense. However, wide variability in temperature response exists between subjects. When temperature is plotted in relation to oxygen consumption expressed as a percentage of each person's max $\dot{V}O_2$ (Fig. 24-3B), the lines move closer together. *It is the relative work load (i.e., the percentage of one's capacity) that determines the change in core temperature with exercise.*[4,26,33,61,70] In general, work in a com-

fortable environment at 50% of max $\dot{V}O_2$ increases temperature to a new steady level of about 37.3°C (99°F), whereas work at 75% of maximum elevates core temperature to 38.5°C (101°F), regardless of the absolute level of oxygen consumption. Thus, at the same percentage of max $\dot{V}O_2$, a fit person generates more energy in exercise yet still has the same core temperature as a less fit counterpart.[61] The extra metabolic heat is dissipated in a larger sweat output by the person working at the higher absolute work load. Of course, at the same workload, the trained person will be exercising with a lower core temperature. More than likely, the resetting of the thermostat at a higher level during exercise is a favorable adjustment that creates an optimal thermal environment for physiologic and metabolic function.

WATER LOSS IN THE HEAT—DEHYDRATION

In a few hours of hard exercise in the heat, water loss or *dehydration* can reach proportions that impede heat dissipation and severely compromise cardiovascular function and work capacity. For an acclimatized person, water loss by sweating may reach a peak of about 3 liters per hour during severe work and average nearly 12 liters (26 lb) on a daily basis.[40]

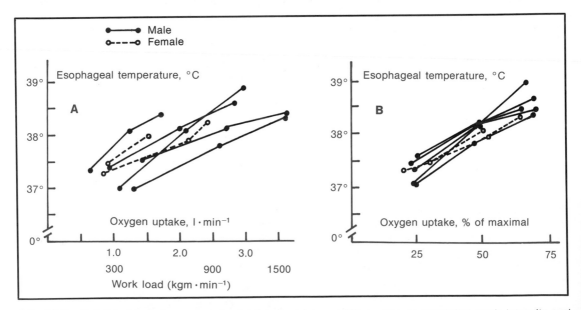

FIG. 24-3. *Relationship between esophagial temperature and (A) oxygen consumption–work intensity and (B) oxygen uptake as a percent of each person's max $\dot{V}O_2$. (From Saltin, B., and Hermansen, L.: Esophagial, rectal, and muscle temperature during exercise. J. Appl. Physiol., 21:1757, 1966.)*

Marathon runners frequently experience fluid losses in excess of 5 liters during competition.[52] For these athletes, the loss represents 6% to 10% of their body weight. Distance running is not the only sport where there are large sweat outputs. Football, basketball, and hockey players may lose similar quantities of fluid in the course of a contest. It has also been reported that high school wrestlers lose 9% to 13% of their preseason body weight prior to certification; the greatest portion of this weight loss comes from voluntarily reducing water intake and excessive sweating just prior to the weigh-in.[71] In the desire to "make weight," high school and collegiate wrestlers usually compete in a dehydrated state.[72]

Fluid loss is particularly apparent during exercise in hot–humid environments. In this situation, the effectiveness of evaporative cooling is thwarted by the high vapor pressure of ambient air. As illustrated in Figure 24-4, there is a linear relationship between sweat rate, both at rest and during exercise, and the air's moisture content.[39] Ironically, the excessive output of sweat in high humidity contributes little to cooling, because evaporation is at a minimum. In this regard, clothing that retards the rapid diffusion and subsequent evaporation of sweat creates an extremely humid microclimate that envelops a large portion of the body. Such clothing "encourages" dehydration and overheating.

Performance Decrements

Body water deficits of only about 1.5 liters are tolerated by adults without an abnormal physiologic response, although a fluid loss equivalent to as little as 1% of body weight is associated with a significant increase in rectal temperature compared to the same exercise with normal hydration.[11,25] When water loss reaches 4% to 5% of body weight, a definite impairment in physical work capacity[53,60] and physiologic function,[9,12,60] is noted. Because a larger portion of water loss through sweating comes from the blood than from other fluid compartments,[2,14,16] circulatory capacity is adversely affected as sweat loss progresses (if water is not continually replenished). This is manifested by a decrease in circulating blood volume, a fall in stroke volume and a compensatory increase in heart rate, and a general deterioration in circulatory efficiency during exercise. In terms of performance, a 48% reduction in walking endurance was noted when subjects were dehydrated to 4.3% of body weight; concurrently, max $\dot{V}O_2$ decreased by 22%.[21] In these same experiments, endurance performance and max $\dot{V}O_2$ were reduced by 22% and 10%, respectively, when dehydration averaged only 1.9% of body weight. *Clearly, dehydration reduces the capability of the circulatory and temperature-regulating systems to meet the metabolic and thermal stress of exercise.*

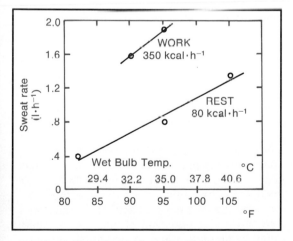

FIG. 24-4. *The effect of humidity (wet-bulb temperature) on sweat rate at rest and during work in the heat. Ambient temperature (dry-bulb) at all times was 43.3°C (110°F). (From Iampietro, P. F.: Exercise in hot environments. In Frontiers of Fitness. Edited by R. J. Shephard. Springfield, Ill., Charles C Thomas, 1971.)*

Use of Diuretics

A greater percentage of water is drawn from the plasma if body water is lost as a result of diuretic-induced dehydration.[12] Thus, wrestlers who use these drugs to lose body water rapidly to "make weight" are at a distinct disadvantage because of a disproportionate reduction in plasma volume and its negative effects on thermoregulation and cardiovascular function. Chemicals to induce vomiting and diarrhea are used by athletes to cause weight loss. Not only does this abuse lead to dehydration, but it may also cause excessive potassium loss with an accompanying muscle weakness. The use of such drugs would clearly give the competitive "edge" to the opponent.

WATER
REPLACEMENT

The primary aim of fluid replacement is to maintain plasma volume so that circulation and sweating can progress at optimal levels. Prevention of dehydration and its consequences can only be achieved with an adequate and strictly adhered to water replacement schedule. This may be "easier said than done," because some coaches and athletes feel that ingesting water hinders performance. Also, in some sports, water intake is actually prohibited. In international marathon competition prior to the 1976 Olympics, drinking fluids was prohibited during the first 10 km of this 42 km race! For wrestlers, dehydration is a "way of life," because young boys and men lose considerable weight to wrestle in a lower weight class. The enlightened exercise specialist must be keenly aware of the importance of proper hydration for thermoregulation, exercise performance, and safety.

Periodic application of cold towels to the forehead and abdomen during exercise or a cold shower prior to exercise in the heat are practical approaches to reducing heat stress.[27] These remedies generally result in a slower exercise heart rate, lower rectal temperature, and reduced fluid loss. The cold treatments cool the blood in the periphery and facilitate heat transfer from the body surface. It must be stressed, however, that the most effective defense against heat is adequate hydration. This is achieved by balancing water loss with water intake, not by pouring water over the head or body.

Practical Recommendations for
Fluid Replacement

Ingestion of "extra" water or *hyperhydration* prior to exercise in the heat provides some protection because it increases sweating during exercise and brings about a significant decrease in core temperature.[32,45] In this regard, it would be wise to consume 400 to 600 ml (13–20 oz.) of cold water 10 to 20 minutes *before* exercising in the heat. This procedure, however, does not replace the need for continual fluid replacement and is not as effective in maintaining thermal balance as consuming an equal volume of water *during* the exercise.[31] *In activities like distance running, matching fluid loss with fluid intake may be virtually impossible because only about 800 ml of fluid can be emptied from the stomach each hour during vigorous exercise.* This is insufficient to match a water loss that may average nearly 2 liters per hour. Consequently, athletes must be carefully monitored during exercise even if they are permitted free access to water.

Studies of fluid absorption indicate that cold fluids (5°C; 41°F) are emptied from the stomach at a significantly faster rate than fluids at body temperature.[15] The volume of fluid in the stomach is also of importance because gastric emptying speeds up for each 100 ml increase in gastric volume up to 600 ml. A volume of about 250 ml (8.5 oz) ingested at 10- to 15-minute intervals is probably a realistic goal because larger volumes tend to produce feelings of a "full stomach." Thus, to obtain a high rate of fluid absorption, the stomach should remain partially filled and the fluid ingested should be relatively cold.

Of considerable importance is the observation that gastric emptying is *retarded* when the ingested fluid contains sugar, whether in the form of glucose, fructose, or sucrose! With intense exercise, even a small amount of carbohydrate blocks fluid movement from the stomach into the intestinal tract.[15] From a practical standpoint, during exercise in the heat, when the need for water greatly exceeds the need for carbohydrate supplementation, glucose in solution hinders water replenishment. Certainly, drinking commercial preparations such as Gatorade, Instant Replay, or Take-Five, which contain 5% glucose, would significantly *retard* the replacement of lost fluid during exercise in the heat. On the other hand, during prolonged exercise in a cool environment, fluid loss from sweating may not be great. Here, a reduction in gastric emptying and fluid uptake can be tolerated and a strong sugar solution (15–30 g per 100 ml water) may be beneficial. One should keep in mind, however, that it may take 20 to 30 minutes for the carbohydrate to reach the muscles after it enters the stomach. The "trade-off" between the composition of the fluid ingested and the rate of gastric emptying must be evaluated on the basis of environmental and metabolic demands. *In terms of survival, fluid replacement is primary during prolonged exercise in the heat.*

Adequacy of Rehydration

Changes in body weight should be used to indicate water loss in exercise and the adequacy of rehydration during and following exercise. Recommendations for fluid intake based on weight loss during exercise are presented in Table 24-1. Although these standards were developed for a 90-minute football practice, they are easily adapted to most exercise situations.

Coaches can have their athletes "weigh-in" before and after practice and insist that weight loss be minimized by periodic water breaks during activity. Water must be available *and* consumed during practice and competition. Because the thirst mechanism is generally an imprecise guide to water needs,[2,40] athletes must be urged to rehydrate themselves. In fact, if rehydration were left entirely to the person's thirst, it could take several days to reestablish fluid balance after severe dehydration.

ELECTROLYTE REPLACEMENT

There is no evidence that electrolyte intake during exercise in the heat improves performance or reduces physiologic strain including muscle cramps. For a fluid loss of less than 2.7 kg (6 lb) in adults, electrolytes are readily replenished by adding a slight amount of salt to the food when the need exists. For example, the addition of the electrolytes sodium and potassium chloride to the drinking water was of minimum value for men and women who were dehydrated due to sweating by about 3% of body weight on five successive days, but who were permitted food and water ad libitum during each daily recovery period.[17]

With prolonged exercise in the heat, sweat loss may deplete the body of 13 to 17 g of salt per day. This amount is about 8 g in excess of that provided in the daily diet. In this case, salt supplements may be necessary, i.e., about $\frac{1}{3}$ of a teaspoon of table salt added to a liter of water. It is doubtful whether potassium supplements are needed because the potassium loss through sweating is negligible except under the most extreme conditions.[18,24] In this case, potassium loss can be replaced by increasing the intake of potassium-rich foods like citrus fruits and bananas. A glass of orange juice or tomato juice replaces almost all of the potassium, calcium, and magnesium excreted in 2 to 3 liters of sweat. For all but unusual cases, dietary modifications and electrolyte conservation by the kidney adequately compensate for electrolyte loss through sweating.

TABLE 24-1. *Recommended fluid availability and intake[a] for a strenuous 90-minute athletic practice*

WEIGHT LOSS		MINUTES BETWEEN WATER BREAK	FLUID PER BREAK		FLUID AVAILABILITY FOR AN 11-PERSON SQUAD	
lbs	(kg)		OZ	(ml)	GALLONS	(LITERS)
8	(3.6)	No practice	—		—	
7½	(3.4)	recommended	—		—	
7	(3.2)	10	8–10	(266)	6½–8	(27.4)
6½	(3.0)	10	8–9	(251)	6½–7	(25.5)
6	(2.7)	10	8–9	(251)	6½–7	(25.5)
5½	(2.5)	15	10–12	(325)	5½–6½	(22.7)
5	(2.3)	15	10–11	(311)	5½–6	(21.8)
4½	(2.1)	15	9–10	(281)	5 –5½	(19.9)
4	(1.8)	15	8–9	(251)	4½–5	(18.0)
3½	(1.6)	20	10–11	(311)	4 –4½	(16.1)
3	(1.4)	20	9–10	(281)	3½–4	(14.2)
2½	(1.1)	20	7–8	(222)	3	(11.4)
2	(0.9)	30	8	(237)	2½	(9.5)
1½	(0.7)	30	6	(177)	1½	(5.7)
1	(0.5)	45	6	(177)	1	(3.8)
½	(0.2)	60	6	(177)	½	(1.9)

[a] Based on an 80% replacement of weight loss.

FACTORS THAT MODIFY HEAT TOLERANCE

Acclimatization to Heat

Tasks that are relatively easy when performed in cool weather become extremely taxing if attempted on the first hot day of spring. The early stages of spring training are often the most hazardous in terms of heat injury, because thermoregulatory mechanisms are not adjusted to the dual challenge of exercise and heat. Repeated exposure of men and women to hot environments, especially when combined with exercise, results in improved capacity for exercise and less discomfort upon heat exposure.[37,38,39] The physiologic adjustments that improve heat tolerance are collectively termed *heat acclimatization*.

As depicted in Figure 24-5, the major acclimatization occurs during the first week of heat exposure and is essentially complete by the end of 10 days.[13,41,65] Only 2 to 4 hours of daily heat exposure are required. In practical terms, the first several exercise sessions in the heat should be light and last about 15 to 20 minutes.

Thereafter, exercise sessions can increase in duration and intensity.

Table 24-2 summarizes the main physiologic adjustments during heat acclimatization. With acclimatization, larger quantities of blood are shunted to cutaneous vessels, so heat moves from the core to the periphery. A more effective distribution of cardiac output is also achieved so that blood pressure remains more stable during exercise. This "circulatory acclimatization" is complemented by a lowered threshold for sweating. Consequently, the cooling process is initiated before temperature increases too markedly. After 10 days of heat exposure, the capacity for sweating is nearly doubled, the sweat becomes more dilute (less salt is lost), and is more evenly distributed on the skin surface.[55] These adjustments in circulation and evaporative cooling enable the heat-acclimatized person to exercise with a lower core temperature and heart rate than an unacclimatized person.[1,7] This lower core temperature might result in less need for blood flow to the skin, thus freeing a greater portion of the cardiac output for distribution to the working muscles. It is important to note that unless the person is well hydrated the acclimatization process is retarded. Also, the major benefits of acclimatization are lost within 2 to 3 weeks after returning to a more temperate environment.[69]

Effects of Training

In a cool environment, exercise-induced "internal" heat stress brings about adjustments in peripheral circulation and evaporative cooling similar to those observed at hot ambient temperatures. This is especially noteworthy during an 8 to 12-week training period at an exercise intensity that exceeds 50% of the person's aerobic capacity. For this reason, well-conditioned men and women generally respond more effectively to a severe heat stress than their sedentary counterparts.[26,28,30] For one thing, training increases the sensitivity of the sweating response so that sweating begins at a lower body temperature. Thus, the trained person stores less heat during the thermal transient phase of exercise and arrives at a thermal steady state sooner and at a lower core temperature than does an untrained counterpart.

As might be expected, however, this form of heat conditioning is much less effective than

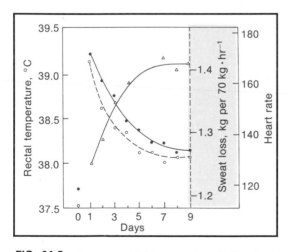

FIG. 24-5. *Average rectal temperature ●, heart rate o, and sweat loss △ during 100-minute daily heat-exercise exposure for 9 consecutive days. On day 0, the men walked on a treadmill at 300 kcal·h⁻¹ in a cool climate. Thereafter, daily exercise was performed in the heat at 48.9°C (26.7°C wet-bulb). (From Lind, A.R., and Bass, D.E.: Optimal exposure time for development of acclimatization to heat. Reprinted from Fed. Proc., 22:704, 1963.)*

TABLE 24-2. *Physiologic adjustments during heat acclimatization*

ACCLIMATIZATION RESPONSE	EFFECT
Improved cutaneous blood flow	Transports metabolic heat from deep tissues to the body's shell
Effective distribution of cardiac output	Appropriate circulation to skin and muscles to meet demands of metabolism and thermoregulation; greater stability in blood pressure during exercise
Lowered threshold for start of sweating	Evaporative cooling begins early in exercise
More effective distribution of sweat over skin surface	Optimum use of effective surface for evaporative cooling
Increased sweat output	Maximizes evaporative cooling
Lowered salt concentration of sweat	Dilute sweat preserves electrolytes in extracellular fluid

acclimatization derived from similar exercise training in the heat.[63,64] *Full heat acclimatization cannot be achieved without actual exposure to heat stress.* Athletes who train and compete in hot weather have a distinct advantage over athletes who train in cool climates but periodically compete in hot weather.

Age and Heat Tolerance

The ability to tolerate and acclimatize to *moderate* heat stress does not appreciably deteriorate with age.[22,37,58] In one experiment, two groups of men and women aged 60 to 93 years were exposed to 70 minutes of heat stress; they progressively exercised at intensities ranging from two to five times the resting metabolism.[37] The relationship between heart rate and work intensity during work in the heat for all subjects is shown in Figure 24-6.

As expected, heart rates were higher for the generally less fit elderly subjects than for the young adults of the same sex. However, the heat imposed no greater physiologic strain upon the older subjects because their body temperature increased an average of 0.3°C compared to 0.2°C for the younger group. The elderly subjects were also tested in the spring and fall to evaluate the extent of natural heat acclimatization during the summer months. After the summer, pulse rates during the standard thermal–work stress were significantly lower for both men and women. In another study,[56] researchers showed that heat-induced stress was no greater when men were evaluated 21 years after initial extensive studies of

heat and exercise tolerance. Not only did the men exhibit the same degree of strain in response to heat as they did when they were younger, but they also acclimatized to about the same extent.

It has been suggested that age is a limiting factor during *vigorous* exercise in excessive heat.[22,34] This age effect is attributed to an apparent delayed onset in sweating with advanc-

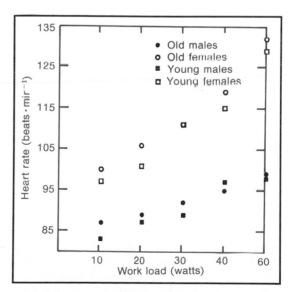

FIG. 24-6. *Heart rate during moderate exercise in the heat for young and old men and women. Dry-bulb ambient temperature was 33.5°C and wet-bulb, 28.5°C. (Adapted from Henshel, A.: The environment and performance. In* Physiology of Work Capacity and Fatigue. *Edited by E. Simonsen. Springfield, Ill., Charles C Thomas, 1971. Courtesy of the publisher.)*

ing years.[37] These conclusions are not supported, however, by findings from competitive runners,[55] because no differentiation could be made between young and middle-aged men in regards to their capacity for temperature regulation during marathon running. Supporting these findings is a report that the capacity for sweating is fully adequate to regulate body temperature during desert walks for men aged 58 to 84 years.[23]

Differences Between Men and Women

The most distinct difference in thermoregulation between men and women is in *sweating*. Women are less prolific sweaters than men. Women start to sweat at higher skin and core temperatures[40]; they also produce less sweat than men for a comparable heat-exercise load,[24] even after acclimatization comparable to that achieved by men.[66] This difference in sweating response occurs even though women possess more heat-activated sweat glands per unit skin area than men.[5]

Despite a lower sweat output, women show heat tolerance similar to that in men at the same exercise level.[6,25] This finding suggests that women rely more on circulatory mechanisms for heat dissipation whereas men make greater use of evaporative cooling. Clearly, the production of less sweat to maintain thermal balance would provide significant protection from dehydration during work at high ambient temperatures.

The sweating response and the ability of women to exercise in the heat does not appear to be related to the *menstrual cycle*.[67] No differences have been noted for untrained, acclimatized young women in skin temperature, core temperature, pulmonary ventilation, oxygen consumption, or sweat rate during exercise at different phases of menstruation.

The available evidence indicates that women can tolerate the physiologic and thermal stress of exercise at least as well as men of *comparable fitness* and *level of acclimatization*.[2a,66a]

Fatness and Heat Stress

Obesity is a liability when working in the heat.[6] Because the specific heat of fat is much greater than that of muscle tissue, excess fat increases the insulatory quality of the body shell and re-tards conduction of heat to the periphery. The large, overfat person also has a relatively small body surface for the evaporation of sweat compared to a leaner, smaller person.

In addition to interfering with heat exchange, excess fat directly adds to the metabolic cost of activities in which the body weight must be moved. When this effect is compounded by the additional weight of football gear, intense competition, and a hot-humid environment, the overfat person is at a distinct disadvantage in terms of heat regulation and physical performance. In fact, fatal heat stroke occurs three and one-half times more frequently in young adults who are excessively overweight than in individuals whose body weight is within reasonable limits.[36]

COMPLICATIONS FROM EXCESSIVE HEAT STRESS: HEAT INJURY

Heat Illness

If the normal signs of heat stress—thirst, tiredness, grogginess, visual disturbances—are not heeded, a series of disabling complications termed *heat illness* can result. The major forms of heat illness in order of increasing severity are heat cramps, heat exhaustion, and heat stroke. There is no clear-cut demarcation between these maladies, because symptoms often overlap. However, when heat illness does occur, immediate action must be taken to relieve the heat stress and rehydrate the person until medical help arrives.

HEAT CRAMPS. During heat exposure, salts can be lost as a result of sweating. If these electrolytes are not replenished, muscle pain and spasm may occur. (The spasms occur most commonly in the calf muscle.) With heat cramps, body temperature is not necessarily elevated. Prevention can usually be assured by providing copious amounts of water and by increasing the daily intake of salt several days *preceding* the period of heat stress; the easiest way is to add a bit more salt to the foods at mealtime.

HEAT EXHAUSTION. This usually develops in unacclimatized people and is often reported during the first heat waves of the summer or during the first hard training session on a hot day. Heat exhaustion is believed to be caused by ineffective circulatory adjustments compounded by a reduction in blood volume due to excessive sweating. Blood usually pools in the dilated peripheral vessels. This drastically reduces the central blood volume necessary to maintain cardiac output. Heat exhaustion is usually characterized by reduced sweating, a weak, rapid pulse, headache, dizziness, and general weakness. Sweating may be reduced somewhat, but body temperature is not elevated to dangerous levels. A person experiencing these symptoms should stop exercising and move to a cooler environment; fluids should be administered.

HEAT STROKE. This is the most serious and complex of the heat stress maladies. *It requires immediate medical attention.* Heat stroke is essentially a failure of the heat regulating mechanisms brought on by excessively high body temperatures. When thermoregulation fails, sweating usually ceases, the skin becomes dry and hot, body temperature rises to dangerous levels, and excessive strain is placed on the circulatory system. If left untreated, the disability progresses and death ensues due to circulatory collapse and eventual damage to the central nervous system. Heat stroke is a medical emergency! While awaiting medical treatment, one must take steps rapidly to lower the elevated core temperature. These include alcohol rubs, ice packs, and whole-body immersion in cold water.

How Hot Is "Too Hot"?

By now it should be clear that factors other than air temperature determine the physiologic strain imposed by heat. These factors include individual variations in body size and fatness, state of training and acclimatization, and external factors such as convective air currents, radiant heat gain, intensity of exercise, amount, type, and color of clothing, and most important, the relative humidity. In fact, several football deaths have been reported when the air temperature was below 75°F (23.9°C) but the relative humidity exceeded 95%.

One way to evaluate the environment in terms of its potential heat challenge is to use a heat stress index, developed by the military, derived from measures of ambient temperature, relative humidity, and radiant heat.[44] The index, termed

the *wet bulb–globe temperature* or *WB–GT* index, is calculated as follows:

$$WB\text{-}GT = 0.1 \times DBT + 0.7 \\ \times WBT + 0.2 \times GT$$

where DBT is the dry-bulb temperature recorded by an ordinary mercury thermometer used for recording air temperature.

WBT is the *wet-bulb temperature* recorded by a similar thermometer except that a wet wick surrounds the mercury bulb that is exposed to rapid air movement. When the relative humidity is high, little evaporative cooling occurs from the wetted bulb, so the temperature of this thermometer is similar to that of the dry-bulb. On a dry day, however, significant evaporation occurs from the wetted bulb and the difference between the two thermometer readings is maximized. A small difference between readings indicates a high relative humidity, whereas a large difference indicates little air moisture and a high rate of evaporation.

GT is the globe temperature recorded by a thermometer whose bulb is enclosed in a metal sphere painted black. The black globe absorbs radiant energy from the surroundings to provide a measure of this important source of heat gain.

Table 24-3 (top) presents WB-GT guidelines that can be applied to athletic activities to reduce the chance of heat injury. These standards apply to lightly clothed humans and do not take into account the specific heat load imposed by uniforms or equipment such as that used in football. For this activity, the lower end of each temperature range would serve as a more prudent guide.

A simple indication of the ambient heat load can also be obtained from the wet-bulb thermometer.[44] This reading evaluates both temperature and humidity. The thermometer is relatively inexpensive and can be purchased at most industrial supply companies. The bottom of Table 24-3 presents recommendations based on wet-bulb temperature (WBT).

SUMMARY

1. Core temperature normally increases during exercise with the magnitude of the rise in temperature determined by the relative stress of a particular work load. This well-regulated temperature adjustment probably creates a favorable environment for physiologic and metabolic function.

TABLE 24-3. *WB-GT for outdoor activities and wet-bulb temperature guide*[a]

WB-GT RANGE		
°F	°C	RECOMMENDATIONS
80–84	26.5–28.8	Use discretion, especially if unconditioned or unacclimatized
85–87	29.5–30.5	Avoid strenuous activity in the sun
88	31.2	Avoid exercise training
WBT RANGE		
°F	°C	RECOMMENDATIONS
60	15.5	No prevention necessary
61–65	16.2–18.4	Alert all participants to problems of heat stress and importance of adequate hydration
66–70	18.8–21.1	Insist that appropriate quantity of fluid be ingested
71–75	21.6–23.8	Rest periods and water breaks every 20 to 30 minutes; limits placed on intense activity
76–79	24.5–26.1	Practice curtailed and modified considerably
80	26.5	Practice cancelled

[a]Modified from Murphy, R.J., and Ashe, W.F.: Prevention of heat illness in football players. J.A.M.A., *194*:650, 1965.

2. Sweating places demands on the body's fluid reserves and creates a relative state of dehydration. If sweating is excessive and fluids are not continually replaced, blood volume falls and core temperature may rise to lethal levels.

3. Exercise in hot, humid environments poses a challenge to temperature regulation because the large sweat loss in high humidity contributes little evaporative cooling.

4. Fluid loss in excess of 4% or 5% body weight significantly impedes heat dissipation and compromises cardiovascular function and work capacity.

5. The primary aim of fluid replacement is to maintain plasma volume so that circulation and sweating can progress at optimal levels. For the ideal replacement schedule during exercise, fluid intake should match fluid loss. This can be effectively monitored by changes in body weight.

6. Although about 800 ml of water can be absorbed from the digestive tract each hour, several factors affect this rate of absorption: (1) colder fluids are absorbed more rapidly than fluids at body temperature, (2) when the stomach is partially filled with fluid, the rate of water absorption is increased, and (3) even small amounts of sugar added to the drinking fluid retard water absorption.

7. The electrolyte loss through sweating is readily replaced by adding a small amount of salt to the food in the daily diet. Except in extreme cases, salt tablets are not recommended.

8. Repeated heat stress initiates thermoregulatory adjustments that result in improved exercise capacity and less discomfort on subsequent heat exposure. This heat acclimatization brings about a favorable distribution of cardiac output and a greatly increased capacity for sweating. Full acclimatization generally occurs in about 10 days of heat exposure.

9. The ability to tolerate and acclimatize to moderate heat stress does not appreciably deteriorate with age.

10. Women seem to be at least as efficient in temperature regulation as men because they produce less sweat while maintaining the same temperature.

11. Various practical heat stress indices make use of ambient temperature, radiant heat, and relative humidity to evaluate the potential heat challenge of an environment to an exercising subject.

References

1. Adams, W. C. et al. Thermoregulation during marathon running in cool, moderate, and hot environments. J. Appl. Physiol., *38:*1030, 1975.

2. Adolph, E. F.: Physiology of Man in the Desert. New York, Interscience, 1947.

2a. American College of Sports Medicine: Opinion statement on: The participation of the female athlete in long-distance running. Med. Sci. Sports., *11:*ix, 1979.

3. Asmussen, E., and Bøje, O.: Body temperature in muscular work. Acta Physiol. Scand., *10:*1, 1945.

4. Åstrand, I.: Aerobic work capacity in men and women with special reference to age. Acta Physiol. Scand. *49* (Suppl. 169):1, 1960.

5. Bar-Or, O. et al.: Distribution of heat-activated sweat glands in obese and lean men and women. Hum. Biol. *40:*235, 1968.

6. Bar-Or, O. et al.: Heat tolerance of exercising obese and lean women. J. Appl. Physiol., *26:*403, 1969.

7. Bass, D. E. et al.: Mechanisms of acclimatization to heat in man. Medicine, *34:*323, 1955.

8. Beaumont, W. van, and Bullard, R. W.: Sweating: its rapid response to muscular work. Science *141:*643, 1963.

9. Buskirk, E. R. et al.: Work performance after dehydration: Effects of physical conditioning and heat acclimatization. J. Appl. Physiol., *12:*189, 1958.

10. Claremont, A. D.: Taking winter in stride requires proper attire. Physician Sportsmed., December: 65, 1976.

11. Claremont, A. D. et al.: Comparison of metabolic, temperature, heart rate and ventilatory responses to exercise at extreme ambient temperatures (0° and 35°C). Med. Sci. Sports, *7:*150, 1975.

12. Claremont, A.D. et al.: Heat tolerance following diuretic induced dehydration. Med. Sci. Sports, *8:*239, 1976.

13. Cleland, T. S. et al.: Acclimatization of women to heat after training. Int. Z. Angew Physiol., *27:*15, 1969.

14. Costill, D. L., and Fink, W. J.: Plasma volume changes following exercise and thermal dehydration. J. Appl. Physiol., *37:*521, 1974.

15. Costill, D. L., and Saltin, B.: Factors limiting gastric emptying during rest and exercise. J. Appl. Physiol., *37:*679, 1974.

16. Costill, D. L., and Sparks, K. E.: Rapid fluid replacement following thermal dehydration. J. Appl. Physiol., *34:*299, 1973.

17. Costill, D. L. et al.: Water and electrolyte replacement during repeated days of work in the heat. Aviation, Space, Environ. Med., *46:*795, 1975.

18. Costill, D. L. et al.: Muscle water and electrolytes following varied levels of dehydration in man. J. Appl. Physiol., *40:*6, 1976.

19. Costill, D. L. et al.: Exercise induced sodium conservation: changes in plasma renin and aldosterone. Med. Sci. Sports, *8:*209, 1976.

20. Craig, A. B., Jr., and Dvorak, M.: Thermal regulation of man exercising during water immersion. J. Appl. Physiol., *25:*28, 1968.

21. Craig, F. N., and Cummings, E. G.: Dehydration and muscular work. J. Appl. Physiol., *21:*670, 1966.

22. Dill, D. B., and Consolazio, C. F.: Responses to exercise as related to age and environmental temperature. J. Appl. Physiol., *17:*645, 1962.

23. Dill, D. B. et al.: Cardiovascular responses and temperatue in relation to age. Aust. J. Sports Med., *7:*99, 1975.

24. Dill, D. B. et al.: Capacity of young males and females for running in desert heat. Med. Sci. Sports, *9:*137, 1977.
25. Drinkwater, B. L.: Thermoregulatory response of women to intermittent work in the heat. J. Appl. Physiol., *41:*57, 1976.
26. Drinkwater, B. L. et al.: Aerobic power as a factor in women's response to work in hot environments. J. Appl. Physiol., *41:*815, 1976.
27. Falls, H. B., and Humphrey, L. D.: Cold water application effects on responses to heat stress during exercise. Res. Quart., *42:*21, 1971.
28. Ferris, E. et al.: Thermoregulatory function in men and women. J. Physiol., *200:*46P, 1969.
29. Fink, W. J. et al.: Leg muscle metabolism during exercise in the heat and cold. Eur. J. Appl. Physiol., *34:*183, 1975.
30. Fox, E. et al.: Effects of football equipment on thermal balance and energy cost during exercise. Res. Quart., *37:*322, 1966.
31. Gisolfi, C. V., and Copping, J. R.: Thermal effects of prolonged treadmill exercise in the heat. Med. Sci. Sports, *6:*108, 1974.
32. Greenleaf, J. E.: Hyperthermia in exercise. *In* International Review of Physiology. Environmental Physiology III, Vol. 20. Edited by D. Robertshaw. Baltimore, University Park Press, 1979.
33. Greenleaf, J. E. et al.: Maximal oxygen uptake, sweating and tolerance to exercise in the heat. Int. J. Biometeorol., *16:*375, 1972.
34. Hellon, R. F. et al.: The physiological reactions of men of two age groups to a hot environment. J. Physiol., *133:*118, 1956.
35. Hemingway, A.: Shivering. Physiol. Rev., *43:*397, 1963.
36. Henshel, A.: Obesity as an occupational hazard. Can. J. Public Health *58:*491, 1967.
37. Henshel, A.: The environment and peformance. *In* Physiology of Work Capacity and Fatigue. Edited by E. Simonsen. Springfield, Ill.: Charles C Thomas, 1971.
38. Hertig, B. A. et al.: Artificial acclimatization of women to heat. J. Appl., Physiol., *18:*383, 1963.
39. Iampietro, P. F.: Exercise in hot environments. *In* Frontiers of Fitness. Edited by R. J. Shepard. Springfield, Ill.: Charles C Thomas, 1971.
40. Leithead, C. S., and Lind, A. R.: Heat Stress and Disorders. London; Cassel and Co., Ltd., 1964.
41. Lind, A. R., and Bass, D. E.: Optimal exposure time for development of acclimatization to heat. Fed. Proc. *22:*704, 1963.
42. Mathews, D. K. et al.: Physiological responses during exercise and recovery in a football uniform. J. Appl. Physiol., *26:*611, 1969.
43. McArdle, W. D. et al.: Metabolic and cardiovascular adjustment to work in air and water at 18, 25, 33°C. J. Appl. Physiol., *40:*85, 1976.
44. Minard, D. et al.: Prevention of heat casualties. J.A.M.A. *165:*1813, 1957.
45. Miroff, S. V., and Bass, D. E.: Effects of overhydration on man's physiological responses to work in the heat. J. Appl. Physiol., *20:*267, 1965.
46. Nadel, E. R.: Thermal and energetic exchanges during swimming. *In* Problems With Temperature Regulation During Exercise. New York, Academic Press, 1977.
47. Nadel, E. R. et al.: Thermoregulatory shivering during exercise. Life Sci. *13:*983, 1973.
48. Nadel, E. R. et al.: Energy exchange of swimming man. J. Appl. Physiol., *36:*465, 1974.
49. Nelms, J. D., and Soper, J. G.: Cold vasodilatation and cold acclimatization in the hands of British fish filleters. J. Appl. Physiol., *17:*444, 1962.
50. Nielsen, B., and Nielsen, M.: On the regulation of sweat secretion in exercise. Acta. Physiol. Scand. *64:*314, 1965.

51. Pugh, L.C.G.E.: A physiological study of channel swimming. J. Clin. Invest. *37:*538, 1960.
52. Pugh, L.C.G.E. et al.: Rectal temperatures, weight losses and sweat rates in marathon running. J. Appl. Physiol. *21:*1251, 1966.
53. Ribisl, P. M., and Herbert, W. G.: Effects of rapid weight reduction and subsequent rehydration upon the physical working capacity of wrestlers. Res. Quart., *41:*536, 1970.
54. Robinson, S.: Physiological adjustments to heat. *In* Physiology of Heat Regulation and the Science of Clothing. Edited by L. H. Newburgh. Philadelphia, W. B. Saunders, 1949.
55. Robinson, S.: Training, acclimatization and heat tolerance. Can. Med. Assoc. J. *96:*795, 1967.
56. Robinson, S. et al.: Acclimatization of older men to work in the heat. J. Appl. Physiol., *20:*583, 1965.
57. Rowell, L. B.: Hepatic clearance of idocyanine green in man under thermal and exercise stesses. J. Appl. Physiol., *20:*384, 1965.
58. Rowell, L. B.: Human cardiovascular adjustment to exercise and thermal stress. Physiol. Rev., *54:*75, 1974.
59. Rowell, L. B. et al.: Splanchnic blood flow and metabolism in heat-stressed man. J. Appl. Physiol., *24:*475, 1968.
60. Saltin, B.: Circulatory response to submaximal and maximal exercise after thermal dehydration. J. Appl. Physiol. *19:*1125, 1964.
61. Saltin, B., and Hermansen, L.: Esophageal, rectal and muscle temperature during exercise. J. Appl. Physiol., *21:*1757, 1966.
62. Smiles, K. A., and Robinson, S. Sodium ion conservation during acclimatization of men to work in the heat. J. Appl. Physiol., *31:*63, 1971.
63. Strydom, N. B. et al.: Comparison of oral and rectal temperatures during work in the heat. J. Appl. Physiol., *8:*406, 1956.
64. Strydom, N. B. et al.: Acclimatization to humid heat and the role of physical conditioning. J. Appl. Physiol., *21.*636, 1966.
65. Taylor, H. L. et al.: Cardiovascular adjustments of man at rest and work during exposure to dry heat. Am. J. Physiol., *139:*583, 1955.
66. Wells, C. L.: Sexual differences in heat stress response. Physician Sportsmed., *5:*70, 1977.
66a. Wells, C. L.: Responses of physically active and acclimatized men and women to exercise in a desert environment. Med. Sci. Sports, *12:*9, 1980.
67. Wells, C. L., and Horvath, S. M.: Responses to exercise in a hot environment as related to the menstrual cycle. J. Appl. Physiol., *36:*299, 1974.
68. Williams, C. G. et al.: Circulatory and metabolic reactions to work in heat. J. Appl. Physiol., *17:*625, 1962.
69. Williams, C. G. et al.: Rate of loss of acclimatization in summer and winter. J. Appl. Physiol., *22:*21, 1967.
70. Wyndham, C. H. et al.: Relation between $\dot{V}O_2$ max and body temperature in hot humid air conditions. J. Appl. Physiol., *29:*45, 1970.
71. Zambraski, E. J. et al.: Iowa wrestling study: urinary profiles of state finalists prior to competition. Med. Sci. Sports, *6:*129, 1974.
72. Zambraski, E. J. et al.: Iowa wrestling study: weight loss and urinary profiles of collegiate wrestlers. Med. Sci. Sports, *8:*105, 1976.

Sport Diving

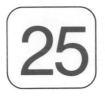

Exploring the subsurface environment is not without risks, even for the well-trained diver.[3a] The diver is exposed to high pressures as well as the possibility of rapid changes in pressure. In fact, these pressure changes can cause fatal lung burst when scuba is used in water as shallow as 6 feet. This and other accidents can be avoided through competent instruction in diving skills and an understanding of preventive measures, symptoms, and dangers. Unfortunately, because skin and scuba diving equipment is so easy to use, many enthusiasts, especially if they are good swimmers, feel that instruction is unnecessary. Unquestionably, safe diving requires thorough knowledge of diving physics and physiology.

As interest in diving increases, pool directors and physical educators are being called upon to initiate, teach, and supervise instructional programs in diving. In the following sections, we outline general principles of diving, as well as potential dangers as a person descends and ascends in the water. Within this framework, emphasis is placed on the relationship between diving depth, pressure, and gas volume, as well

as on the potentially toxic effects of the various gases respired in diving. With this background, persons involved in aquatic instruction can better understand the inherent dangers in the sport and evaluate the safety of instruction currently in practice.

PRESSURE–VOLUME RELATIONSHIPS AND DIVING DEPTH

Diving Depth and Pressure

Because water is essentially noncompressible, the water pressure against the diver's body increases directly with the depth of the dive. This pressure is the result of two forces: (1) the weight of the column of water directly above, and (2) the weight of the atmosphere at the surface. As shown in Table 25-1, a column of fresh water exerts a force of one sea level atmosphere or 760 mm Hg (14.7 lb per square inch) for each 33 ft (10 m) one descends below the water's surface. (Because salt water is more dense than fresh water, a depth of about 32 ft

TABLE 25-1. *Relationship of depth in water to pressure and volume*

DEPTH		PRESSURE		HYPOTHETICAL LUNG VOLUME	INSPIRED AIR	
(ft)	(m)	(ATMOSPHERE)	(mm HG)	(ml)	Po_2	Pn_2
Sea level		1	760	6000	159	600
33	10	2	1520	3000	318	1201
66	20	3	2280	2000	477	1802
100	30	4	3040	1500	636	2402
133	40	5	3800	1200	795	3003
166	50	6	4560	1000	954	3604
200	60	7	5320	857	1113	4204
300	90	10	7600	600	1590	6006
400	120	13	9880	461	2068	7808
500	150	16	12160	375	2545	9610
600	180	19	14440	316	3022	11412

corresponds to the pressure equivalent of one atmosphere in ocean diving.) Consequently, a person diving to a depth of 33 ft is exposed to a pressure of 2 atmospheres—1 atmosphere due to the weight of the ambient air at the surface and the other due to the weight of the column of water itself. Diving from sea level to a depth of 66 ft (20 m) exposes the diver to an absolute pressure equal to 3 atmospheres; at 99 ft (30 m) the pressure is 4 atmospheres, and so on. Clearly, considerable pressure is exerted at relatively short distances below the surface.

Because the tissues of the body are largely water, they too are incompressible and thus are not especially susceptible to the increased external pressure in diving. However, the body also contains air-filled cavities—notably the lungs, respiratory passages, and sinus and middle-ear spaces. Volume and pressure in these spaces can be greatly modified by any increase or decrease in diving depth. *Unless adjustments are made to equalize the rapid and significant pressure changes in diving, pain, injury, and even death can occur.*

Diving Depth and Gas Volume

In accordance with *Boyle's law,* the volume of any gas varies inversely with the pressure on it. Thus, if the pressure is doubled, the volume is halved; conversely, reducing the pressure by half causes the volume of any gas to expand to twice its previous size.

As shown in Table 25-1 and illustrated in Figure 25-1, if a diver fills his or her lungs with 6 liters of air at sea level and descends to a depth of 33 ft, the lung volume is compressed to 3 liters; diving an additional 33 ft to a depth of 66 ft (where the external pressure is now 3 atmospheres), the original 6-liter lung volume is reduced one-third to 2 liters. In fact, at a depth of 166 ft (50 m), the lung volume is compressed to about 1 liter, simply due to the force of water acting against the air-filled chest cavity. For most of us, any further increase in diving depth would cause the air volume in the respiratory tract to become so small as to result in serious damage to the chest wall and lung tissue. If the diver returns to the surface the air volume re-expands to its original 6-liter volume. Of great significance to the scuba diver who breathes pressurized air is the fact that 6 liters of air in the lungs at a depth of 33 ft will expand to 12 liters when brought to the surface. This same 6-liter volume at 166 ft will occupy 36 liters at sea level pressure! *If this "extra" air is not permitted to escape via the nose or mouth as the diver ascends, the lung tissue will rupture under the force of expanding gases.*

SNORKELING AND BREATHHOLD DIVING

A common form of recreation and sport is swimming at the surface of the water with fins, mask, and snorkel. This "skin diving" is especially popular for spear-fishing and exploring shallow areas of clear water. The snorkel is a J-shaped tube about 15 in. (38 cm) long that allows the swimmer to breathe continually with the face immersed in water. The swimmer periodically takes a full breath of air and dives beneath the water for a closer look. After about 30 seconds, the carbon dioxide level in the blood increases, the diver senses the need to breathe and quickly surfaces. This activity is basically an extension of swimming and is limited entirely by the swimmer's breathhold ability.

Limits to Snorkel Size

Novice skin divers often speculate that if only the snorkel were longer, it would certainly be possible to swim deeper in the water and still breathe ambient air through the top of the snorkel. In fact, many beginners feel they would be able to sit at the pool bottom and breathe through a garden hose extending up to the pool deck. Although the idea of a longer snorkel is intriguing, two factors must be considered: (1) the increased water pressure on the chest cavity as the swimmer descends beneath the water, and (2) the increase in pulmonary dead space brought on by enlarging the snorkel.

INSPIRATORY CAPACITY IN RELATION TO DEPTH. When breathing through a snorkel, the diver must inspire air at atmospheric pressure. At a depth of about 3 ft (1 m), the compressive force of water against the chest cavity is so large that the inspiratory muscles are usually unable to overcome external pressure and expand thoracic dimensions. Consequently, inspiration is impossible unless air is supplied at a pressure sufficient to counter the compressive force of water at the particular depth. This is the principle of scuba that is discussed fully in a later section.

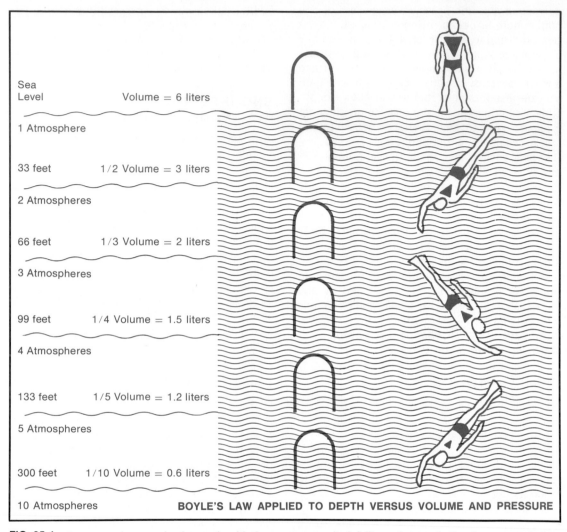

Sea Level   Volume = 6 liters

1 Atmosphere

33 feet   1/2 Volume = 3 liters

2 Atmospheres

66 feet   1/3 Volume = 2 liters

3 Atmospheres

99 feet   1/4 Volume = 1.5 liters

4 Atmospheres

133 feet   1/5 Volume = 1.2 liters

5 Atmospheres

300 feet   1/10 Volume = 0.6 liters

10 Atmospheres   **BOYLE'S LAW APPLIED TO DEPTH VERSUS VOLUME AND PRESSURE**

FIG. 25-1. *Any gas volume varies inversely with the pressure on it. A 6-liter volume, whether in an open bell or in the flexible chest cavity, is compressed to 3 liters in 33 feet of water. This is simply because the external pressure has been doubled. At 99 feet or 4 atmospheres, the gas is reduced to 25% of its original volume, or 1.5 liters.*

SNORKEL SIZE IN RELATION TO PULMONARY DEAD SPACE. Not all of the inspired air enters the alveoli. About 150 ml of each breath fill the nose, mouth, and other nondiffusable portions of the respiratory tract. The snorkel adds to the volume of this anatomic dead space.

Ideally, the snorkel should be about 15 in. long with an inside diameter of five-eighths to three-quarters inch.[8] For healthy people this additional dead space of approximately 150 ml poses no special problems because adequate alveolar ventilation can be maintained by a slight increase in the depth of breathing. Any further increase in snorkel size, however, significantly increases the dead space and encroaches on one's capacity for alveolar ventilation. Adequate gas exchange becomes impossible when the dead space reaches about 60% of the lung volume.

Breathhold Diving

If a person takes a full inspiration of ambient air, about 1 liter of oxygen is brought into the lungs. If the breath is then held, 600 to 700 ml of oxygen in the lungs can be utilized to sustain metabolism before the partial pressures of arterial oxygen and carbon dioxide signal the need for renewed breathing. With some training, most of us can breathhold for about 1 minute. During this time, arterial P_{O_2} drops to about 60 mm Hg whereas P_{CO_2} rises to 50 mm Hg. With exercise, breathhold time is greatly reduced, because oxygen consumption and carbon dioxide production increase directly with the severity of the activity. During breathhold diving, especially if preceded by hyperventilation, certain factors must be considered that may extend the breathhold period yet significantly increase the danger of the dive.

HYPERVENTILATION AND BREATHHOLD DIVING: BLACKOUT. The problem of sudden loss of consciousness or *blackout* is unique to skin diving and usually occurs in divers who attempt to extend the duration of a dive beyond reasonable limits. The cause is probably either a critical reduction in oxygen, an increase in carbon dioxide, or the combined effects of both.

The breakpoint for breathhold usually corresponds to an increase in arterial P_{CO_2} to about 50 mm Hg. For some people, however, it is possible to "ignore" the stimulus and continue to breathhold until carbon dioxide reaches levels that cause severe disorientation and even blackout.[2] With hyperventilation prior to breathhold, arterial P_{CO_2} may decrease from its normal value of 40 mm Hg to 20 or 15 mm Hg. This elimination of carbon dioxide significantly extends the duration of breathhold until the arterial P_{CO_2} increases to a level to stimulate ventilation.

The attempt to extend breathhold time in diving, however, is not without serious risks.[2,3,6] If a skin diver hyperventilates at the surface prior to a dive, arterial P_{CO_2} is reduced and the potential length of the breathhold is extended. The diver now takes a full inhalation and descends beneath the water. Alveolar oxygen continually moves into the blood to be delivered to the working muscles. Due to the previous hyperventilation, carbon dioxide levels remain low and the diver is essentially "free" from the urge to breathe. Concurrently, as the diver goes deeper, the external water pressure compresses the thorax. This increased pressure maintains a relatively high P_{O_2} within the alveoli. Thus, even though the absolute quantity of oxygen in the lungs is lowered (as oxygen moves into the blood during the dive), adequate

pressure is maintained to load hemoglobin as the dive progresses. Now, as the diver senses the need to breathe and begins the ascent, significant reversals in pressure occur. As water pressure on the thorax decreases and lung volume expands, the partial pressure of alveolar oxygen is reduced proportionately. In fact, as the diver nears the surface, the alveolar P_{O_2} may be so low that dissolved oxygen actually leaves the blood and flows into the alveoli! In this situation, the diver may suddenly lose consciousness before reaching the surface.

Hyperventilation should not be used in the water environment. Aside from the fact that prolonged breathhold may result in a dangerous reduction in arterial P_{O_2}, other physiologic effects must be considered:

1. A *normal quantity of arterial carbon dioxide* is necessary to maintain the acid–base balance of the blood. This is mediated by the release of H^+ as carbonic acid is formed from the union of carbon dioxide and water. By reducing the blood's carbon dioxide content through hyperventilation, the H^+ concentration is lowered, causing the blood to become more *alkaline*.

2. Arterial P_{CO_2} also provides a continuous stimulus for the dilation of small arteries in the brain. The elimination of carbon dioxide during hyperventilation can reduce cerebral blood flow and cause dizziness or even loss of consciousness. This would obviously create a dangerous situation in the water.

DEPTH LIMITS WITH BREATHHOLD DIVING: Thoracic Squeeze. The body's air cavities are subjected to tremendous compressive forces as the skin diver progresses deeper beneath the water. In general, if the lung volume is compressed below 1.0 to 1.5 liters (residual lung volume), internal and external pressures are unable to equalize and *lung squeeze* occurs. This effect of excessive hydrostatic pressure can cause extensive damage to respiratory tissue.

There is considerable variability among individuals as to the safe depth for breathhold diving without danger of lung squeeze. This critical depth is generally determined by the ratio of the diver's total lung volume to residual lung volume; this ratio usually averages about 4:1 at the surface. *There is no danger from lung squeeze if the lung volume remains greater than the residual volume.* This is because sufficient air remains in the lungs and rigid respiratory passages to equalize pressure and prevent damage due to compression. For most of us, this critical depth is usually about 100 ft. If the lung volume during a dive is reduced below residual volume—that is, if the ratio of total to residual volume is less than 1.00—the pulmonary air pressure becomes less than the external water pressure. This unequalized pressure creates a relative vacuum within the lungs that can cause serious damage to alveolar tissue. In severe cases of lung squeeze, blood is literally sucked from the pulmonary capillaries through the alveoli into the lungs. In this situation, the diver actually drowns in his or her own blood. Further increases in depth cause compression fractures of the ribs as the chest cavity begins to cave in from the external pressure.

OTHER PROBLEMS. If internal and external pressures are unable to equalize, problems other than lung squeeze limit the depth of any dive. For example, if air at ambient pressure remains trapped in the middle ear (due to inflamed tissue or a mucous plug) and cannot equilibrate with air from the lungs, the hydrostatic pressure will cause the eardrum to move inward and eventually to rupture. This can occur even at relatively shallow depths.

The sinuses are also a source of difficulty for the skin diver. Air that is compressed in the lungs by the external force of water attempts to move into the paranasal sinuses. Inflamed and irritated sinuses due to infection have extremely narrow openings and are often unable to equilibrate with small pressure change. This creates a relative vacuum in these cavities and distorts the shape of the involved tissue causing intense sinus pain. In severe cases, fluid and blood move into the sinuses in an attempt to fill the vacuum. Problems arising from a diver's inability to equalize pressure are also common in scuba diving and are examined in the sections that follow.

SCUBA DIVING

In our discussion of snorkeling, it was noted that at depths below 1 m, the inspiratory muscles are unable to overcome the compressive force of water against the chest cavity. To counteract this external force, air under pressure must be supplied from an external source so that inspiratory action is possible. *The self-contained underwater breathing apparatus* or scuba is the most common apparatus used for this purpose. The scuba system is strapped to the diver's chest or back and consists of a tank of compressed air and a regulator with a hose and mouthpiece or full face mask. Two basic scuba designs are in use: (1) the popular open-circuit system, and (2) the closed-circuit system that is especially useful for military operations and special applications using mixed gases.

Open-Circuit Scuba

The typical open-circuit scuba system is illustrated in Figure 25-2. *This is the only form of scuba that should be used in sport diving!* For most diving purposes, the tanks are constructed of steel or aluminum and contain 1000 to 2000 liters of air compressed to pressures of about 2200 pounds per square inch (p.s.i.). One tank supplies enough air for $\frac{1}{2}$ to 1 hour at moderate depths. The compressed air flows through a regulator valve that reduces the tank pressure to the "ambient" pressure at a particular depth. A slight negative pressure is created as the diver begins inspiration. This causes the demand valve to open and release air to the diver at a pressure about equal to the external pressure of the water. On exhalation, the inspiratory valves close and the exhaled air is discharged into the water.

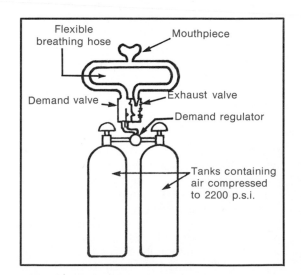

FIG. 25-2. *Open-circuit scuba system.*

Open-circuit scuba is not without its drawbacks. Because expired air generally contains about 16% to 17% oxygen, the open-circuit system is wasteful because about 75% of the total oxygen in the tank is ultimately exhaled into the water. In addition, a significant mass of air must be supplied to the diver at increased depths to provide the appropriate tidal volume for adequate pulmonary ventilation. As an extreme example, the equivalent of 50 liters of air at sea level must be pumped to a diver at 300 ft to provide a 5-liter volume! This effect of pressure greatly limits the length of time one can remain at a great depth before the air in the scuba tank is depleted.

Figure 25-3 shows the theoretical time limit for a diver doing similar work at various depths. These theoretical times are based on a completely filled standard tank and a 60-ft per minute rate of ascent and descent. For example, a single tank with 71.2 cubic ft of air compressed to 2200 p.s.i. normally supplies a 70-minute dive near the surface. At a depth of 33 ft, however, this tank supplies enough air for 35 minutes, whereas at 3 atmospheres or 66 ft, the diving time is reduced by one-third to about 23 minutes.

Closed-Circuit Scuba

The closed-circuit underwater breathing apparatus operates in the same manner as the closed-circuit spirometer described in Chapter 8. A small cylinder of pure oxygen feeds into a bellows or bag from which the diver breathes. This breathing bag acts as a pressure regulator. Appropriate valves in the breathing mask direct the exhaled gas through a cannister containing soda lime that absorbs carbon dioxide and passes the carbon dioxide-free gas back to the diver. The cylinder of oxygen replenishes the oxygen used in metabolism. Consequently, oxygen is continually rebreathed, and the only gas lost is that used to supply the metabolic requirements of the dive. With only a small cylinder of oxygen, the diver can remain submerged for several hours. The system also provides for an almost completely silent and "bubble-free" operation in contrast to open-circuit diving systems.

Two main problems exist with closed-circuit scuba: (1) Serious injury can occur should the carbon dioxide output exceed its rate of absorption or should the absorbent fail altogether. With a faulty rebreathing system, the diver may not receive warning symptoms and can drown as a result of being anesthetized by carbon dioxide. (2) High concentrations of oxygen, especially when breathed under pressure, have a variety of adverse effects on physiologic functions. In fact, at greater than 2 atmospheres of pressure, oxygen becomes a deadly poison. This phenomenon is discussed more fully in the section on "oxygen poisoning."

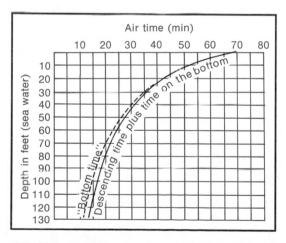

FIG. 25-3. *Theoretical air time for a single tank containing 71.2 cubic feet of air. The solid line includes the time spent while descending (at a rate of 60 ft·min⁻¹) plus the time on the bottom; the dashed line represents only "bottom time."*

SPECIAL PROBLEMS BREATHING GASES AT HIGH PRESSURES

Underwater breathing systems must supply air or other gas mixtures at sufficient pressure to overcome the force of water against the diver's chest. At 66 ft or 3 atmospheres of pressure, for example, the respired gas must be delivered at approximately 2280 mm Hg (3 × 760 mm Hg), whereas at 200 feet the gas is delivered at a pressure of 5320 mm Hg. In the sections that follow, we consider the specific dynamics of breathing gases at high pressures and examine their effects on bodily functions as well as on the physical responses of gas to abrupt pressure changes. In regard to this latter objective, Figure 25-4 summarizes the main hazards of scuba diving that result from improper equalization of pressure within the body's air spaces (and diving mask) in response to changes in external pressure.

Air
Embolism

An air volume breathed underwater expands in direct proportion to the reduction in external pressure as the diver ascends toward the surface. Air breathed at a depth of 33 ft doubles in volume if brought to the surface. This expand-ing air vents freely if normal breathing contin-ues during the ascent. However, if a diver takes a full breath at this depth but fails to exhale while ascending to the surface, the progressive and rapid expansion of gas eventually ruptures the lungs before he or she reaches the surface. The potential for lung burst is quite real, be-cause many beginning divers react to a per-ceived danger by filling their lungs and then "holding their breath" while rapidly swimming to the surface. This particular diving hazard is not necessarily related to deep dives. Accidents

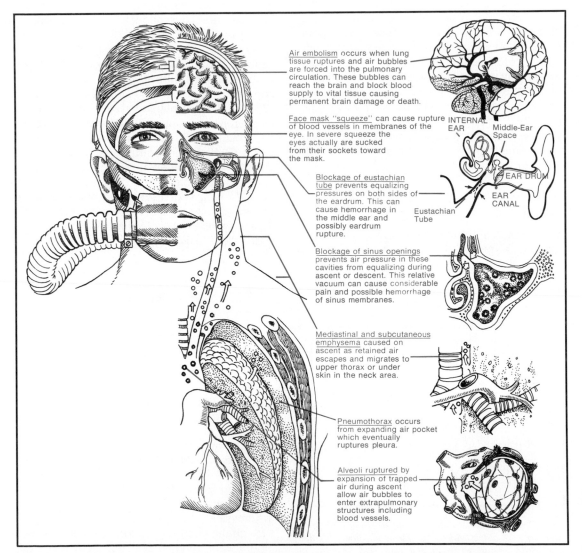

FIG. 25-4. *Hazards in scuba diving due to inability to equalize internal and external pressure.*

caused by breathhold ascent with scuba frequently occur near the surface where the changes in pressure have the greatest effect on the expanding lung volume. *A full inhalation in 6 ft of water can cause serious overdistension of lung tissue during ascent if the diver does not exhale on the way up.* In fact, fatal *air embolism* has occurred in swimming pools as shallow as 8 feet for an inexperienced diver using scuba.[4]

If the expansion of air in the respiratory tract causes lung tissue to rupture, air bubbles may be forced into the pulmonary venous system. These bubbles or *emboli* are then carried to the heart and passed into the systemic circulation. Because the diver is usually in the head up, vertical position on ascent, the bubbles move upward in the body. Eventually, they become lodged in the small arterioles or capillaries and restrict the blood supply to vital tissue. General symptoms of air embolism include confusion, weakness, dizziness, and blurred vision. Severe blockage of pulmonary, coronary, and cerebral circulation causes collapse, unconsciousness, and frequently death. The only effective treatment for air embolism is rapid decompression to reduce the size of the bubbles and to force them into solution in order to open the plugged vessels. Even with rapid, expert treatment, approximately 16% of air embolism victims die.

Pneumothorax: Lung Collapse

Often, when lung tissue ruptures and air is forced through the alveoli, it migrates laterally to burst through the pleural sac covering the lungs.[4] This causes an air pocket to form in the chest cavity outside the lungs between the chest wall and lung tissue. Continued expansion of this trapped air during ascent causes the ruptured lung to collapse and the heart and other organs to be pushed out of their normal positions. Treatment for this condition of *pneumothorax* often requires surgical intervention in which a syringe is used to "extract" the air bubble.

To eliminate the danger of air embolism and pneumothorax, all divers must be instructed to ascend slowly and breathe normally when using scuba gear. It is imperative that the diver's lungs be free of any disease that could lead to the trapping of air and make it difficult for alveolar pressure to equalize during ascent.

Mask Squeeze

Prior to a dive, air in the face mask or goggles is at the same pressure as ambient air at the surface. A considerable pressure differential develops between the inside and outside of the mask as the diver progresses beneath the water. This creates a relative vacuum within the mask. If this pressure does not equilibrate, there is a tendency for the eyes to bulge out or "squeeze" from their sockets, and the surrounding capillaries to rupture. This is a serious problem for divers who wear goggles because *there is no way to equalize the pressure within the air cavity of the goggles.* With a face mask, however, the nose is also encased within the mask. With scuba, the inspired air is automatically adjusted to the outside water pressure. Thus, periodically exhaling through the nose into the mask balances the pressures on both sides of the face mask. In breathhold diving, air in the lungs becomes compressed and can be passed through the nose to equalize the mask pressure.

Aerotitis: Middle-Ear Squeeze

Another significant problem encountered by the diver is equalizing the air space within the *eustachian tubes*, the passages that connect the middle ear with the back of the throat. These mucus-lined passages are relatively narrow and generally resist air flow. In healthy individuals, the tubes are clear so that changes in external pressure against the eardrum can be equalized by the same pressure transmitted from within the lungs through the eustachian tubes. In both skin and scuba diving (as well as in air travel in nonpressurized aircraft), middle-ear pressure can usually be equalized by blowing gently against closed nostrils. Swallowing, yawning, or moving the jaws from side to side is also helpful in "popping the ears."

With an upper respiratory infection, the eustachian tube membranes swell and produce mucus that may plug these air passages. The greatest difficulty is usually experienced in equalizing middle-ear pressure during descent because a change in pressure against the outer surface of the eardrum is not readily met by an equal force from the interior. In diving, the pressure changes are considerable compared to those experienced in air travel. The diver can suffer severe pain in only a few feet of water because the eardrum becomes stretched and moves inward toward the plugged canal. With further pressure disequilibrium, the relative vacuum in the middle ear causes tissue to hemorrhage. In fact, when the eustachian tubes are totally blocked, the eardrums rupture and water rushes into the middle ear, which is at a considerably lower pressure.

NEVER DIVE WITH EARPLUGS! For the same reasons outlined previously, *earplugs should never be worn while diving*. The external water pressure will push the ear plug deep into the external ear canal. If a pocket of ambient air is trapped between the plug and eardrum, the eardrum may rupture outward during descent. People who have respiratory disease, perforated eardrums, or temporary blockage of the eustachian tubes due to infection, should not dive. In the latter case, diving can be resumed again when the infection subsides and the ear canal clears.

AEROSINUSITIS. As mentioned in our discussion of breathhold diving, inflamed, congested sinuses prevent the air pressure in these cavities from equalizing during descent or ascent. If sinus air pressure does not equalize during descent, the air in these spaces remains at atmospheric pressure while external pressure increases. This relative vacuum creates "sinus squeeze," which causes bleeding in the sinus membranes as blood moves in to equalize the pressure differential.

Nitrogen Narcosis:
"Raptures of the Deep"

During the dive, the total pressure of the respired gas increases in direct proportion with the depth of the dive. Likewise, the partial pressure of each gas in the breathing mixture increases so that at 33 ft the partial pressure of nitrogen is double the sea level value, i.e., 1200 mm Hg. With each additional 33 ft, the partial pressure of nitrogen increases by 600 mm Hg—at a depth of 200 ft, the inspired P_{N_2} is about 4200 mm Hg. Thus, at each successive depth, a gradient exists for the net flow of nitrogen across the alveolar membrane into the blood and eventually into the tissues, with which it equilibrates. At 66 ft, for example, all tissues will eventually contain about three times as much nitrogen as they did before the dive.

An increase in the pressure and quantity of dissolved nitrogen causes physical and mental reactions characterized by a general state of euphoria not unlike alcohol intoxication. This has been termed *"raptures of the deep."* In fact, this effect at a depth of 100 ft is likened to the feelings one often experiences after drinking a martini on an empty stomach; at 200 ft the feelings are similar to the effects of two or three martinis. Eventually, high nitrogen levels produce a numbing or anesthetic effect on the central nervous system, the symptoms of which are collectively termed *nitrogen narcosis*. This affects thought processes to the extent that a diver may feel that the scuba gear is unnecessary and may actually remove it and swim deeper instead of toward the surface.

As nitrogen diffuses slowly into the body tissues, the narcosis effect is dependent not only on depth but also on the duration of the dive. Although great individual variation in sensitivity exists, a mild narcosis usually appears after an hour or more at a depth of 100 to 130 ft. *This is usually the maximum recommended depth range for recreational scuba divers.* The treatment for nitrogen narcosis simply requires that the diver ascend to a shallower depth—recovery is usually immediate and complete.[8]

Decompression Sickness:
The Bends

Decompression sickness or the "bends" occurs when dissolved nitrogen moves out of solution and forms bubbles in body tissues and fluids. It is caused by a diver ascending to the surface too rapidly after a deep, prolonged dive. Because nitrogen reaches equilibrium slowly in many tissues, especially fatty tissues, it leaves the body slowly. If the diver ascends at a prescribed, relatively slow rate, however, all of the body's excess dissolved nitrogen has sufficient time to diffuse from the tissues into the blood and be eliminated through the lungs. If the ascent is too rapid and the external pressure against the diver's body is reduced dramatically, the excess nitrogen begins to escape from the dissolved state and eventually forms bubbles in the tissues. This effect is not unlike the formation of carbon dioxide bubbles in carbonated beverages when the cap is removed. As long as the cap is in place, the gas is under pressure and remains in the dissolved state.

When the cap is removed, the pressure is suddenly reduced and bubbles form.

Diving at 100 ft for up to 30 minutes, for example, is the upper limit before sufficient nitrogen is dissolved to pose danger from the bends. About 18 minutes duration is the limit at 130 ft, whereas almost an hour can be spent at 60 ft without danger of decompression sickness. If the diver exceeds the depth-duration recommendations for compressed-air diving shown in Figure 25-5,[9] the ascent to the surface must be accomplished in stages. Such pauses or decompression stops give sufficient time for excess nitrogen to diffuse from the tissues via the blood to exit through the lungs without bubbles forming.[8] For example, a dive to 100 ft for 50 minutes requires one 2-minute decompression stop at 20 ft and another 24-minute stop at 10 ft.

The evidence is overwhelming that bubbles within the vascular circuit initiate the complications responsible for decompression injury. With the exception of bubbles forming in central nervous tissue, the primary bubbles occur in the venous and arterial vascular bed.[1] Symptoms of decompression sickness usually appear within 4 to 6 hours after the dive. However, if decompression procedures have been severely violated, e.g., when a diver runs out of air and ascends rapidly, symptoms may appear immediately and progress to paralysis within minutes.[7] The most common symptoms of inadequate decompression are dizziness, itchy skin, and pain in the legs and arms, especially in the "tight" tissues such as ligaments and tendons. The degree of injury depends on the size of the bubbles and where they are formed. Bubbles in the lungs can cause choking and asphyxia, whereas bubbles in the brain and coronary arteries block blood flow. The bubbles deprive these vital tissues of oxygen and nutrients and cause subsequent cellular damage and death. Central nervous system "bends" is relatively common and especially serious because it can cause permanent neural damage if treatment is delayed.

Treatment for the bends involves the lengthy process of recompression in a small chamber to force the nitrogen gas back into solution. This step is followed by slow *decompression* so that the expanding gas has sufficient time to leave the body as the diver is brought back to the "surface."

For the sport diver, the chances are slim of having a recompression chamber nearby. This makes it imperative that the recommendations for diving depth and duration not be exceeded.[9]

Oxygen Poisoning

In general, when the inspired P_{O_2} exceeds 2 atmospheres or 1520 mm Hg, the diver becomes highly susceptible to *oxygen poisoning*.[5] For this reason, closed-circuit scuba systems that use pure oxygen place severe restrictions on both the depth and length of a dive. At depths greater than 25 feet, the use of pure oxygen is not recommended except in extraordinary circumstances (Table 25-2).

High oxygen pressures affect bodily functions in several ways: (1) a high P_{O_2} directly irritates respiratory passages and eventually induces bronchopneumonia if exposure is continued; (2) at pressures of about 2 atmospheres, oxygen tends to constrict cerebral blood vessels and has a profound effect on central nervous system function; and (3) high pressures of inspired oxygen may also cause dysfunction by affecting carbon dioxide elimination. Specifically, a high inspired P_{O_2} may force sufficient oxygen into solution in the plasma to supply the metabolic needs of the diver. Oxygen is therefore returned in combination with hemoglobin so that carbon dioxide elimination via hemoglobin is greatly reduced.

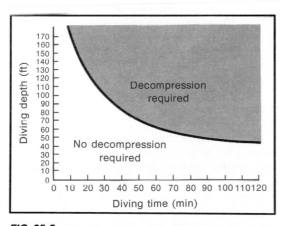

FIG. 25-5. *Zero decompression limits. Any single dive falling on the left side of the curve requires no decompression as long as the rate of ascent does not exceed 60 ft per minute. Dives on the right side of the line require a decompression period, the specifics of which can be obtained from Navy Standard Decompression Tables.*[9]

TABLE 25-2. *United States Navy recommended depth–time limits breathing pure oxygen during working dives*

Normal Operations[a]		
Depth (ft)	(m)	Time (minutes)
10	3.0	240
15	4.6	150
20	6.1	110
25	7.6	75
Exceptional Operations		
Depth (ft)	(m)	Time (minutes)
30	9.2	45
35	10.7	20
40	12.2	10

[a]No symptoms of oxygen poisoning were noted at these depths and durations.

The treatment for oxygen poisoning consists of breathing air at sea-level pressure.

Carbon Monoxide Poisoning

Carbon monoxide is a lethal gas that combines with hemoglobin 200 times more readily than oxygen. Thus, tissue hypoxia can easily occur with only a small quantity of carbon monoxide in the inspired mixture. This becomes a special problem in deep dives because the partial pressures of all gases in the breathing mixture (including the impurities) increase greatly.

Contaminants from automotive and industrial exhausts, including carbon monoxide and oxides of sulfur, may be high in urban areas. For this reason, it is not advisable to fill scuba tanks when an air pollution alert is in effect.[8] Aside from the contaminants present in free air, carbon monoxide and oil impurities can also be added during the operation of the gasoline or diesel engine compressor. This potential source of contamination can be eliminated by placing the engine's exhaust downstream from the air intake that provides the compressed air.

SUMMARY

1. The underwater diver is exposed to high pressures and to the possibility of rapid changes in pressures. The diver can suffer severe injury and even death unless adjustments are made to equalize pressures in the body's air-filled cavities.

2. Snorkel size is limited by two factors: (1) the underwater depth at which the skin diver can generate sufficient inspiratory force to breathe, and (2) the additional pulmonary dead space created by the snorkel's volume.

3. Hyperventilation increases breathhold time but can also contribute to underwater blackout. This extremely dangerous consequence of hyperventilation is probably brought on by a critical reduction in oxygen, an abnormal increase in carbon dioxide, acid–base imbalance, or the combined effects of all these factors.

4. The maximum depth for breathhold diving is generally determined by the point at which the diver's lung volume is compressed to residual volume. Below this critical depth, internal and external pressures are unable to equalize and lung squeeze results.

5. Because scuba systems supply breathing mixtures at great depths and pressures, specific hazards result from improper equalization of pressure in the lungs, sinus, and middle-ear spaces. The most significant dangers are from air embolism, pneumothorax, mask and middle-ear squeeze, and aerosinusitis.

6. Gases breathed at high pressures move across the pulmonary membrane and eventually dissolve and equilibrate in all fluids and tissues of the body. High tissue pressures of oxygen and nitrogen have profound effects on physiologic function. Because of these problems, the maximum recommended depth for breathing compressed air is generally about 100 ft.

7. As a scuba diver ascends toward the surface, a gradient is created for the net flow of nitrogen from the body fluids into the lungs. If the ascent is too rapid, the excess nitrogen that cannot exit via the lungs escapes from the dissolved state and forms bubbles in the tissues. This extremely painful condition is termed the bends.

References

1. Behnke, A. R.: Decompression sickness: advances and interpretations. Aerosp. Med., *42:*255, 1971.
2. Craig, A. B., Jr.: Causes of loss of consciousness during underwater swimming. J. Appl. Physiol., *16:*583, 1961.
3. Craig, A. B., Jr.: Summary of 58 cases of loss of consciousness during underwater swimming and diving. Med. Sci. Sports, *8:*171, 1976.
3a. Craig, A. B., Jr.: Principles and problems of underwater diving. Physician Sportsmed., *8:*72, 1980.
4. Kindwall, E. P.: Medical aspects of sport scuba diving. Aqua Notes *3:*1, 1976.
5. Lambertsen, C. J.: Effects of oxygen at high partial pressure. *In* Handbook of Physiology. Edited by W. O. Fenn and H. Rahn. Washington, D. C., American Physiological Society, 1965.
6. Lanphier, E. H., and Rahn, H.: Alveolar gas exchange during breathhold diving. J. Appl. Physiol., *18:*471, 1963.
7. Strauss, R. H., and Yount, D. E.: Decompression sickness. Am. Sci., *65:*598, 1977.
8. The NOAA Diving Manual. U.S. Department of Commerce, Washington, D.C., National Oceanic and Atmospheric Administration.
9. U.S. Navy Diving Manual. Department of Navy, Washington, D.C., 1970.

SECTION VI

Body Composition, Energy Balance, and Weight Control

An accurate appraisal of body composition provides an important basis for formulating an intelligent program of total fitness. The frequently used standard—the age-height-weight tables— is of limited value in evaluating physique, for it is now well established that overweight and overfat are not the same thing. This point is clearly illustrated with athletes. Many of these individuals are quite muscular and in excess of some average weight for their age and height, but otherwise lean in terms of body composition. For such people, a weight loss program is unnecessary and may even be harmful to sports performance. On the other hand, it is possible to be "average" for body weight yet still possess an undesirable excess of body fat. In this situation, a weight loss or body composition modification program may be desirable. Of even greater importance is the need for effective weight control among adults who suffer the insidious consequences of physical inactivity and overeating. For these people, body fat eventually exceeds even the most liberal limits for normalcy and should be reduced. To this end, diet *plus* exercise can play an important role.

In this section we discuss body composition—its assessment, and differences between men and women, trained and untrained. We also deal with topics relevant to obesity and weight-control programs using diet and exercise.

Body Composition
Assessment

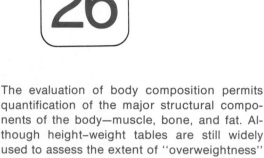

The evaluation of body composition permits quantification of the major structural components of the body—muscle, bone, and fat. Although height–weight tables are still widely used to assess the extent of "overweightness" based on age and "frame size," such tables do not provide information with regard to the relative composition or quality of an individual's body weight. Someone may weigh much more than the average weight-for-height standards based on insurance company statistics, yet still be "underfat" in terms of the body's total quantity of fat. The "extra" weight could simply be additional muscle mass. According to the popular, height–weight tables, assuming a "large" frame size, the desirable body weight range for a 21-year-old professional football player who is 74 in. tall and weighs 255 lb, is 173 to 194 pounds. Based on the latest data from the United States Public Health Service and Nutrition Examination Survey,[31] the average weight for 18- to 24-year-old males who are 74 in. tall is 188 lb. Using either set of criteria, the player is clearly "overweight" and by conventional standards should reduce his body weight at least 61 lb just to achieve the upper limit of the desirable weight range! He must reduce an additional 6 lb to match his "average" American male counterpart based on the Health and Nutrition Survey.

If the player followed these guidelines, it is a good bet he would no longer be playing football and might even jeopardize his overall health by undertaking a crash or bizarre diet that prohibited the proper intake of essential nutrients. Although many larger-sized persons are indeed "overweight," they are not necessarily too fat and do not necessarily need to reduce. The total fat content of the football player was only 12.7% of his body weight compared with 15.0% body fat typically reported for young, male nonathletes.[22,41] This player's body fat was *below* that normally found in the general population, even though he weighed much more than the average. Such observations were made in the early 1940s on 25 football players, 17 of whom were found unfit for military service because they were overweight and presumably too fat or obese.[1,40] However, a careful evaluation of each player's body composition revealed that the so-called excess weight was due primarily to muscular hypertrophy. The term overweight refers only to body weight in excess of some standard, usually the mean weight for a given stature. Being above some "average," "ideal," or "desirable" body weight based on height–weight tables should not necessarily dictate whether or not someone goes on a reducing regime. A more desirable alternative to the height–weight tables is to determine the body composition by one of several laboratory or field techniques. In this chapter, we review various methods for body composition assessment.

COMPOSITION OF THE HUMAN BODY

The three major structural components of the human body include muscle, fat, and bone. Because there are marked sex differences in body composition, a convenient basis for evaluation and comparison is to employ the concept proposed by Behnke of the *reference man* and *reference woman*.[3] Figure 26-1 depicts the gross composition for a reference man and woman in terms of muscle, fat, and bone. This theoretical model is based upon the average

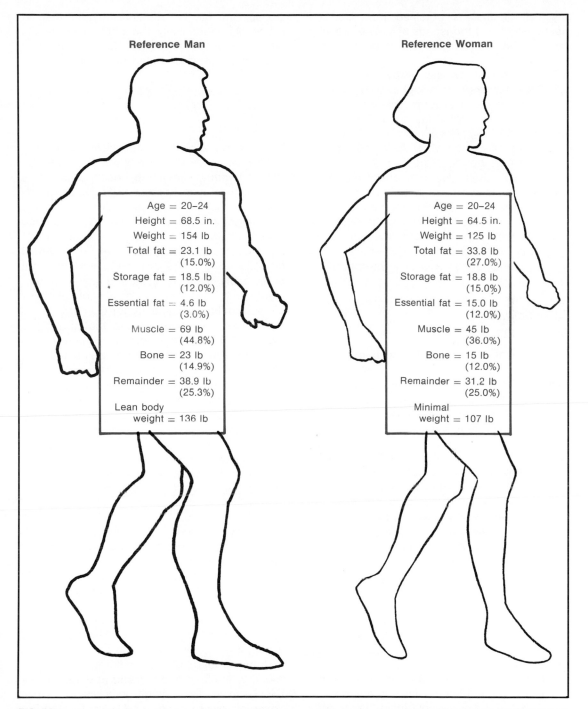

FIG. 26-1. *Behnke's theoretical model for a reference man and woman. The mean values for 13 circumference measures and 8 skeletal diameters, including proportionality constants for the reference man and woman and comparisons with various groups, are presented in the Behnke and Wilmore monograph.*[3]

physical dimensions obtained from detailed measurements of thousands of individuals who were subjects in large-scale anthropometric surveys.

The reference man is taller by 4 in., heavier by 29 lb; his skeleton weighs more (23 vs. 15 lb); and he has a larger muscle mass (69 vs. 45 lb) and lower total fat content (23.1 vs. 33.8 lb) than the reference female. These sex differences exist even when the amount of fat, muscle, and bone are expressed as a percentage of body weight. The concept of reference standards does not mean that men and women should strive to achieve the body composition of the reference models, nor that the reference man and woman are in fact "average." The models are useful as a frame of reference for statistical comparison and data interpretation.

Essential and Storage Fat

The total amount of body fat exists in two depots or storage sites. The first depot, termed *essential fat,* is the fat stored in the marrow of bones as well as in the heart, lungs, liver, spleen, kidneys, intestines, muscles, and lipid-rich tissues throughout the central nervous system. This fat is required for normal physiologic functioning. In the female, essential fat also includes *sex-specific* or *sex-characteristic* fat. It is not at all clear whether this fat depot is expendable or serves as reserve storage. The mammary glands and pelvic region are probably primary storage sites for this fat, although the precise quantitative amounts are unknown. The contribution of breast weight to the body's total body fat content was estimated to be no higher than 4% for women who varied in body fat content from 14% to 35%.[25] This must mean that sites other than the breasts contribute a larger proportion of sex-specific fat, perhaps in the lower body region, which includes the pelvis and thighs.

The other major fat depot, the *storage fat,* consists of fat that accumulates in adipose tissue. This nutritional reserve includes the fatty tissues that protect the various internal organs from trauma, as well as the larger subcutaneous fat volume deposited beneath the skin surface. Although the proportional distribution of storage fat in males and females is similar (12% in males, 15% in females), the total quantity of essential fat in females, which includes the sex-specific fat, is four times higher than in males. More than likely, the additional essential fat is biologically important for child-bearing and other hormone-related functions.

Minimal Standards for Leanness

There seems to be a biologically lower limit beyond which a person's body weight cannot be reduced without impairing health status. This lower limit in men is referred to as *lean body weight* and is calculated as body weight minus the weight of storage fat. For the reference man, the lean weight is equivalent to 136 lb; this includes approximately 3% or 4.1 lb essential fat. According to Behnke,[2] this amount of fat presumably is a lower limit, and any encroachment into this reserve may impair normal physiologic function or capacity for exercise.

In our studies of professional football players (1975–1979 New York Jets; 1976–1978 Dallas Cowboys; 1979–1980 Miami Dolphins and New Orleans Saints), values of fatness as low as 1.0% of body weight have been recorded for several defensive backs. This corresponds to the body weight with essentially no storage fat. Any further reduction in fatness would encroach on the essential fat stores and could impair optimal health.

Similar low values of body fat have been reported for champion male athletes, chiefly world-class marathon runners, and some conscientious objectors who voluntarily reduced their body fat stores during a prolonged experiment with semistarvation.[26] The low fat levels of marathon runners, which ranged from about 1% to 8% of body weight,[35] probably reflects an adaptation to the severe training requirements of prolonged distance running. A minimal fat level permits a more effective gradient for the rapid tranfer of metabolic heat produced during high-intensity exercise.

Considerable individual differences also are found in the lean body weight of different athletes, with values ranging from a low of 106 lb in some jockeys to a high of 248 lb in an All-Pro football defensive lineman and Olympic champion discus thrower.

MINIMAL WEIGHT. In contrast to the lower limit of body weight of males, which includes 3% essential fat, the lower limit of body weight for the reference female includes 12% essential fat.

This theoretical limit is termed *minimal weight,* and for the reference woman it is equivalent to 107 lb. In general, the leanest women in the population do not have body fat levels below about 10% to 12% of body weight. This probably represents the lower limit of fatness for most women in good health. *This concept of minimal weight in females that incorporates about 12% essential fat is equivalent to lean body weight in males that includes 3% essential fat.*

It should be emphasized that the concept of female minimal weight is based on theoretical considerations, with little actual data other than the fact that in carefully conducted experiments values lower than 10% body fat are rarely reported. Data from female distance runners constitute an exception,[44] where a value of 5.9% body fat was reported for one runner who weighed 52.6 kg. Although some measurement error is to be expected, this value is well below the limits for minimal weight specified by the Behnke model. Corroboration of such findings with a larger sample will probably result in modification of the lower limits of minimal weight.

CALCULATION OF MINIMAL WEIGHT. Behnke has proposed a relatively simple method for estimating a woman's minimal weight based on bone diameter measurements.[3] If body weight is lower than the computed minimal weight, then the woman is clearly underweight and should not reduce body weight further without

medical supervision. The following equation is used to calculate minimal weight:

$$\text{Minimal weight} = (D/33.5)^2 \times h_{dm} \times 0.111$$

where D is the sum of eight bone diameters, h_{dm} is height in decimeters, and 33.5 and 0.111 are constants.

The example shown in Table 26-1 illustrates the computation of minimal weight in a young, thin-appearing female who weighed 38.7 kg (85.3 lb) and was 65.6 in. tall (166.7 cm or 16.67 dm). The eight bone diameter measurements were taken according to standard procedures.[3] Clearly, by Behnke's standards, this woman would be classified as *underweight,* since her body weight of 38.7 kg is about 8% below her recommended minimal weight.

Underweight and Thin

The terms underweight and thin are not necessarily synonomous. In fact, in some cases they describe physical conditions that differ considerably. Measurements in our laboratories in Michigan and Massachusetts have focused on the structural characteristics of apparently "thin" females.[24b] Subjects were initially screened subjectively as appearing thin or "skinny." The 26 women then underwent a thorough anthropometric evaluation that included the measurement of skinfolds, circumferences, and bone diameters, and the determination of body fat and lean body weight by hydrostatic weighing. (These techniques are discussed in detail in the following sections.)

The results were unexpected in that the percent body fat of these women averaged 18.2%, which is about 7 percentage units below the average value of 25% body fat typically reported for college-aged women. The other striking finding was the lack of significant differences in four trunk and four extremity bone diameter measurements between the thin-appearing women and 174 women who averaged 25.6% fat and 31 women who averaged 31.4% fat. Thus, appearing thin or skinny does not necessarily mean that skeletal frame size is diminutive or that the body's total fat content is excessively low, as would be the case for the lower limits for minimal weight and essential fat proposed by Behnke.

Based on our studies, we believe that three criteria can be used to designate a female who

TABLE 26-1. *Procedure for computing a woman's minimal weight*

DIAMETER	MEASUREMENT, CM
Biacromial	34.4
Chest	23.8
Bi-iliac	22.7
Bitrochanteric	29.8
Knees[a]	16.1
Ankles[a]	11.5
Elbows[a]	11.1
Wrists[a]	10.0
	Sum = 159.4

[a]Sum of right and left sides

Step 1. Compute D, which is the sum of the 8 diameters. Note that the last 4 measurements represent the sum of the right and left sides.
Step 2. Substitute in the equation for minimal weight.

$$\begin{aligned}\text{Minimal weight} &= (D/33.5)^2 \times h_{dm} \times 0.111 \\ &= (159.4/33.5)^2 \times 16.67 \times 0.111 \\ &= 41.9 \text{ kg}\end{aligned}$$

is underweight: (1.) body weight lower than minimal weight calculated from skeletal measurements as outlined on page 371; (2.) body weight lower than the 20th percentile by height-for-age;[31] (3.) percent body fat lower than 17%.

The underweight female can be classified as one of three types:

Type 1. Characterized by a low lean body weight. This person is preanorexic, nutritionally deficient, and amenorrhea (failure to menstruate) is present.

Type II. Characterized by an average lean body weight and low fat. This person is physically active with normal menses.

Type III. Characterized by a high lean body weight and low fat. This person has extensive experience in athletics and strenuous physical training with weight lifting. Amenorrhea frequently occurs during training and competition; normal menses usually returns with detraining and lack of competition.[12a]

Further studies are required to refine and establish the body fat and lean body weight boundaries for the Type I, II, and III underweight female.

COMMON TECHNIQUES FOR ASSESSING BODY COMPOSITION

Two general procedures are used to evaluate body composition: (1) direct, i.e., chemical analysis of the animal carcass and human cadaver, and (2) indirect, i.e., hydrostatic weighing and skinfold and circumference measurements. Other indirect techniques are discussed in detail in technical publications.[4,7,9,10] Although the direct methods provide the theoretical validity for the indirect procedures, it is the indirect techniques that enable the exercise specialist to assess the fat and lean components of living persons.

The following section presents three indirect procedures for assessing body composition. The first describes the application of Archimedes' principle to *hydrostatic weighing*. With this method, percent body fat is computed from body density (the ratio of body weight to body volume). The other procedures involve the prediction of body fat from skinfold and girth measurements.

Archimedes' Principle of Hydrostatic Weighing

The Greek mathematician Archimedes is attributed with discovering the physical principle that serves as the basis of body composition evaluation. When King Hieron asked Archimedes to determine the gold content of his crown, he was in fact asking for an analysis of a two-component system of gold and some other metal that was supposedly diluting the crown's gold content. In solving this problem, Archimedes reasoned that the volume of water that overflowed his bath when he entered was equal to the volume of his submerged body. He also reasoned that an object either submerged or floating in water is buoyed up by a counterforce that equals the weight of water displaced. This buoyant force helps support the submerged object against the downward pull of gravity. Thus an object is said to lose weight in water. *Because the object's loss of weight in water equals the weight of the volume of water it displaces, its specific gravity* can be defined as the ratio of weight in air divided by its loss of weight in water.*

$$\frac{\text{Specific}}{\text{gravity}} = \frac{\text{Weight in air}}{\substack{\text{Loss of weight in water} \\ \text{(wt. in air minus wt. in water)}}}$$

Archimedes used quantities of silver and gold each having the same weight as the crown. When the silver and gold were submerged in a container filled with water, each caused a different volume to overflow. When the crown was submerged, it displaced more water than the gold but less than the silver. Thus, Archimedes deduced that the King's gold crown was indeed composed of both gold *and* silver.

---

* The specific gravity can be thought of as an object's degree of "heaviness" in relation to its volume. Objects of the same volume may, of course, vary considerably in density, density being defined as weight per unit volume (density = weight ÷ volume). The volume of 1 g of water occupies exactly one cubic centimeter at a temperature of 39.2° F (4° C). Its density would be 1 g per cubic centimeter, or $1 \text{ g} \cdot \text{cc}^{-1}$. Because the density of water is greatest at 39.2° F, increasing the temperature would increase the volume of 1 g of water and decrease its density. It is necessary, therefore, to correct the volume of an object weighed in water in terms of the water's density at the weighing temperature. The temperature effect distinguishes density from specific gravity.

VALIDITY OF HYDROSTATIC WEIGHING FOR ESTIMATING BODY FAT. There is both direct and indirect experimental evidence that establishes the validity of hydrostatic weighing for estimating body fat content. In Behnke's early studies of Navy divers,[40] 64 subjects were placed into two groups based on their body density. The mean difference between the groups in body weight and body volume was 12.4 kg and 13.29 liters, respectively. The ratio of these average differences (Δ weight ÷ Δ volume), was 0.933 g · ml⁻¹, a value within the densitometric range of 0.92 to 0.96 g · ml⁻¹ for human adipose tissue. Thus, the difference in body weight between the high- and low-density groups was equivalent to the density of adipose tissue. When the density of a group of heavy but lean pro football players was determined by hydrostatic weighing, the players had an average density of 1.080 g · ml⁻¹ and an average lean body weight that was 20 kg higher than that of the divers. As Behnke has stated,[3] "Here indeed was a presumptive demonstration that fat could be separated from bone and muscle in vivo or 'the silver from the gold' by application of a principle renowned in antiquity."

The upper and lower limits of body density in the population are approximately 0.93 g · ml⁻¹ in the very obese and 1.10 g · ml⁻¹ in the leanest males. This coincides nicely with the 1.10 density value of fat-free (or lean) samples of homogenized whole body tissues in small mammals.[29] Experiments with hamsters have confirmed the intrinsic relationships between the fat and nonfat components of the total body mass and provide strong support for the validity of the hydrostatic technique for the estimation of body fat from body density.[27]

COMPUTING BODY DENSITY. According to Archimedes' principle, if an object weighs 75 kg in air and 3 kg when submerged in water, the loss of weight in water of 72 kg is equal to the weight of the displaced water. Because the density of water at any temperature is known, the volume of water displaced can easily be computed. In the example, 72 kg of water is equal to 72 liters of 72,000 cubic centimeters (1 g of water = 1 cc in volume). If the water temperature is 4° C, there would be no correction factor. Refer to Appendix E for the correction factors at higher temperatures. The density of the person, computed as weight ÷ volume, would be 75,000 g ÷ 72,000 cc, or 1.0416 g · cc⁻¹. The laboratory procedures for measuring body density are discussed on pages 374–376. Once the body density is known, the next step is to convert the density value to percentage of body fat.

COMPUTING PERCENT BODY FAT. The percentage of fat in the body can be determined from a simple equation that incorporates density.* The simplified "Siri equation" is obtained by substituting 0.90 g · cc⁻¹ and 1.10 g · cc⁻¹ for the densities of fat and lean tissue, respectively.

$$D = \frac{F + L}{(F/f) + (L/l)}$$

Because the density of the whole system equals the sum of its parts, $F + L = 1$.

$$D = \frac{1}{(F/f) + (L/l)}$$

By rearranging terms, the proportional contribution of F becomes:

$$F = \frac{1}{D} \times \frac{f \times l}{(l - f)} - \frac{f}{(l - f)}$$

Its derivation by Berkeley scientist Dr. William Siri[37] is:

$$\text{Percent body fat} = \frac{495}{\text{Density}} - 450$$

This equation was derived from a two-compartment model of the body consisting of fat and lean tissues. Fat extracted from adipose tissue has a density of 0.90 g · ml⁻¹ at 36° C, whereas fat-free tissue has a density of approximately 1.10 g · ml⁻¹. Each of these densities remains relatively constant even with large individual variations in total body fat.

In the previous example, in which weight and volume were equal to 75 kg and 72 liters, respectively, the density of 1.0416 g · cc⁻¹ when converted to percent fat by the Siri equation equals 25.23%.

$$\text{Percent fat} = \frac{495}{1.0416} - 450$$
$$= 25.23$$

It should be noted that several formulas other than Siri's equation have been devised to estimate body fat from density.[8,36] The basic difference between the formulas is generally less

---

*An algebraic expression that incorporates the densities of the fat and fat-free tissues can be represented by D, the density of the whole system, where F and L are the fat and lean tissue components, each with densities f and l, respectively. The object is to solve for F.

than about 1% within a range of body fat of 4% to 30%:

COMPUTING THE WEIGHT OF FAT. The weight of the body's fat content is computed by multiplying percent fat by body weight.

Fat weight = (Percent fat/100) × body weight
= .2523 × 75 kg
= 18.92 kg

Further calculations could be done to subdivide the total fat weight for this person into essential and storage fat. For a female with about 12% essential fat, there would be 9.0 kg of essential fat (0.12 × 75 kg) and a remainder of 9.9 kg of storage fat (0.132 × 75 kg); for a male with 3% essential fat and 22.2% storage fat (based on the above percent fat of 25.2), the corresponding values for essential and storage fat would be 2.3 and 16.5 kg, respectively. Clearly, if a man and a woman have the same percent body fat, the man could be considered "fatter" because a larger percentage of his body fat is in the form of storage fat. Because each gram of fat contains about 9 kcal (9000 kcal per kg), a rough approximation can also be made of the potential energy stored in each fat depot. For storage fat, the values would be 81,000 kcal for the female and 148,500 kcal for the male; for essential fat, the values would 89,100 and 20,700 kcal for the woman and man, respectively.

COMPUTING FAT-FREE BODY WEIGHT. Fat-free body weight is calculated by subtracting the weight of fat from body weight.

Fat-free body weight = Body weight
                     − Fat weight
= 75 kg − 18.92 kg
= 56.1 kg

Measurement of Body Volume

The principle discovered by Archimedes is applied to measurement of body volume in one of two ways: (1) water displacement, or (2) underwater weighing. Body volume must be measured accurately because small variations in volume can have a substantial effect on the density calculation and, hence, on the computed values for percent fat and lean body weight. Dr. Behnke and his Navy collaborators were the first scientists to make detailed measurements of body volume that included a correction for the volume of air in the lungs. Their pioneering work in the late 1930s with Navy divers and athletes provided the basis for techniques presently in use.

WATER DISPLACEMENT. The volume of an object submerged in water can be measured by the corresponding rise in the level of water within a container. With this technique, the rise of water is measured in a thin tube secured to the side of a tank. This finely calibrated tube permits accurate volume measurements. When the volume of the body is measured in this manner, the volume of air remaining in the subject's lungs during submersion must be considered. This residual volume is usually determined before the subject enters the tank and is subtracted from the total body volume determined by water displacement.

UNDERWATER WEIGHING. With this procedure, body volume is computed as the difference between body weight measured in air and weight measured during water submersion. *Body volume is equal to the loss of weight in water with the appropriate temperature correction for the density of water.* Figure 26-2 illustrates the procedure used in one of our laboratories to measure body volume by underwater weighing.

The subject's body weight is first determined in air on a balance scale accurate to ± 50 g. A diver's belt is usually secured around the waist of fatter-appearing subjects to ensure that they do not float upward during submersion. (The underwater weight of this belt and chair weight is determined beforehand and is subtracted from the subject's total weight under water.) The subject, who wears a thin nylon swim suit, sits in a lightweight, plastic tubular chair suspended from the scale and submerged beneath the surface of the water. A swimming pool can serve the same purpose as the tank, and the scale and chair assembly can be suspended from a support at the side of the pool. In the tank, water temperature is maintained at about 95° F, which is close to the subject's skin temperature. Water temperature is recorded in order to correct for the density of water at the weighing temperature.

The subject makes a forced maximal exhalation as the head is lowered under water. The breath is held for about 5 seconds while underwater weight is recorded on a sensitive scale

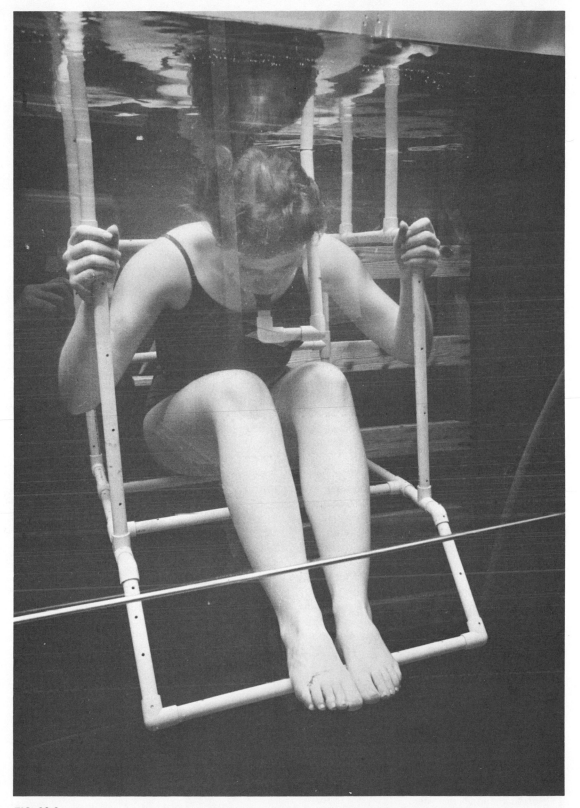

FIG. 26-2. *Measuring body volume by the seated underwater weighing method. Prone and supine methods can also be used for underwater weighing. We use a snorkel during such procedures and measure residual air volume at the time of underwater weighing following a maximal exhalation. (Photo courtesy of Department of Exercise Science, University of Massachusetts.)*

accurate to $\pm$ 10 g or on a force transducer system with digital readout. The underwater weighing procedure is repeated 8 to 12 times, because subjects "learn" to expel more air from their lungs with each additional underwater trial. We use an average of the last two or three weighings because these trials represent the subject's "true" underwater weight with minimal intraindividual variation.[21] Although some researchers select the highest score in the series of weighings,[42] we would like to emphasize that this procedure does not yield the most dependable or reliable score, because it may contain a variable and unknown error source. The same reasoning applies to the selection of any high score in a consecutive series of measures, as, for example, in designating a single oxygen uptake score measured during a functional capacity test such as *the* maximal oxygen uptake. As was the case with the water displacement method, residual volume must be subtracted from total body volume determinations. Reproducibility of body volume scores measured several times on the same day or on consecutive days is always high, with the test–retest reliability coefficient usually above r = 0.94.[15,19]

CALCULATION OF BODY COMPOSITION FROM BODY WEIGHT, BODY VOLUME, AND RESIDUAL LUNG VOLUME. Data from actual measurements on two professional football players who were "All-Pro" and played on Super Bowl teams are given in Table 26-2. Both athletes were weighed without the diver's belt.

The conventional formula for density is mass $\div$ volume, where density is expressed in $g \cdot cc^{-1}$, and mass and volume in kilograms and liters, respectively. Mass (Ma) is determined by weighing in air. The difference between Ma and submerged weight (Mw) is equal to the body volume when the appropriate water temperature correction (Dw) is applied. Because the air

remaining in the lungs at the time of underwater weighing also contributes to buoyancy, this volume must be subtracted from the total body volume.

The formula for calculating the density of the body (D_b) is:

$$D_b = \frac{Mass}{Volume} = \frac{Ma}{\dfrac{(Ma - Mw)}{Dw} - RV}$$

For ease in computation, the formula can be rewritten as:

$$D_b = Ma \times Dw / (Ma - Mw - RV \times Dw)$$

Using the body density formula and incorporating the equations in the previous sections for percent fat, fat weight, and fat-free body weight, the results shown in Table 26-3 were obtained for the two athletes.

Skinfold and Circumference Measurements

Hydrostatic weighing and water displacement are two of the most accurate methods of measuring body density currently available for assessing the body's total fat content. When proper laboratory facilities are unavailable, alternative but simple procedures to predict body fatness can be used. Two of these procedures, the measurement of *subcutaneous skinfold fat* and of *girths* or *circumferences,* require relatively inexpensive equipment. Although it is more difficult to obtain accurate skinfold measurements, circumferences are easy to take, and accuracy can be achieved with a minimum of practice.

MEASUREMENT OF SUBCUTANEOUS SKINFOLD FAT. The rationale for skinfold measurements is based on the fact that approximately one-half of the body's total fat content is located in the

TABLE 26-2. *Measurements of two professional football players using underwater weighing method*

VARIABLE	SYMBOL	DEFENSIVE LINEMAN	RUNNING BACK
Body weight, kg	Ma	121.73	97.37
Net underwater weight, kg	Mw	7.39	6.52
Water temperature correction	Dw	.99336	.99336
Residual lung volume, liters	RV	1.213	1.374

TABLE 26-3. *Body composition of two professional football players determined by underwater weighing*

RESULTS	DEFENSIVE LINEMAN	RUNNING BACK
Total body volume, liters	113.89	90.08
Body density, $g \cdot ml^{-1}$	1.0688	1.0809
Percent fat[a]	13.14	7.95
Fat weight, kg	16.00	7.74
Fat free body weight, kg	105.73	89.63

[a] Siri equation[37]

fat depots directly beneath the skin and this is closely related to total fat. By 1930, a special pincer-type caliper was used to measure subcutaneous fat at selected sites on the body with relative accuracy. The caliper works on the same principle as the micrometer used to measure distance between two points. The procedure for measuring skinfold thickness is to grasp firmly with the thumb and forefinger a fold of skin and subcutaneous fat, pulling it away from the underlying muscular tissue following the natural contour of the skinfold. Constant tension is exerted by the pincer arms of the calipers at their point of contact with the skin. The thickness of the double layer of skin and subcutaneous tissues is then read directly from the caliper dial and recorded in millimeters.

The most common areas for taking skinfold measurements are at the triceps and subscapula, and at the suprailiac, abdominal, and upper thigh sites. All measures are taken on the right side of the body with the subject standing. A minimum of two or three measurements are made at each site, and the average value is used as the skinfold score. When skinfolds are measured for research purposes, the investigator has usually had considerable experience and is consistent in duplicating values for the same subject made on the same day, consecutive days, or even weeks apart. Figure 26-3 shows the anatomic location of the five most frequently measured skinfold sites: (1.) triceps—vertical fold measured at the midline of the upper arm halfway between the tip of the shoulder and the tip of the elbow; (2.) subscapula—oblique fold measured just below the bottom tip of the scapula; (3.) suprailiac—slightly oblique fold measured just above the hip bone. The fold is lifted to follow the natural

diagonal line at this point; (4.) abdomen—vertical fold measured 1 in. to the right of the umbilicus; and (5.) thigh—vertical fold measured at the midline of the thigh, two-thirds of the distance from the knee cap to the hip.

USEFULNESS OF SKINFOLD SCORES. There are two ways in which skinfolds can be used. The first is to sum the five skinfold scores as an indication of the relative degree of fatness among individuals. The "sum of skinfolds" can also be used to reflect changes in fatness "before" and "after" a physical conditioning program. Changes in individual skinfold values as well as the total score can then be evaluated on either an absolute or percentage basis.

From the skinfold data shown in Table 26-4, obtained from a 22-year-old female college student prior to and following a 16-week exercise program, the following observations are made: (1.) The largest changes in skinfold thickness occurred at the suprailiac and abdominal sites. (2.) The triceps showed the largest decrease and the subscapular, the smallest decrease when changes were expressed in percentages. (3.) The total reduction in subcutaneous skinfold fat at the five sites was 16.6 mm or 12.6% of the "before" condition.

The second way to use skinfolds is in conjunction with mathematical equations designed to *predict* body density or percent body fat. These equations are "population specific"[17a] and predict fatness fairly accurately in samples of subjects similar to those from which the equations were derived. The predicted value of fatness for an individual is usually within 3% to 5% of the body fat based on body density measurements determined by hydrostatic weighing or water displacement.

As a result of several experiments conducted

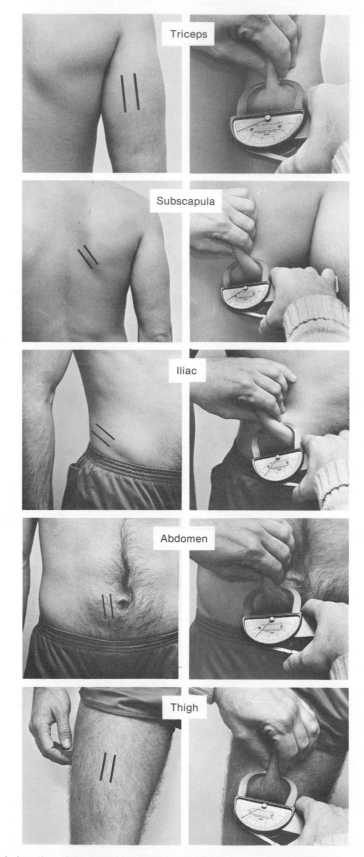

FIG. 26-3. *Anatomic location of the five skinfold sites. All skinfolds are measured in the vertical plane except at the subscapula and iliac, which are oblique.*

TABLE 26-4. *Changes in selected skinfolds for a young woman during a 16-week exercise program*

SKINFOLDS, MM	BEFORE	AFTER	ABSOLUTE CHANGE	PERCENT CHANGE
Triceps	22.5	19.4	−3.1	−13.8
Subscapular	19.0	17.0	−2.0	−10.5
Suprailiac	34.5	30.2	−4.3	−12.8
Abdomen	33.7	29.4	−4.3	−12.8
Thigh	21.6	18.7	−2.9	−13.4
Sum	131.3	114.7	−16.6	−12.6

in our laboratories, equations have been developed to predict body fat from triceps and subscapula skinfolds.[22,23] The equations most useful for predicting total body fat in young women and men are:

Young women, ages 17 to 26 years
Percent body fat = .55(A) + .31(B) + 6.13
Where A = triceps skinfold, mm
B = subscapula skinfold, mm

Young men, ages 17 to 26 years
Percent body fat = .43(A) + .58(B) + 1.47
Where A = triceps skinfold, mm
B = subscapula skinfold, mm

Using the actual skinfold data of the young woman who participated in the 16-week physical conditioning program, we can compute her percent body fat prior to and following the conditioning program using the equation for women just presented. Substituting the pre-training values for triceps (22.5 mm) and subscapula (19.0 mm) skinfolds, percent body fat equals 24.4%.

$$\text{Percent body fat} = .55(A) + .31(B) + 6.13$$
$$= .55\ (22.5) + .31\ (19.0) + 6.13$$
$$= 12.38 + 5.89 + 6.13$$
$$= 24.4\%$$

Substituting the values for triceps (19.4 mm) and subscapula (17.0 mm), the post-training value for percent body fat is computed in a similar fashion.

$$\text{Percent body fat} = .55\ (19.4) + .31\ (17.0) + 6.13$$
$$= 10.67 + 5.27 + 6.13$$
$$= 22.1\%$$

The determination of percent body fat, prior to and following a conditioning and weight control program, provides a convenient means for evaluating alterations in body composition that often are independent of changes in body weight.

Although the use of skinfolds to predict percent body fat has been widely used in the allied health professions, a major drawback is that the person taking the measurements must have considerable experience with the proper techniques in order to obtain consistent skinfold values. Because there are no standards by which to compare the results between different investigators from diverse geographic regions, it is almost impossible to determine which sets of skinfold data are in fact "correct." Thus, prediction equations developed by a particular researcher (which may be highly valid for the sample measured) may be almost useless to predict accurately the body fat for an individual when another person takes the skinfolds. The *error* in predicting body fat could be plus or minus 200% or higher![24a]

Even when a different approach to body fat prediction that incorporates surface area with skinfolds is used,[24] there is still the basic limitation imposed by technique. Despite this limitation, the surface area formulation may provide valid estimates of body fat for different populations.[24] The basic equation is:

$$\text{Percent Fat} = \frac{\Sigma \text{skinfolds}}{3F \times k(sf)}$$

where Σskinfolds is the sum of 3, 4, or 5 skinfolds, usually triceps, subscapular, suprailiac, abdomen, or thigh; 3F = 3$\sqrt{\text{weight}/\text{height}}$ (where weight is in kg and height is in dm); and k(sf) = Σskinfolds/3F × % fat. The % fat is based on a criterion method such as underwater weighing, and is based on the observed average for the general group or population (of a particular age, sex, state of training, or sport). Thus, different k(sf) constants are required for diverse populations. For example, consider the mean values for a population that represents relatively sedentary young men: height = 18.42 dm; weight = 72.16 kg; skinfolds = 67.3 mm; % fat = 15.3. The k(sf) constant is calculated as

$$k(sf) = \frac{67.3}{3\sqrt{3.9175 \times 15.3}} = 0.741$$

By knowing the k(sf) constant, the percent body fat for any similar individual can now be computed with the basic equation. If weight = 74.0 kg, height = 17.52 dm, and the sum of 5 skinfolds = 57.5 mm, then percent fat for this particular young man is computed as follows:

$$Percent\ Fat = \frac{\Sigma skinfolds}{3F \times k(sf)}$$

$$Percent\ Fat = \frac{57.5}{6.166 \times 0.741}$$

$$Percent\ Fat = 12.58\%$$

We believe this method of computing percent body fat warrants further study, especially in younger age groups where estimates of body composition are desirable. This procedure may provide more useful information than the percentile norm method recently advocated as part of the revised AAHPERD Youth Fitness Test.

MEASUREMENT OF CIRCUMFERENCES. A cloth or flexible steel or plastic measuring tape should be used. The tape is applied lightly to the skin surface so that the tape is taut but not tight. This procedure avoids skin compression, which produces lower than normal scores. Duplicate measurements should be taken at each site and the average used as the circumference score. The anatomic landmarks for the various circumferences for young and older men and women are (1.) abdomen—1 in. above the umbilicus; (2.) buttocks—maximum protrusion with the heels together; (3.) right thigh—upper thigh just below the buttocks; (4.) right upper arm—arm straight, palm up, and extended in front of the body, measured at the midpoint between the shoulder and the elbow; (5.) right forearm—maximum circumference with the arm extended in front of the body with palm up; and (6.) right calf—widest circumference midway between the ankle and knee.

Different prediction equations have been developed for each sex and age group. It must be emphasized that the equations developed for these subgroups, although cross-validated

on different samples with good results,[23] nevertheless seem to be population specific and should *not* be used for predicting fatness in individuals (1) who appear very thin or very fat, (2) who are members of athletic teams, or (3) who have been involved for a number of years in strenuous sports or weight training.

USEFULNESS OF CIRCUMFERENCE MEASUREMENTS. The best procedure to determine fatness is to use the water immersion or displacement technique, or other laboratory methods such as isotopic dilution[5] or potassium-40 counting.[16] The circumference-based prediction equations are most useful in ranking or ordering individuals within a group according to their relative fatness. If one uses the equations and constants presented in Tables 26-5 to 26-9 for young and older men and women, the error in predicting an individual's body fat is ± 2.5% to 4.0%. These relatively low prediction errors make the equations particularly useful to those without access to laboratory facilities, especially since the measurements are easy to take and a tape measure is inexpensive.

PREDICTING BODY FAT FROM CIRCUMFERENCES. The various sites measured in individuals of different sexes and ages are indicated in Table 26-9.

From the appropriate table (Tables 26-5 to 26-9), one can substitute the corresponding constants, A, B, and C in the formula shown at the bottom of the table. Two addition steps and two subtraction steps are required. The following five-step example shows how to calculate percent fat, fat weight, and lean body weight for a 21-year-old man who weighed 174 pounds:

Step 1. The upper arm, abdomen, and right forearm circumferences were measured with a cloth tape and recorded to the nearest one-fourth inch.
Upper arm = 11.5 in. (29.21 cm)
Abdomen = 31.0 in. (78.74 cm)
Right forearm = 10.75 in. (27.30 cm)

Step 2. The three constants A, B, and C corresponding to the three circumference measures were determined from Table 26-5.
Constant A, corresponding to 11.5 in., = 42.56
Constant B, corresponding to 31.0 in., = 40.68
Constant C, corresponding to 10.75 in., = 58.37

TABLE 26-5. *Conversion constants to predict percent body fat for* ***young men***

UPPER ARM			ABDOMEN			FOREARM		
IN	CM	CONSTANT A	IN	CM	CONSTANT B	IN	CM	CONSTANT C
7.00	17.78	25.91	21.00	53.34	27.56	7.00	17.78	38.01
7.25	18.41	26.83	21.25	53.97	27.88	7.25	18.41	39.37
7.50	19.05	27.76	21.50	54.61	28.21	7.50	19.05	40.72
7.75	19.68	28.68	21.75	55.24	28.54	7.75	19.68	42.08
8.00	20.32	29.61	22.00	55.88	28.87	8.00	20.32	43.44
8.25	20.95	30.53	22.25	56.51	29.20	8.25	20.95	44.80
8.50	21.59	31.46	22.50	57.15	29.52	8.50	21.59	46.15
8.75	22.22	32.38	22.75	57.78	29.85	8.75	22.22	47.51
9.00	22.86	33.31	23.00	58.42	30.18	9.00	22.86	48.87
9.25	23.49	34.24	23.25	59.05	30.51	9.25	23.49	50.23
9.50	24.13	35.16	23.50	59.69	30.84	9.50	24.13	51.58
9.75	24.76	36.09	23.75	60.32	31.16	9.75	24.76	52.94
10.00	25.40	37.01	24.00	60.96	31.49	10.00	25.40	54.30
10.25	26.03	37.94	24.25	61.59	31.82	10.25	26.03	55.65
10.50	26.67	38.86	24.50	62.23	32.15	10.50	26.67	57.01
10.75	27.30	39.79	24.75	62.86	32.48	10.75	27.30	58.37
11.00	27.94	40.71	25.00	63.50	32.80	11.00	27.94	59.73
11.25	28.57	41.64	25.25	64.13	33.13	11.25	28.57	61.08
11.50	29.21	42.56	25.50	64.77	33.46	11.50	29.21	62.44
11.75	29.84	43.49	25.75	65.40	33.79	11.75	29.84	63.80
12.00	30.48	44.41	26.00	66.04	34.12	12.00	30.48	65.16
12.25	31.11	45.34	26.25	66.67	34.44	12.25	31.11	66.51
12.50	31.75	46.26	26.50	67.31	34.77	12.50	31.75	67.87
12.75	32.38	47.19	26.75	67.94	35.10	12.75	32.38	69.23
13.00	33.02	48.11	27.00	68.58	35.43	13.00	33.02	70.59
13.25	33.65	49.04	27.25	69.21	35.76	13.25	33.65	71.94
13.50	34.29	49.96	27.50	69.85	36.09	13.50	34.29	73.30
13.75	34.92	50.89	27.75	70.48	36.41	13.75	34.92	74.66
14.00	35.56	51.82	28.00	71.12	36.74	14.00	35.56	76.02
14.25	36.19	52.74	28.25	71.75	37.07	14.25	36.19	77.37
14.50	36.83	53.67	28.50	72.39	37.40	14.50	36.83	78.73
14.75	37.46	54.59	28.75	73.02	37.73	14.75	37.46	80.09
15.00	38.10	55.52	29.00	73.66	38.05	15.00	38.10	81.45
15.25	38.73	56.44	29.25	74.29	38.38	15.25	38.73	82.80
15.50	39.37	57.37	29.50	74.93	38.71	15.50	39.37	84.16
15.75	40.00	58.29	29.75	75.56	39.04	15.75	40.00	85.52
16.00	40.64	59.22	30.00	76.20	39.37	16.00	40.64	86.88
16.25	41.27	60.14	30.25	76.83	39.69	16.25	41.27	88.23
16.50	41.91	61.07	30.50	77.47	40.02	16.50	41.91	89.59
16.75	42.54	61.99	30.75	78.10	40.35	16.75	42.54	90.95
17.00	43.18	62.92	31.00	78.74	40.68	17.00	43.18	92.31
17.25	43.81	63.84	31.25	79.37	41.01	17.25	43.81	93.66
17.50	44.45	64.77	31.50	80.01	41.33	17.50	44.45	95.02
17.75	45.08	65.69	31.75	80.64	41.66	17.75	45.08	96.38
18.00	45.72	66.62	32.00	81.28	41.99	18.00	45.72	97.74
18.25	46.35	67.54	32.25	81.91	42.32	18.25	46.35	99.09
18.50	46.99	68.47	32.50	82.55	42.65	18.50	46.99	100.45
18.75	47.62	69.40	32.75	83.18	42.97	18.75	47.62	101.81
19.00	48.26	70.32	33.00	83.82	43.30	19.00	48.26	103.17
19.25	48.89	71.25	33.25	84.45	43.63	19.25	48.89	104.52
19.50	49.53	72.17	33.50	85.09	43.96	19.50	49.53	105.88
19.75	50.16	73.10	33.75	85.72	44.29	19.75	50.16	107.24
20.00	50.80	74.02	34.00	86.36	44.61	20.00	50.80	108.60
20.25	51.43	74.95	34.25	86.99	44.94	20.25	51.43	109.95
20.50	52.07	75.87	34.50	87.63	45.27	20.50	52.07	111.31

TABLE 26-5. *continued*

UPPER ARM			ABDOMEN			FOREARM		
IN.	CM	CONSTANT A	IN.	CM	CONSTANT B	IN.	CM	CONSTANT C
20.75	52.70	76.80	34.75	88.26	45.60	20.75	52.70	112.67
21.00	53.34	77.72	35.00	88.90	45.93	21.00	53.34	114.02
21.25	53.97	78.65	35.25	89.53	46.25	21.25	53.97	115.38
21.50	54.61	79.57	35.50	90.17	46.58	21.50	54.61	116.74
21.75	55.24	80.50	35.75	90.80	46.91	21.75	55.24	118.10
22.00	55.88	81.42	36.00	91.44	47.24	22.00	55.88	119.45
			36.25	92.07	47.57			
			36.50	92.71	47.89			
			36.75	93.34	48.22			
			37.00	93.98	48.55			
			37.25	94.61	48.88			
			37.50	95.25	49.21			
			37.75	95.88	49.54			
			38.00	96.52	49.86			
			38.25	97.15	50.19			
			38.50	97.79	50.52			
			38.75	98.42	50.85			
			39.00	99.06	51.18			
			39.25	99.69	51.50			
			39.50	100.33	51.83			
			39.75	100.96	52.16			
			40.00	101.60	52.49			
			40.25	102.23	52.82			
			40.50	102.87	53.14			
			40.75	103.50	53.47			
			41.00	104.14	53.80			
			41.25	104.77	54.13			
			41.50	105.41	54.46			
			41.75	106.04	54.78			
			42.00	106.68	55.11			

Note: Percent fat = Constant A + Constant B − Constant C − 10.2

Step 3. Percent body fat was computed by substituting the appropriate constants in the formula shown at the bottom of Table 26-5.

$$\text{Percent fat} = \text{Constant A} + \text{Constant B} - \text{Constant C} - 10.2$$
$$= 42.56 + 40.68 - 58.37 - 10.2$$
$$= 83.24 - 58.37 - 10.2$$
$$= 24.87 - 10.2$$
$$= 14.7\%$$

Step 4. Weight of fat = Percent fat/100 × Body weight

$$\text{Weight of fat} = 14.7/100 \times 174 \text{ lb}$$
$$= 0.147 \times 174 \text{ lb}$$
$$= 25.6 \text{ lb}$$

Step 5. Fat-free body weight = Body weight − Weight of fat

$$\text{Fat-free body weight} = 174 \text{ lb} - 25.6 \text{ lb}$$
$$= 148.4 \text{ lb}$$

What is Average for Percent Body Fat?

Considerable data are available concerning the average body composition of various groups of men and women of different ages and fitness levels. Because there has been no systematic evaluation of the body fat content of representative samples from the general population, there are no precise norms or standards for comparison purposes. The best that can be done is to present the mean values of body fat for young and older men and women in Table 26-10, including plus or minus one unit of variation, the standard deviation. This gives some idea of the spread about the average body fat in each of the studies for 68% of the people in the sample measured.

It is evident from the mean values in Table 26-10 that with increasing age body fat increases in both sexes. This average change does not necessarily mean the trend should be

TABLE 26-6. *Conversion constants to predict percent body fat for **older men***

BUTTOCKS			ABDOMEN			FOREARM		
IN.	CM	CONSTANT A	IN.	CM	CONSTANT B	IN.	CM	CONSTANT C
28.00	71.12	29.34	25.50	64.77	22.84	7.00	17.78	21.01
28.25	71.75	29.60	25.75	65.40	23.06	7.25	18.41	21.76
28.50	72.39	29.87	26.00	66.04	23.29	7.50	19.05	22.52
28.75	73.02	30.13	26.25	66.67	23.51	7.75	19.68	23.26
29.00	73.66	30.39	26.50	67.31	23.73	8.00	20.32	24.02
29.25	74.29	30.65	26.75	67.94	23.96	8.25	20.95	24.76
29.50	74.93	30.92	27.00	68.58	24.18	8.50	21.59	25.52
29.75	75.56	31.18	27.25	69.21	24.40	8.75	22.22	26.26
30.00	76.20	31.44	27.50	69.85	24.63	9.00	22.86	27.02
30.25	76.83	31.70	27.75	70.48	24.85	9.25	23.49	27.76
30.50	77.47	31.96	28.00	71.12	25.08	9.50	24.13	28.52
30.75	78.10	32.22	28.25	71.75	25.29	9.75	24.76	29.26
31.00	78.74	32.49	28.50	72.39	25.52	10.00	25.40	30.02
31.25	79.37	32.75	28.75	73.02	25.75	10.25	26.03	30.76
31.50	80.01	33.01	29.00	73.66	25.97	10.50	26.67	31.52
31.75	80.64	33.27	29.25	74.29	26.19	10.75	27.30	32.27
32.00	81.28	33.54	29.50	74.93	26.42	11.00	27.94	33.02
32.25	81.91	33.80	29.75	75.56	26.64	11.25	28.57	33.77
32.50	82.55	34.06	30.00	76.20	26.87	11.50	29.21	34.52
32.75	83.18	34.32	30.25	76.83	27.09	11.75	29.84	35.27
33.00	83.82	34.58	30.50	77.47	27.32	12.00	30.48	36.02
33.25	84.45	34.84	30.75	78.10	27.54	12.25	31.11	36.77
33.50	85.09	35.11	31.00	78.74	27.76	12.50	31.75	37.53
33.75	85.72	35.37	31.25	79.37	27.98	12.75	32.38	38.27
34.00	86.36	35.63	31.50	80.01	28.21	13.00	33.02	39.03
34.25	86.99	35.89	31.75	80.64	28.43	13.25	33.65	39.77
34.50	87.63	36.16	32.00	81.28	28.66	13.50	34.29	40.53
34.75	88.26	36.42	32.25	81.91	28.88	13.75	34.92	41.27
35.00	88.90	36.68	32.50	82.55	29.11	14.00	35.56	42.03
35.25	89.53	36.94	32.75	83.18	29.33	14.25	36.19	42.77
35.50	90.17	37.20	33.00	83.82	29.55	14.50	36.83	43.53
35.75	90.80	37.46	33.25	84.45	29.78	14.75	37.46	44.27
36.00	91.44	37.73	33.50	85.09	30.00	15.00	38.10	45.03
36.25	92.07	37.99	33.75	85.72	30.22	15.25	38.73	45.77
36.50	92.71	38.25	34.00	86.36	30.45	15.50	39.37	46.53
36.75	93.34	38.51	34.25	86.99	30.67	15.75	40.00	47.28
37.00	93.98	38.78	34.50	87.63	30.89	16.00	40.64	48.03
37.25	94.61	39.04	34.75	88.26	31.12	16.25	41.27	48.78
37.50	95.25	39.30	35.00	88.90	31.35	16.50	41.91	49.53
37.75	95.88	39.56	35.25	89.53	31.57	16.75	42.54	50.28
38.00	96.52	39.82	35.50	90.17	31.79	17.00	43.18	51.03
38.25	97.15	40.08	35.75	90.80	32.02	17.25	43.81	51.78
38.50	97.79	40.35	36.00	91.44	32.24	17.50	44.45	52.54
38.75	98.42	40.61	36.25	92.07	32.46	17.75	45.08	53.28
39.00	99.06	40.87	36.50	92.71	32.69	18.00	45.72	54.04
39.25	99.69	41.13	36.75	93.34	32.91	18.25	46.35	54.78
39.50	100.33	41.39	37.00	93.98	33.14			
39.75	100.96	41.66	37.25	94.61	33.36			
40.00	101.60	41.92	37.50	95.25	33.58			
40.25	102.23	42.18	37.75	95.88	33.81			
40.50	102.87	42.44	38.00	96.52	34.03			
40.75	103.50	42.70	38.25	97.15	34.26			
41.00	104.14	42.97	38.50	97.79	34.48			
42.25	104.77	43.23	38.75	98.42	34.70			
41.50	105.41	43.49	39.00	99.06	34.93			

TABLE 26-6. *continued*

BUTTOCKS			ABDOMEN		
IN.	CM	CONSTANT A	IN.	CM	CONSTANT B
41.75	106.04	43.75	39.25	99.69	35.15
42.00	106.68	44.02	39.50	100.33	35.38
42.25	107.31	44.28	39.75	100.96	35.59
42.50	107.95	44.54	40.00	101.60	35.82
42.75	108.58	44.80	40.25	102.23	36.05
43.00	109.22	45.06	40.50	102.87	36.27
43.25	109.85	45.32	40.75	103.50	36.49
43.50	110.49	45.59	41.00	104.14	36.72
43.75	111.12	45.85	41.25	104.77	36.94
44.00	111.76	46.12	41.50	105.41	37.17
44.25	112.39	46.37	41.75	106.04	37.39
44.50	113.03	46.64	42.00	106.68	37.62
44.75	113.66	46.89	42.25	107.31	37.87
45.00	114.30	47.16	42.50	107.95	38.06
42.25	114.93	47.42	42.75	108.58	38.28
45.50	115.57	47.68	43.00	109.22	38.51
45.75	116.20	47.94	43.25	109.85	38.73
46.00	116.84	48.21	43.50	110.49	38.96
46.25	117.47	48.47	43.75	111.12	39.18
46.50	118.11	48.73	44.00	111.76	39.41
46.75	118.74	48.99	44.25	112.39	39.63
47.00	119.38	49.26	44.50	113.03	39.85
47.25	120.01	49.52	44.75	113.66	40.08
47.50	120.65	49.78	45.00	114.30	40.30
47.75	121.28	50.04			
48.00	121.92	50.30			
48.25	122.55	50.56			
48.50	123.19	50.83			
48.75	123.82	51.09			
49.00	124.46	51.35			

Note: Percent Fat = Constant A + Constant B − Constant C − 15.0

interpreted as being "normal," because studies have shown that participation in vigorous physical activities after age 35 can retard the "average" increase in body fatness.[14,18,28] Higher fat values could be in part due to the fact that aging causes the skeleton to become demineralized and porous, thereby reducing the body density because of the decrease in bone density. Adaptation to a more sedentary life style and concomitant reduction in the level of daily physical activity would also cause the relative increase in body fat. This would occur even if the daily caloric consumption remained the same.

Desirable Body Weight

Although large quantities of body fat are undesirable for good health and fitness, precise statements cannot be made as to an optimum level of body fat or body weight for a particular individual. More than likely, this optimum varies from person to person and is greatly influenced by a variety of genetic factors. Based on data from active young adults and competitive athletes, however, it does appear that it would be desirable to maintain body fat at about 15% of body weight *or less* for men, and 25% *or less* for women. This "optimal" or desirable body weight can be computed (based on a desired body fat level) as follows:

$$\text{Desirable body weight} = \frac{\text{Lean body weight}}{1.00 - \% \text{ fat desired}}$$

Suppose a 200 lb man who is 20% body fat wishes to know the weight he should attain so that this new lower body weight would contain

TABLE 26-7. *Conversion constants to predict percent body fat for **young women***

ABDOMEN			THIGH			FOREARM		
IN.	CM	CONSTANT A	IN.	CM	CONSTANT B	IN.	CM	CONSTANT C
20.00	50.80	26.74	14.00	35.56	29.13	6.00	15.24	25.86
20.25	51.43	27.07	14.25	36.19	29.65	6.25	15.87	26.94
20.50	52.07	27.41	14.50	36.83	30.17	6.50	16.51	28.02
20.75	52.70	27.74	14.75	37.46	30.69	6.75	17.14	29.10
21.00	53.34	28.07	15.00	38.10	31.21	7.00	17.78	30.17
21.25	53.97	28.41	15.25	38.73	31.73	7.25	18.41	31.25
21.50	54.61	28.74	15.50	39.37	32.25	7.50	19.05	32.33
21.75	55.24	29.08	15.75	40.00	32.77	7.75	19.68	33.41
22.00	55.88	29.41	16.00	40.64	33.29	8.00	20.32	34.48
22.25	56.51	29.74	16.25	41.27	33.81	8.25	20.95	35.56
22.50	57.15	30.08	16.50	41.91	34.33	8.50	21.59	36.64
22.75	57.78	30.41	16.75	42.54	34.85	8.75	22.22	37.72
23.00	58.42	30.75	17.00	43.18	35.37	9.00	22.86	38.79
23.25	59.05	31.08	17.25	43.81	35.89	9.25	23.49	39.87
23.50	59.69	31.42	17.50	44.45	36.41	9.50	24.13	40.95
23.75	60.32	31.75	17.75	45.08	36.93	9.75	24.76	42.03
24.00	60.96	32.08	18.00	45.72	37.45	10.00	25.40	43.10
24.25	61.59	32.42	18.25	46.35	37.97	10.25	26.03	44.18
24.50	62.23	32.75	18.50	46.99	38.49	10.50	26.67	45.26
24.75	62.86	33.09	18.75	47.62	39.01	10.75	27.30	46.34
25.00	63.50	33.42	19.00	48.26	39.53	11.00	27.94	47.41
25.25	64.13	33.76	19.25	48.89	40.05	11.25	28.57	48.49
25.50	64.77	34.09	19.50	49.53	40.57	11.50	29.21	49.57
25.75	65.40	34.42	19.75	50.16	41.09	11.75	29.84	50.65
26.00	66.04	34.76	20.00	50.80	41.61	12.00	30.48	51.73
26.25	66.67	35.09	20.25	51.43	42.13	12.25	31.11	52.80
26.50	67.31	35.43	20.50	52.07	42.65	12.50	31.75	53.88
26.75	67.94	35.76	20.75	52.70	43.17	12.75	32.38	54.96
27.00	68.58	36.10	21.00	53.34	43.69	13.00	33.02	56.04
27.25	69.21	36.43	21.25	53.97	44.21	13.25	33.65	57.11
27.50	69.85	36.76	21.50	54.61	44.73	13.50	34.29	58.19
27.75	70.48	37.10	21.75	55.24	45.25	13.75	34.92	59.27
28.00	71.12	37.43	22.00	55.88	45.77	14.00	35.56	60.35
28.25	71.75	37.77	22.25	56.51	46.29	14.25	36.19	61.42
28.50	72.39	38.10	22.50	57.15	46.81	14.50	36.83	62.50
28.75	73.02	38.43	22.75	57.78	47.33	14.75	37.46	63.58
29.00	73.66	38.77	23.00	58.42	47.85	15.00	38.10	64.66
29.25	74.29	39.10	23.25	59.05	48.37	15.25	38.73	65.73
29.50	74.93	39.44	23.50	59.69	48.89	15.50	39.37	66.81
29.75	75.56	39.77	23.75	60.32	49.41	15.75	40.00	67.89
30.00	76.20	40.11	24.00	60.96	49.93	16.00	40.64	68.97
30.25	76.83	40.44	24.25	61.59	50.45	16.25	41.27	70.04
30.50	77.47	40.77	24.50	62.23	50.97	16.50	41.91	71.12
30.75	78.10	41.11	24.75	62.86	51.49	16.75	42.54	72.20
31.00	78.74	41.44	25.00	63.50	52.01	17.00	43.18	73.28
31.25	79.37	41.78	25.25	64.13	52.53	17.25	43.81	74.36
31.50	80.01	42.11	25.50	64.77	53.05	17.50	44.45	75.43
31.75	80.64	42.45	25.75	65.40	53.57	17.75	45.08	76.51
32.00	81.28	42.78	26.00	66.04	54.09	18.00	45.72	77.59
32.25	81.91	43.11	26.25	66.67	54.61	18.25	46.35	78.67
32.50	82.55	43.45	26.50	67.31	55.13	18.50	46.99	79.74
32.75	83.18	43.78	26.75	67.94	55.65	18.75	47.62	80.82
33.00	83.82	44.12	27.00	68.58	56.17	19.00	48.26	81.90
33.25	84.45	44.45	27.25	69.21	56.69	19.25	48.89	82.98
33.50	85.09	44.78	27.50	69.85	57.21	19.50	49.53	84.05

TABLE 26-7. *continued*

ABDOMEN			THIGH			FOREARM		
IN.	CM	CONSTANT A	IN.	CM	CONSTANT B	IN.	CM	CONSTANT C
33.75	85.72	45.12	27.75	70.48	57.73	19.75	50.16	85.13
34.00	86.36	45.45	28.00	71.12	58.26	20.00	50.80	86.21
34.25	86.99	45.79	28.25	71.75	58.78			
34.50	87.63	46.12	28.50	72.39	59.30			
34.75	88.26	46.46	38.75	73.02	59.82			
35.00	88.90	46.79	29.00	73.66	60.34			
35.25	89.53	47.12	29.25	74.29	60.86			
35.50	90.17	47.46	29.50	74.93	61.38			
35.75	90.80	47.79	29.75	75.56	61.90			
36.00	91.44	48.13	30.00	76.20	62.42			
36.25	92.07	48.46	30.25	76.83	62.94			
36.50	92.71	48.80	30.50	77.47	63.46			
36.75	93.34	49.13	30.75	78.10	63.98			
37.00	93.98	49.46	31.00	78.74	64.50			
37.25	94.61	49.80	31.25	79.37	65.02			
37.50	95.25	50.13	31.50	80.01	65.54			
37.75	95.88	50.47	31.75	80.64	66.06			
38.00	96.52	50.80	32.00	81.28	66.58			
38.25	97.15	51.13	32.25	81.91	67.10			
38.50	97.79	51.47	32.50	82.55	67.62			
38.75	98.42	51.80	32.75	83.18	68.14			
39.00	99.06	52.14	33.00	83.82	68.66			
39.25	99.69	52.47	33.25	84.45	69.18			
39.50	100.33	52.81	33.50	85.09	69.70			
39.75	100.96	53.14	33.75	85.72	70.22			
40.00	101.60	53.47	34.00	86.36	70.74			

Note: Percent = Constant A + Constant B − Constant C − 19.6

10% body fat. The computations would be:

$$\text{Fat weight} = 200 \text{ lb} \times .20 = 40 \text{ lb}$$
$$\text{Lean body weight} = 200 \text{ lb} - 40 \text{ lb} = 160 \text{ lb}$$
$$\text{Desirable body weight} = \frac{160 \text{ lb}}{1.00 - .10}$$
$$= \frac{160 \text{ lb}}{.90}$$
$$= 177.8 \text{ lb}$$

$$\text{Desirable fat loss} = \text{Present body weight} - \text{Desirable body weight}$$
$$= 200 \text{ lb} - 177.8 \text{ lb}$$
$$= 22.2 \text{ lb}$$

If this man lost 22.2 lb of body fat, his new body weight of 177.8 lb would have a fat content equal to 10% of body weight.

SUMMARY

1. Standard age-height-weight tables reveal little about an individual's body composition, which, at any given weight and height, may vary considerably. It is possible to be overweight and *not* overfat.

2. Total body fat can be thought of as existing in two depots: essential fat and storage fat. Essential fat is the fat present in bone marrow, nerve tissue, and the various organs; it is generally required for normal physiologic function. Storage fat is the energy reserve that accumulates mainly as adipose tissue beneath the skin.

3. True sex differences appear to exist for quantities of essential fat. Although storage fat values for men and women average 12% to 15% of body weight, the essential fat differences are large, averaging 12% and 3% of body weight for women and men, respectively. This difference is probably related to child-bearing and hormonal functions.

4. It appears that a person cannot reduce below the essential fat level and still maintain good health.

5. The two most popular *indirect* methods for body composition assessment are hydro-

TABLE 26-8. *Conversion constants to predict percent body fat for **older women***

ABDOMEN			THIGH			CALF		
IN.	CM	CONSTANT A	IN.	CM	CONSTANT B	IN.	CM	CONSTANT C
25.00	63.50	29.69	14.00	35.56	17.31	10.00	25.40	14.46
25.25	64.13	29.98	14.25	36.19	17.62	10.25	26.03	14.82
25.50	64.77	30.28	14.50	36.83	17.93	10.50	26.67	15.18
25.75	65.40	30.58	14.75	37.46	18.24	10.75	27.30	15.54
26.00	66.04	30.87	15.00	38.10	18.55	11.00	27.94	15.91
26.25	66.67	31.17	15.25	38.73	18.86	11.25	28.57	16.27
26.50	67.31	31.47	15.50	39.37	19.17	11.50	29.21	16.63
26.75	67.94	31.76	15.75	40.00	19.47	11.75	29.84	16.99
27.00	68.58	32.06	16.00	40.64	19.78	12.00	30.48	17.35
27.25	69.21	32.36	16.25	41.27	20.09	12.25	31.11	17.71
27.50	69.85	32.65	16.50	41.91	20.40	12.50	31.75	18.08
27.75	70.48	32.95	16.75	42.54	20.71	12.75	32.38	18.44
28.00	71.12	33.25	17.00	43.18	21.02	13.00	33.02	18.80
28.25	71.75	33.55	17.25	43.81	21.33	13.25	33.65	19.16
28.50	72.39	33.84	17.50	44.45	21.64	13.50	34.29	19.52
28.75	73.02	34.14	17.75	45.08	21.95	13.75	34.92	19.88
29.00	73.66	34.44	18.00	45.72	22.26	14.00	35.56	20.24
29.25	74.29	34.73	18.25	46.35	22.57	14.25	36.19	20.61
29.50	74.93	35.03	18.50	46.99	22.87	14.50	36.83	20.97
29.75	75.56	35.33	18.75	47.62	23.18	14.75	37.46	21.33
30.00	76.20	35.62	19.00	48.26	23.49	15.00	38.10	21.69
30.25	76.83	35.92	19.25	48.89	23.80	15.25	38.73	22.05
30.50	77.47	36.22	19.50	49.53	24.11	15.50	39.37	22.41
30.75	78.10	36.51	19.75	50.16	24.42	15.75	40.00	22.77
31.00	78.74	36.81	20.00	50.80	24.73	16.00	40.64	23.14
31.25	79.37	37.11	20.25	51.43	25.04	16.25	41.27	23.50
31.50	80.01	37.40	20.50	52.07	25.35	16.50	41.91	23.86
31.75	80.64	37.70	20.75	52.70	25.66	16.75	42.54	24.22
32.00	81.28	38.00	21.00	53.34	25.97	17.00	43.18	24.58
32.25	81.91	38.30	21.25	53.97	26.28	17.25	43.81	24.94
32.50	82.55	38.59	21.50	54.61	26.58	17.50	44.45	25.31
32.75	83.18	38.89	21.75	55.24	26.89	17.75	45.08	25.67
33.00	83.82	39.19	22.00	55.88	27.20	18.00	45.72	26.03
33.25	84.45	39.48	22.25	56.51	27.51	18.25	46.35	26.39
33.50	85.09	39.78	22.50	57.15	27.82	18.50	46.99	26.75
33.75	85.72	40.08	22.75	57.78	28.13	18.75	47.62	27.11
34.00	86.36	40.37	23.00	58.42	28.44	19.00	48.26	27.47
34.25	86.99	40.67	23.25	59.05	28.75	19.25	48.89	27.84
34.50	87.63	40.97	23.50	59.69	29.06	19.50	49.53	28.20
34.75	88.26	41.26	23.75	60.32	29.37	19.75	50.16	28.56
35.00	88.90	41.56	24.00	60.96	29.68	20.00	50.80	28.92
35.25	89.53	41.86	24.25	61.59	29.98	20.25	51.43	29.28
35.50	90.17	42.15	24.50	62.23	30.29	20.50	52.07	29.64
35.75	90.80	42.45	24.75	62.86	30.60	20.75	52.70	30.00
36.00	91.44	42.75	25.00	63.50	30.91	21.00	53.34	30.37
36.25	92.07	43.05	25.25	64.13	31.22	21.25	53.97	30.73
36.50	92.71	43.34	25.50	64.77	31.53	21.50	54.61	31.09
36.75	93.35	43.64	25.75	65.40	31.84	21.75	55.24	31.45
37.00	93.98	43.94	26.00	66.04	32.15	22.00	55.88	31.81
37.25	94.62	44.23	26.25	66.67	32.46	22.25	56.51	32.17
37.50	95.25	44.53	26.50	67.31	32.77	22.50	57.15	32.54
37.75	95.89	44.83	26.75	67.94	33.08	22.75	57.78	32.90
38.00	96.52	45.12	27.00	68.58	33.38	23.00	58.42	33.26
38.25	97.16	45.42	27.25	69.21	33.69	23.25	59.05	33.62
38.50	97.79	45.72	27.50	69.85	34.00	23.50	59.69	33.98

TABLE 26-8. *continued*

ABDOMEN			THIGH			CALF		
IN.	CM	CONSTANT A	IN.	CM	CONSTANT B	IN.	CM	CONSTANT C
38.75	98.43	46.01	27.75	70.48	34.31	23.75	60.32	34.34
39.00	99.06	46.31	28.00	71.12	34.62	24.00	60.96	34.70
39.25	99.70	46.61	28.25	71.75	34.93	24.25	61.59	35.07
39.50	100.33	46.90	28.50	72.39	35.24	24.50	62.23	35.43
39.75	100.97	47.20	28.75	73.02	35.55	24.75	62.86	35.79
40.00	101.60	47.50	29.00	73.66	35.86	25.00	63.50	36.15
40.25	101.24	47.79	29.25	74.29	36.17			
40.50	102.87	48.09	29.50	74.93	36.48			
40.75	103.51	48.39	29.75	75.56	36.79			
41.00	104.14	48.69	30.00	76.20	37.09			
41.25	104.78	48.98	30.25	76.83	37.40			
41.50	105.41	49.28	30.50	77.47	37.71			
41.75	106.05	49.58	30.75	78.10	38.02			
42.00	106.68	49.87	31.00	78.74	38.33			
42.25	107.32	50.17	31.25	79.37	38.64			
42.50	107.95	50.47	31.50	80.01	38.95			
42.75	108.59	50.76	31.75	80.64	39.26			
43.00	109.22	51.06	32.00	81.28	39.57			
43.25	109.86	51.36	32.25	81.91	39.88			
43.50	110.49	51.65	32.50	82.55	40.19			
43.75	111.13	51.95	32.75	83.18	40.49			
44.00	111.76	52.25	33.00	83.82	40.80			
44.25	112.40	52.54	33.25	84.45	41.11			
44.50	113.03	52.84	33.50	85.09	41.42			
44.75	113.67	53.14	33.75	85.72	41.73			
45.00	114.30	53.44	34.00	86.36	42.04			

Note: Percent fat = Constant A + Constant B − Constant C − 18.4

TABLE 26-9. *Variations in body sites measured by the circumference method, depending on age and sex*

AGE (YEARS)	SEX	SITE MEASURED		
		A	B	C
18–26	M	Right upper arm	Abdomen	Right forearm
	F	Abdomen	Right thigh	Right forearm
27–50	M	Buttocks	Abdomen	Right forearm
	F	Abdomen	Right thigh	Right forearm

static weighing and prediction methods from skinfolds and circumferences. Hydrostatic weighing involves the determination of body density and subsequent calculations of percent body fat assuming a constant density for human fat and fat-free tissues. Lean body weight is calculated by subtracting fat weight from body weight.

6. The prediction methods employ equations developed from relationships between selected skinfolds or circumference measures and body density or percent fat. These equations are "population specific" in that they are most accurate with subjects similar to those from which the equations were derived. A valid surface area formula based on height, weight, and skinfolds can be used to estimate body composition in diverse population groups of different ages.

TABLE 26-10. *Average values of percent body fat for younger and older women and men from selected studies*

STUDY	AGE RANGE	HEIGHT, CM	WEIGHT, KG	PERCENT FAT[a]	68% VARIATION LIMIT
Younger women					
Sloan, 1962[39]	17–25	165.0	55.5	22.9	17.5–28.5
Young, 1962[45]	16–30	167.5	59.0	28.7	24.6–32.9
Katch and Michael, 1968[20]	19–23	165.9	58.4	21.9	17.0–26.9
Wilmore and Behnke, 1970[43]	17–29	164.9	58.6	25.5	21.0–30.1
Clauser et al, 1972[12]	17–22	164.1	55.8	28.7	22.3–35.3
Katch and McArdle, 1973[22]	17–26	160.4	59.0	26.2	23.4–33.3
Pollock et al., 1975[33]		166.1	57.5	24.6	
Diaz, 1978[13]	18–26	165.0	57.4	25.5	21.1–30.0
Older women					
Chen, 1953[11]	31–45	163.3	60.7	28.9	25.1–32.8
	43–68	160.0	60.9	34.2	28.0–40.5
Young, 1963[46]	30–40	164.9	59.6	28.6	22.1–35.3
	40–50	163.1	56.4	34.4	29.5–39.5
Pollock et al., 1975[33]	33–50			29.7	23.1–36.5
Younger men					
Brozek and Keys, 1951[6]	17–26	177.8	69.1	11.8	5.9–11.8
Pascale, 1956[32]	17–25	172.4	68.3	13.5	8.3–18.8
Myhre and Kessler, 1966[30]	18–23	180.1	75.5	12.6	8.7–16.5
Sloan, 1967[38]	18–26	176.1	70.6	10.3	1.9–19.0
Wilmore and Behnke, 1968[41]	16–31	175.7	74.1	15.2	6.3–24.2
Katch and McArdle, 1973[22]	17–26	176.4	71.4	15.0	8.9–21.1
Jackson and Pollock, 1977[17]	18–24	179.9	74.6	13.4	7.4–19.4
Older men					
Myhre and Kessler, 1966[30]	24–38	179.0	76.6	17.8	11.3–24.3
	40–48	177.0	80.5	22.3	16.3–28.3
Pollock et al., 1976[34]	27–50			23.7	17.9–30.1
Jackson and Pollock, 1977[17]	27–59	180.0	85.3	27.1	23.7–30.5

[a]Percent body fat was computed from density by the Siri equation.[37]

References

1. Behnke, A.R. et al.: The specific gravity of healthy men. J.A.M.A. *118:*495, 1942.
2. Behnke, A.R.: New concepts in height-weight relationships. *In* Obesity. Edited by N. Wilson, Philadelphia, F.A. Davis, 1969.
3. Behnke, A.R., and Wilmore, J.H.: Evaluation and Regulation of Body Build and Composition. Englewood Cliffs, N.J., Prentice-Hall, 1974.
4. Body Composition in Animals and Man. Washington, D.C., National Academy of Sciences, Publication 1598, 1968.
5. Boling, E.A., and Lipkind, J.B.: Body composition and serum electrolyte concentrations. J. Appl. Physiol., *18:*943, 1963.

6. Brozek, J., and Keys, A.: The evaluation of leanness–fatness in man: Norms and interrelationships. Br. J. Nutr. *36:*32, 1951.

7. Brozek, J., and Henschel, A.: Techniques for Measuring Body Composition. Washington, D.C., National Academy of Sciences—National Research Council, 1961.

8. Brozek, J. et al.: Densitometric analysis of body composition: Revision of some quantitative assumptions. Ann. N.Y. Acad. Sci., *110:*113, 1963.

9. Brozek, J. (Ed.): Body composition. Parts 1 and 2. Ann. N.Y. Acad. Sci., *110:*1, 1963.

10. Brozek, J. (Ed.): Human Body Composition. Approaches and Applications. Oxford, Pergamon Press, 1965.

11. Chen, K.P.: Report on measurement of total body fat in American women on the basis of specific gravity as an evaluation of individual fatness and leanness. J. Formosan Med. Assoc. *52:*271, 1953.

12. Clauser, C.E. et al.: Anthropometry of air force women. AMRL-TR-70-5. Wright Patterson Air Force Base, Ohio, 1972.

12a. Dale, E.D. et al.: Menstrual dysfunction in distance runners. Obstet. Gynecol., *54:*47, 1979.

13. Diez, E.D.: Relation of anthropometric measures to body fatness in college-age women. Unpublished M.S. Thesis. University of Illinois, Urbana-Champaign, 1978.

14. Dill, D.B. et al.: Training: youth and age. Ann. N.Y. Acad. Sci., *134:*760, 1966.

15. Durnin, J.V.G.A.: Replicability of measurements of density of the human body as determined by underwater weighing. J. Appl. Physiol., *15:*142, 1960.

16. Forbes, G.B., and Hursh, J.B.: Age and sex trends in lean body mass calculated from K^{40} measurements: with a note on the theoretical basis for the procedure. Ann. N.Y. Acad. Sci., *110:*255, 1963.

17. Jackson, A.S., and Pollock, M.L.: Prediction accuracy of body density, lean body weight, and total body volume equations. Med. Sci. Sports, *9:*197, 1977.

17a. Jackson, A.S. et al.: Generalized equations for predicting body density of women. Med. Sci. Sports., *12:*175, 1980.

18. Kasch, F.W., and Wallace, J.P.: Physiological variables during 10 years of endurance exercise. Med. Sci. Sports, *8:*5, 1976.

19. Katch, F.I. et al.: Estimation of body volume by underwater weighing: description of a simple method. J. Appl. Physiol. *23:*811, 1967.

20. Katch, F.I., and Michael, E.D.: Prediction of body density from skinfold and girth measurements of college females. J. Appl. Physiol., *25:*92, 1968.

21. Katch, F.I.: Practice curves and errors of measurement in estimating underwater weight by hydrostatic weighing. Med. Sci. Sports, *1:*212, 1969.

22. Katch, F.I., and McArdle, W.D.: Prediction of body density from simple anthropometric measurements in college-age men and women. Hum. Biol. *45:*445, 1973.

23. Katch, F.I., and McArdle, W.D.: Validity of body composition prediction equation for college men and women. Am. J. Clin. Nutr., *28:*105, 1975.

24. Katch, F.I. et al.: Estimation of body fat from skinfolds and surface area. Hum. Biol. *51:*411, 1979.

24a. Katch, F.I., and Katch, V.L.: Measurement and prediction errors in body composition assessment and the search for the perfect prediction equation. Res. Quart. for Exercise and Sport. *51:*249, 1980.

24b. Katch, F.I. et al.: The underweight female. Physician Sportsmed. *8:*55, 1980.

25. Katch, V.L. et al.: Contribution of breast volume and weight to body fat distribution in females. Am. J. Phys. Anthropol., *53:*93, 1980.

26. Keys, A. et al.: The Biology of Human Starvation. Minneapolis, University of Minnesota Press, 1950.

27. Kodama, A.A.: In vivo and in vitro determinations of body fat and body water on the hamster. J. Appl. Physiol., *31:*218, 1971.
28. Lewis, S. et al.: Body composition of middle-aged female endurance athletes. *In Biomechanics of Sports and Kinanthropometry,* Vol. 6. Edited by F. Landry and W.A.R. Orban. Miami, Florida, Symposia Specialists, 1978.
29. Morales, M. F. et al: Studies on body composition: II. Theoretical considerations regarding the major body tissue compartments with suggestions for application to man. J. Biol. Chem., *158:*677, 1945.
30. Myhre, L.G., and Kessler, W.V.: Body density and potassium 40 measurements of body composition as related to age. J. Appl. Physiol., *21:*1251, 1966.
31. National Center for Health Statistics. Weight by height and age of adults 18-74 years: United States, 1971-74. Vital and Health Statistics. Advance Data. Public Health Service. No. 14. Washington, D.C., U.S. Government Printing Office, November 30, 1977.
32. Pascale, L.R. et al.: Correlations between thickness of skin-folds and body density in 88 soldiers. Hum. Biol. *28:*165, 1956.
33. Pollock, M.L. et al.: Prediction of body density in young and middle-aged women. J. Appl. Physiol., *38:*745, 1975.
34. Pollock, M.L. et al.: Prediction of body density in young and middle-aged men. J. Appl. Physiol., *40:*300, 1976.
35. Pollock, M.L. et al.: Body composition of elite class distance runners. Ann. N.Y. Acad. Sci., *301:*361, 1977.
36. Rathbun, E.W., and Pace, N.: Studies on body composition. 1. Determination of body fat by means of the body specific gravity. J. Biol. Chem., *158:*667, 1945.
37. Siri, W.E.: Gross composition of the body. *In* Advances in Biological and Medical Physics, Vol. IV, Edited by J.H. Lawrence and C.A. Tobias. Academic Press, New York, 1956.
38. Sloan, A.W.: Estimation of body fat in young men. J. Appl. Physiol., *23:*311, 1967.
39. Sloan, A.W. et al.: Estimation of body fat in young women. J. Appl. Physiol., *17:*967, 1962.
40. Welham, W.C., and Behnke, A.R.: The specific gravity of healthy men. J.A.M.A.: *188:*498, 1942.
41. Wilmore, J.H., and Behnke, A.R.: Predictability of lean body weight through anthropometric assessment in college men. J. Appl. Physiol., *25.*349, 1968.
42. Wilmore, J.H.: The use of actual, predicted and constant residual volumes in the assessment of body composition by underwater weighing. Med. Sci. Sports, *1:*87, 1969.
43. Wilmore, J. H., and Behnke, A.R.: An anthropometric estimation of body density and lean body weight in young women. Am. J. Clin. Nutr., *23:*267, 1970.
44. Wilmore, J.H., and Brown, C.H.: Physiological profiles of women distance runners. Med. Sci. Sports, *6:*178, 1974.
45. Young, C.M. et al.: Predicting specific gravity and body fatness in young women. J. Am. Diet. Assoc., *40:*102, 1962.
46. Young, C.M. et al.: Body composition of "older" women. J. Am. Diet. Assoc., *43:*344, 1963.

Physique, Performance, and Physical Activity

27

body comp → body fat + lean body wgt

The evaluation of body composition provides an excellent opportunity to partition the gross size of a person into two major structural components—body fat and lean body weight. As discussed in Chapter 26, the physique of the adult *man* differs considerably from that of the *woman*. The male is generally taller, heavier, and has a larger muscle mass. He possesses less total fat, has a heavier skeletal (bone) mass, and is larger in bone width and circumference size than his female counterpart. Differences in physique are also pronounced when comparisions are made between sports participants of the same sex such as Olympic competitors, track and field specialists, wrestlers, and football players. Aside from describing physique in relation to sports category and level of competition, some experiments have focused on the effects of different forms of sports training and exercise on the body composition of men and women. In this chapter, we take a closer look at the physiques of champion athletes in various sports and evaluate the relative effects of diet and exercise in modifying body composition.

PHYSIQUE OF CHAMPION ATHLETES

Many anthropometric studies have been made of champion athletes. In this section, we focus on four groups: (1) Olympic specialists, (2) endurance runners, (3) collegiate and professional football players, and (4) high school wrestlers.

Olympic Specialists

Early studies of Olympic competitors revealed that physique was related to a high level of achievement in certain sports.[6,13] Tables 27-1 and 27-2 list the anthropometric characteristics of male and female competitors, respectively, who participated in the 1964 Tokyo and 1968 Mexico City Olympics.[7,10] Lean body weight and percent body fat were estimated from bone diameter measures and height to show relative differences in body composition among the different sports specialists.[3]

SEX DIFFERENCES. For the men, basketball players, rowers, and weight throwers were the tallest and heaviest competitors; they also possessed the largest amount of lean body weight and percent body fat. For example, weight throwers in both Olympiads averaged 30% body fat, whereas 94 marathon and 133 long-distance runners averaged an exceptionally low 1.6% body fat. The biggest discrepancy in body composition within a particular sports category was noted between the Tokyo wrestlers, who averaged 12.7% body fat, and the wrestlers in Mexico City, who averaged only 1.2% body fat. This difference is even more remarkable because the age, height, and lean body weight of both groups of wrestlers were very similar.

For female Olympic athletes, the most striking observation is their relatively low body fat values. Except for the weight throwers, who averaged about 31% body fat, the other sports

Sex diff in physique
facial diff

TABLE 27-1. *Age, body size, and body composition of male athletes in selected events who competed in the Tokyo and Mexico City Olympics*[a]

EVENT	SPECIALTY	OLYMPICS	N	AGE YEARS	HEIGHT CM	WEIGHT KG	LBW[b] KG	BODY FAT[c] %
Sprinters	100–200 m; 4 x 100 m; 110-m hurdles	Tokyo	172	24.9	178.4	72.2	64.9	10.1
		Mexico City	79	23.9	175.4	68.4	62.8	8.2
Long-distance runners	3000–5000–10,000 m;	Tokyo	99	27.3	173.6	62.4	61.5	1.4
		Mexico City	34	25.3	171.9	59.8	60.1	−0.5
Marathoners	26 miles, 365 yards	Tokyo	74	28.3	170.3	60.8	59.2	2.7
		Mexico City	20	26.4	168.7	56.6	58.1	2.7
Decathlon		Tokyo	26	26.3	183.2	83.5	68.5	18.0
		Mexico City	8	25.1	181.3	77.5	67.1	13.4
Jumpers	High, long, triple jump	Tokyo	89	25.3	181.5	73.2	67.2	8.2
		Mexico City	14	23.5	182.8	73.2	68.2	6.8
Weight throwers	Shot, discus, hammer	Tokyo	79	27.6	187.3	101.4	71.6	29.4
		Mexico City	9	27.3	186.1	102.3	70.7	30.9
Swimmers	Free, breast, back, butterfly, medley	Tokyo	450	20.4	178.7	74.1	65.1	12.1
		Mexico City	66	19.2	179.3	72.1	65.6	9.0
Basketball		Tokyo	186	25.3	189.4	84.3	73.2	13.2
		Mexico City	63	24.0	189.1	79.7	73.0	8.4
Gymnastics	All events	Tokyo	122	26.0	167.2	63.3	57.0	9.9
		Mexico City	28	23.6	167.4	61.5	57.2	7.0
Wrestling	Bantam and featherweight	Tokyo	29	27.3	163.3	62.3	54.4	12.7
		Mexico City	32	22.5	166.1	57.0	56.3	1.2
Rowing	Single and double skulls; pairs, fours, eights	Tokyo	357	25.0	186.0	82.2	70.6	14.1
		Mexico City	85	24.3	185.1	82.6	69.9	15.4

[a] Adapted from De Garay, A.L., Levine, L., and Carter, J.E.L.: Genetic and Anthropological Studies of Olympic Athletes, New York, Academic Press, 1974 and from Hirata K.: Physique and age of Tokyo Olympic champions. J. Sports Med. Phys. Fitness 6:207–222, 1966.
[b] Calculated by Behnke's method described in reference 3; LBW = $h^2 \times 0.204$, where h = height, decimeters.
[c] Body fat = (body weight − LBW)/body weight × 100

groups were very close to the average body fat of 13.1% for all 676 female participants in both Olympics.

RACIAL DIFFERENCES. Racial differences in physique have also been observed among Olympic competitors and may be significant in terms of athletic performance.[20] Black sprinters and high jumpers, for example, have longer limbs and narrower hips than their white counterparts. From a mechanical perspective, a black sprinter with leg and arm size identical to that of a white sprinter would have a lighter, shorter, and slimmer body to propel. This might confer a more favorable power to body weight ratio for black athletes at any given size compared to white competitors. A relatively greater power output would be advantageous in jumping events and in all sprint running events in which generating rapid energy for short periods

is crucial for successful performance. This advantage may be diminished somewhat in the various throwing events. These activities are not totally dependent on speed of body movement, but also require skill and a large absolute power output to propel the projectile. In contrast to whites and blacks, Asian athletes have short legs relative to their upper body size. This might confer some advantage in the very short and longer distance races, as well as in weight lifting. In fact, successful weight lifters of all races have relatively short arms and legs for their height compared to other groups of athletes.

Female Long-Distance Runners

Table 27-3 presents data for height, weight, and body composition of 11 female long-distance

TABLE 27-2. *Age, body size, and body composition of female athletes in selected events who competed in the Tokyo and Mexico City Olympics*[a]

EVENT	SPECIALTY	OLYMPICS	N	AGE (YEAR)	HEIGHT (CM)	WEIGHT (KG)	LBW[b] (KG)	BODY FAT[c] (%)
Sprinters	100–200 m; 100-m hurdles	Tokyo	85	22.7	166.0	56.6	49.6	12.4
		Mexico City	28	20.7	165.0	56.8	49.0	13.7
Jumpers	High, long, triple jump	Tokyo	56	23.6	169.5	60.2	51.7	14.1
		Mexico City	12	21.5	169.4	56.4	51.7	8.4
Weight throwers	Shot, discus, hammer	Tokyo	37	26.2	170.4	79.0	52.3	33.8
		Mexico City	9	19.9	170.9	73.5	52.6	28.5
Swimmers	Free, breast, back, butterfly, medley	Tokyo	272	18.6	166.3	59.7	49.8	16.6
		Mexico City	28	16.3	164.4	56.9	48.6	14.5
Diving	Spring, high	Tokyo	65	18.5	160.9	54.1	46.6	13.9
		Mexico City	7	21.1	160.4	52.3	46.3	11.5
Gymnastics	All events	Tokyo	102	22.7	157.0	52.0	44.4	14.7
		Mexico City	21	17.8	156.9	49.8	44.3	11.0

[a] Adapted from De Garay, A.L., Levine, L., and Carter, J.E.L.: Genetic and Anthropological Studies of Olympic Athletes, New York, Academic Press, 1974 and from Hirata, K.: Physique and age of Tokyo Olympic champions. J. Sports Med. Phys. Fitness 6:207–222, 1966.
[b] Calculated by Behnke's method described in reference 3; LBW (lean body weight) = $h^2 \times 0.18$, where h = height, decimeters.
[c] Body fat = (body weight − LBW)/body weight × 100

runners of national and international caliber.[26] The runners averaged 15.2% body fat (determined by underwater weighing), which is considerably lower than the average value of about 26% reported for sedentary females of the same age, height, and weight.[12] Compared to other female athletes, the runners have a lower average fat value than collegiate basketball players (20.9%),[18] competitive gymnasts (15.5%),[17] younger distance runners (18%),[13] swimmers (20.1%),[11] or tennis players (22.8%).[11]

Interestingly, the average percent body fat for these runners is the same as the 15% average generally reported for males, and is close to the quantity of essential fat proposed by Behnke in his model for the "reference woman." In fact, the body fat of several of the female distance runners described in Table 27-3 was within the

TABLE 27-3. *Body composition of female long-distance runners*[a]

SUBJECTS	AGE (YEAR)	HEIGHT (CM)	WEIGHT (KG)	LBW (KG)	BODY FAT (KG)	BODY FAT (%)
1[b]	24	172.7	52.6	49.5	3.1	5.9
2[c]	26	159.8	71.5	46.2	25.3	35.4
3[d]	28	162.6	50.7	47.6	3.1	6.1
4	31	171.5	52.0	47.3	4.7	9.0
5	33	176.5	61.2	50.8	10.4	17.0
6	34	166.4	52.9	44.8	8.1	15.2
7	35	168.4	55.0	48.7	6.3	11.6
8	36	164.5	53.1	44.3	8.8	16.6
9	36	182.9	61.5	50.4	11.1	18.1
10	36	182.9	65.4	55.7	9.7	14.8
11	37	154.9	53.6	44.0	9.6	18.0
Average	32.4	169.4	57.2	48.1	9.1	15.2

[a] From Wilmore, J.H., and Brown, C.H.: Physiological profiles of women distance runners. Med. Sci. Sports, 6:178, 1974.
[b] World's best time in marathon (2:49:40) as of 1974.
[c] World's best time in 50-mile run (7:05:31); established 18 months after the body composition evaluation.
[d] Noted U.S. distance runner. Five consecutive national and international crosscountry championships.

range of values reported for topflight male distance runners. According to Behnke's "reference woman," however, the leanest women in the population have sex-specific essential fat equal to about 12% to 14% of body weight. This apparent discrepancy between the estimated fat content of some distance runners and Behnke's theoretical lower limit for body fat in women requires further study. It is also difficult to explain the relatively high body fat content of one of the best runners and indicates that other factors can override the obvious limitations to distance running imposed by excess fat.

Male Distance Runners

The body composition of male middle and long-distance runners and eight elite marathoners is shown in Table 27-4. The high caliber of the athletes is indicated by the fact that the group included Prefontaine (former American record holder in the 800- and 1500-m runs) and Shorter (1976 Olympic Gold Medalist). For comparative purposes, we have also presented data for a typical sample of untrained college-aged men.

For both groups of runners, body fat values were extremely low, considering that the quantity of essential fat is about 3% of the body weight. Clearly, these endurance runners are at the lowest end of the lean-to-fat continuum for topflight athletes. Apparently, this physique characteristic is a prerequisite for success in distance running. This makes sense for several reasons. For one thing, the body's ability to dissipate metabolic heat during running is of primary importance in maintaining thermal balance during competition. Excess fat thwarts heat dissipation. Also, excess body fat is "dead weight" that adds directly to the energy cost of running. This would definitely hinder the distance runner who must maintain a high level of steady rate aerobic metabolism for a prolonged period of time.

In terms of body structure, elite distance runners are also generally smaller in circumferences and bone diameters than untrained males.[6] One could consider these structural differences, especially the bone diameters, to be "genetic." *The best long-distance runners inherit a physique that is slight of build, not only in terms of height but also in skeletal dimensions. When this physique is blended with a lean body composition, highly developed aerobic system, and the proper psychologic attitude for prolonged, intensive training, the proper ingredients certainly exist for a champion!*

Football Players

The first detailed body composition analyses of football players vividly demonstrated the inadequacy of determining a person's "optimal" weight from standards based on height and weight.[22] Specifically, football players as a group had a body fat content that averaged only 10.4% of body weight, whereas lean body weight averaged 81.3 kg (179.3 lb). Certainly the men were heavy, but they were *not* fat. The *heaviest* lineman weighed 118 kg (260 lb, 17.4% body fat, 215 lb lean body weight), whereas the *fattest* lineman had 23.2% body fat at a body weight of 115.4 kg (252 lb). The player with the least fat was a defensive back; for his weight of 82.3 kg (182 lb), body fat was 3.3% with a lean body weight of 79.6 kg (175 lb).

Table 27-5 presents a clearer picture of the average values for height, weight, percent body fat, and lean body weight of *college*[23] and pro-

TABLE 27-4. *Anthropometric characteristics of elite male distance runners*

VARIABLE	MIDDLE-LONG DISTANCE[a] (N = 11)	MARATHON[a] (N = 8)	COLLEGE MEN[b] (N = 54)
Height (cm)	176.0	176.8	176.4
Weight (kg)	63.1	62.1	71.4
Body fat (%)	5.0	4.3	15.3
Body fat (kg)	3.21	2.73	10.92
LBW (kg)	59.9	59.4	60.5

[a] Data from Pollock, M.L. et al.: Body composition of elite class distance runners. Ann. N.Y. Acad. Sci. *301*:361, 1977.
[b] Data from Katch, F.I., and McArdle, W.D.: Prediction of body density from simple anthropometric measurements in college-age men and women. Hum. Biol., *45*:445, 1973.

TABLE 27-5. *Comparison of body composition between collegiate and professional football players grouped by position*[a]

POSITION	LEVEL	N	HEIGHT (CM)	WEIGHT (KG)	BODY FAT (%)	LBW (KG)
Defensive	St. Cloud[b]	15	178.3	77.3	11.5	68.4
backs	USC[c]	15	183.0	83.7	9.6	75.7
	Pro[d]	26	182.5	84.8	9.6	76.7
Offensive	St. Cloud	15	179.7	79.8	12.4	69.6
backs and	USC	18	185.6	86.1	9.9	77.6
receivers	Pro	40	183.8	90.7	9.4	81.9
Linebackers	St. Cloud	7	180.1	87.2	13.4	75.4
	USC	17	185.6	98.8	13.2	85.8
	Pro	28	188.6	102.2	14.0	87.6
Offensive	St. Cloud	13	186.0	99.2	19.1	79.8
linemen and	USC	25	191.1	106.5	15.3	90.3
tight ends	Pro	38	193.0	112.6	15.6	94.7
Defensive	St. Cloud	15	186.6	97.8	18.5	79.3
linemen	USC	13	191.1	109.3	14.7	93.2
	Pro	32	192.4	117.1	18.2	95.8
Total	St. Cloud	65	182.5	88.0	15.0	74.2
	USC	88	186.6	96.6	11.4	84.6
	Pro	164	188.1	101.5	13.4	87.3
	Dallas-Jets[e]	107	188.2	100.4	12.6	87.7

[a] Suggested grouping from reference 25.
[b] Data from Wickkiser, J.D., and Kelley, J.M.: The body composition of a college football team. Med. Sci. Sports, 7:199, 1975
[c] USC data courtesy of Dr. Robert Girandola, University of Southern California, Los Angeles, 1978.
[d] Data from Wilmore, J.H. et al: Football pros' strengths—and CV weakness—charted. Physician Sportsmed. 4:45, 1976.
[e] Data from Katch, F.I., and Katch, V.L.: Body composition of the Dallas Cowboys and New York Jets Football teams. Unpublished data, 1978.

fessional[25] players grouped by position. Two groups of collegiate players are represented: (1) the St. Cloud State College, Minnesota, players who were candidates for spring practice, and (2) teams from the University of Southern California (USC), 1973 to 1977, who were National Champions and participants in two Rose Bowls. For comparison, there are two groups of professional players. The first consists of 164 players from 14 teams in the National Football League (NFL); veteran players comprised 69% of this sample and rookies, 31%. The second group were 107 members of the 1976–1978 Dallas Cowboys and New York Jets football teams.

One would generally expect professional players to be larger in body size at each position than a representative group of college players. Although this was true for the comparison with the St. Cloud players, the USC players were similar in physique to the professionals. With the exception of defensive linemen, the USC players at each position had almost the same body fat content, although they tended to weigh less than the National Football League players at each position. For the all-important component of lean body weight, the USC players were no more than 4.4 kg lighter than the "pros" at each position. In fact, the average defensive lineman in the NFL outweighed his

USC counterpart in lean tissue by only 1.8 kg. However, the total body weight of the pro linemen was significantly heavier than that of the USC counterparts. This difference was due largely to the fact that the professional linemen possessed 18.2% body fat whereas collegians were leaner at 14.7%. *Considered in total, one can conclude that at the highest levels of collegiate competition, the body size and composition of college and professional players are similar.*

High School Wrestlers

Wrestlers represent a unique group of athletes who undergo both severe training and acute weight loss. Despite warnings from medical[2] and professional[1] groups regarding rapid weight loss, most high school and college wrestlers lose considerable weight a few days before or on the day of competition. This is done with the hope of gaining a competitive advantage by wrestling in a lower weight category. This process of "making weight" usually occurs by combining food restriction and dehydration, either through fluid deprivation or exercising in a hot environment while wearing plastic or rubber garments. To reduce the possibility of injury from acute weight loss and de-

hydration, the American College of Sports Medicine recommends that each wrestler's body composition be assessed several weeks prior to the competitive season to determine an acceptable minimal wrestling weight.[1] Some researchers advocate more stringent evaluation, and they propose a series of measures on each athlete to determine more precisely the body composition changes that accompany weight loss. *A lower limit of 5% body fat is proposed as the lowest acceptable level for safe wrestling competition.*

PHYSICAL CHARACTERISTICS OF HIGH SCHOOL WRESTLERS. The physical characteristics of two groups of high school wrestlers are presented in Table 27-6.[5] The "certified" Iowa and Minnesota wrestlers were assigned to wrestle at one of 12 different weight categories; the "champion" wrestlers competed in the State or Conference finals. Except for age and skinfolds, there was little difference in the physical characteristics of the Iowa and Minnesota certified and champion wrestlers. As reflected by the skinfold measures, however, the champions were considerably leaner than their less successful teammates. Since differences in body weight were small between groups, the elite wrestlers actually competed at a heavier lean body weight. This may have contributed greatly to their success in a particular weight class.

TABLE 27-6. *Anthropometric comparisons between certified and champion Iowa and Minnesota high school wrestlers*[a]

MEASUREMENT	CERTIFIED WRESTLERS		CHAMPION WRESTLERS	
	IOWA (N = 484)	MINN (N = 245)	IOWA (N = 382)	MINN (N = 164)
Age (years)	15.9	16.8	17.8	17.4
Height (cm)	169.9	172.0	171.7	172.5
Weight (kg)	64.3	65.3	64.6	64.7
Chest diameter (cm)	26.8	26.5	27.7	26.6
Chest depth (cm)	19.0	16.8	19.2	17.3
Bitochanteric diameter (cm)	31.0	31.4	31.1	31.5
Ankles diameter[b] (cm)	14.3	14.3	14.0	14.3
Skinfolds (mm)				
Scapula	8.4	7.9	6.4	6.8
Triceps	8.6	9.1	6.0	5.6
Suprailiac	13.3	12.3	9.1	7.5
Abdominal	13.1	12.2	8.6	8.3
Thigh	10.8	13.6	7.7	8.3
Sum of 5 skinfolds	54.2	55.1	37.8	36.5

[a]From Clarke, K.S.: Predicting certified weight of young wrestlers: a field study of the Tcheng-Tipton method. Med. Sci. Sports, 6:52, 1974.

[handwritten margin notes: ↓ body wgt / ↓ body fat / ↓ skinfold]

WEIGHT LOSS RECOMMENDATIONS FOR WRESTLERS. Prior to the season's start, suppose a high school wrestler who wishes to compete in the lowest possible weight category compatable with good health and performance[19] weighs 70 kg; body composition assessment reveals that he has 15% body fat. A prudent recommendation for weight loss would be that which would lower body fat content no lower than 5% of body weight.[21] For this young man, the proposed weight loss would therefore be 10% of his body weight or about 7 kg, resulting in a final body weight of 63 kg. With increased training and moderate caloric restriction, a weight loss of 1 kg per week is a reasonable objective. Thus, in about 7 weeks, the desired weight loss will be achieved and the wrestler can effectively compete in the 145-lb weight class.

EFFECTS OF TRAINING ON BODY COMPOSITION

[handwritten: –duration]

In this section, we look at the effectiveness of walking, jogging, and cycling in modifying the body composition of young and middle-aged adults. These findings have special meaning to physical educators and others involved in leading exercise programs, because of the important role exercise can play in effective weight control.

Ten-Week Jogging Program

Table 27-7 shows changes in physique for men aged 17 to 59 years who jogged 3 days a week for 10 weeks.[24] The average distance run by the end of 10 weeks was 84.4 km (51.8 miles), or about 2.8 km or 1.7 miles a day. Body composition changes did occur but they were relatively small. Because lean body weight did not change, the decrease in body weight was due to a *reduction in percent body fat* from pretest (18.9%) to post-test (17.8%) values, which represented a fat loss of 1.07 kg. The reduction in individual skinfold values paralleled the decrease in body fat.

It is possible that this small reduction in body fat was due to (1) the relatively short duration of the jogging program and (2) the average body fat of the group prior to training was only slightly greater than the average for college-aged men. As such, these men could not be considered overfat and in need of greatly reducing body size.

Walking–Running Program for Different Durations

[handwritten margin notes: ↓ body wgt (except 15 / ↓ changes in body fat / ↓ skinfolds / ↓ waist girth]

The duration of exercise has an effect on fat loss with training. Table 27-8 shows the changes in body fat (predicted from skinfolds) for three groups of men who trained walking

TABLE 27-7. *Body composition changes resulting from a 10-week jogging program*[a]

VARIABLE	PRETRAINING	POST TRAINING	DIFFERENCE
Weight (kg)	79.59	78.58	− 1.01[b]
Body fat (%)	18.88	17.77	− 1.11[b]
Body fat (kg)	15.03	13.96	− 1.07
LBW (kg)	64.56	64.62	0.06
Skinfolds (mm)			
Triceps	11.5	11.1	− 0.4
Scapula	16.3	15.1	− 1.2[b]
Suprailiac	24.9	24.4	1.5
Mid axillary	17.3	14.3	− 3.0[b]
Abdominal	24.4	23.5	− 0.9
Thigh	16.9	16.0	− 0.9[b]
Chest	12.7	11.5	− 1.2[b]
Circumferences (cm)			
Waist	84.8	84.4	− 0.8[b]
Abdomen	88.2	87.7	− 0.5

[a] From Wilmore, J.H. et al.: Body composition changes with a 10-week program of jogging. Med. Sci. Sports, 2:113, 1970.
[b] Statistically significant.

TABLE 27-8. *Effects of three training durations of walking and running on body composition changes*[a]

	CONTROL (N = 16)			15 MINUTE (N = 14)		30 MINUTE (N = 17)		45 MINUTE (N = 12)	
				TRAINING GROUP					
VARIABLE	PRE	POST		PRE	POST	PRE	POST	PRE	POST
Body weight (kg) ✓	72.1	73.2		76.9	76.3	80.6	78.9	70.9	69.9
Body fat (%) ✓	12.5	13.0		13.7	13.2	14.2	13.6	13.2	12.0
Sum of skinfolds (mm) ✓	73.8	79.6		83.0	77.0	90.0	83.8	77.5	67.0
Waist girth (cm) ✓	82.7	84.9		84.3	82.8	88.2	86.1	83.6	81.8
Distance run per workout (miles)	week 4			1.56		2.89		4.13	
	8			1.54		2.95		4.46	
	13			1.79		3.19		4.82	
	17			1.75		3.24		5.06	
Total time of exercise (min:s)	week 4			14:58		30:25		41:18	
	8			14:11		28:40		42:48	
	13			15:51		29:43		43:19	
	17			14:53		30:12		42:27	
Training heart rate (beats · min^{-1})	week 4			179		175		174	
	8			179		174		169	
	13			182		175		177	
	17			180		175		175	
Intensity (% of max HR)	week 4			89.4		83.8		84.5	
	8			89.8		73.4		81.0	
	13			94.0		90.1		89.5	
	17			92.5		90.2		88.1	

[a]From Milesis, C.A. et al.: Effects of different durations of physical training on cardiorespiratory function, body composition, and serum lipids. Res. Quart., 47:716–725, 1976.

and running for either 15, 30, or 45 minutes per workout.[14] Also included are the distance run and the total duration of the weekly workouts, training heart rate, body weight, the sum of skinfolds (chest, axilla, triceps, abdomen, suprailiac, anterior thigh), and waist circumference.

Compared to the control group that remained unchanged over the 20-week training period, the three exercise groups significantly decreased their body fat, skinfolds, and waist girth. Body weight was also significantly lowered with exercise except for the 15-minute group, whose weight remained stable. When comparisons were made between the three groups, the 45-minute training group lost a greater percentage of body fat than either the 30- or 15-minute exercise groups. *This was attributed to the greater calorie-burning effect of the longer exercise period.*

Two-Year Program of Calisthenics and Jogging

Figure 27-1 displays the effects of a 2-year calisthenics and jogging program on the body composition of seven middle-aged men.[4] Comparative data are also presented for six men measured at the same 6-month intervals who did not take part in the exercise program. The exercisers participated in a supervised program 3 days a week. Initially, they walked and jogged for 10 minutes; thereafter, they jogged for 30 to 35 minutes. The average distance covered increased from 2.4 to 12.1 km per week, and the total mileage run per subject after 2 years of training averaged 1188 km or 738 miles.

Compared with control subjects, whose body compositions remained relatively constant during the 2-year period, the exercisers after the

[handwritten: walking 40-60min]

first year significantly reduced their body weight (5.7%), sum of skinfolds (27.4%), and girth measurements (3.1%). Thereafter, there was little further change in body weight and body composition. *These findings show that calisthenics and jogging can significantly alter the physique of previously sedentary 40- to 60-year-old men.* The changes were paralleled by a 25% improvement in aerobic capacity assessed by a maximal oxygen uptake test.

Walking, Running, and Bicycling

[handwritten: ↓ body wgt, body fat skinfold thickness + girth.]

When the relative training effects of walking, running, or bicycling on body composition are evaluated, each mode of exercise is found to reduce significantly body weight, body fat, skinfold thickness, and girths. In addition, there is generally *no selective effect of running, walking, or bicycling; each training mode is equally effective in altering body composition.*

Frequency of Training

[handwritten: at least 3 days of traing/wk → changes in body comp — threshold of 300 kcal — 20-30 min mod-vergorous running, swimming, bicycling]

Researchers have summarized the body composition changes for 148 subjects in six studies designed to investigate optimal training frequency.[15] Training consisted of either running or walking and was conducted for 30 to 47 minutes a day for 20 weeks; exercise intensity was always maintained at 80% to 95% of maximum heart rate. Training 2 days a week did not change body weight, skinfolds, or percent body fat. Training 3 and 4 days a week significantly decreased body weight, skinfolds, and percent body fat. Subjects who trained 4 days a week reduced their body weight and skinfold fat significantly more than the 3-day per week group. However, reductions in percent body fat were similar for both groups.

Within the framework of these findings, it appears that at least 3 days of training per week are required to bring about changes in body composition through exercise. There is some indication that more frequent training may even

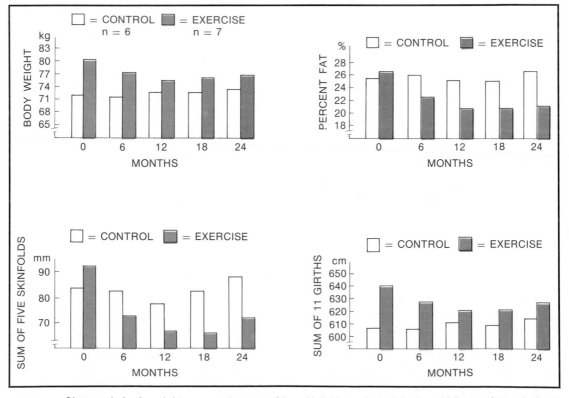

FIG. 27-1. *Changes in body weight, percent fat, sum of five skinfolds, and 11 girths for middle-aged men during a 2-year exercise program. (From Carter, J.E.L., and Phillips, W.H.: Structural changes in exercising middle-aged males during a 2 year period. J. Appl. Physiol., 27:787, 1969.)*

be more effective. *More than likely,* this effect is probably the direct result of the added caloric stress provided by the extra training. In addition, the calorie-burning effect of each exercise session should reach a threshold of about 300 kcal.[16] This is generally achieved with 20 to 30 minutes of moderate to vigorous running, swimming or bicycling, or walking programs of 40 to 60 minutes duration.

EFFECTS OF DIET AND EXERCISE ON BODY COMPOSITION DURING WEIGHT LOSS

The addition of exercise to the program of weight control may favorably modify the composition of the weight lost. To evaluate this possibility, a caloric deficit of 500 calories per day was maintained by each of three groups of adult women during a 16-week period of weight loss.[27] The diet group reduced daily food intake by 500 kcal, whereas women in the exercise group increased their energy output by 500 kcal through participation in a supervised walking and exercise program 5 days a week. The women using diet plus exercise created their daily 500 kcal deficit by reducing food intake by 250 kcal and increasing energy output by 250 kcal through exercise. Figure 27-2 illustrates the changes in body weight, percent body fat, and lean body weight for the three groups. In terms of weight loss, there was no significant difference between the three groups because each group lost approximately 5 kg. This finding shows that as long as a caloric deficit is created body weight will be reduced, regardless of the method used to create the imbalance. In terms of reducing body fat, however, combining diet and exercise was the most effective approach to weight loss. Expressed as a percent of initial fatness, the diet plus exercise group reduced by 13.1%; the exercisers reduced by 12.6% and the diet group reduced body fat by 9.3%. The most interesting observation concerned lean body weight. Although the exercise and combination groups *increased* their lean body weight by 0.9 and 0.5 kg respectively, the dieters *lost* 1.1 kg of lean tissue! It might be argued that this lean tissue loss was due to a reduced protein intake during food restriction. However, the women in the diet group had an average protein intake of 71.3 g per day, which would be more than ade-

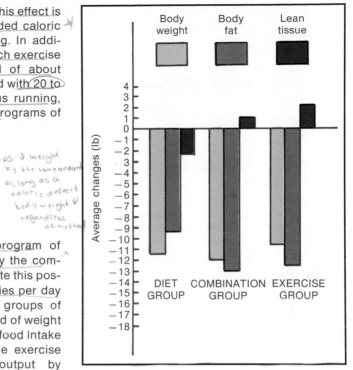

FIG. 27-2. *Changes in body weight, body fat, and lean body weight for the diet, exercise, and combination groups. (From Zuti, W.B., and Golding, L.A.: Comparing diet and exercise as weight reduction tools. Physician Sportsmed., 4:49, 1976.)*

quate to prevent a protein deficit. *Although more research in this area is needed, it does appear that when weight is reduced by diet alone, more lean tissue is lost (and less fat) than when a similar weight loss occurs following the appropriate use of exercise.*

GAINING WEIGHT

Gaining weight for athletes poses a unique problem that is not easily resolved. Weight gain per se is a relatively easy and often enjoyable task brought about by imbalancing the body's energy balance in favor of a greater caloric intake. For a sedentary person, an excess intake of 3500 kcal results in a body weight gain of about 0.5 kg. This is because the excess calories are stored as body fat. Weight gain for athletes, however, must be in the form of lean body weight, specifically muscle mass. It is generally agreed that this form of weight gain can only be accomplished if an increased caloric intake is accompanied by an appropriate program of muscular work.[19] Although endurance exercise can increase lean body weight slightly,[16] the body composition change is frequently accompanied by a loss in body weight due to fat loss. This weight loss is probably the result of the calorie-burning and appetite-depressing effects of the endurance exercise.

Heavy muscular overload (strength training) supported by a prudent diet appears to be an effective means to increase muscle mass and strength. If all the "extra" calories consumed were used for muscle growth during strength training, then 2000 to 2500 extra kcal from a well-balanced diet are required for each 0.5 kg increase in lean tissue. In a practical sense, 700 to 1000 kcal added to the daily diet supply the nutrients to support a 0.5- to 1.0-kg gain in lean tissue as well as the energy requirements of the training.[8] This ideal situation presupposes that all extra calories are used to synthesize lean tissue. Variation from this ideal depends on many factors including the type, intensity, and frequency of training and the hormonal characteristics of the athlete. A male or female athlete with a relatively high androgen-estrogen ratio probably increases lean tissue to a greater extent than a similarly trained athlete with lower androgen production.[9] One means to verify whether the combination of training and increased food intake is increasing lean tissue (and not body fat) is to monitor regularly body weight and body fat. This can be accomplished in the laboratory with hydrostatic weighing or in the "field" with the simple techniques of skinfold and circumference measurements.

SUMMARY

1. Body composition assessment has revealed that athletes generally have physique characteristics unique to their specific sport. For example, field-event athletes have relatively large quantities of lean tissue and a high percent body fat, whereas long-distance runners have the least amount of lean body weight and fat weight.

2. Physique characteristics blended with highly developed physiologic support systems provide important ingredients for a champion performance.

3. Body composition analysis of football players reveals they are among the heaviest and often leanest of all sportsmen. As a group, football players average 10.4% body fat and possess a lean body weight of 81.3 kg. At the highest levels of competition, collegiate and professional football players are similar in body size and composition.

4. Wrestlers should probably not be permitted to compete with a body fat level below 5%.

5. Continuous exercise, because of its calorie-burning effects, can be an effective tool for weight reduction. Of course, the greater the caloric expenditure, the greater the potential for weight loss. This effect is independent of mode of exercise, as long as there is sufficient caloric deficit caused by the exercise. At least 3 training days a week is required.

6. Twenty to 30 minutes of moderately strenuous running, bicycling, or swimming, or 40 to 60 minutes of walking will stimulate fat loss. This threshold amount of exercise generally represents about a 300-kcal increase in daily energy expenditure.

7. A combination of diet and exercise offers the greatest flexibility for achieving a negative caloric balance and desirable weight loss. The inclusion of exercise with diet in a weight-loss program provides protection against the loss of lean tissue. This results in greater fat weight loss than would be achieved by diet alone.

8. For athletes, weight gain must be in the form of lean body weight, i.e., muscle mass. Increased caloric intake plus strength training seems to increase muscle mass and strength effectively. Ideally, 700 to 1000 extra kcal per day support a 0.5- to 1.0-kg gain in lean tissue and training energy requirements. Realistically, individual physiologic variations and training factors also affect weight gain. For this reason, body weight and body fat should be monitored on a regular basis.

References

1. Amercian College of Sports Medicine: Weight loss in wrestlers. Med. Sci. Sports, *8*:xi, 1976.
2. American Medical Association Committee on the Medical Aspects of Sports: Wrestling and weight control. J.A.M.A. *201*:541, 1967.
3. Behnke, A.R., and Wilmore, J. H.: *Evaluation and Regulation of Body Build and Composition.* Englewood Cliffs, N.J., Prentice Hall, 1974.
4. Carter, J.E.L., and Phillips, W. H.: Structural changes in exercising middle-aged males during a 2-year period. J. Appl. Physiol., *27*:787, 1969.
5. Clarke, K. C.: Predicting certified weight of young wrestlers: a field study of the Tcheng–Tipton Method. Med. Sci. Sports, *6*.52, 1974.
6. Cureton, T. K.: *Physical Fitness of Champion Athletes.* Urbana, Ill., University of Illinois Press, 1951.
7. De Garay, A. L. et al.: Genetic and Anthropological Studies of Olympic Athletes. New York, Academic Press, 1974.
8. Fahey, T. D., and Brown, C.: The effects of an anabolic steroid. Med. Sci. Sports, *5*:272, 1973.
9. Harris, D. V.: The female athlete: Strength, endurance and performance. *In* Toward an Understanding of Human Performance. Edited by E. J. Burke. Ithaca, N.Y., Mouvement Publications, 1977.
10. Hirata, K.: Physique and age of Tokyo Olympic champions. J. Sports Med. Phys. Fitness, *6*:207, 1966.
11. Katch, F. I. et al.: Effects of physical training on the body composition and diet of females. Res, Quart , *40*·99, 1969.
12. Katch, F. I., and McArdle, W. D.: Prediction of body density from simple anthropometric measurements in college-age men and women. Hum. Biol., *45*:445, 1973.
13. Kohlraush, W.: Zusammenhang von Korperform und Leistung. Ergebnisse der anthropometrischen Messungen an der Athleten der Amsterdamer Olympiade. Int. Z. Angew. Physiol., *2*:187, 1970.
14. Milesis, C. A. et al.: Effects of different durations of physical training on cardiorespiratory function, body composition, and serum lipids. Res. Quart., *47*:716, 1976.
15. Pollock, M. L. et al.: Frequency of training as a determinant for improvement in cardiovascular function and body composition of middle-aged men. Arch. Phys Med. Rehabil., *56*:141, 1975.
16. Pollock, M. L., and Jackson, A.: Body composition: Measurement and changes resulting from physical training. *In* Toward an Understanding of Human Performance. Edited by E. J. Burke. Ithaca, N.Y., Mouvement Publications, 1977.
17. Sinning, W. E., and Lindberg, G. D.: Physical characteristics of college age women gymnasts. Res. Quart., *43*:226, 1972.
18. Sinning, W. E.: Body composition, cardiorespiratory function, and rule changes in women's basketball. Res. Quart., *44*:313, 1973.
19. Smith, N. J.: Gaining and losing weight in athletics. J.A.M.A., *236*:149, 1976.
20. Tanner, J. M.: The Physique of the Olympic Athlete. London, George Allen and Unwin, Ltd. 1964.
21. Tcheng, T., and Tipton, C. M.: Iowa wrestling study: Anthropometric measurements and the prediction of a "minimal" body weight for high school wrestlers. Med. Sci. Sports, *5*:1, 1973.

22. Welham, W. C., and Behnke, A. R.: The specific gravity of healthy men. J.A.M.A., *118:*498, 1942.
23. Wickkiser, J. D., and Kelly, J. M.: The body composition of a college football team. Med. Sci. Sports, *7:*199, 1975.
24. Wilmore, J. H. et al.: Body composition changes with a 10-week program of jogging. Med. Sci. Sports, *2:*113, 1970.
25. Wilmore, J. H., and Haskell, W. L.: Body composition and endurance capacity of professional football players. J. Appl. Physiol., *33:*564, 1972.
26. Wilmore, J. H., and Brown, C. H.: Physiological profiles of women distance runners. Med. Sci. Sports, *6:*178, 1974.
27. Zuti, W. B., and Golding, L. A.: Comparing diet and exercise as weight reduction tools. Physician Sportsmed., *4:*49, 1976.

Obesity and
Weight Control

28

Obesity

It is indeed unfortunate that in our modern era of technologic and scientific achievement, where man has walked on the moon, developed surgical procedures to prolong and enhance the quality of life, and discovered many of the secrets of molecular interaction, there is no adequate explanation for a seemingly simple question; "Why do people become too fat and what can be done to prevent it?" About 50 million men and 60 million women between the ages of 18 and 79 are "too fat" and need to reduce excess weight.[1,22] This amounts to about 377 million kg of excess fat for men and 667 million kg for women, or a total of 1044 million kg (2297 million lb) for the United States adult population! If the overfat men and women dieted by consuming 600 fewer calories each day to reduce to a "normal" value of body fat (achievable in 68 days for men and 101 days for women), the reduced caloric intake would equal 5.7 trillion calories. Translating this into fossil fuel energy and considering such factors as the energy required to plant, cultivate, harvest, feed, process, transport, wholesale, retail, acquire, store, and cook the food, the annual energy savings would be equal to that required to supply the residential electric demands of Boston, Chicago, San Francisco, and Washington, D.C., or 1.3 billion gallons of gasoline to fuel 900,000 autos per year.

Until recently, the major cause of obesity was believed to be overeating. However, if gluttony and overindulgence were the only factors associated with an increase in body fat, the easiest way to permanently reduce would surely be to cut back on food. Of course, if it were that simple, obesity would soon be eliminated as a major health problem. There are obviously other factors operative such as genetic, environmental, and social influences. However, it is difficult to partition the cause(s) of obesity into distinct categories because the cause(s) probably overlap. However, it seems fairly certain that the treatment procedures devised so far, whether they be diets, surgery, drugs, psychologic methods, or exercise, either alone or in combination, have not been particularly successful in solving the problem on a *long-term* basis. There is optimism, nonetheless, that as researchers continue to investigate the many facets of obesity, as well as to test and quantify various treatment modalities, significant progress can be made to conquer this major health problem.

This section deals with various aspects of obesity, including (1) measurement and risk factors, (2) comparison of fat cell size and number in normal and obese persons before and after weight gain and reduction, (3) development of adipose cellularity in animals and humans, and (4) modification of adipose cellularity by diet and exercise.

HEALTH RISKS
OF OBESITY

Although there is little agreement as to the exact cause(s) of obesity, there is considerable information regarding the associations between obesity and a number of health risks.[4,5] What is not clear is whether obesity per se causes the risks or simply is a by-product of a particular medical condition. The following are health-related correlates of obesity: (1) impairment of cardiac function due to an increase in the heart's mechanical work,[3] and to left ventricular dysfunction[1,2,19]; (2) hypertension[6,12,40]; (3) diabetes[41,42,47]; (4) renal disease[46]; (5) gallbladder disease[31,35]; (6) pulmonary respiratory diseases[10]; (7) problems in administration of anesthetics during surgery[45]; (8) osteoarthritis, degenerative joint disease, and gout[44]; (9) endometrial cancer[8]; and (10) abnormal plasma lipid and lipoprotein concentrations[18,20,37].

CRITERION OF OBESITY:
HOW FAT IS TOO FAT?

A person's fat content is generally evaluated in terms of the percentage of body weight that is fat (percent body fat) or in relation to the size and number of individual fat cells.

Percent Body
Fat

Obesity can be defined as excessive enlargement of the body's total quantity of fat. However, where do we draw the line between what is considered normal and what is obese? In Chapter 26, we suggested a "normal" range of body fat in adult men and women—an "average" value for body fat plus or minus one unit of variation. For men and women aged 17 to 50, this variation unit is approximately 5% body fat. Using this statistical boundary, "overfatness" would then correspond to body fat that exceeds the average value plus 5%. For example, in young men whose body fat averages 15% of body weight, the borderline for obesity would be 20% body fat. For older men whose average fatness is approximately 25%, obesity would be defined as a body fat content in excess of 30%. For young women aged 17 to 27, obesity would

correspond to a body fat content above 30%; for older women, age 27 to 50, the borderline between the average and obesity would be about 37% body fat. We emphasize, however, that just because the "average" value for percent body fat tends to increase with age, this should *NOT* dictate that people should expect to get fatter as they grow older. We believe that the criterion for what is considered "too fat" should be that established for younger men and women—above 20% for men and above 30% for women. In this way, "average" population values do not become the reference standard and subsequently accepted as "normal."

> *Standards for Overfatness:*
> Men—above 20%;
> Women—above 30%

Fat Cell Size and Number:
Hypertrophy versus Hyperplasia

Another way to determine and classify obesity is to measure the size and number of fat cells. Adipose tissue increases in two ways: Existing fat cells are enlarged or filled with more fat—a process called *fat cell hypertrophy,* or the total number of fat cells is increased—a process called *fat cell hyperplasia.*

A variety of techniques are used to study adipose cellularity in both humans and animals. One technique involves sucking small fragments of subcutaneous tissue into a syringe with a needle inserted directly into a fat depot. These tissue fragments are usually sampled from the back of the arm at the triceps, the subscapular region, the buttocks, and the lower abdomen. The tissue is then treated chemically so the fat cells can be isolated and counted.

Once the number of fat cells is determined for a known weight of fat tissue, the average quantity of fat per cell is determined by dividing the quantity of fat in the sample by the total number of fat cells present. If total body fat is known, a good estimate can then be made of the total number of fat cells in the body. For example, if an individual weighs 88 kg and is 13% body fat determined by the underwater weighing method outlined in Chapter 26, total fat weight equals 11.4 kg (0.13×88 kg). The total number of fat cells in the body is determined by dividing 11.4 kg by the average content of fat per cell. For example, if the average fat cell contained 0.60 μg of fat, then there would be 19 billion fat cells in the body.

$$\text{Total number of fat cells} = \frac{\text{Weight of body fat}}{\text{Fat content per cell}}$$

In one of our laboratories,[12a,b] needle biopsy and photomicrographic techniques are used to extract and measure the average size of fat cells at selected sites in the body. After the fat sample is obtained, it is prepared for sizing by appropriate biochemical methods[13,30] and photographed for later projection as a slide on a large screen that permits measuring cell diameters with a light-emitting pen that interfaces with a computer. At least 200 cells are measured per site. Figure 28-1 depicts fat cells from the abdominal area in an endurance trained athlete and middle-aged male executive. Once the mean diameter of the cells is known, the fat content per cell is determined by the appropriate volume conversion, $\pi \times \text{radius}^3$. For the

middle-aged subject, whose total fat content was 17.02 kg (196 lb and 19.1% body fat) with 0.73 μg of lipid per cell, the total number of cells was estimated to be 23.3 billion (17.02 kg $\div$ 0.73 μg).

ADIPOSE CELLULARITY

Comparison of Fat Cellularity in Normal and Obese Individuals

Several comparative studies of adipose cellularity in obese and nonobese humans show conclusively that fat accumulation in the obese occurs either by storing larger quantities of fat in existing adipose cells (hypertrophy), new fat cell formation (hyperplasia), or by both hypertrophy and hyperplasia.

Figure 28-2 compares body weight, total fat content, and cellularity in 25 subjects, 20 of

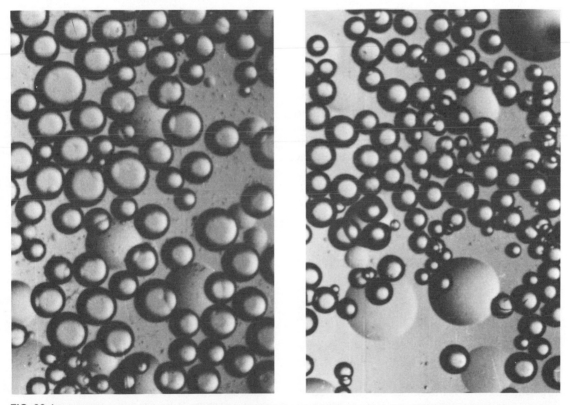

FIG. 28-1. *Photomicrograph of fat cells biopsied from the abdominal region. The larger fat cells (left) were from a sedentary, middle-aged executive. The smaller cells (right) were taken from an endurance trained, experienced marathoner. The large, spherical structures in the background are lipid droplets. (Courtesy of the Muscle Biochemistry Laboratory, Department of Exercise Science, University of Massachusetts.)*

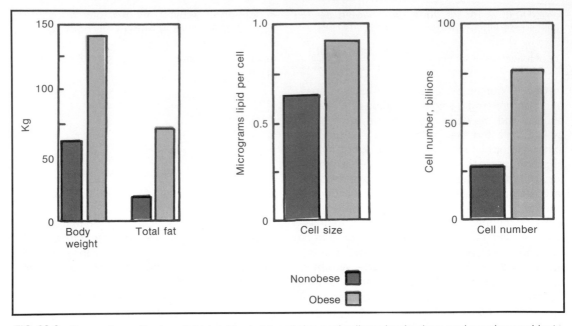

FIG. 28-2. *Comparison of body weight, total body fat, cell size, and cell number in obese and nonobese subjects. (Modified from Hirsch, J., and Knittle, J.: Cellularity of Obese and Non-obese Human Adipose Tissue. Fed. Proc., 29:1518, 1970.)*

whom were clinically classified as obese. The body weight of the obese subjects averaged more than twice that of the nonobese, and their total fat content was nearly three times larger than that of the leaner group. In terms of cellularity, the average fat content per cell was about 35% greater in the obese, whereas the total *number* of fat cells was approximately three times greater than that of the nonobese (75 compared to 27 billion). These results illustrate dramatically that the major structural difference in adipose tissue cellularity between the obese and nonobese is in cell number.

The importance of fat cell number in obesity can be further illustrated by relating total fat content to both cell size and cell number. Most available research suggests that fat cells may reach some biologic upper limit. Once this size is reached, cell number becomes the key factor in determining any further extent of obesity. Even if fat cells could double in size, this would still not account for the large difference in the total fat content of the obese as compared to normal individuals. The excessive quantity of adipose tissue in obesity must, therefore, occur by the process of fat cell hyperplasia. For comparison, a nonobese person has approximately

25 to 30 billion fat cells, whereas the number of fat cells in the "extremely obese" may be as high as 260 billion![7]

Effects of Weight Reduction

When obese adults reduce body size, there is a decrease in fat cell size but no change in the cell number. If normal body weight and body fatness are achieved, then individual fat cells shrink and actually become smaller in size than the fat cells of nonobese individuals. Figure 28-3 depicts the results of weight reduction in obese subjects on adipose cellularity.

In this study, 19 obese adults reduced their body weight from 328 to 227 lb by the end of the first stage of the experiment. The average number of fat cells before weight reduction was approximately 75 billion and remained essentially unchanged even after reducing by 101 pounds. Fat cell size, on the other hand, was reduced from 0.9 to 0.6 μg of fat per cell, a decrease of 33%. When subjects attained normal body weight by reducing 62 more pounds, cell number again remained unchanged but cell size continued to shrink to about one-third the

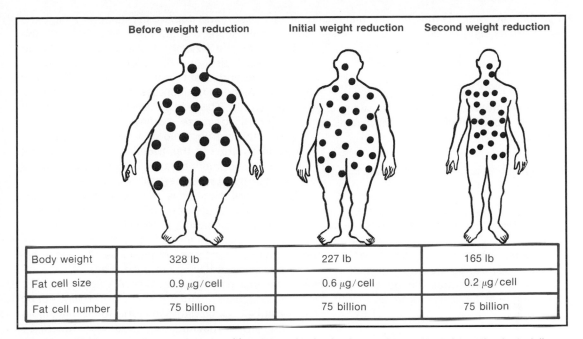

	Before weight reduction	Initial weight reduction	Second weight reduction
Body weight	328 lb	227 lb	165 lb
Fat cell size	0.9 μg/cell	0.6 μg/cell	0.2 μg/cell
Fat cell number	75 billion	75 billion	75 billion

FIG. 28-3. *Changes in adipose cellularity with weight reduction in obese subjects. (Data from Hirsch, J.: Adipose Cellularity in Relation to Human Obesity.* In *Advances in Internal Medicine, Vol. 17. Edited by G. H. Stollerman. Copyright © 1971 by Year Book Medical Publisher, Inc. Used by permission.) Drawings from Katch, F. I., and McArdle, W. D.: Nutrition, Weight Control, and Exercise. Boston, Houghton Mifflin, 1977.*

size of the fat cells of normal, nonobese subjects. The major structural change in adipose cellularity following weight loss in adults is a shrinkage in fat cell *size* with *no change* in cell *number.*

These findings suggest that the formerly obese person is not really "cured" of his or her obesity, at least in terms of the total number of fat cells present. There is no doubt that formerly obese patients have an extremely difficult time maintaining their new body size.[26,43]

Effects of Weight Gain

An interesting series of studies was conducted on the development of obesity.[39] Adult male volunteers with an initial average body fat content of 15% deliberately increased their caloric intake three times above normal to about 7000 kcal per day for a period of 40 weeks. For a typical subject, body weight increased 25%, and body fat doubled from 14.6% to 28.2% of body weight. Consequently, of the 28 lb gained during the period of overeating, 23 were caused by increased deposition of body fat.

In a similar experiment with nonobese subjects with no previous personal or family history of obesity, voluntary overeating produced an average increase in body weight of 36 lb.[38] In comparing cell size and number before and after the 4-month experiment, the average fat cell had increased substantially in size with no change in cell number. When caloric intake was reduced and subjects achieved their normal weight, total body fat declined and the original size of the fat cells was restored. These results indicate that when adults get fatter as a result of overeating, they are filling or enlarging existing adipose cells rather than creating new ones.

There is some indication that *extreme* fat development in adults may modify adipose cellularity.[24] This is because there is an upper limit to fat cell size beyond which hypertrophy fails to occur; this limit is reached when the cell contains about 1.0 μg of lipid per cell (normal is about 0.5–0.6 μg). In the massively obese (60% body fat; above 170% of normal weight), almost all the fat cells have attained their hypertrophic limit and more cells are recruited from the preadipocyte pool to increase cell number.[24] Thus, in maturity-onset severe obesity, where the already fat adult becomes fatter, hypercellularity may accompany the greatly increasing size of the existing fat cells.

FAT CELL DEVELOPMENT

The development of adipose tissue during growth has been studied in both animals and humans.

Animal Studies

The most extensive studies of adipose cellularity have been conducted with rats, because these mammals have a relatively short life span, and various diets and exercise regimens can be studied easily during the growth cycle.

Figure 28-4 illustrates the general upward-trending curves for body weight, fat weight, and

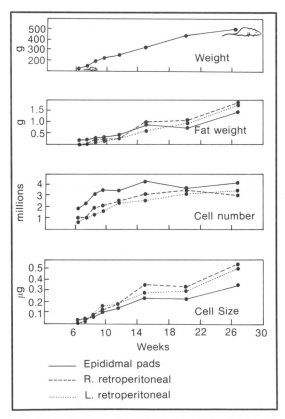

FIG. 28-4. *Changes in body weight, fat weight, cell number, and cell size during the first 5 months of growth in rats. (From Hirsch, J., and Han, P. W.: Cellularity of rat adipose tissue: Effects of growth, starvation, and obesity. J. Lipid Res., 10:77, 1969).*

fat cell size and number in rats during the first 5 months of life. It should be noted that both the number and size of fat cells increased during weeks 6 through 16. As the animals became heavier and total body fat increased, there was a corresponding increase in the *size* of the fat cells only. The additional increase in body fat occurred because existing cells became filled with fat, not because new fat cells developed.

In contrast to this traditional view regarding the development of fat cells, some investigators argue that under certain conditions adult adipose cell number is *not* permanently fixed.[17] When adult rats were fed highly palatable diets so that they gained both weight and fat significantly, cell size increased to a maximum level; the further increase in the mass of adipose tissue occurred by an increase in adipocyte number that persisted even after weight loss. The researchers postulated that cell size may not be infinitely expandable and that once maximum cell size is reached, and food continues to be available, a response to proliferate new fat cells may be triggered. The increased cell number at this point would constitute a failure of adipocyte regulation that leads to obesity.

Human Studies

In one study,[23] adipose cellularity was established for 34 infants and children who ranged in age from a few days to age 13. Fat cell size in newborn infants and children up to the age of 1 year was about one-fourth the size of adult fat cells. Fat cell size tripled during the first 6 years with little further increase in size to age 13. Although several studies have determined adipose cellularity in childhood and adolescence,[9,21] there is still a scarcity of data on changes in adipose cell size during this growth period. We may reasonably assume, however, that cell size increases during this period because cell size in adulthood is significantly larger than cell size at age 13 or in late adolescence.

Cell number increases fairly rapidly during the first year of life, being about three times greater at this point than at birth. It is believed that most of the fat cells existing prior to birth are formed during the last trimester of pregnancy. Beyond age 1, cell number increases gradually to the age of about 10. Like cell size, there is significant cell hyperplasia during the growth spurt in adolescence until adulthood; thereafter, there is generally little further increase in cell number.

Obese adults who significantly increase their already large adipose tissue mass appear to be an exception to this general rule. Reports indicate that moderately obese subjects have significantly higher than normal cell size, whereas cell number is only slightly elevated.[24] Cell size reaches a maximum value of about 1.0 μg triglyceride per cell in persons almost twice their normal weight. Once maximum cell size occurs, further increases in adiposity occur by increases in the number of fat cells.

CAN ADIPOSE TISSUE CELLULARITY BE MODIFIED?

Although the precise causes for fat cell development are poorly understood, it does appear that certain practices can affect body fat. In humans, for example, nutritional practices of the mother during pregnancy may modify the body composition of the developing fetus. A weight gain by the mother in excess of 40 lb was associated with a significantly larger skinfold thickness of the offspring than that in a woman who followed a recommended weight gain during pregnancy.[44a] Bottle feeding and the early introduction of solid food may also be associated with the development of obesity. Conversely, breast feeding, allowing the infant to set the limits to food consumption, and a delayed introduction to solid food may prevent overfeeding, the development of poor eating habits, and subsequent obesity.

Research in animals suggests that alterations in fat cell size and number can be achieved in two ways: (1) modification of early nutrition and (2) exercise.

Effects of Diet

In one well-designed study,[29] rats were distributed at birth so that some mothers had large litters of 22 animals and others smaller litters of 4 animals. After weaning at 21 days, both groups of animals had unlimited access to food. Six animals in each group were then sacrificed at 5, 10, 15, and 20 weeks of age. At weaning and after each subsequent 5-week period, the body weight of animals from large

(calorically deprived) litters was significantly lower than that of the other group, suggesting that early nutritional deprivation resulted in the permanent stunting of growth, even though both groups of animals had free access to food after weaning.

In both groups of animals, fat weight increased from weaning to 20 weeks of age, the dramatic differences occurring in animals reared in small litters, especially at weeks 15 and 20. These relative differences were larger than the differences observed in body weight for the same period. Figure 28-5 shows that in terms of cell size and number, the nutritionally deprived animals had fewer and smaller fat cells at all age intervals than animals reared in small litters.

At 5 and 10 weeks of age, the height of the rectangles is greater than the base, indicating that the proliferation of fat cells made a greater contribution to adipose mass than to cell size. For the 15- and 20-week periods, the shape of the bar approaches a square, indicating that cell size plays an increasingly important role in the development of adipose tissue. An interest-

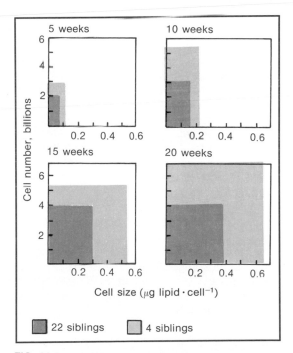

FIG. 28-5. *Changes in cell size and number in animals raised in small and large litters. (Adapted from Knittle, J., and Hirsh, J.: Effect of early nutrition on the development of rat epididymal fat pads: Cellularity and metabolism. J. Clin. Invest., 47:2091, 1968.)*

ing comparison is seen in the two shaded areas of the bar that represent animals raised in large and small litters. The total area of the bar represents the fat depot of the overnourished animals raised in small litters; the darker area represents that of the undernourished animals, with the difference in shading illustrating the difference in depot size between the two groups. By 15 weeks of age, the underfed group reached a definite plateau in fat cell number. Cell number continued to increase in the overfed, small-litter animals. In both groups, cell size increased progressively during the experimental period. These data certainly suggest that there may be a critical time during the growth period when a permanent modification in adipose tissue cellularity can occur.

Though extrapolation from rat experiments to humans is difficult, some striking similarities in adipose tissue development between humans and rats are worth noting. As shown in a previous section, extremely obese humans show a large increase in the *number* of fat cells and, to a lesser extent, an increase in the *size* of individual fat cells. When obese adults lose body weight, the number of fat cells remains unaltered and the decrease in total body fat is achieved almost exclusively by a reduction in fat cell size. The same process seems to take place in studies of adult rats. When adult rats are deprived of food, the decrease in body weight that occurs is only temporary and is rapidly reinstated upon refeeding. In such animals, the weight loss is due to a decrease in fat cell size with no corresponding change in cell number. Overfeeding of *adult* animals produces an increase in total body fat, but as with humans, this increase is usually brought about by "stuffing" of cells with fat rather than by an increase in cell number. The exception occurs when adipocyte size reaches a maximum; further increases in adipose mass occur by additional proliferation of fat cells.[17,24] Furthermore, when the fat content of adult humans is reduced, cell size shrinks accordingly only to expand again when the body's content of fat is restored. The number of existing or newly added fat cells remains constant.

Effects of Physical Activity

Several experiments have been done to evaluate the influence of exercise in modifying adipose cellularity. Figure 28-6 summarizes the results of studies with young rats with free access to food who were forced to swim in plastic barrels 6 days a week for 14 to 16 weeks.[32] The exercise sessions were gradually lengthened until the animals were swimming for 360 minutes. Two adult groups of rats remained sedentary; one group had free access to food and water; the other group was food restricted to maintain body weight at the same level as the exercise group.

The results were convincing; animals given unlimited food but forced to exercise for 15 weeks gained weight more slowly and had a lower final body weight than sedentary, freely eating rats. Because both groups consumed the same number of calories each day, the lower rate of weight gain in the exercisers could be attributed to the increased caloric requirements of the exercise. It was also shown that the total fat content of the nonexercise group was about four times higher than the fat content of the freely eating exercise group. Table 28-1 is a comparison of adipose cellularity in the three groups. The exercise intervention program during the growth period resulted in a significant reduction in total body fat due to a decrease in both cell size *and* number.

The total fat content of the sedentary, food-restricted group was lower than that of the sedentary animals who could eat ad libitum. Reducing food intake resulted in a reduction in cell size and cell number. When the body fat of the food restricted and exercised animals was

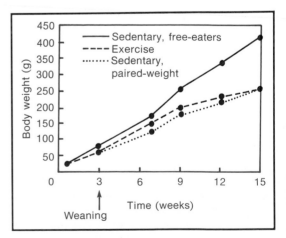

FIG. 28-6. *Effects of exercise and food restriction on body weight of rats. (From Oscai, L. et al.: Effects of exercise and of food restriction on adipose tissue cellularity. J. Lipid Res., 13:588, 1972.)*

TABLE 28-1. *Adipose cell size and number in exercising and sedentary rats*[a]

GROUP	BODY WEIGHT (g)	CELL NUMBER PER FAT PAD (BILLIONS)	FAT CELL SIZE, (μg)
Exercise	260	4.46	0.286
Sedentary, freely eating	418	6.89	0.462
Sedentary, pair weighted	266	5.72	0.319

[a] Adapted from Oscai, L. et al.: Exercise or food restriction: Effect on adipose tissue cellularity, Am. J. Physiol., *277*:901, 1974.

compared, the exercisers had fewer fat cells and less fat per cell, even though the final body weights of both groups were approximately equal. The results demonstrated that exercise performed *early* during the growth period depressed the growth of new fat cells. In a follow-up experiment,[33] the fat-retarding effects of exercise or diet early in an animal's life were studied to determine whether either would reduce fat accumulation in adulthood.

Three groups of animals were used: an exercise group, a sedentary group with free access to food and water, and a sedentary group with restricted food intake. Exercise and food restriction were terminated after 28 weeks. Several animals from each group were then sacrificed and the groups compared for growth, body fat, and adipose cell size and number. The remaining animals were subjected to 34 weeks of sedentary living without exercise and were allowed unlimited food and water. The animals were then sacrificed and the groups compared for body weight, cell size, and cell number. The data in Figure 28-7 and Table 28-2 show that the exercised animals had lower body weights at 28 weeks of age than the other groups.

During the next 34 weeks of inactivity, the previously exercised animals continued to maintain a lower body weight than the sedentary animals. Thus, the 28-week exercise program performed earlier in life caused a reduction in body weight that was still evident at the end of the experiment. Comparing cell size and number at the end of the training period revealed that the exercised group had *fewer* and *smaller* fat cells than either sedentary group of animals. These results were in agreement with the previous experiment.

Table 28-2 contains a comparison of the total fat content, cell number, and cell size of the three groups after 62 weeks. The exercise

group had a lower final body weight and reduced total body fat content than their sedentary counterparts, as well as significantly *fewer* fat cells in later life than animals in the other groups. Twenty-six weeks of exercise, begun early in life and then terminated, retarded the expansion and proliferation of fat cells during the growth period to adulthood—even though the exercise period was followed by 34 weeks of inactivity.

If these findings can be applied to humans, it is possible that the introduction of a diet and/or exercise program during the early stages of growth may aid in controlling the proliferation of new fat cells and the filling up of previously dormant ones. Programs of exercise and weight control begun later in life and maintained thereafter can be effective in lowering the body's total quantity of fat. As far as we

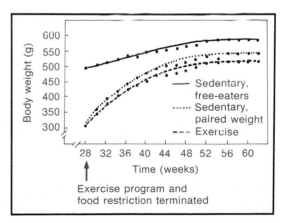

FIG. 28-7. *Effects of 28 weeks of exercise and food restriction on body weight in rats followed by no exercise with unlimited access to food. (Data from Oscai, L. et al.: Exercise or food restriction: Effect on adipose tissue cellularity. Am. J. Physiol., 227:901, 1974.)*

TABLE 28-2. *Comparison of total fat and adipose cellularity in rats at 62 weeks of age*[a]

GROUP	TOTAL FAT WEIGHT (g)	CELL NUMBER PER FAT PAD (BILLIONS)	ADIPOSE CELL DIAMETER (μ)
Exercisers	116	4.23	131
Sedentary, food restricted	123	5.24	137
Sedentary, freely eating	162	5.82	134

[a] Data from Oscai, L. et al.: Exercise or food restriction: Effect on adipose tissue cellularity. Am. J. Physiol., 277:901–904, 1974.

know, however, it is only cell size and *not* cell number than can be reduced. If exercise or dietary intervention is discontinued, then the existing adipose tissue mass is likely to increase again by expansion of the cellular volume. Early *prevention* of obesity through exercise and diet, rather than *correction* of obesity once it is present, may be the most effective method to curb the grossly "overfat" condition so common in teenagers and adults.[1]

SUMMARY

1. Obesity is usually defined in terms of excessive quantities of total body fat. There is no biologic reason for men and women to get fatter as they grow older. Therefore, the standards for overfatness for all adult men and women should be that established for younger adults, namely, men—above 20%, women—above 30% body fat.

2. Another classification for obesity is based on the size and number of fat cells. Before adulthood, body fat increases in two ways: by enlargement of individual fat cells, termed fat cell *hypertrophy,* or by an increase in the total number of fat cells, termed fat cell *hyperplasia.* Fat cells probably reach some biologic upper limit in size, so that cell number becomes the key factor determining the extent of obesity.

3. The number of fat cells becomes stable sometime before adulthood; any weight gain or loss thereafter is usually related to a change in the size of the individual cells.

4. Increases in the number of fat cells appear to involve three critical periods: the last trimester of pregnancy, the first year of life, and the adolescent growth spurt prior to adulthood.

5. Dietary restriction and exercise have influenced fat cell development in animals. These effects are most prominent during early growth when the rate of fat cell division can be retarded.

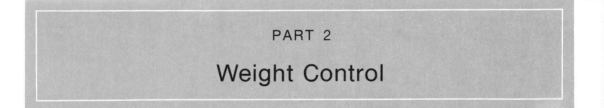

PART 2

Weight Control

The body weight of most adults fluctuates only slightly during the year, even though the annual food intake averages close to 2000 lb. The relative constancy in body weight is impressive when one considers that a slight but consistent increase in food intake can cause weight to increase substantially if there is no compensatory alteration in daily energy expenditure. However, the fact that the weight of most adults fluctuates only slightly illustrates the body's exquisite regulatory control in balancing caloric intake with daily energy expenditure. If the total calories ingested as food exceed the daily energy requirements, the excess calories are stored as fat in adipose tissue. To prevent an increase in weight and fat because of a caloric disequilibrium, an effective program of weight control must establish a balance between energy input and energy output.

ENERGY BALANCE IN THE BODY: INPUT VERSUS OUTPUT

A review of the scientific literature dealing with weight loss in obese persons reveals that initial success in modifying body composition has little relation to the long-term effects of maintaining desired body size and shape. This has been demonstrated in studies concerned with follow-up measurements of participants in weight reduction programs where caloric intake was carefully regulated and monitored. In one survey of studies dealing with weight control management during a 10-year period,[43] the dropout rate varied from 20% to 80%. Of those who remained in a program, no more than 25% lost as much as 20 lb and only 5% lost 40 lb or more. Such statistics indicate that long-term success in maintaining a low-calorie diet is extremely difficult; it is especially difficult in the relaxed atmosphere of one's home where there is ready access to food.

The *energy balance equation* states that body weight remains constant when caloric intake equals caloric expenditure. Any imbalance on the energy output or input side of the equation causes the body weight to change.

Energy input = Energy output → Stable
body weight
Energy input > Energy output → Increase in
body weight
Energy input < Energy output → Decrease in
body weight

Three ways to "unbalance" the energy balance equation are to (1) reduce caloric intake *below* daily energy requirements, (2) maintain regular food intake and *increase* caloric output through additional physical activity *above* daily energy requirements, and (3) combine methods (1) and (2) by *decreasing* daily food intake and *increasing* daily energy expenditure.

When considering the sensitivity of the energy balance equation in regulating overall energy balance, we note that if caloric intake exceeds output by 100 kcal per day, the surplus number of calories consumed in a year would be 365 days × 100 kcal or 36,500 kcal. Because one pound of body fat contains about 3500 kcal (each pound of adipose tissue is about 87% fat or 395 g × 9 kcal · g^{-1} = 3555 kcal per pound), this is equivalent to a gain of 10.4 lb of fat in one year. On the other hand, if daily food intake is reduced just 100 kcal and energy expenditure is increased 100 kcal by jogging 1 mile each day, then the caloric deficit is equivalent to a reduction of about 21 lb of fat in one year!

DIETING FOR WEIGHT CONTROL

This approach to weight loss creates a disequilibrium in the energy balance equation by reducing energy intake. If an obese woman who consumes 2800 calories daily and maintains body weight at 175 pounds wishes to lose weight, she must maintain her regular level of activity but reduce daily food intake to 1800 calories to create a 1000-calorie deficit. In 7 days, the caloric deficit created would equal 7000 calories, the caloric equivalent of 2 lb of body fat. Actually, considerably more than 2 lb would be lost during the first week of caloric restriction because the body's carbohydrate stores would be used up first. This stored nutrient contains fewer calories and much more water than does fat. For this reason, short periods of caloric restriction often prove encouraging to the dieter but result in a large percentage of water and carbohydrate loss per unit of weight reduction with only minimal decrease in body fat. Then, as weight loss continues, a larger proportion of body fat is used for energy to supply the caloric deficit created by food restriction. To reduce fat by another 3 pounds, the reduced caloric intake of 1800 calories would have to be maintained for another 10.5 days. If she held to this diet, body fat would theoretically be reduced at a rate of 1 lb every 3.5 days. Although the mathematics of weight loss through caloric restriction are straightforward, they depend upon several basic assumptions that, if violated, reduce the effectiveness of weight loss through dieting.

For example, dieting frequently causes lethargy and thus reduces the daily activity level. In addition, as body weight decreases, the energy cost of moving the body is reduced proportionately. Consequently, the energy output side of the "energy balance equation" becomes smaller. Also, physiologic changes may occur during caloric restriction that can affect the rate at which weight loss occurs. One such change is in the resting metabolic rate. With semistarvation, both body weight and resting energy output decline. Interestingly, this decrease is greater than the decrease in body weight. This actually conserves energy and causes the diet to be less effective. This "slowing up" of the theoretical weight loss curve often leaves the dieter frustrated and discouraged.

Starvation Diets

A starvation diet may be recommended in some cases of massive obesity in which body fat exceeds 50% of body weight. Such diets are usually prescribed for up to 3 months, but only as a "last resort" prior to undertaking more extreme medical approaches that include various surgical treatments[11,16,34] and that are closely supervised, usually in a hospital setting.[14,15,25,36] The possible advantages and disadvantages of prolonged fasting can be summarized as follows:

Advantages

1. Severe feelings of hunger become depressed in about 7 days and craving for food decreases.
2. There is an initial rapid decrease in body weight, with slower yet progressive decreases in weight when fasting is maintained for 1 or 2 months.
3. The observed weight loss may convince the patient that compulsive eating behaviors can be controlled, thus reversing the patient's usual positive caloric balance.
4. Fasting may be "easier" than adhering to a less severe, semistarvation diet.

Disadvantages

1. Some patients experience a dramatic decrease in blood pressure when assuming an upright position (postural hypotension). Typical symptoms are dizziness and fainting.
2. Possible development of gout, a metabolic disorder in which there is an increased concentration of uric acid in the blood serum. This can lead to recurrent attacks of acute arthritis that usually last for several hours, but can continue for days or weeks if no treatment is given. Also, there may be acute inflammation and swelling of tissues.

3. Development of anemia (low blood hemoglobin concentration). Lethargy and depressed physical activity are often present.
4. Impairment of kidney and renal function.
5. Loss of hair.
6. Muscle irritability and cramping.
7. Emotional disturbances.
8. Reduction in capability for physical activity.
9. Generalized state of malnutrition.

If a person fasts even for several days and then attempts to exercise, deterioration in performance as well as fatigue are likely to occur. Since adequate carbohydrates are not consumed in the starvation diet, the glycogen storage depots in the liver and muscles are reduced to low levels and may cause impairment in most tasks requiring a sustained muscular effort.

Daily medications are usually prescribed and include calcium carbonate or antihistamines for nausea; bicarbonate of soda and potassium chloride to maintain consistency in body fluids; mouthwash and sugar-free chewing gum for bad breath (due to high level of fat metabolism) that is present as long as fasting persists, and various bath oils for dry skin. Clearly, for most individuals starvation is *not* an "ultimate diet" or proper approach to weight control. Furthermore, the success rate of prolonged fasting is poor.[26] Over a 7.3-year follow-up period in 121 patients, much of the reduced weight was maintained for the first 12 to 18 months. The tendency to regain weight was independent of length of fast (up to 2 months), extent of weight loss (up to 41.4 kg), or age at onset of obesity. Return to original weight occurred in 50% within 2 to 3 years, and only 7 patients remained at their reduced weights. Figure 28-8 shows these rather depressing observations.

Minnesota Semistarvation Experiments

From November, 1944 through September, 1946, one of the most interesting series of experiments in human nutrition was undertaken by the Laboratory of Physiological Hygiene at the University of Minnesota.[28] These experiments were designed to quantify the biologic and psychologic effects of prolonged severe undernutrition imposed on thousands of people living in Europe during World War II.

The experiment was conducted in three phases: *Phase I* was a 12-week control period

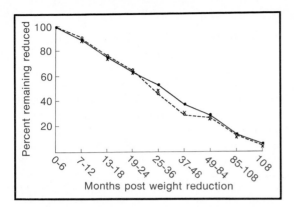

FIG. 28-8. *Percent of patients remaining at reduced weights at various time intervals following accomplished weight loss. Solid line represents 60 subjects with obesity onset before age 21; broken line, 42 subjects with obesity onset after age 21. (From Johnson, D., and Drenick, E. J.: Therapeutic fasting in morbid obesity. Arch. Intern. Med., 137:1381, 1977. Copyright 1977, American Medical Association.)*

during which subjects had access to a normal diet that averaged 3492 kcal per day. During this time, caloric intake was balanced with caloric expenditure so that body weight as well as numerous other physiologic functions would stabilize. The measurements during this period served as the reference point for determining the effects of semistarvation and subsequent rehabilitation. *Phase 2* was a 24-week period of semistarvation in which the daily caloric intake was reduced by 45% of control values to 1570 kcal. *Phase 3* was a 12-week rehabilitation period in which caloric intake was gradually increased to control values. There was an additional 8-week period of rehabilitation during which measurements were made on a selected group of subjects and a final follow-up on a few subjects from 8 to 12 months after the recovery period.

The subjects were 32 men in good physical condition. They lived in special testing facilities where daily food intake, exercise, and work routines were carefully monitored by a full-time staff that included physicians, exercise scientists, dietitians, chemists, statisticians, psychologists, and various technical and administrative staff. Each subject's weight loss was carefully planned to reduce to about 24% of initial body weight by the end of the 24-week semistarvation period. To accomplish this, the metabolic re-

quirement of each subject was determined from the daily caloric intake required to maintain body weight during the last 2 weeks of the control period. Food intake and physical activity were adjusted during semistarvation to produce the necessary weight loss. Food intake was carefully regulated by dietitians who made precise measurements of the number of calories ingested. Two meals a day were served and consisted of 3 basic menus repeated in rotation. The major food items were whole-wheat bread, potatoes, cereals, turnips, and cabbage, with only small quantities of meat or dairy products. If the weight loss for an individual during any one week fell short or increased above his predicted weight loss, the servings of bread or potatoes were adjusted the following week to bring the body weight back to the desired value. In this way, despite the decrease in resting metabolism that occurs with weight reduction, weight loss could still be made to coincide with that predicted from the energy balance equation.

During the first 12 weeks of semistarvation, body fat declined 11.6 lb from an average of 13.9% of body weight (21.1 lb of fat) to 7.5% (9.5 lb of fat). Concurrently, body weight decreased 25.4 lb from 152.5 lb to 127.1 lb. During the subsequent 12 weeks on the low-calorie diet, there was a further decline in body weight to 118 lb. Percent body fat dropped to 5.2%, which represented 6.1 lb of the total body weight. In addition, the average *decrease in muscle mass* was intermediate between the decrease in body weight and decrease in body fat. These data vividly show that *both* fat and lean tissue are lost during weight loss from severe caloric restriction.

At the completion of the semistarvation period, subjects were placed in one of four groups of eight men. During the first 6 weeks of rehabilitation, the average daily caloric intake for the four groups was 1931, 2245, 2675, and 2924 kcal. During the next 6 weeks, the average intake of calories was increased by approximately 1100 kcal per day per group. For the following 8-week period, one group remained at the laboratory and was permitted to eat food ad libitum. During the first 2 weeks of unlimited food, daily calorie intake reached as high as 7000 to 10,000 kcal. It then dropped and leveled off during the remaining 6 weeks to about 3200 to 4500 kcal per day.

The Minnesota experiments illustrate the severe alterations in body composition that can result from a prolonged period of caloric restriction. Many people are able to tolerate some special 1000-calorie diet for a week or so within the comfort of their own home. However, the severe physical and psychologic stresses encountered by the Minnesota subjects, under the best of laboratory conditions, with a 1570-kcal diet leads us to question seriously the chances the "average" person has for success with such long-term caloric deprivation, independent of their body fat content.

EXERCISE FOR WEIGHT CONTROL

Increased caloric output through exercise provides a significant option for unbalancing the energy balance equation to bring about weight loss. Only recently, however, has this approach to weight control come to prominence.[17a] Two arguments have generally been raised against the exercise approach. One is the belief that exercise inevitably causes an increase in appetite so that any caloric deficit is rapidly made up by a proportionate increase in food intake. The second argument is that the calorie-burning effects of exercise are so small that a reasonable use of exercise would make only a small "dent" in the body's fat reserves compared to the approach using starvation or semistarvation. We shall take a closer look at these two misconceptions.

Exercise and Food Intake

In considering the effects of exercise on appetite and food consumption, a distinction should be made between the type and duration of the exercise. People such as lumberjacks, farm laborers, and endurance athletes, who perform hard, physical labor for prolonged periods, consume about twice the daily calories (4000 to 7000 kcal) than more sedentary counterparts (2000 to 3000 kcal). Under such circumstances, the high caloric intakes are required to balance the extremely high daily caloric requirements, especially for many athletes who spend considerable time each day in vigorous physical training. Table 28-3 lists the estimated daily caloric intake of various international-caliber athletes. It should be emphasized that athletes who achieve at this level often spend 8 hours a day in training. It should be noted that endurance athletes like marathon runners, cross-country skiers, and cyclists consume about 6000 kcal each day, yet are among the leanest people in the world! Obviously, this extreme caloric intake is required just to meet the energy requirements of their training.

When considering the dietary intake for people who train for relatively short periods, the apparent appetite-stimulating effect of exercise is noticeably reduced. This occurred for college women whose daily caloric intake was evaluated before and after a season of competi-

TABLE 28-3. *Estimated daily caloric intake for athletes in various sport activities*

SPORT	AVERAGE BODY WEIGHT (kg)	ESTIMATED DAILY KCAL INTAKE
Cross-country skiing	67.5	6105
Bicycle racing	68.0	5995
Canoe racing	75.0	5995
Marathon racing	68.0	5940
Soccer	74.0	5885
Field hockey (men)	75.0	5720
Handball (European)	75.0	5610
Basketball	75.0	5610
Ice hockey	68.0	5390
Gymnastics (men)	67.0	5000
Sailing	74.0	5170
Fencing	73.0	5000
Sprinting (track)	69.0	4675
Boxing (middle and welter weight)	63.5	4675
Diving	61.0	4620
Pole vault	73.0	4620

tive swimming and tennis.[27] Swim workouts were conducted daily for 2 hours from January to May. Total distance swum each day was 2000 to 4000 m during January and March and 1000 to 2000 m in April and May. The workouts for the tennis players consisted of 10 minutes of rope-skipping, 45 minutes of organized practice and games, followed by a half-mile jog. Rope-skipping and jogging were discontinued after January. Average daily caloric intake was assessed for each woman before and after the 5-month training and competitive season by a 7-day dietary inventory.

The average caloric intake of the swimmers, shown in Table 28-4, remained about 15% higher than that of the tennis players during the training and competitive seasons. Within each group, there were insignificant changes in caloric intake or food composition before and after the experiment. In terms of body composition, there was no change for both groups in body weight, percent body fat, and lean body weight.

Caloric Stress of Physical Activity

A common misconception about the role of increased exercise in programs of weight reduction concerns the calorigenic effects of regular exercise. It has been argued that an inordinate amount of exercise must be performed just to lose one pound of body fat, as for example, chopping wood for 10 hours, playing golf for 20 hours, performing mild calisthenic exercises for 22 hours, or playing Ping-Pong for 28 hours or volleyball for 32 hours. From a different perpective, however, golf played only 2 hours (about 350 kcal per day), 2 days per week (700 kcal) would take about 5 weeks to reduce 1 lb of fat. Assuming one could play year round, devoting 2 days a week to this form of exercise would result in a 10-lb loss of fat during the

year, provided that the food intake remained fairly constant. *The calorie-expending effects of exercise are cumulative, whether the deficit occurs rapidly or systematically over a longer period.*

In determining the caloric cost of various physical activities, the assumption is made that the energy cost is fairly constant among people of a particular body size. In Chapter 8, we stated that the energy cost data for most physical activities were averages often based on few observations. A wide range of values is therefore possible because of individual differences in performance style and technique, and environmental factors that include terrain, temperature, and wind resistance, as well as the intensity of participation.

The values of energy expenditure for physical activities presented in Appendix C should not be considered absolute. These are "average" values, applicable under "average" conditions when applied to the "average" person of a given body weight. However, these gross values do provide a relative approximation of energy expenditure for establishing the appropriate caloric cost of different physical activities.

DIET PLUS EXERCISE: THE IDEAL COMBINATION

For men and women, combinations of exercise and diet offer considerably more flexibility in achieving a negative caloric balance and accompanying fat loss than either exercise alone or diet alone. In fact, the addition of exercise to the program of weight control may facilitate a more permanent weight loss than would total reliance on caloric restriction.

How can an obese person, utilizing exercise *and* diet while attempting to maintain a prudent weight loss of about 1 lb a week, reduce body weight by 20 pounds? Under these conditions, even under the best circumstances, 20 weeks

TABLE 28-4. *Average kcal intake of swimmers and tennis players before and after a 5-month training and competitive season*[a]

GROUP	CALORIES BEFORE	AFTER	PROTEIN (g) BEFORE	AFTER	FATS (g) BEFORE	AFTER	CARBOHYDRATES (g) BEFORE	AFTER
Swimmers	2091	2065	80.8	71.8	92.3	90.0	247.9	240.6
Tennis players	1811	1797	78.1	74.2	78.9	78.8	192.6	195.2

[a] From Katch, F.I. et al.: Effects of physical training on the body composition and diet of females. Res. Quart., 40:99, 1969.

would be required to achieve a 20-lb fat loss. With this goal, the average *weekly* deficit would have to be 3500 calories whereas the *daily* deficit must be 500 calories.

One-half hour of moderate exercise (about 350 "extra" calories) performed 3 days a week adds 1050 calories to the weekly caloric deficit. Consequently, the weekly caloric intake would have to be reduced by only 2400 calories instead of 3500 calories in order to lose the desired 1 lb of fat each week. If the number of exercise days is increased from three to five, food intake need only be reduced by 250 calories each day. If the duration of the 5-day per week workouts were prolonged from 30 minutes to 1 hour, then no reduction in food intake would be necessary for weight loss to occur, because the required 3500 caloric deficit would have been created entirely through exercise.

Clearly, physical activity can be used effectively by itself or in combination with mild dietary restriction to bring about an effective loss of body fat. Either approach is likely to produce fewer of the feelings of intense hunger and other psychologic stress that occur with a program of weight loss that relies exclusively on caloric restriction. Perhaps of equal or greater significance is the fact that the use of exercise in a weight-reducing program provides protection against a loss in lean tissue.[48] Thus, more of the weight loss will be *fat loss.*

FACTORS AFFECTING WEIGHT LOSS

When caloric intake is below the daily energy requirement, the initial decrease in body weight occurs primarily from water loss and corresponding depletion of the body's carbohydrate reserves; with further weight loss, a larger proportion of body fat is metabolized to supply the caloric deficit created by restricting food intake or increasing physical activity.

Figure 28-9 shows the percentage composition of the average daily weight loss for water, protein, and fat during 24 days on a 1000-kcal-per-day carbohydrate diet and $2\frac{1}{2}$ hours of prescribed exercise. In the first 3 days of caloric deficit, 70% of the weight loss could be attributed to water loss. The contribution of water to weight loss became progressively less as the caloric deficit continued and represented only 19% of the weight loss during days 11 to 13. At the same time, fat loss accelerated from 25% to 69% during this period. From day 21 to day 24,

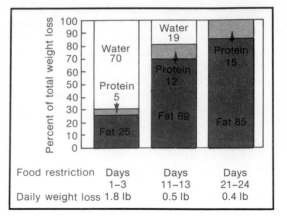

FIG. 28-9. *Percentage composition of weight loss at the start, middle, and end of 24 days of food restriction (1000 kcal per day) plus enforced exercise of 2.5 hours per day. (From Grande, F.: Nutrition and energy balance in body composition studies. In Techniques for Measuring Body Composition. Washington, D. C., National Academy of Sciences-National Research Council, 1961.)*

85% of the weight loss was due to a reduction in body fat with no corresponding increase in water loss. The contribution of protein to weight loss increased from 5% initially to 12% during days 11 to 13 and to 15% by the end of the observation period.

Figure 28-10 shows the relationship between the proportion of water, protein, and fat lost and the amount of water consumed during the first few days of caloric restriction. The left bar is the same as that shown in Figure 28-9 for days 1 to 3. In this experiment, subjects had unlimited access to water. The middle bar represents the compositional loss in weight for six men who also subsisted on the 1000-kcal carbohydrate diet, but with daily water intake restricted to 1800 ml. The bar at the right displays the average weight loss for six men who consumed an identical diet, but whose daily water intake was further reduced to 900 ml. Water restriction during the first 3 days significantly increased the proportion of water loss and decreased the proportion of fat loss, especially in subjects who consumed the least water. Although more total weight was lost when daily water intake was 900 ml per day, this additional loss in weight could be attributed to water loss. Regardless of whether or not fluid intake was restricted, the total quantity of fat lost was essentially *the same.*

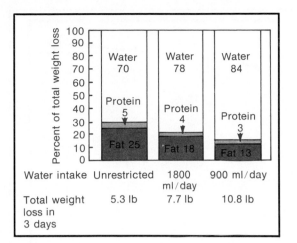

FIG. 28-10. *Percentage composition of weight loss during the first 3 days on a 1000-kcal carbohydrate diet with water intake unrestricted and reduced to 1800 ml and 900 ml per day. (From Grande, F.: Nutrition of energy balance in body composition studies. In Techniques for Measuring Body Composition. Washington, D. C., National Academy of Sciences-National Research Council, 1961.)*

Figure 28-11 illustrates the important concept that the caloric equivalent of weight loss increases as a function of increasing the duration of caloric restriction. *This is the major reason why it is crucial to maintain a sustained caloric deficit for extended periods because shorter periods cause a larger percentage of water and carbohydrate loss per unit of weight reduction with only a minimal decrease in body fat.* It should be noted that the caloric equivalent per kg of weight loss more than doubles after 2 months as compared to the first four or five days.

The results of the aforementioned studies, in which various approaches to establishing a caloric imbalance have been evaluated, are as follows:

1. Exercise combined with dietary restriction appears to be a more valid approach for achieving a negative caloric balance as compared with exercise or diet alone.
2. During the first few days of weight reduction, the rapid weight loss is due primarily to a loss in body water and carbohydrates; at least 2 months of weight reduction is associated with a substantially greater loss of fat per unit of weight loss.
3. Water intake should not be restricted when beginning a weight reduction program because this can precipitate dehydration but no additional fat loss.
4. Undesirable psychologic and medically related problems may occur with prolonged caloric restriction maintained below minimal energy requirements.
5. Weight loss by diet alone also causes a significant loss of muscle mass. Exercise appears to protect against lean tissue losses; thus, more of the weight loss is fat loss.

SUMMARY

1. There are three ways to unbalance the energy balance equation and bring about weight loss: (1) reduce caloric intake below daily energy expenditure, (2) maintain regular food intake and increase energy output, and (3) combine methods 1 and 2 by decreasing food intake and increasing energy expenditure.

2. Long-term weight control through dietary restriction is generally successful less than 20% of the time.

3. A caloric deficit of 3500 kcal created either through diet or exercise is the equivalent to the calories in 1 pound of adipose tissue.

4. Dieting for weight loss can be effective if done properly. The disadvantages of semistarvation, however, are significant and include a loss of lean body tissue, lethargy, possible malnutrition and metabolic disorders, and a decrease in the basal energy expenditure. Some of these factors actually conserve energy and cause the diet to be less effective.

5. The calorie-expending effects of exercise are cumulative, so that a little exercise performed routinely has a dramatic effect over time. The role of exercise in appetite suppression or stimulation is unclear. Over time, most athletes eventually consume enough calories to counterbalance caloric expenditure—but many of these athletes are the leanest in the world.

6. Combinations of exercise and diet offer a flexible and effective approach to weight control. Exercise enhances the mobilization and utilization of fat, thus increasing fat weight loss, and at the same time retards losses in lean tissue.

7. The rapid weight loss during the first few days of caloric deficit is due primarily to a loss in body water and carbohydrates. Continued weight reduction is associated with a greater loss of fat per unit of weight loss.

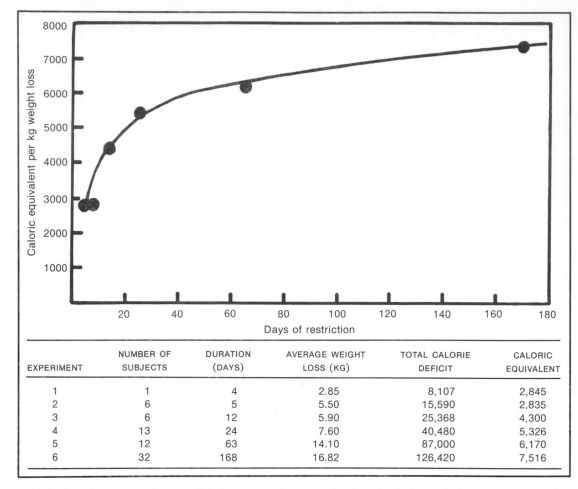

EXPERIMENT	NUMBER OF SUBJECTS	DURATION (DAYS)	AVERAGE WEIGHT LOSS (KG)	TOTAL CALORIE DEFICIT	CALORIC EQUIVALENT
1	1	4	2.85	8,107	2,845
2	6	5	5.50	15,590	2,835
3	6	12	5.90	25,368	4,300
4	13	24	7.60	40,480	5,326
5	12	63	14.10	87,000	6,170
6	32	168	16.82	126,420	7,516

FIG. 28-11. *Caloric equivalent of weight loss in relation to the duration of calorie restriction. Each datum point represents an experiment summarized in the accompanying legend. (Adapted from Grande, F.: Nutrition and energy balance in body composition studies. In Techniques for Measuring Body Composition. Washington, D. C., National Academy of Sciences-National Research Council, 1961.)*

References

1. Abraham, S., and Johnson, C.L.: Prevalence of severe obesity in adults in the United States. Am. J. Clin. Nutr., *33*:364, 1980.
1a. Alexander, J.K. et al.: Observations on some clinical features of extreme obesity with particular references to the cardiorespiratory effects. Am. J. Med., *32*:512, 1962.
2. Alexander, J.K., and Pettigrove, J.R.: Obesity and congestive heart failure. Geriatrics *22*:101, 1967.
3. Alexander, J.K., and Peterson, K.L.: Cardiovascular effects of weight reduction. Circulation *45*:310, 1972.

4. Angel, A.: 1. Pathophysiologic changes in obesity. Can. Med. Assoc. J., *119:*1401, 1978.

5. Angel, A., and Roncari, D.A.K.: Medical complications of obesity. *Can. Med. Assoc. J., 119:*1408, 1978.

6. Backman, L. et al.: Cardiovascular function in extreme obesity. Acta Med. Scand., *193:*437, 1972.

7. Bjorntrop, P. et al.: Effect of an energy reduced dietary regimen in relation to adipose tissue cellularity in obese women. Am. J. Clin. Nutrition. *28:*445, 1975.

8. Blitzer, P.H. et al.: Association between teenage obesity and cancer in 56,111 women. *Prev. Med., 5:*20, 1976.

9. Brook, C.G.D., and Lloyd, J.K.: Adipose cell size and glucose tolerance in obese children and effects of diet. *Arch. Dis. Child., 48:*301, 1973.

10. Burwell, C.S. et al.: Extreme obesity associated with alveolar hypoventilation—a Pickwickian syndrome. *Am. J. Med., 21:*811, 1956.

11. Campbell, J.M.: Jejunoileal bypass as a treatment of morbid obesity. *Ann. Intern Med. 75:*377, 1971.

12. Chaing, B.N. et al.: Overweight and hypertension: A review. Circulation *39:*403, 1969.

12a. Clarkson, P.M. et al.: Regional odyrose cellularity and reliability of odipose cell size determination. Am. J. Clin. Nutr., *33:*2245, 1980.

12b. Clarkson, P.M. et al.: A comparison of four methods to measure fat cell size. Am. J. Clin. Nutr. *34:*2287, 1981.

13. DiGirolamo, M. et al.: A simple method to determine fat cell size and number in four mammalian species. *Am. J. Physiol., 221:*850, 1971.

14. Drenick, E.J. et al.: Prolonged starvation as a treatment for severe obesity. J.A.M.A., *187:*100, 1964.

15. Drenick, E.J. *Editor:* Weight reduction by prolonged fasting. *In:* Bray, G.A. (ed.) *Obesity in Perspective.* Bethesda, MD. United States Department of Health, Education and Welfare, 1975.

16. Faloon, W.W (ed.): Conference on jejunolleostomy for obesity. *Am. J. Clin. Nutr. 30:*1, 1977.

17. Faust, I.M. et al.: Diet induced adipocyte number increase in adult rats: A new model of obesity. Am. J. Physiol., *235:*279, 1978.

17a. Foreyt, J.P., et al: Weight control and nutrition education programs in occupational settings. Public Health Reports, *95:*127, 1980.

18. Goldstein, J.L. et al.: Hyperlipidemia in coronary heart disease. Lipid levels in 500 survivors of myocardial infarction. J. Clin. Invest., *52:*1533, 1973.

19. Gordon, T., and Kannel, W.B.: The effects of overweight on cardiovascular diseases. Geriatrics *28:*80, 1973.

20. Gordon, T. et al.: Diabetes, blood lipids, and the role of obesity in coronary heart disease risk for women. Ann. Intern. Med., *87:*393, 1977.

21. Hagar, A. et al.: Adipose tissue cellularity in obese school girls before and after dietary treatment. Am. J. Clin. Nutr., *31:*68, 1978.

22. Tannon, B.M., and Lohman, T.G.: The energy cost of overweight in the United States. Am. J Public Health *68:*765, 1978.

23. Hirsch, J., and Knittle, J.: Cellularity of obese and non-obese human adipose tissue. *Fed. Proc., 29:*1518, 1970.

24. Hirsch, J., and Batchelor, B.R.: Adipose tissue cellularity in human obesity. Clin. Endocrinol. Metab., *5:*299, 1976.

25. Innes, J.A. et al.: Long term follow-up of therapeutic starvation. *Br. Med. J., 2:*356, 1974.

26. Johnson, D. and Drenick, E.J.: Therapeutic fasting in morbid obesity. *Arch. Intern. Med., 137:*1381, 1977.

27. Katch, F.I. et al.: Effects of physical training on the body composition and diet of females. *Res. Q., 40:*99, 1969.

28. Keys, A. et al.: *The Biology of Human Starvation.* University of Minnesota Press. Minneapolis, Minn. 1970.

29. Knittle, J. and Hirsch, J.: Effect of early nutrition on the development of rat epididymal fat pads; cellularity and metabolism. *J. Clin. Invest. 47:*2901, 1968.
30. LaVau, J.: Reliable photomicrographic method of determining fat cell size and number: Application to dietary obesity. *Proc. Soc. Exp. Biol. Med. 156:*251, 1977.
31. Mabee, T.M. et al.: The mechanism of increased gallstone formation in obese human subjects. Surgery, *79:*460, 1976.
32. Oscai, L. et al.: Effects of exercise and of food restriction on adipose tissue cellularity. *J. Lipid Res. 13:*588, 1972.
33. Oscai, L. et al.: Exercise or food restriction: Effect on adipose tissue cellularity. *Am. J. Physiol. 227:*901, 1974.
34. Parfitt, A.M.: Metabolic bone disease after intestinal bypass for treatment of obesity. *Ann. Intern. Med., 89:*193, 1978.
35. Rimm, A.A. et al.: Disease and obesity in 73,532 women. Obesity Bariatric Med. *1:*77, 1972.
36. Rooth, G. and Carlstrom, S.: Therapeutic fasting. *Acta Med. Scand., 187:*455, 1970.
37. Rössner, S., and Hallberg, D.: Serum lipoproteins in massive obesity. Acta Med. Scand., *204:*103, 1978.
38. Salans, L.B. et al.: Experimental obesity in man: Cellular character of the adipose tissue. *J. Clin. Invest. 50:*1005, 1971.
39. Sims, E.A.H. and Horton, E.S.: Endocrine and metabolic adaptation to obesity and starvation. *Am. J. Clin. Nutr. 21:*1455, 1968.
40. Stamler, R. et al.: Weight and blood pressure. Findings in hypertension screening of 1 million Americans. J.A.M.A., *240:*1607, 1978.
41. Stern, J.S., and Hirsch, J.: Obesity and pancreatic function. *In* Handbook of Physiology, Section 1. Endocrinology, Vol. 1. Edited by D. Steener and N. Frankel. Washington, D.C., American Physiological Society, 1972.
42. Stern, J.S. et al.: Pancreatic insulin release and peripheral tissue resistance in Zucker obese rats fed high and low carbohydrate diets. Am. J. Physiol., *228:*543, 1975.
43. Stunkard, A.J. and McLaren-Hume, M.: The results of treatment of obesity: A review of the literature and report of a series. *Arch. Intern. Med. 103:*79, 1959.
44. Thorn, G.W. et al.: Harrison's Principles of Internal Medicine, 8th ed. New York, McGraw-Hill Book Co., 1977.
44a. Udall, J.G. et al.: Interaction of maternal and neonatal obesity. *Pediatrics 62:*17, 1978.
45. Warner, W.A.: The obese patient and anesthesia. J.A.M.A., *205:*102, 1968.
46. Weisinger, J.R. et al.: The nephrotic syndrome: A complication of massive obesity. Ann. Intern. Med., *50:*233, 1974.
47. West, K.: Epidemiology of Diabetes and Its Vascular Lesions. New York, Elsevier, 1978.
48. Zuti, W.B., and Golding, L.A.: Comparing diet and exercise as weight reduction tools. Physician Sportsmed., *4:*49, 1976.

SECTION VII
Aging and Health-Related
Aspects of Exercise

There is no question that the physiology and performance capabilities of older people generally differ from those of younger adults. It is unknown, however, the extent to which these differences are due to true biologic aging, or are the result of sociologic constraints that alter the life styles and activity opportunities for people as they grow older. If an active life style is continued into later years, a relatively high level of function is retained and vigorous activities can be engaged in safely and successfully.

Aside from the positive effects of exercise in maintaining physiologic function, it now appears that physical activity is protective against the ravages of coronary heart disease. Although the precise mechanism for protection remains unknown, physical inactivity is now considered a heart disease risk factor. More specifically, the chance for mortality from heart disease is generally two to three times greater in sedentary people than in physically active counterparts. Clearly, evolution has not kept pace with automation, and people who are physically active—either in their job or leisure time—have less chance of contracting heart disease; if they do, their survival rates are higher.

The recommendations for physical activity and reconditioning should not be formulated from some arbitrarily devised standards based on chronologic age. Rather, knowledge of past and present activity experiences plus a careful evaluation of the person's adaptability to a standard exercise task must provide the framework for the intelligent formulation of activity programs.

Exercise, Aging, and Cardiovascular Disease

29

In this chapter, we explore several aspects of the aging process with special reference to exercise and its relation to cardiovascular disease.

Aging and Physiologic Function

Physiologic and performance measures generally improve rapidly during childhood and reach a maximum between the late teens and 30 years of age. Functional capacity then declines with age. Figure 29-1 shows the decline in various functional measures plotted as the percentage deviation from typical values for a 30-year-old person. Although all measures decline with age, not all decline at the same rate. Nerve conduction velocity, for example, declines only 10% to 15% from 30 to 80 years of age, whereas resting cardiac index (ratio of cardiac output to surface area) declines 20% to 30%; maximum breathing capacity at age 80 is about 40% that of a 30-year-old. In addition, some functions (such as ventilation) that show only a moderate aging effect at rest may show dramatic changes under the stress of exercise. Because long-term exercise studies on the same subjects are lacking, it is not known whether long-term exercise participation can change the actual rate of decline in physiologic function or "override" deterioration in function that normally occurs with increasing age. In the following sections, we discuss the relationship of age to several physiologic measures important to exercise performance.

Muscular Strength

Maximum strength of men and women is generally achieved between the ages of 20 and 30 years[22a], at the time when muscular cross-sectional area is usually the largest. Thereafter, there is a progressive decline in strength for most muscle groups. This is due primarily to a reduced muscle mass that reflects a loss of total muscle protein brought about by inactivity, aging, or both. Indirect evidence indicates that habitual physical training facilitates protein retention and thus delays the strength decrement with aging.[14,18a]

Neural Function

The cumulative effects of aging on central nervous system function are exhibited by a 37% decline in the number of spinal cord axons, a 10% decline in nerve conduction velocity, and a significant loss in the elastic properties of connective tissue.[4,29a] These changes may partially explain the age-related decrement in neuromuscular performance as assessed by both simple and complex reaction and movement times.[7a,30a] When reaction time is partitioned into a central processing time and muscle contraction time, it is the central processing time that is most affected by the aging process. Thus, aging affects the ability to detect a stimulus and process the information to produce a response. Since reflexes, such as the knee jerk

426

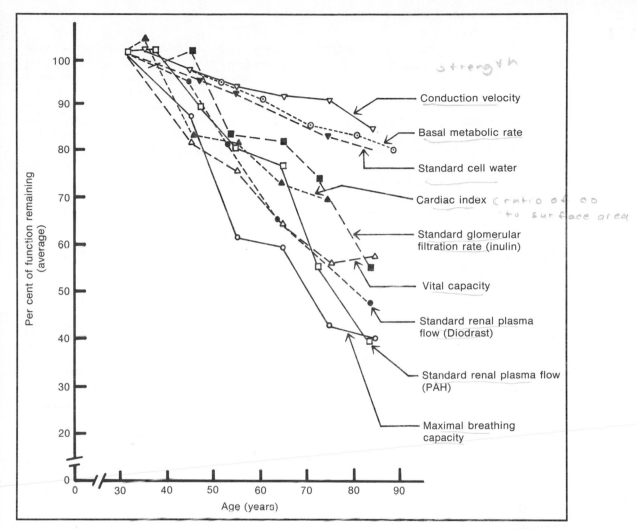

strength

Conduction velocity

Basal metabolic rate

Standard cell water

Cardiac index (ratio of CO to surface area)

Standard glomerular filtration rate (inulin)

Vital capacity

Standard renal plasma flow (Diodrast)

Standard renal plasma flow (PAH)

Maximal breathing capacity

FIG. 29-1. *Decline in various human functional capacities and physiologic measurements. Values are adjusted so that the value at age 30 equals 100% (Originally published in Can. Med. Assoc. J., 96:836, March 1967.)*

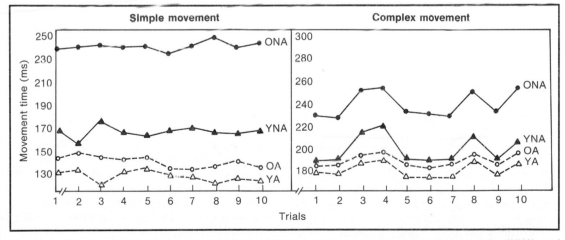

FIG. 29-2. *Simple and complex movement time in young active (YA), old active (OA), young nonactive (YNA), and old nonactive (ONA) subjects. Note that in both simple and complex movement tasks, the movement time is slower for the old and young nonactive individuals than in the young and old active individuals. (From Spirduso, W.W.: Reaction and movement time as a function of age and physical activity level. J. Gerontol., 30:435, 1975.)*

427

reflex, do not involve processing in the brain, they are less affected by the aging process than voluntary responses, i.e., reaction and movement times.[7b] As shown in Figure 29-2, movement times for simple and complex tasks were significantly slower for older subjects than for younger counterparts of the same activity level. *In all instances, however, the active groups (be they young or old) moved significantly faster than a corresponding age group that was less active.* These observations suggest that an active life-style may significantly and positively affect movement time at any age. It is tempting to speculate that the biologic aging of certain neuromuscular functions can be somewhat retarded by regular participation in physical activity.

Cardiovascular Function

The progressive decline in maximal oxygen uptake after age 25 was discussed in Chapter 11. This is due largely to various age-related decrements in physiologic functions related to oxygen transport. One well-documented change in cardiovascular function is a decline in the maximal heart rate. This apparent age-effect is progressive with advancing years and appears to occur to the same extent in both active and sedentary men and women. A rough approximation of the change in maximal heart rate with age is expressed by the following relationship:

max HR (beats · min^{-1}) = 220 − age (years)

As a consequence of a lower maximum heart rate, maximum cardiac output is reduced with age. Also contributing to this reduced blood flow capacity is a reduction in the heart's stroke volume, which may reflect changes in myocardial contractility. Other age-related changes in the cardiovascular system include a reduction in peripheral blood flow capacity. This may be due to a decrease in the capillary-to-muscle fiber ratio and a reduction in arterial cross-sectional area.[24a]

Whether the preceding changes in cardiovascular function are a direct result of the aging process per se or of a lack of habitual physical activity has not been determined. In fact, sedentary living may bring about losses in functional capacity that are as great as the effects of aging itself. Results from training studies suggest that regular exercise enables older individ-

uals to retain cardiovascular functioning much above age-paired sedentary subjects.[9,15] When previously active middle-aged men followed a regular endurance exercise program over a 10-year period, the usual 9% to 15% decline in work capacity and maximal aerobic power was forestalled.[15] In fact, at age 55, these active men had maintained the same values for blood pressure, body weight, and max $\dot{V}O_2$ that they had had when measured at age 45.

Body Composition

In the Western world, the average 35-year-old male will gain 0.2 to 0.8 kg of fat each year until the fifth or sixth decade of life.[24] Figure 29-3 clearly shows this trend in percent body fat for men and women of different ages.

After age 60, there is a reduction in total body weight despite increasing body fat. This is partly explained by the fact that in the upper age group many of the grossly overweight people have died, so there are just not many heavy subjects to be measured. Also, lean body weight does tend to decrease with age. This is largely due to the aging skeleton becoming demineralized and porous; concurrently, the quantity of muscle mass is reduced. Whether or not regular physical activity can retard these changes in body density with age is unknown.

A major limitation of age-trend studies is that the same subjects are not followed over time, but rather different subjects in different age categories are evaluated at the same time. From these *cross-sectional* data, one attempts to generalize as to expected age-related changes for an individual. Sometimes these generalizations are misleading, especially in attempts to make inferences concerning age trends for individual growth patterns. For example, today's 70 and 80-year-olds are generally shorter than 20-year-old college students. This does not necessarily mean that we get shorter as we grow older (although this does happen to some extent). Rather, the young adults of this generation are better nourished than their 80-year-counterparts were at the age of 20 and thus achieve optimal growth. In terms of body fat changes, the limited longitudinal data from the same subjects tend to support the trends noted in cross-sectional studies.[6] When the fat content of 27 adult men was studied over a 12-year-span from age 32 to 44 years, the deposition of body fat increased with age. Of the 27

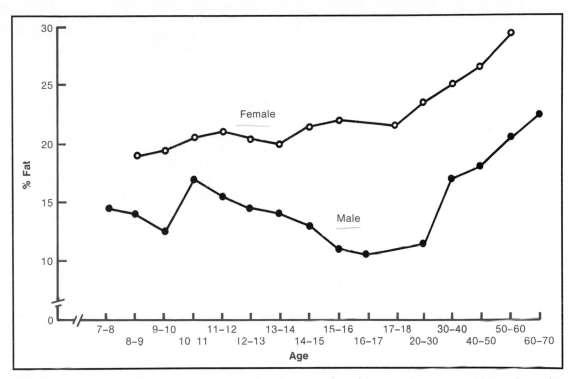

FIG. 29-3. *Body composition changes as a function of age. (From Parizkova, J.: Body composition and exercise during growth and development. In Physical Activity: Human Growth and Development. Edited by G.L. Rarick. New York, Academic Press, 1974.)*

men studied, only 4 did not gain in body fat. Fat weight increased an average of 6.5 kg which was equal to the total gain in body weight over the 12 years.[6]

Osteoporosis is a major problem in aging. This condition results in a loss of bone mass, increased bone porosity, and a decrease in the thickness of bone cortex. For people over 60 years of age, these alterations in aging bone can reduce the bone mass by 30% to 50%.[5] Water loss in normal calcified bone may also reflect cellular loss. These changes in body density may invalidate the equations underlying the use of hydrostatic weighing and may result in gross inaccuracies in determining body fat content in older individuals.

TRAINABILITY AND AGE

Regular vigorous physical activity produces physiologic improvements regardless of age. Of course, the magnitude of the changes depends on several factors including initial fitness status, age, and the specific type of training.[25]

With regard to the age factor, it appears that older individuals are not able to improve their strength and endurance capacity to the same extent as younger people.[28] The reasons for this decreased "trainability" are not well understood. It is probably the result of a general decline in neuromuscular function as well as of an age-related impairment in the cell's capability for protein synthesis and chemical regulation.

Figure 29-4 shows the improvement to be expected from physical conditioning for people of different ages in relation to their initial fitness level at the start of training. Essentially, when a person, young or old, has a relatively high functional capacity at the start of training, there is less room for improvement compared to someone who starts at a lower level and has considerable room for improvement. At the same time, ability to improve appears to be age-related; older persons can expect less improvement when they begin to train later in life than younger counterparts who start training at the same initial level of fitness. For both young and old, however, significant training improvements can be expected.

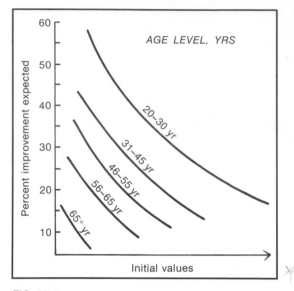

FIG. 29-4. *Theoretical representation of the improvement that might be expected with conditioning relative to age and initial level of functioning.*

EXERCISE AND LONGEVITY

Because older fit individuals have many of the functional characteristics of younger people, one could argue that improved physical fitness may help retard the aging process and thus offer some protection to health in later life.

Regular Exercise and Longevity

In one of the first studies of the possible beneficial influence of sport and regular exercise on prolonging life,[12] it was shown that former Harvard oarsmen exceeded their predicted longevity by 5.1 years per man. Earlier studies showed similar but more modest results.[2] However, these studies were plagued with methodologic problems, including inadequate record keeping, small sample size, improper statistical procedures for estimating expected longevity, and an inability to account for other important factors such as socioeconomic background, body type, cigarette smoking, and family background. One group of researchers attempted to overcome many of these limitations in their study of the diseases and longevity of former college athletes.[21] Because collegiate athletes usually have a longer involvement in

habitual physical activity prior to entering college than nonathletes, and since they *may* remain more physically active after college,[22] this seemed to be an excellent group to study in order to provide insight concerning exercise and longevity.

Figure 29-5 shows that there was essentially no difference in the longevity of the exathletes as compared to that of their nonathletic counterparts. Some degree of equality in genetic background existed between the groups, because the average age at death of grandparents, parents, and siblings of exathletes and nonathletes was also similar. These findings suggest that participation in athletics as a young adult does not necessarily ensure increased longevity. It is still possible, however, that *regular* physical activity *throughout life* offers protection in terms of health and longevity.

Aging and Activity Patterns

If habitual physical activity helps retard the aging process, it would certainly be an important reason to increase the leisure-time activities of older people. Figure 29-6 shows the amount of time spent in occupational as well as active leisure pursuits for 1600 males aged 16 to 69 years.[22] With the older men, there is a slight decrease in the number of hours spent in occupational activities. There is also a significant and progressive decrease in the amount of time devoted to leisure-time activities. Clearly, older-aged groups spend less time in daily physical activity.[3,34]

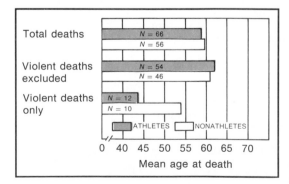

FIG. 29-5. *Age at death of athletes and nonathletes. None of the differences between the groups are statistically significant. (From Montoye, J.H. et al.: The Longevity and Morbidity of College Athletes. Indianapolis, Ind., Phi Epsilon Kappa, 1957.)*

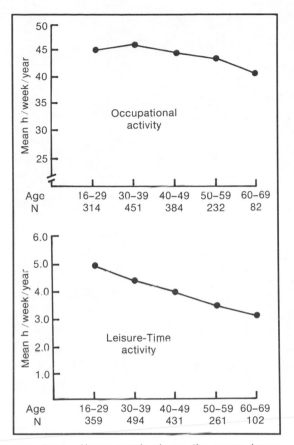

FIG. 29-6. *Upper graph shows the mean hours worked in occupational activity; the lower graph shows the hours per week per year spent in leisure-time activities. Both are drawn as a function of age (N represents the number of people studied).(From Montoye, H.J.: Physical Activity and Health: An Epidemiologic Study on an Entire Community. Englewood Cliffs, Prentice-Hall, Inc., N. J., © 1975, p. 20. Adapted by permission of Prentice-Hall, Inc., Englewood Cliffs, New Jersey.)*

The reasons why people become less active as they get older are complex and require further study. Several approaches, however, can be followed to help alleviate the trend toward sedentary living observed in adulthood. For one thing, children and adults of all ages should be taught active recreational and sport skills that can be *maintained* throughout life. Opportunities must also be provided for the present "senior citizens" to retain and maintain active life-styles. Increasing one's opportunity for exercise and physical activity will reap positive social, psychologic, and physical benefits throughout life.

CORONARY HEART DISEASE

Coronary heart disease (CHD) generally involves degenerative changes in the intima or inner lining of the larger arteries that supply the heart muscle. These vessels become congested with either lipid-filled plaques or fibrous scar tissue or both. This change progressively reduces the capacity for blood flow and causes the myocardium to become *ischemic*—that is, poorly supplied with oxygen due to reduced blood flow. Figure 29-7 shows the progressive occlusion of an arterial wall with a buildup of calcified fatty substances in the process of *atherosclerosis*. In this degenerative process, the roughened, hardened lining of the coronary artery frequently causes the slowly flowing blood to clot. This blood clot or *thrombus* may plug one of the smaller coronary vessels. In such cases, a portion of the heart muscle dies and the person is said to have suffered a heart attack or *myocardial infarction*. If the blockage is not too severe but blood flow is still reduced below the heart's requirement, the person may experience temporary chest pains termed *angina pectoris*. These pains are usually felt during exertion, because this causes the greatest demand for myocardial blood flow. Such anginal attacks provide painful and dramatic evidence of the importance of adequate oxygen supply to this vital organ.

CHD has reached epidemic proportions throughout the United States and most technologically advanced societies. Beginning at age 30 for men and age 40 for women, CHD is the single largest cause of death in the Western world. For example, about twice as many people die from CHD as from cancer. As depicted in Figure 29-8, after age 35 in males and 45 in females, the chance of dying from CHD increases progressively and dramatically. Between ages 55 and 65, about 13 of every 100 men and about 6 of every 100 women die from coronary artery disease.

Almost all people show some evidence of coronary artery disease, and it can be severe in seemingly healthy young adults. Actually, the disease probably starts early in life, because fatty streaks are common in the coronary arteries of children by the age of 5 years. There seems to be little harm, however, unless there is marked narrowing of the arteries. *At rest, blood supply to the heart becomes deficient only when obstruction of the coronary vessels*

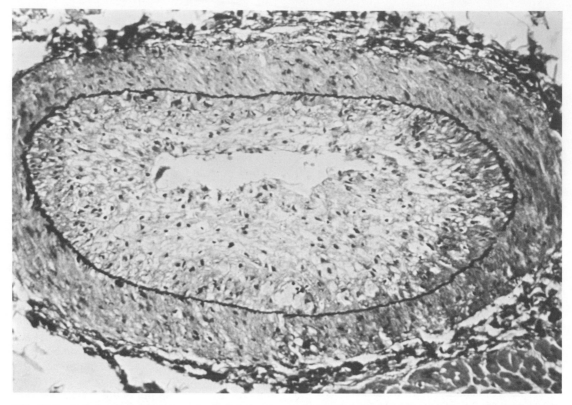

FIG. 29-7. *Deterioration of a normal artery is seen as atherosclerosis develops and begins depositing fatty substances, roughening the center. The clot then forms and plugs the artery, depriving the heart muscle of vital blood. The result is a heart attack.*

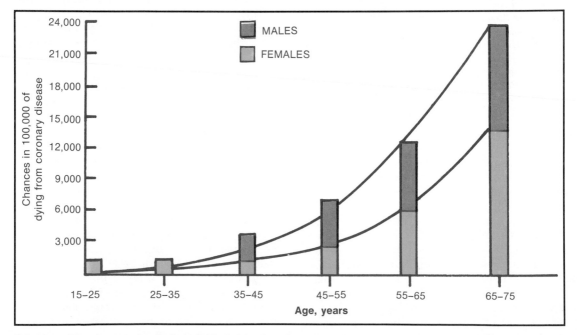

FIG. 29-8. *The chance of a single individual dying from coronary atherosclerosis. (Data from the American Heart Association.)*

reaches 80%. In fact, at least 50% to 70% occlusion must take place before the disease can be clinically detected. Generally, death occurs from CHD when there is advanced obstruction in several major vessels supplying the myocardium.

The mechanism by which fatty-type deposits or plaques develop is poorly understood. Many feel this lumpy thickening of the arterial wall begins as a fatty streak on the vessel's inner lining. It is often argued that this process is in some way mediated by consuming a diet high in cholesterol and saturated fats. The deposition of fatty material eventually leads to calcification and fibrotic changes so that the arterial walls become narrower, rigid, and hard, making blood flow more difficult. It has also been suggested that changes in cellular characteristics of the vessel's smooth muscle wall initiate the athersclerotic process. These changes cause cellular mutation of smooth muscle cells and proceed in a manner similar to the development of a benign tumor. This abnormal cell division may be triggered by environmental factors such as diet, cigarette smoking, and high blood pressure. The proliferating cells ultimately lead to the characteristic changes in the vascular wall associated with fatty accumulation and plaque formation.[5a]

Coronary Heart Disease
Risk Factors

Significant information has been provided as to the natural history and dynamics of heart disease. Various personal characteristics and environmental factors have been identified over the past 30 years that appear to make individuals more susceptible to CHD. The following is a list of the more frequently implicated *CHD risk factors:* (1) age and sex; (2) elevated blood lipids; (3) hypertension; (4) cigarette smoking; (5) physical inactivity; (6) obesity; (7) diabetes mellitus; (8) diet; (9) heredity; (10) personality and behavior patterns; (11) high uric acid levels; (12) pulmonary function abnormalities; (13) race; (14) electrocardiographic abnormalities during rest and exercise; and (15) tension and stress.

It is difficult to determine quantitatively the importance of a single CHD risk factor in comparison to any other because many of the factors are interrelated. For example, blood lipid abnormalities, diabetes, heredity, and obesity often go hand-in-hand. One research study reported that men living in Ireland consumed more saturated fat than their blood brothers who lived in the United States, yet the former had a much lower incidence of CHD.[31] This protection was attributed to higher physical activity levels for those living in Ireland. Similar findings of high saturated fat intake, high physical activity, and low incidence of CHD have been reported for Masai tribesmen of East Africa[19] and farm laborers in Georgia.[20] Compounding such observations is the often observed finding that physical training generally lowers body weight and body fat. Also, certain groups are generally exposed to less psychologic stress because of the nature of their occupation or cultural setting.

In the following sections, we discuss blood lipid abnormalities, obesity, cigarette smoking, and physical inactivity as potent CHD risk factors. Hypertension, another important risk factor, was discussed in Chapter 15. These factors were chosen because they have received the greatest public attention. All (with perhaps the exception of obesity) are powerful and consistent predictors in assessing one's chances for developing heart disease. It must be noted, however, that although these factors are closely associated with CHD, the associations do not necessarily infer causality. It still remains to be shown that risk factor modification offers effective protection from the disease. Until definite proof is demonstrated, however, logic causes us to assume that elimination or reduction of one or more risk factors will cause a corresponding decrease in the probability of contracting CHD.

BLOOD LIPID ABNORMALITIES. An increased fat (lipid) level in the blood is termed *hyperlipidemia.* Cholesterol and triglycerides are the two most common lipids associated with this CHD risk. These fats do not circulate freely in the blood plasma, but rather are transported in combination with a carrier protein to form a *lipoprotein.* Table 29-1 lists the four different lipoproteins, their approximate density, and percent composition in the blood. Serum cholesterol represents the total cholesterol contained in the different lipoproteins. Although it is proper to refer to hyperlipidemia, it is more meaningful to evaluate and discuss the different types of *hyperlipoproteinemia.*

The precise mechanism by which elevated blood lipids affect the development of CHD is almost totally unknown. Nevertheless, the over-

TABLE 29-1. *Approximate composition of lipoproteins in the blood*

	CHYLOMICRONS	VERY LOW DENSITY LIPOPROTEINS (VLDL: PREBETA)	LOW-DENSITY LIPOPROTEINS (LDL: BETA)	HIGH-DENSITY LIPOPROTEINS (HDL: ALPHA)
Density	0.95	0.95–1.006	1.006–1.019	1.063–1.210
Protein (%)	0.5–1.0	5–15	25	45–55
Lipid (%)	99	95	75	50
Cholesterol (%)	2–5	10–20	40–45	18
Triglyceride (%)	85	50–70	5–10	2
Phospholipid (%)	3–6	10–20	20–25	30

whelming evidence seems to link high levels of blood lipids with increased incidence of CHD. In many cases, these elevated lipids are related to consuming diets high in saturated fats and cholesterol.

The distribution of cholesterol among the various *types* of lipoproteins may be a more powerful predictor of heart disease than simply the total *quantity* of plasma lipids. Specifically, a high level of high-density lipoproteins (HDL, which comprise the smallest portion of lipoproteins but contain the largest quantity of protein) is associated with a lower heart disease risk, whereas elevated levels of the low-density lipoproteins (LDL and VLDL) represent an increased risk. Although much controversy exists as to the precise role of lipoproteins in heart disease, it is generally believed that the LDL and VLDL are means for transporting fat throughout the body for delivery to the cells, including those of the smooth muscle walls of the arteries. Here it ultimately becomes involved in the artery-narrowing process of atherosclerosis. Whereas LDL is targeted for peripheral tissue, HDL may reflect the removal aspect of lipid dynamics by promoting the movement of cholesterol from peripheral tissues (including arterial walls) for transport to the liver where it is excreted through bile synthesis.[20b,30b] It is also possible that HDL may retard cholesterol buildup in cells by directly blocking their uptake of LDL. Research is currently progressing to clarify whether HDL is truly protective and what factors can raise them. It is encouraging from an exercise perspective that HDL levels are elevated in endurance athletes and may be favorably altered in sedentary people who engage in vigorous aerobic training.[11a,19a]

OBESITY. Although excess body fatness has received great notoriety as a CHD risk factor, existing evidence suggests only a modest relationship, or that the relation is codependent with such factors as hypertension, diabetes mellitus, and cigarette smoking.[18] Autopsy studies have *not* revealed a strong association between body fatness per se and the degree of atherosclerosis.[30,32] Similar findings using different methods to evaluate coronary function have also been reported.[8,17] Research indicates, however, that overfat individuals are often hypertensive and have elevated serum lipid levels. Weight loss and accompanying fat reduction generally normalize cholesterol and triglyceride levels and have a beneficial effect on blood pressure. Although being too fat may not be a primary CHD risk factor, its role as a secondary and contributing factor in heart disease cannot be denied.

CIGARETTE SMOKING. *Cigarette smoking may be one of the best predictors of CHD.* In fact, the probability of death from heart disease for smokers is almost twice as great as for nonsmokers. *The increase in death rate from heart disease among women in this country almost parallels their increased consumption of cigarettes.* Surprisingly, this CHD risk is associated with more deaths than the excess mortality of cigarette smokers due to lung cancer!

It is generally observed that the smoking risk acts independently of other risk factors. At the same time, however, if other risk factors are present, cigarette smoking accentuates their influence. If smoking is stopped, the risk of CHD generally returns to that of nonsmokers, although this may not always be the case.[10a]

PHYSICAL INACTIVITY. Information on the role of physical activity in protecting one from CHD is sometimes contradictory but generally encouraging. Aside from the fact that physically active people generally have fewer clinical symptoms of heart disease, when a heart attack does strike, their chances for survival are much greater than are those of their inactive counterparts.[10] These findings must be viewed with caution, however, for several reasons. For one thing, comparisons are often made between active and sedentary people with the assumption that other factors (blood lipids, hypertension, cigarette smoking, occupational status, body fatness) are essentially equal. This assumption is frequently not met. It is also possible that people with strong constitutions who are "destined" to live longer select active occupations or leisure-time pursuits. Likewise, as people detect certain symptoms of CHD, they move into a sedentary job or life-style. Thus, at the time of death, they are rated as being inactive. Equally important in research of this nature is the difficulty encountered in obtaining an objective and quantified statement of a person's activity level, both on the job and during leisure time. Activity classifications are generally subjective, broad, and leave much room for error.

It has been suggested that many of the conclusions concerning the singular beneficial effects of exercise "outrun" the facts.[17] Although the data on physical inactivity and CHD generally fall short of critical "proof," there is certainly *no* evidence that the prudent use of exercise is harmful. In fact, the major bulk of research on animals and humans indicates that regular exercise may operate against CHD in a variety of beneficial ways to:

1. *Improve myocardial circulation and metabolism,* which may protect the heart from hypoxic stress; this includes enhanced vascularization, as well as modest increases in cardiac glycogen stores and glycolytic capacity that could be beneficial when the heart's oxygen supply is compromised.
2. *Enhance the mechanical or contractile properties* of the myocardium; this may enable the conditioned heart to maintain or increase contractility during a specific challenge.
3. *Establish more favorable blood clotting* characteristics and other hemostatic mechanisms.
4. *Normalize the blood lipid profile.*

5. *Favorably alter heart rate* and blood pressure so that the work of the myocardium is significantly reduced at rest and during exercise.
6. *Achieve a more desirable body composition.*
7. *Establish a more favorable neural-hormonal balance* that may conserve oxygen for the myocardium.
8. *Provide a favorable outlet* for psychologic stress and tensions.

In light of these findings, most physicians and exercise specialists prescribe exercise as a preventive and rehabilitative health measure.

Risk Factors In Children

Several studies have documented multiple CHD risk factors in young children.[11,33] The prevalence of risk factors for active and apparently healthy boys and girls aged 7 to 12 years is shown in Table 29-2. Obesity and a family history of heart disease were the two most frequently occurring risk factors.[11] A relatively large percentage of children also showed abnormally high blood lipids. Of the total group, 65% had at least one or two risk factors whereas 31% had three or more! As is generally the case with adults, the association between body fatness and serum lipid levels becomes readily apparent with subjects classified as obese; the fattest children generally have the highest levels of cholesterol and triglycerides.

In view of the prevalence of CHD risk factors in some children, plus autopsy observations of young adults and children, it seems likely that heart disease has its origins in childhood. Whether risk factor identification in children is linked to premature heart disease remains to be shown. Equally important is the question of whether "risk intervention" in these children will improve their health outlook. Certainly, if regular physical activity can modify or at least stabilize the risk factor profile *and* if this protects against CHD, then all children should be encouraged and taught to pursue active lifestyles.

EXERCISE STRESS TESTING

Without doubt, vigorous aerobic exercise increases the functional capacity of the circulatory system. In addition, it is now generally ac-

TABLE 29-2. *Prevalence of CHD risk factors in boys and girls aged 7 to 12*[a]

RISK FACTOR	PREVALENCE		TOTAL	N	PERCENT IN TOTAL SAMPLE
	MALE	FEMALE			
Obesity (>20% body fat)	10	4	14	47	30
Low work capacity (<31 ml · kg^{-1} · min^{-1})	3	1	4	34	12
Elevated blood lipids					
Cholesterol (>200 mg%)	1	3	4	38	10
Triglycerides (>100 mg%)	4	3	7	38	18
Liproprotein classification					
Type II	1	1	2	38	5
Type IV	4	3	7	38	18
Family history of CHD	7	5	12	47	26

[a]From Gilliam, T. et al.: Prevalence of coronary heart disease risk factors in active children, 7 to 12 years of age. Med. Sci. Sports, *9:* 21, 1977. Copyright 1977, the American College of Sports Medicine. Reprinted by permission.

cepted that this type of exercise can serve important protective and rehabilitative functions in the battle against CHD. However, the potential therapeutic and fitness benefits of exercise should be viewed in perspective. For a sedentary person, for example, a sudden burst of strenuous exercise could place an inordinate strain on the cardiovascular system. This risk can be considerably reduced with proper medical evaluation, which should minimally include a thorough personal health and family history and physical examination. The physical examination should emphasize signs and symptoms of cardiovascular disease including blood pressure, resting 12-lead ECG, cardiac murmurs and dysrhythmias, edema, blood analysis, and chronic lung disease. For many people, an important part of the medical evaluation is the *exercise stress test.*

The term "stress test" is generally used to describe the systematic use of exercise for two main purposes: (1) for ECG observations and (2) to evaluate the adequacy of physiologic adjustments to metabolic demands that exceed the resting requirement. The test can be a single-stage test such as the *Master "2-step"* bench stepping test in which the work load remains constant throughout the exercise period. In recent years, however, multistage bicycle and treadmill tests have become increas-

ingly popular. These tests are *graded* in terms of physical work. They include several levels of 3 to 5 minutes of submaximal exercise and may often bring the person to a self-imposed fatigue level called the *maximum physical working capacity* or *PWC max.* The submaximal work levels allow work to be increased in small increments until ischemic manifestations such as anginal pain or ST-segment deviations make their appearance. This provides for a more precise manipulation of work load and gives a reliable and quantitative index of the person's functional impairment if heart disease is detected. This enhances the accuracy of diagnosis and subsequent exercise prescription. For most screening purposes, the test need not be maximal, but it is desirable to bring a person to at least 85% of the age-predicted maximal heart rate.

A resting electrocardiogram should precede the exercise test. The ECG establishes that the person can safely engage in graded exercise, and also provides the important baseline against which the exercise results can be compared. For diagnostic purposes, the stress test provides the means for obtaining important electrocardiographic information. The exercise ECG often picks up signs of subtle coronary disease including myocardial ischemia and cardiac rhythm disorders. Stress testing is limited, however, by its inability to show the extent and specific location of the disease. Also, 25% to 40% of the people with relatively advanced CHD demonstrate *false negative* readings in that a patient has a normal stress test but an abnormal coronary angiogram (see page 438).

For the person with documented cardiovascular disease, the exercise stress test provides an objective and reliable means to define the patient's limitations and capacity for physical activity and to evaluate specific therapy. This aspect of stress testing also provides the basis for prudent exercise prescription for healthy and coronary-prone adults as well as for patients with CHD. In fact, with proper clearance, it is not out of the question for individuals with documented CHD to train safely for *and* complete marathon runs![16]

Why Be Stress Tested?

There are at least six reasons to include stress testing in an overall CHD evaluation:

1. *To establish,* from ECG observations, a diagnosis of overt heart disease and also to screen for possible "silent" coronary disease in seemingly normal men and women. Approximately 30% of the people with confirmed coronary artery disease will have normal resting electrocardiograms. During relatively intense exercise, however, about 80% of these abnormalities will be uncovered.
2. *To reproduce and assess* exercise related chest symptoms. In many instances, individuals over the age of 40 suffer chest or related pain in the left shoulder or arm on physical exertion. Proper electrocardiographic analysis during an exercise stress test helps to identify myocardial abnormalities and provide a more precise diagnosis of exercise-induced pain.
3. *To screen candidates* for preventive and cardiac rehabilitative exercise programs. Stress test results can then be used to design an exercise program that is within the person's current functional capacity and health status with emphasis on intensity, frequency, duration, and type of exercise. Repeated testing aids in evaluating one's progress in the exercise intervention program as well as in determining the need for safe program modification.

4. *To detect* an abnormal blood pressure response. It is not uncommon to find individuals with a normal resting blood pressure who show higher than normal increases in systolic blood pressure with exercise. This exercise hypertension may signify developing cardiovascular complications.
5. *To monitor* responses to various therapeutic interventions (drug, surgical, dietary) designed to improve cardiovascular functioning. For example, the success of coronary bypass surgery can be detected by a patient's adjustment to exercise and his or her ability to successfully reach a target exercise heart rate without complications.
6. *To define* the functional aerobic capacity and evaluate its degree of deviation from normal standards.

Who Should Be Stress Tested?

Table 29-3 shows a classification system by age and health status for screening and supervisory procedures to be used in conjunction with an exercise stress test. The prudent rules are:

1.   *If a person is less than 35 years of age* and has no previous history of cardiovascular disease and no known primary risk factors (and has had a medical evaluation within the past 2 years), it is generally acceptable to begin an exercise program without special medical clearance. These people may also be stress tested for purposes of functional evaluation and for preparing the exercise prescription by a trained exercise specialist.

2.   *If a person is younger than 35 years of age* but has evidence of CHD or a significant combination of risk fators, he or she should be medically cleared prior to embarking on an exercise program. This should include a graded exercise test under the supervision of a physician.

3.   *For all adults above 35 years of age,* medical evaluation is advised prior to any major increase in exercise habits. This medical evaluation should include an ECG monitored before, during, and in recovery from a graded exercise test and supervised by a physician.

These standards conform to policies and practices of the American College of Sports Medicine and the American Medical Association.[1]

TABLE 29-3. *Classification by age and health status for men and women who require different screening and supervisory procedures prior to and during a stress test*

AGE	PATIENT HEALTH STATUS	EVALUATION AND REQUIRED MEDICAL CLEARANCE	12-LEAD RESTING ECG	PERSONNEL INVOLVED DURING STRESS TEST
<35	No known primary CHD risk factors;[a] may have secondary CHD risk factors[b]	During past 2 years, signed statement	Not required	No test required
35–40	No known primary CHD risk factors; may have secondary CHD risk factors	During past 2 years, signed statement	Required	Exercise technician; exercise physiologist; M.D. in area
>40	No known primary CHD risk factors; may have secondary CHD risk factors	During past 2 years, signed statement	Required	Exercise technician; exercise physiologist; M.D. in area
Any age	Documented CHD: hypertension; suspected CHD	During past 2 years, signed statement	Required	Exercise technician; exercise physiologist; M.D. conducting test

[a]Primary risk factors: Hypertension, hyperlipidemia, cigarette smoking.
[b]Secondary risk factors: Family history, obesity, physical inactivity, diabetes mellitus, hyperglycemia.

Exercise-Induced Indicators of CHD

Several clues to CHD become especially apparent during exercise, for this creates the greatest demand on coronary blood flow.

ANGINA PECTORIS. Approximately 30% of the initial manifestations of CHD take the form of chest-related pain called angina pectoris. This is a temporary but painful condition that indicates that coronary blood flow (oxygen supply) has momentarily reached a critically low level. This *myocardial ischemia* (usually the result of restricted coronary circulation brought about by coronary atherosclerosis) stimulates sensory nerves in the walls of the coronary arteries and myocardium itself. The resulting pain or discomfort is generally felt in the upper chest region, although it is frequently characterized by a sensation of pressure or constriction in the left shoulder, neck, jaw, or left arm. Many people also report sensations of "being smothered" during an angina episode. In addition to pain, cardiac performance is also impaired with angina. This depressed myocardial function is accompanied by reduced cardiac output, reduced stroke volume, and generally impaired contractility of the left ventricle. After a few minutes of rest, the pain usually subsides with no permanent damage being done to the heart muscle.

ELECTROCARDIOGRAPHIC DISORDERS. Alterations in the heart's normal pattern of electric activity are often indicative of insufficient oxygen supply to the myocardium. However, these electric "clues" are rarely observed until the metabolic (and blood flow) requirements are increased above the resting level. In some instances, oxygen insufficiency causes the T wave of the ECG to invert. The most important electrocardiographic indication of coronary insufficiency is horizontal *ST-segment depression*. This is shown in Figure 29-9 in relation to the ST segment of a normal electrocardiogram.

Although it is not known why the ST segment becomes depressed, this deviation from normal is closely correlated with other indicators of CHD including coronary artery narrowing as measured by coronary *angiography* and *radioisotope scintigraphy*. Angiography is generally considered the most sensitive reference of CHD. With this technique, an opaque fluid is cast into the coronary circulation so that a series of roentgenographic pictures can be taken of the vessels. *This provides for a relatively precise determination of the location and degree of occlusion in the coronary arteries.* The newer scintigraphic technique uses radio nuclides (usually containing radioactive potassium, particularly thallium-201) that are distributed throughout the heart muscle in proportion to regional myocardial blood flow. The scintillation camera thus gives an image of myocardial perfusion.

Those individuals with significant ST-segment depression usually have severe and extensive obstruction of the coronary arteries. This generally involves a reduction of more than 70% of the normal opening of one or more coronary vessels. In addition, the amount of ST-segment depression is directly related to the chances of dying from CHD. In one study, persons with 1- to 2-mm ST-segment depression during exercise had a 4.6-fold increase in mortality, whereas those with more than 2-mm depression had a 19.1-fold greater chance of dying.[26]

CARDIAC RHYTHM ABNORMALITIES. Although exercise can bring out abnormalities in the ST segment of the electrocardiogram, it also provides an effective way to observe both normal and abnormal cardiac rhythm. One significant alteration in cardiac rhythm (*arrhythmia*) with exercise is the occurrence of *premature ventricular contractions* or *PVCs*. In this situation, the ventricles demonstrate disorganized electric activity. They are not stimulated by the normal passage of the wave of depolarization through the atrioventricular node. Rather, portions of the ventricle become spontaneously depolarized. This shows up on the electrocardiogram as an "extra ventricular beat" or QRS complex that occurs without being preceded by a P wave that indicates atrial depolarization.

PVCs in exercise generally herald the presence of severe ischemic atherosclerotic heart disease, often involving two or three major cor-

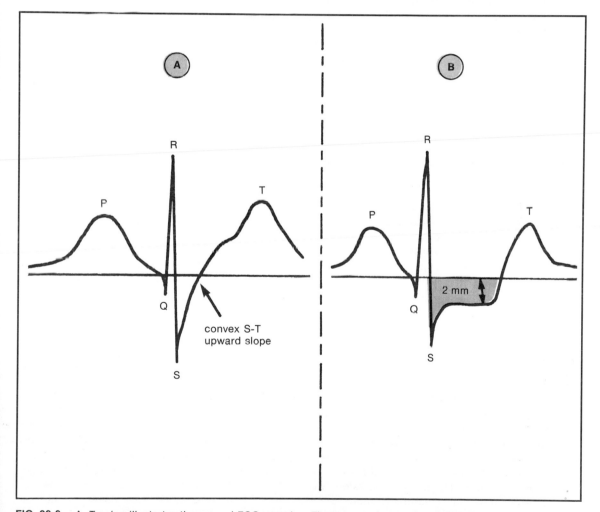

FIG. 29-9. A, *Tracing illustrates the normal ECG complex. The arrow points to the slightly convex and upward-sloping ST-segment.* B, *Tracing shows an abnormal horizontal ST-segment depression (shaded area) of 2 mm measured from a stable baseline.*

onary vessels. In fact, this specific electric instability of the myocardium has a greater predictive value than ST-segment depression for the diagnosis of CHD. The incidence of sudden death due to *ventricular fibrillation* is generally about six to ten times as high in a group with frequent PVCs as in heart disease patients without this abnormality. With fibrillation, the ventricles are unable to contract in a unified manner. As a result, blood is not effectively pumped and cardiac output falls dramatically.

OTHER INDICES OF CHD. Two useful nonelectrocardiographic indices of possible CHD are the blood pressure and heart rate responses to exercise. During a graded exercise test, there is a normal, progressive increase in systolic blood pressure from about 120 mm Hg to 160 to 190 mm Hg at peak exercise. The change in diastolic pressure is generally less than 10 mm Hg. For some individuals, however, strenuous exercise may cause the systolic blood pressure to rise well above 200 mm Hg, whereas the diastolic pressure can increase to 100 to 150 mm Hg. This abnormal hypertensive response can be a significant clue to cardiovascular disease.

The inability of blood pressure to increase with exercise can also reflect cardiovascular malfunction. For example, failure of the systolic blood pressure to increase by at least 20 or 30 mm Hg during graded exercise may reflect diminished cardiac reserve. Rapid, large increase in heart rate (tachycardia) early in exercise is often a harbinger of cardiac problems. Likewise, abnormally low exercise heart rates may reflect unhealthy function of the heart's sinus node. Also, the inability of the heart rate to increase during exercise, especially when accompanied by extreme fatigue, may be indicative of cardiac strain and heart disease.

Multilevel Graded Exercise Test Versus Single-Level Test

The exercise electrocardiogram often picks up signs of subtle CHD, especially myocardial ischemia and cardiac rhythm disorders. A multistage exercise test with progressively increasing work loads is generally more effective than a single work bout (such as the Master Two-Step test) for revealing latent ischemic heart disease. In establishing a diagnosis of CHD, the graded exercise test should include at least several 3- to 5-minute levels of submaximal exercise with the option of bringing the person to a self-imposed maximum work level.

With small increments of exercise, the precise physiologic correlates (heart rate, blood pressure, oxygen consumption, and work level) of the ischemic manifestations of anginal pain, ECG abnormalities, or dysrhythmias can be identified and interpreted. This multilevel approach to stress testing enhances the accuracy of diagnosis and is most desirable in determining a person's functional capacity or degree of improvement. To improve confidence in a negative diagnosis for CHD via stress testing, it is desirable to bring the person to at least 85% of the age-predicted maximum heart rate. Also, the progressive picture of the aerobic and cardiovascular adjustment to graded work provides the important basis for formulating the exercise prescription.

Is Stress Testing Safe?

For men who show clinical evidence of heart disease, the yearly death rate is 2% to 12%. This broad variation in expected mortality is directly related to the number and severity of diseased coronary arteries. In general, however, if a person has had a previous myocardial infarction or episode of angina, the risk of having another episode or dying is increased 10 to 30 times above normal. This raises some question as to the advisability of stress testing adults, especially patients who have had myocardial infarctions or who have demonstrated other heart disease symptoms or significant risk profiles.

One research group reported that in about 170,000 submaximum and maximum stress tests only 16 high-risk but apparently healthy patients suffered coronary episodes during testing.[27] This represented about one person per 10,000 or about 0.01% of the total group. Other researchers determined that the risk of having a coronary episode for apparently healthy middle-aged adults was 1 in 3000 during a *maximum* stress test.[20a] This amounts to a risk that is 6 to 12 times normal for most middle-aged adults. For patients with documented heart disease, the risk in stress testing may increase to as much as 30 to 60 times normal. In fact, in one study, five cases of cardiac arrest were reported following exercise in men with prior myocardial infarctions or angina pectoris.[13]

If patients with documented CHD were excluded from stress testing, it is estimated that this testing would cause about one fatality every 10 to 20 years in a population of 5 million.[29] Despite these rather comforting statistics, there are instances where stress testing should *not* be undertaken. Patients with recent myocardial infarctions (4 to 6 weeks) should not be stress tested, although some cardiologists show evidence that symptom-limited stress testing is safe for patients without evidence of congestive heart failure as soon as 3 weeks after a myocardial infarction.[8a] Patients with cardiac infections such as myocarditis or pericarditis or those with signs of unstable angina, heart block, congestive heart failure, or extreme arterial hypertension (systolic blood pressure > 200 mm Hg, diastolic pressure > 110 mm Hg) should not undergo an exercise stress test because the risks encountered by such exercise are generally not outweighed by the potential benefits.

Guidelines for Stress Testing

The following guidelines should be used for stopping a stress test. Each of these symptoms generally indicates extreme cardiovascular strain that could be dangerous to the patient being exercised.

1. *Repeated presence* of premature ventricular contraction (PVCs)
2. *Progressive* angina pain
3. *Presence* of ST-segment depression of 2.0 mm or more
4. *An extremely rapid increase* in heart rate that may reflect a severely compromised cardiovascular response
5. *Failure* of heart rate or blood pressure to increase with progressive exercise or *progressive drop* in systolic blood pressure with increasing work load
6. *An increase* in diastolic pressure of 20 mm Hg or more, or a rise above 110 mm Hg
7. *Headache,* blurred vision, pale, clammy skin, faintness, or extreme breathlessness

Persons exhibiting these responses require further medical evaluation and should be excluded from unsupervised exercise programs pending such study. Those patients who complete the stress test without significant ECG responses or other evidence of CHD can be medically cleared for unsupervised exercise that does not exceed the intensity of exercise reached during the test.

Exercise Prescription

Prior to starting an exercise program, it is generally advisable for adults to obtain *medical clearance.* Although this term is frequently used loosely, specific evaluations must be made of the prospective exerciser. Minimally, these include a thorough personal health and family history and physical examination. This in itself, however, is a crude assessment. Young adults with significant CHD risk profiles and older adults above age 35 to 40 years are also urged to obtain an electrocardiogram, preferably one administered during graded exercise. The person who has suffered a coronary infarction *must* be medically cleared and should be at least 2 months postinfarction before starting a training program.

Heart rate and oxygen uptake data also obtained during the stress test are used to formulate the exercise prescription; this is an individualized exercise program based on the person's current fitness and health status, with emphasis on intensity, frequency, duration, and type of exercise. This is important because many people who start exercising do not recognize their limitations and may exercise above a safe level. Even group exercise programs that require medical clearance are limited in that all members exercise at about the same work level (walk, jog, or swim at the same speed) with little attention paid to individual differences.

IMPROVEMENTS IN CHD PATIENTS. Many cardiac patients can expect to improve their functional capacity to a degree comparable to a healthy person of the same age. In some instances, even clinical symptoms such as ECG abnormalities are improved or even eliminated. This is related to the fact that many individuals respond to exercise training with physiologic adjustments that actually *reduce* the work of the heart at any given external work load. For example, reduced exercise heart rate and blood pressure (two major determinants of myocardial oxygen consumption) and improved myocardial contractility reduce myocardial effort. This delays the onset of anginal pain allowing work of greater intensity and duration. This seems to be a primary benefit for anginal patients, because the threshold at which pain develops is generally at the same level of heart rate and systolic pressure before and after training. For individuals whose occupations predominantly require arm work, this musculature should be exercised in training, because many of the benefits of physical conditioning are highly specific and generally not transferable from one muscle group to another.

THE PROGRAM. Exercise programs for preventive purposes as well as for rehabilitation are most effective when they are individualized. The exercises prescribed usually consist of a slow but steady program of general movements that stimulate cardiovascular improvement, such as walking, jogging, running, cycling, rope skipping, swimming, or rhythmic calisthenics. However, any other endurance-type sport activity that the person enjoys will be equally effective in the long run.

The guidelines for making decisions concerning frequency, duration, and intensity of training were discussed in Chapter 20. *For physical conditioning of adult groups, exercise should generally be performed at least three times a week for 20 to 40 minutes each exercise session.* Longer and more frequent exercise will reap greater benefits, but the relatively small extra improvement may not be worth the time invested. Big muscle endurance activities should be performed at 60% to 80% of the person's working capacity or oxygen intake capacity as measured on the stress test. This "target zone" will put the person above the threshold level for a training effect, yet ensure that he or she is not unduly stressed by the training program. Ideally, the personalized exercise prescription should include a recommendation for weight loss and dietary modification (if necessary), as well as warm-up and cool-down exercises and a developmental strength program. Some heart disease patients show a reduced heart rate response to exercise with a corresponding reduction in maximum heart rate.[25a] For these individuals, the use of target heart rates based on and age-predicted maximum will grossly overestimate the appropriate training intensity. These observations argue for exercise testing each patient to a symptom-limited maximum and then formulating the exercise prescription based on the actual heart rate data.

In certain instances, exercise reconditioning should be conducted under the supervision of a qualified physician. Adults in this category include postmyocardial infarction and coronary bypass patients as well as those with documented angina pectoris and ECG abnormalities during graded exercise. This supervision does not necessarily mean direct eye contact with the physician. However, the exercise program should be based on an exercise prescription formulated from a stress test. Ideally, the program should be monitored by well-trained exercise specialists or other allied health personnel, and emergency resuscitation equipment should be readily available.

PRACTICAL ILLUSTRATION. Figure 29-10 shows the oxygen uptake–heart rate relationship for a 65-year-old man who performed graded exercise on a bicycle ergometer. The man was able to exercise for 12 minutes with 3-minute work increments. His maximum heart rate was 146 beats per minute, which was 95% of his age-predicted maximum heart rate of 155 beats per minute; the peak $\dot{V}O_2$ on the test was 24.6 ml $\cdot$ kg^{-1} $\cdot$ min^{-1} (2.13 liters $\cdot$ min^{-1}).

Eighty percent of this subject's peak $\dot{V}O_2$ is about 19 ml $\cdot$ kg^{-1} $\cdot$ min^{-1}, whereas 60% is equivalent to 14 ml $\cdot$ kg^{-1} $\cdot$ min^{-1}. The shaded area in Figure 29-10 corresponds to the appropriate exercise heart rates that constitute his specific "training-sensitive zone" (Chap. 20, p. 275). Because oxygen consumption is not easily measured in training, the exercise heart rate provides a convenient and valid substitute by which to establish an appropriate training intensity. As noted in the exercise stress test data, any exercise heart rate between 111 and 126 beats per minute will place this man in the appropriate training zone. He can exercise in relative comfort and safety. By maintaining a fairly stable training heart rate, the work of the heart stays essentially constant from workout to workout. For these reasons, the exercise heart rate is generally used in writing the exercise prescription because it is a highly individualized tool for estimating and regulating the severity of exercise.

Table 29-4 illustrates a 10-week exercise prescription for the man whose data appear in Figure 29-10. After the second week, the approximate energy output levels that are within the training sensitive zone range from 14 to 20 ml $\cdot$ kg^{-1} $\cdot$ min^{-1}; this is equivalent to 4.0 to 5.8 METs. (A MET is a unit of resting energy metabolism equivalent to an oxygen consumption of about 3.5 ml $\cdot$ kg^{-1} $\cdot$ min^{-1}). After about 3

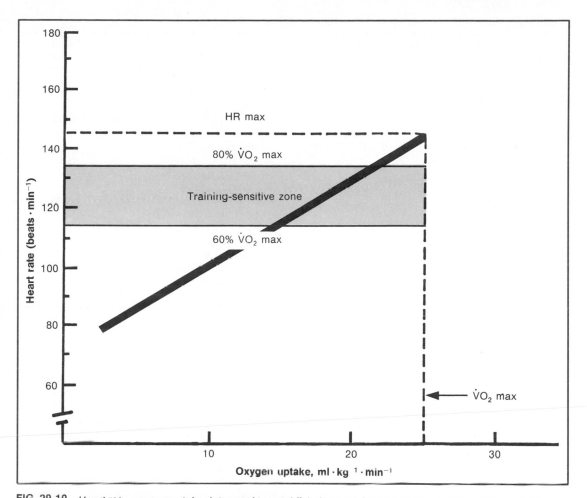

FIG. 29-10. *Heart rate-oxygen uptake data used to establish the "training sensitive zone" for a 65-year-old man. The blue area represents the appropriate exercise heart rate zone to bring about aerobic fitness improvements. The solid line represents the HR $\dot{V}O_2$ line from the bicycle test.*

months on the reconditioning program, the stress test is repeated. This provides an objective means for evaluating the patient's progress and making appropriate adjustments in the training program.

SUMMARY

1. Physiologic and performance capability generally declines after about 30 years of age. The rates of decline in the various functions differ, however, and are significantly influenced by many factors, including level of physical activity. It appears that regular physical training enables older persons to retain higher levels of functional capacity, especially cardiovascular function.

2. Regardless of age, regular vigorous physical activity produces measurable physiologic improvements. The magnitude of these improvements depends on many factors including initial fitness status, age, and type and amount of training.

3. Participation in vigorous activity early in life probably contributes little to increased longevity or health in later life. It is likely, however, that an active life-style *throughout life* provides significant health benefits.

4. Coronary heart disease (CHD) is the single largest cause of death in the Western world. The pathogenesis of this disease involves degenerative changes in the inner lining of the arterial wall resulting in progressive occlusion. The mechanism for the development of coronary atherosclerosis is poorly understood.

5. Numerous factors have been identified

TABLE 29-4._Example of a personalized aerobic exercise prescription_

WEEK	ESTIMATED $\dot{V}O_2$ (ml·kg⁻¹·min⁻¹)	PERCENT PEAK $\dot{V}O_2$	MET LEVEL	EXERCISE LEVEL	DURATION (MIN)	DISTANCE (MILES)
1	12.3	50	3.5	Walk at 3 mph (20 min per mile)	12	0.6
2	13.0	54	3.7	Walk at 3 mph	15	0.75
3	14.0	58	4.0	Walk at 4 mph (15 min per mile)	20	1.3
4	15.0	62	4.3	Walk–jog at 4.3 mph (14 min per mile)	20	1.4
5	16.0	66	4.6	Walk–jog at 4.5 mph (13 min: 20 s per mile)	20	1.5
6	17.0	70	4.9	Walk–jog at 4.7 mph (12 min: 40 s per mile)	20	1.6
7	18.0	74	5.1	Walk–jog at 5 mph (12 min per mile)	20	1.7
8	19.0	78	5.4	Walk–jog at 5 mph	25	2.1
9	19.0	78	5.4	Walk–jog at 5.5 mph (11 min per mile)	25	2.3
10	20.0	82	5.8	Walk–jog 5.5 mph	30	2.7

that make individuals more susceptible to developing CHD. The major risk factors are age and sex, elevated blood lipids, hypertension, cigarette smoking, obesity, physical inactivity, diet, heredity, and ECG abnormalities during rest and exercise.

6. Many CHD risk factors can be modified by proper nutrition, exercise, and weight control programs. It is generally assumed that this "risk intervention" improves an individual's health outlook.

7. Stress testing provides the means to evaluate objectively physiologic capacity and observe heart function during exercise. This is important because the stress test often picks up subtle signs of coronary artery disease that would normally remain undetected under resting conditions. These CHD indicators include angina pectoris, cardiac rhythm disorders, ECG abnormalities, and an abnormal blood pressure response.

8. Stress testing is relatively safe provided that appropriate guidelines are followed. Results from graded exercise tests provide valuable information for clearing individuals to begin exercising and also for individualizing the exercise prescription.

9. Many cardiac patients can improve their functional capacity to the same extent as a healthy person of the same age.

References

1. American College of Sports Medicine: Guidelines for Exercise Stress Testing. Lea & Febiger, Philadelphia, 1975.
2. Andersen, W.G.: Further studies on the longevity of Yale athletes. Med. Times, *44:*75, 1916.
3. Baley, J.A.: Recreation and the aging process. Res. Quart. *26:*1, 1955.
4. Barrett, J.H.: Gerontological Psychology, Springfield, Ill., Charles C Thomas, 1972.
5. Behnke, A., and Wilmore, J.: Evaluation and Regulation of Body Build and Composition. Englewood Cliffs, N.J., Prentice-Hall, 1974.
5a. Benditt, E.P.: The origin of atherosclerosis. Sci. Am., Feb., 74, 1977.
6. Chien, S. et al.: Longitudinal measurements of blood volume and essential body mass in human subjects. J. Appl. Physiol. *39:*818, 1975.
7. Clarke, D.H.: Adaptations in strength and muscular endurance resulting from exercise. *In* Exercise and Sport Science Reviews, Edited by J. Wilmore. New York, Academic Press, 1973.
7a. Clarkson, P.M.: The effect of age and activity level on simple and choice fractionated response time. Eur. J. Appl. Physiol., *40:*17, 1978.
7b. Clarkson, P.M.: The relationship of age and level of physical activity with the fractionated components of patellar reflex time. J. Gerontol., *33:*650, 1978.
8. Cramer, K. et al.: Coronary angiographic findings in correlation with age, body weight, blood pressure, serum lipids and smoking habits. Circulation, *33:*888, 1966.
8a. Davidson, D.M., and DeBusk, R.E.: Prognostic value of a single exercise test 3 weeks after uncomplicated myocardial infarction. Circulation *61:*236, 1980.
9. DeVries, H.A.: Physiological effects of an exercise training regimen upon men aged 52-88. J. Gerontol., *25:*325, 1970.
10. Frank, C.W. et al.: Physical inactivity as a lethal factor in myocardial infarction among men. Circulation, *34:*1022, 1966.
10a. Friedman, G.D., and Siegelaub, M.S.: Changes after quitting cigarette smoking. Circulation, *61:*716, 1980.
11. Gilliam, T. et al.: Prevalence of coronary heart disease risk factors in active children, 7-12 years of age. Med. Sci. Sports, *9:*21, 1977.
11a. Hartung, G.H. et al.: Relation of diet to HDL cholesterol in middle-aged marathon runners, joggers, and inactive men. N. Engl. J. Med., *302:*357, 1980
12. Hill, A.B.: Cricket and its relation to the duration of life. Lancet 2:949, 1927.
13. Irving, J.D., and Bruce, R.A.: Exertional hypotension and postexertional ventricular fibrillation in stress testing. Am. J. Cardiol., *39:*849, 1977.
14. Karvonen, M.J.: Age and performance in athletes. Arbeitsphysiologie, *16:*110, 1955.
15. Kasch, F.W.: The effects of exercise on the aging process. Physician Sportsmed. *4:*64, 1976.
16. Kavanagh, T. et al.: Marathon running after myocardial infarction. J.A.M.A. *229:*1602, 1974.
17. Keys, A.: Physical activity and the epidemiology of CHD. *In* Physical Activity and Aging. Medicine and Sport. Edited by D. Brunner. Baltimore, University Park Press, 1970.
18. Keys, A.: Coronary heart disease: The global picture. Atherosclerosis, *22:*149, 1975.
18a. Kroll, W., and Clarkson, P.M.: Age, isometric knee extension strength, and fractionated resisted response time. Exp. Aging Res., *4:*389, 1978.
19. Mann, G.V. et al.: Physical fitness and immunity to heart disease in Masai. Lancet 2:1308, 1965.
19a. Martin, R.P. et al.: Blood chemistry and lipid profiles of elite distance runners. Ann. N.Y. Acad. Sci., *301:*346, 1977.

20. McDonough, J.R. et al.: Coronary heart disease among Negroes and Whites in Evans County Georgia. J. Chronic Dis., *18:*443, 1965.

20a. McDonough, J.R., and Bruce, R.A.: Maximal exercise testing in assessing cardio-vascular function. J.S.C. Med. Assoc., *65:*26, 1969.

20b. Miller, A.J., and Miller, N.E.: Plasma high-density lipoprotein concentration and development of ischemic heart disease. Lancet, *1:*16, 1975.

21. Montoye, H.J. et al.: The Longevity and Morbidity of College Athletes. Indianapolis, Phi Epsilon Kappa, 1957.

22. Montoye, H.J.: Physical Activity and Health: An Epidemiologic Study of an Entire Community. Englewood Cliffs, N.J., Prentice-Hall, 1975.

22a. Montoye, H.J., and Lamphiear, D.E. Grip and arm strength in males and females, age 10 to 69. Res. Q., *48:*109, 1977.

23. Morris, J.N. et al: Incidence and prediction of ischaemic heart-disease in London busmen. Lancet 2:553, 1966.

24. Parizkova, J.: Body composition and exercise during growth and development. *In* Physical Activity: Human Growth and Development. Edited by G.L. Rarick. New York, Academic Press, 1974.

24a. Pariskova, J. et al.: Body composition, aerobic capacity and density of muscle capillaries in young and old men. J. Appl. Physiol., *31:*323, 1971.

25. Pollock, M.L. et al.: Effects of walking on body composition and cardiovascular function of middle-aged men. J. Appl. Physiol., *30:*126, 1971.

25a. Powles, A.C.P. et al.: Reduced heart rate response to exercise in ischemic heart disease: The fallacy of the target heart rate in exercise testing. Med. Sci. Sports, *11:*227, 1979.

26. Robb, G.P., and Marks, H.H.: Latent coronary artery disease determination, its presence and severity by the exercise electrocardiogram. Am. J. Cardiol., *13:*603, 1964.

27. Rochmis, P., and Blackburn, H.: Exercise tests. A survey of procedures, safety and litigation experience in approximately 170,000 tests. J.A.M.A., *217:*1060, 1971.

28. Saltin, B. et al.: Physical training in sedentary middle-aged and older men. II. Oxygen uptake, heart rate, and blood lactate concentration at submaximal and maximal exercise. Scand. J. Clin. Lab. Invest., *24:*323, 1969.

29. Shephard, R.J.: Do risks of exercise justify costly caution? Physician Sportsmed., *5:*58, 1977.

29a. Shock, N.W.: Physical activity and the rate of aging. Can. Med. Assoc. J., *96:*836, 1967.

30. Spain, D.M. et al.: Weight, body type, and prevalence of atherosclerotic heart disease in males. Am. J. Med. Sci., *245:*63, 1963.

30a. Spirduso, W.W.: Reaction and movement time as a function of age and physical activity level. J. Gerontol., *30:*435, 1975.

30b. Toll, A. and Small, D.M.: Current concepts: Plasma high density lipoproteins. N. Engl. J. Med., *229:*1232, 1978.

31. Trulson, M.F. et al.: Comparisons of siblings in Boston and Ireland. J. Am. Diet. Assoc., *45:*225, 1964.

32. Wilkins, R.H. et al.: Autopsy studies in atherosclerosis. Part 3. Distribution and severity of atherosclerosis in the presence of obesity, hypertension, nephrosclerosis, and rheumatic heart disease. Circulation, *20:*527, 1959.

33. Wilmore, J.W., and McNamera, J.J.: Prevalence of coronary heart disease risk factors in boys 8 to 12 years of age. J. Ped., *84:*527, 1974.

34. Zborowski, M., and Eyde, L.: Aging and social participation. J. Gerontol., *17:*424, 1962.

Appendix A

The Metric System

Most measurements in science are expressed in terms of the metric system. This system uses units that are related to one another by some power of 10. The prefix "centi" means one-hundredth, "milli" means one-thousandth, whereas the prefix "kilo" is derived from a word that means one thousand. In the following sections, we show the relationship between metric units and English units of measurement that are relevant to the material presented in this book. Also presented are some common expressions of work, energy, and power.

Units of Length

METRIC UNIT	EQUIVALENT METRIC UNIT	EQUIVALENT ENGLISH UNIT
meter (m)	100 cm 1000 mm	39.37 in. (3.28 ft; 1.09 yd)
centimeter (cm)	0.01 m 10 mm	0.3937 in.
millimeter (mm)	0.001 m 0.1 cm	0.03937 in.

Units of Weight

METRIC UNIT	EQUIVALENT METRIC UNIT	EQUIVALENT ENGLISH UNIT
kilogram (kg)	1000 g 1,000,000 mg	35.3 oz (2.2046 lb)
gram (g)	0.001 kg 1000 mg	0.0353 oz
milligram (mg)	0.000001 kg 0.001 g	0.0000353 oz

Units of Volume

METRIC UNIT	EQUIVALENT METRIC UNIT	EQUIVALENT ENGLISH UNIT
liter (l)	1000 ml	1.057 qt
milliliter (ml) or cubic centimeter (cc)	0.001 l	0.001057 qt

Temperature

To convert a Fahrenheit temperature to centigrade:
$$°C = (°F - 32)/1.8$$

To convert a centigrade temperature to Fahrenheit:
$$°F = (1.8 \times °C) + 32$$

With the Fahrenheit scale, the freezing point of water is 32° F and the boiling point, 212° F. On the centigrade scale, the freezing point of water is 0° C and the boiling point is 100° C.

Units of Speed

MPH	$KM \cdot HR^{-1}$	$M \cdot S^{-1}$	MPH	$KM \cdot HR^{-1}$	$M \cdot S^{-1}$
1	1.6	0.47	11	17.7	5.17
2	3.2	0.94	12	19.3	5.64
3	4.8	1.41	13	20.9	6.11
4	6.4	1.88	14	22.5	6.58
5	8.0	2.35	15	24.1	7.05
6	9.6	2.82	16	25.8	7.52
7	11.2	3.29	17	27.4	7.99
8	12.8	3.76	18	29.0	8.46
9	14.4	4.23	19	30.6	8.93
10	16.0	4.70	20	32.2	9.40

Common Expressions of Work, Energy, and Power

WATTS
1 watt $= 0.73756$ ft-lb $\cdot s^{-1}$

1 watt $= 0.01433$ kcal $\cdot min^{-1}$

1 watt $= 1.341 \times 10^{-3}$ hp
        or 0.0013 hp

1 watt $= 6.12$ kg $\cdot min^{-1}$

KILOCALORIES (KCAL)
1 kcal $= 3086$ ft-lb

1 kcal $= 426.8$ kg

1 kcal $= 3087.4$ ft-lb

1 kcal $= 1.5593 \times 10^{-3}$ hp $\cdot h^{-1}$

FOOT-POUNDS (FT-LB)
1 ft-lb $= 3.2389 \times 10^{-3}$ kcal

1 ft-lb $= 0.13825$ kg

1 ft-lb $= 5.050 \times 10^{-3}$ hp $\cdot h^{-1}$

Appendix B*

Nutritive Value of Commonly Used Foods

Explanation of the Table

The foods have been arranged in alphabetical order. The weight of the food is given in grams (g) as well as in ounces (oz), followed by the approximate measure of the food and its description. The next columns present the caloric value of the food (kcal); the number of grams of protein, fat, and carbohydrates; and the number of milligrams of calcium, iron, ascorbic acid, thiamin, riboflavin, and vitamin-A activity expressed in international units (IU). Page 474 lists the caloric value of alcoholic beverages, and pages 474 to 477 list the caloric value of specialty items purchased at selected fast-food chain stores. The abbreviation *tr* indicates that only a trace of a food nutrient is present.

Equivalents by Weight

1 pound (16 ounces)	= 454 grams
1 ounce	= 28.4 grams
$3\frac{1}{2}$ ounces	= 100 grams

Equivalents by Volume

1 quart	= 4 cups
1 cup	= 8 fluid ounces
	= $\frac{1}{2}$ pint
	= 16 tablespoons
2 tablespoons	= 1 fluid ounce
1 tablespoon	= 3 teaspoons
1 pound regular margarine or butter	= 4 sticks
	= 2 cups
1 pound whipped butter or margarine	= 6 sticks
	= two 8-ounce containers

---

*Data from B. K. Watt and A. L. Merrill, *Composition of Foods—Raw, Processed and Prepared,* U.S. Department of Agriculture, Washington, D.C., 1963; *Nutritive Value of Foods,* Home and Garden Bulletin no. 72, rev, U.S. Department of Agriculture, Washington, D.C., 1971.

FOOD	WEIGHT		APPROXIMATE MEASURE AND DESCRIPTION	KCAL
	G	OZ		
Alcoholic beverages (*see* page 474)				
Apples, raw	150	5.3	1 apple, about 3 per lb.	70
Apple, baked	130	4.6	1 medium apple, 2½ in. dia.	120
Apple brown betty	115	4.0	½ cup	175
Apple juice (sweet cider)	124	4.3	½ cup, bottled or canned	60
Apple pie (*see* pies)				
Applesauce, canned sweetened	128	4.5	½ cup	115
Apricots, fresh raw (as purchased)	114	4.0	3 apricots, about 12 per lb.	55
Apricots, canned	130	4.6	½ cup or 4 medium halves, 2 tbsp. juice (syrup pack)	110
Apricots, dried, stewed	108	3.8	½ cup (scant) or 8 halves, 2 tbsp. juice, sweetened	135
Apricot nectar (peach and pear nectar have similar values)	125	4.4	½ cup	70
Asparagus, cooked, green	73	2.6	½ cup, 1½- to 2-in. lengths	15
Avocado, raw (as purchased)	142	5.0	½ avocado, 3⅛ in. dia., pitted and peeled	185
Bacon, broiled or fried	15	0.5	2 slices, cooked crisp (20 slices per lb., raw)	90
Bacon, Canadian, cooked	43	1.5	3 slices, cooked crisp	100
Bananas, raw (as purchased)	175	6.1	1 medium banana	100
Bavarian cream, orange	99	3.5	½ cup	210
Bean sprouts, mung, cooked	63	2.2	½ cup, drained	18
Beans, green snap, cooked	63	2.2	½ cup	15
Beans, dry, green lima, cooked	144	5.0	¾ cup	195
Beans, immature, green lima, cooked	85	2.8	½ cup	95
Beans, dry, red kidney, canned	191	6.7	¾ cup	173
Beans, dry, white, canned with tomato sauce, without pork	196	6.9	¾ cup	233
Beans, dry, white, canned with tomato sauce and pork	191	6.7	¾ cup	233
Beef, corned, canned	85	3.0	3 slices, 3 × 2 × ¼ i	185
Beef, corned hash, canned	85	3.0	½ cup (approx.)	155
Beef, dried or chipped	57	2.0	4 thin slices, 4 × 5 in.	115
Beef, hamburger, broiled	85	3.0	1 patty, 3 in. dia. (regular ground beef)	245
Beef, heart, braised	85	3.0	2 round slices, 2½ in. dia., ½ in. thick	160

PROTEIN G	FAT G	CARBOHYDRATE G	CALCIUM MG	IRON MG	VITAMIN-A ACTIVITY IU	ASCORBIC ACID MG	THIAMIN MG	RIBOFLAVIN MG
tr	tr	18	8	0.4	50	3	0.04	0.02
tr	tr	30	8	0.4	50	3	0.04	0.02
2	4	34	21	0.7	115	2	0.07	0.05
tr	tr	15	8	0.8	—	1	0.01	0.03
tr	tr	31	5	0.7	50	2	0.03	0.02
1	tr	14	18	0.5	2890	10	0.03	0.04
1	tr	29	14	0.4	2255	5	0.03	0.03
2	tr	34	26	1.5	2287	3	tr	0.04
1	tr	19	12	0.3	1190	4	0.02	0.02
2	tr	3	15	0.5	655	19	0.12	0.13
3	19	7	11	0.7	315	15	0.12	0.22
5	8	1	2	0.5	0	—	0.08	0.05
18	12	tr	13	2.2	0	0	0.62	0.12
1	tr	26	10	0.8	230	12	0.06	0.07
2	10	30	27	0.1	627	54	0.10	0.05
2	tr	4	11	0.6	15	4	0.06	0.07
1	tr	4	32	0.4	340	0	0.05	0.06
12	1	37	41	4.2	—	—	0.19	0.08
7	1	17	40	2.2	240	15	0.16	0.09
11	1	32	56	3.5	8	—	0.10	0.08
12	1	45	133	3.9	120	4	0.14	0.07
12	5	37	104	3.5	248	4	0.15	0.06
22	10	0	17	3.7	20	—	0.01	0.20
7	10	9	11	1.7	—	—	0.01	0.08
19	4	0	11	2.9	—	—	0.04	0.18
21	17	0	9	2.7	30	—	0.07	0.18
27	5	1	5	5.0	20	1	0.21	1.04

FOOD	WEIGHT G	OZ	APPROXIMATE MEASURE AND DESCRIPTION	KCAL
Beef liver (*see* liver)				
Beef loaf				
(*see* meat loaf)				
Beef potpie, baked	227	7.9	1 pie, $4\frac{1}{4}$ in. dia.	560
Beef, pot roast, cooked	85	3.0	1 piece, $4 \times 3\frac{3}{4} \times \frac{1}{2}$ in.	245
Beef roast, oven-cooked	85	3.0	2 slices, $6 \times 3\frac{1}{4} \times \frac{1}{8}$ in., relatively lean	165
Beef steak, broiled	85	3.0	1 piece, $3\frac{1}{2} \times 2 \times \frac{3}{4}$ in., relatively fat, no bone	330
Beef stroganoff, cooked	130	4.6	$\frac{1}{2}$ cup	250
Beef tongue, braised	85	3.0	7 slices, $2\frac{1}{4} \times 2\frac{1}{4} \times \frac{1}{8}$ in.	210
Beets, cooked	85	3.0	$\frac{1}{2}$ cup, diced	28
Beverages, alcoholic				
(*see* page 474)				
Beverages, cola-type	185	6.5	about $\frac{3}{4}$ cup	75
Beverages, ginger ale	240	8.4	1 cup	75
Biscuits, baking powder	28	1.0	1 biscuit, 2 in. dia. (enriched flour)	105
Blackberries, raw	72	2.5	$\frac{1}{2}$ cup	45
Blueberries, raw	70	2.5	$\frac{1}{2}$ cup	45
Bluefish, cooked	85	3.0	1 piece, $3\frac{1}{2} \times 2 \times \frac{1}{2}$ in.	135
Bologna (*see* sausage)				
Bouillon cubes	4	0.1	1 cube, $\frac{5}{8}$ in.	5
Bran flakes	26	0.9	$\frac{3}{4}$ cup, 40% bran, (thiamin and iron added)	80
Bread, Boston brown	48	1.7	1 slice, $3 \times \frac{3}{4}$ in.	100
Bread, cracked wheat	25	0.9	1 slice, 18 slices per lb. loaf	65
Bread, French or Vienna	20	0.7	1 slice, $3\frac{1}{4} \times 2 \times 1$ in. (enriched flour)	60
Bread, Italian	20	0.7	1 slice, $3\frac{1}{4} \times 2 \times 1$ in. (enriched flour)	55
Bread, light rye	25	0.9	1 slice, 18 slices per lb. loaf ($\frac{1}{3}$ rye, $\frac{2}{3}$ wheat)	60
Bread, pumpernickel	34	1.2	1 slice, $3\frac{1}{4} \times 2 \times 1$ in. (dark rye flour)	85
Bread, raisin	25	0.9	1 slice, 18 slices per lb. loaf	65
Bread, white firm crumb (enriched)	23	0.8	1 slice, 20 slices per lb. loaf	65
Bread, white soft crumb (enriched)	25	0.9	1 slice, 18 slices per lb loaf	70
Bread, white soft crumb (enriched), toasted	22	0.8	1 slice, 18 slices per lb loaf	70
Bread, white soft crumb (unenriched)	25	0.9	1 slice, 18 slices per lb loaf	70
Bread, whole wheat firm crumb	25	0.9	1 slice, 18 slices per lb loaf	60
Bread crumbs	25	0.9	$\frac{1}{4}$ cup, dry grated	98

PROTEIN G	FAT G	CARBOHYDRATE G	CALCIUM MG	IRON MG	VITAMIN-A ACTIVITY IU	ASCORBIC ACID MG	THIAMIN MG	RIBOFLAVIN MG
23	33	43	32	4.1	1860	7	0.25	0.27
23	16	0	10	2.9	30	—	0.04	0.18
25	7	0	11	3.2	10	—	0.06	0.19
20	27	0	9	2.5	50	—	0.05	0.16
17	18	6	41	2.6	395	2	0.12	0.29
18	14	tr	6	1.9	—	—	0.04	0.25
1	tr	6	12	0.5	15	5	0.03	0.04
0	0	19	—	—	0	0	0	0
0	0	19	—	—	0	0	0	0
2	5	13	34	0.4	tr	tr	0.06	0.06
1	1	10	23	0.7	145	15	0.03	0.03
1	1	11	11	0.7	70	10	0.02	0.04
22	4	0	25	0.6	40	—	0.09	0.08
1	tr	tr	—	—	—	—	—	—
3	1	21	19	9.3	0	0	0.11	0.05
3	1	22	43	0.9	0	0	0.05	0.03
2	1	13	22	0.3	tr	tr	0.03	0.02
2	1	11	9	0.4	tr	tr	0.06	0.04
2	tr	11	3	0.4	0	0	0.06	0.04
2	tr	13	19	0.4	0	0	0.05	0.02
3	0	19	30	0.8	0	0	0.08	0.05
2	1	13	18	0.3	tr	tr	0.01	0.02
2	1	12	22	0.6	tr	tr	0.06	0.05
2	1	13	21	0.6	tr	tr	0.06	0.05
2	1	13	21	0.6	tr	tr	0.05	0.05
2	1	13	21	0.2	tr	tr	0.02	0.02
3	1	12	25	0.8	tr	tr	0.06	0.03
3	1	18	31	0.9	tr	tr	0.06	0.08

FOOD	WEIGHT		APPROXIMATE MEASURE AND DESCRIPTION	KCAL
	G	OZ		
Broccoli, cooked	78	2.7	$\frac{1}{2}$ cup, stalks cut into $\frac{1}{2}$-in. pieces	20
Brussels sprouts, cooked	78	2.7	$\frac{1}{2}$ cup or 5 medium sprouts	28
Buns (see rolls)				
Butter	14	0.5	1 tbsp or $\frac{1}{8}$ stick	100
Cabbage, cooked	73	2.6	$\frac{1}{2}$ cup, cooked short time in little water	15
Cabbage, raw	45	1.6	$\frac{1}{2}$ cup, finely shredded	10
Cabbage, raw, Chinese	38	1.3	$\frac{1}{2}$ cup, 1-in. pieces	5
Cake, angel food (from mix)	53	1.9	1 piece, $\frac{1}{12}$ of 10-in.-dia. cake	135
Cake, Boston cream pie	69	2.4	1 piece, $\frac{1}{12}$ of 8-in.-dia. pie (unenriched flour)	210
Cake, plain chocolate-iced cupcake (from mix)	36	1.3	1 cupcake, $2\frac{1}{2}$ in. dia.	130
Cake, plain uniced cupcakes (from mix)	25	0.9	1 cupcake, $2\frac{1}{2}$ in. dia.	90
Cake, 2-layer devil's food with chocolate icing (from mix)	69	2.4	1 piece (mix), $\frac{1}{16}$ of 9-in.-dia. cake	235
Cake, fruit, dark	15	0.5	1 slice, $\frac{1}{30}$ of 8-in.-long loaf (enriched flour)	55
Cake, pound	30	1.1	1 slice, $2\frac{3}{4} \times 3 \times \frac{5}{8}$ in. (unenriched flour)	140
Cake, sponge	66	1.4	1 piece, $\frac{1}{12}$ of 10-in.-dia. cake (unenriched)	195
Cake, 2-layer white with chocolate icing	71	2.5	1 piece, $\frac{1}{16}$ of 9-in.-dia. cake	250
Candy, caramels	28	1.0	4 small	115
Candy, plain chocolate	28	1.0	1 bar, $3\frac{3}{4} \times 1\frac{1}{2} \times \frac{1}{4}$ in.	145
Candy, chocolate with almonds	51	1.8	1 bar, $5\frac{1}{3} \times 1\frac{7}{8} \times \frac{1}{3}$ in.	265
Candy, chocolate creams	28	1.0	2 pieces, $1\frac{1}{4}$ in. dia. (base), $\frac{5}{8}$ in. thick	110
Candy, chocolate fudge	28	1.0	1 piece, $1\frac{1}{4} \times 1\frac{1}{4} \times 1$ in.	115
Candy, hard	28	1.0	6 pieces, 1 in. dia., $\frac{1}{4}$ in. thick	110
Candy, peanut brittle	28	1.0	1 piece, $3\frac{1}{4} \times 2\frac{1}{2} \times \frac{1}{4}$ in.	125
Cantaloupes	385	13.5	$\frac{1}{2}$ melon, 5 in. dia.	60
Carrots, raw grated	55	1.9	$\frac{1}{2}$ cup grated	23
Carrots, raw whole or strips	50	1.8	1 carrot, $5\frac{1}{2}$ in. long, or 25 thin strips	20
Carrots, cooked	73	2.6	$\frac{1}{2}$ cup diced	23
Catsup, tomato (see tomato)				
Cauliflower, cooked	60	2.1	$\frac{1}{2}$ cup flowerets	13
Celery, raw diced	50	1.8	$\frac{1}{2}$ cup	8
Celery, raw whole	40	1.4	1 stalk, large outer, 8 in. long	5
Cheese, blue (Roquefort type)	28	1.0	$\frac{3}{4}$-in. sector or 3 tbsp	105

PROTEIN G	FAT G	CARBOHYDRATE G	CALCIUM MG	IRON MG	VITAMIN-A ACTIVITY IU	ASCORBIC ACID MG	THIAMIN MG	RIBOFLAVIN MG
3	1	4	68	0.6	1940	70	0.07	0.16
4	1	5	25	0.9	405	68	0.06	0.11
tr	12	tr	3	0	470	0	—	—
1	tr	3	32	0.2	95	24	0.03	0.03
1	tr	3	22	0.2	60	21	0.03	0.03
1	tr	1	16	0.3	55	10	0.02	0.02
3	tr	32	50	0.2	0	0	tr	0.06
4	6	34	46	0.3	140	tr	0.02	0.08
2	5	21	47	0.3	60	tr	0.01	0.04
1	3	14	40	0.1	40	tr	0.01	0.03
3	9	40	41	0.6	100	tr	0.02	0.06
1	2	9	11	0.4	20	tr	0.02	0.02
2	9	14	6	0.2	80	0	0.01	0.03
5	4	36	20	0.8	300	tr	0.03	0.09
3	8	45	70	0.4	40	tr	0.01	0.06
1	3	22	42	0.4	tr	tr	0.01	0.05
2	9	16	65	0.3	80	tr	0.02	0.10
4	19	25	102	1.4	70	0	0.07	0.25
1	4	20	—	—	—	0	—	—
1	4	21	22	0.3	tr	tr	0.01	0.03
0	tr	28	6	0.5	0	0	0	0
2	4	21	11	0.6	10	0	0.03	0.01
1	tr	14	27	0.8	6540	63	0.08	0.06
1	tr	6	21	0.4	6050	5	0.03	0.03
1	tr	5	18	0.4	5500	4	0.03	0.03
1	tr	5	24	0.5	7610	5	0.04	0.04
2	tr	3	13	0.4	35	33	0.06	0.05
1	tr	2	20	0.2	120	5	0.02	0.02
tr	tr	2	16	0.1	100	4	0.01	0.01
6	9	1	89	0.1	350	0	0.01	0.17

| FOOD | WEIGHT | | APPROXIMATE MEASURE AND DESCRIPTION | KCAL |
	G	OZ		
Cheese, cheddar (American), cubed	28	1.0	1 cube, $1\frac{1}{8}$ in.	115
Cheese, cheddar (American), grated	7	0.3	1 tbsp	30
Cheese, creamed cottage	61	2.1	$\frac{1}{4}$ cup (made from skim milk)	65
Cheese, uncreamed cottage	28	1.0	2 tbsp (made from skim milk)	25
Cheese, cream	16	0.5	1 tbsp	60
Cheese, Swiss (domestic)	28	1.0	1 slice, $7 \times 4 \times \frac{1}{8}$ in.	105
Cheese foods, cheddar	28	1.0	2 round slices, $1\frac{5}{8}$ in. dia., $\frac{1}{4}$ in. thick or 2 tbsp	90
Cheese sauce	60	2.1	$\frac{1}{4}$ cup	110
Cheese soufflé	79	2.8	$\frac{3}{4}$ cup	200
Cheesecake	162	5.7	$\frac{1}{10}$ of 9-in.-dia. cake	400
Cherries, raw sweet	130	4.6	1 cup with stems	80
Cherries, raw West Indian (acerola)	11	0.4	2 medium cherries	3
Chick peas, dry raw (garbanzos)	105	3.7	$\frac{1}{2}$ cup	380
Chicken, broiled	85	3.0	3 slices, flesh only	115
Chicken, canned	85	3.0	$\frac{1}{3}$ cup boned meat	170
Chicken, creamed	99	3.5	$\frac{1}{2}$ cup	222
Chicken breast, fried	94	3.3	$\frac{1}{2}$ breast with bone	155
Chicken drumstick, fried	59	2.1	1 drumstick with bone	90
Chicken pie (see poultry potpie)				
Chili con carne with beans, canned	188	6.5	$\frac{3}{4}$ cup	250
Chili con carne without beans, canned	191	6.7	$\frac{3}{4}$ cup	383
Chili powder	15	0.5	1 tbsp hot red peppers, dried and ground	50
Chili sauce	17	0.6	1 tbsp, mainly tomatoes	20
Chocolate, bitter (baking chocolate)	28	1.0	1 square	145
Chocolate candy (see candy)				
Chocolate-flavored milk drink	250	8.8	1 cup (made with skim milk)	190
Chocolate morsels	15	0.5	30 morsels or $1\frac{1}{2}$ tbsp	80
Chocolate syrup	40	1.4	2 tbsp	80
Chop suey, cooked	122	4.3	$\frac{3}{4}$ cup	325
Clams, canned	85	3.0	$\frac{1}{2}$ cup or 3 medium clams	45
Cocoa, beverage	182	6.3	$\frac{3}{4}$ cup (made with milk)	176
Coconut, dried shredded, sweetened	16	0.6	$\frac{1}{4}$ cup	85
Coconut, fresh shredded	33	1.2	$\frac{1}{4}$ cup	113
Codfish, dried	51	1.8	$\frac{1}{2}$ cup	190
Coffee cake, frosted	79	2.8	1 piece, $3 \times 3 \times 1\frac{1}{4}$ in.	260
Cole slaw	60	2.1	$\frac{1}{2}$ cup	50
Cookies, brownies	26	0.9	1 piece, $1\frac{7}{8} \times 1\frac{7}{8} \times \frac{5}{8}$ in.	145
Cookies, chocolate chip	11	0.4	1 cookie, $2\frac{1}{4}$ in. diameter	60
Cookies, coconut bar chews	11	0.4	1 cookie, $3 \times \frac{7}{8} \times \frac{1}{3}$ in.	55
Cookies, oatmeal with raisins and nuts	11	0.4	1 cookie, $2\frac{1}{8}$ in. diameter	65

PROTEIN G	FAT G	CARBOHYDRATE G	CALCIUM MG	IRON MG	VITAMIN-A ACTIVITY IU	ASCORBIC ACID MG	THIAMIN MG	RIBOFLAVIN MG
6	10	2	206	0.3	368	0	0.02	0.13
2	2	tr	52	0.1	90	0	tr	0.03
8	3	2	58	0.2	105	0	0.02	0.15
5	tr	1	26	0.1	tr	0	0.01	0.08
1	6	tr	10	tr	250	0	tr	0.04
8	8	1	262	0.3	320	0	tr	0.11
6	6	2	160	0.2	280	0	tr	0.16
5	9	4	156	0.1	337	1	0.02	0.14
10	16	7	210	1.0	826	1	0.08	0.23
15	23	35	128	0.8	958	1	0.08	0.33
2	tr	20	26	0.5	130	12	0.06	0.07
—	—	1	1	—	—	100	—	0.01
22	5	64	97	7.5	tr	2	0.58	0.19
20	2	0	8	1.4	80	—	0.05	0.16
18	10	0	18	1.3	200	3	0.03	0.11
20	12	6	84	1.1	445	1	0.04	0.20
25	5	1	9	1.3	70	—	0.04	0.17
12	4	tr	6	0.9	50	—	0.03	0.15
14	11	23	60	3.2	113	—	0.06	0.14
20	29	11	73	2.7	285	—	0.04	0.23
2	2	8	40	2.3	9750	2	0.03	0.17
tr	tr	4	3	0.1	240	3	0.02	0.01
3	15	8	22	1.9	20	0	0.01	0.07
8	6	27	270	0.5	210	3	0.10	0.40
1	4	10	5	0.3	tr	0	tr	tr
tr	tr	22	6	0.6	—	—	—	—
19	20	16	43	2.9	85	17	0.11	0.13
7	1	2	47	3.5	—	—	0.01	0.09
7	8	20	215	0.7	293	2	0.07	0.34
1	6	8	3	0.3	0	0	0.01	0.01
1	12	3	4	0.6	0	1	0.02	0.01
41	2	0	25	1.8	0	0	0.04	0.23
4	11	37	25	1.0	477	0	0.12	0.13
1	4	5	24	0.3	40	25	0.03	0.03
2	9	17	12	0.5	231	—	0.03	0.04
1	3	7	4	0.2	81	—	0.01	0.01
tr	2	9	7	0.3	76	0	0.01	0.01
1	4	6	5	0.3	18	tr	0.04	0.02

FOOD	WEIGHT		APPROXIMATE MEASURE AND DESCRIPTION	KCAL
	G	OZ		
Cookies, sugar, plain	9	0.3	1 cookie, $2\frac{1}{2}$ in. diameter	40
Corn, sweet, cooked	140	4.9	1 ear, 5 in. long	70
Corn, sweet, canned	128	4.5	$\frac{1}{2}$ cup, solids and liquid	85
Corn grits, cooked	163	5.7	$\frac{2}{3}$ cup, enriched and degermed	85
Corn muffins	40	1.4	1 muffin, $2\frac{3}{8}$ in. dia., enriched flour and enriched degermed meal	125
Corned beef (see beef)				
Corned beef hash (see beef)				
Cornflakes	33	1.2	$1\frac{1}{3}$ cup (added nutrients)	133
Cornmeal, dry	138	4.8	1 cup, white or yellow, enriched and degermed	500
Cow peas (see peas)				
Crabmeat, canned	85	3.0	$\frac{1}{2}$ cup flakes	85
Crackers, graham, plain	14	0.6	2 medium or 4 small	55
Crackers, saltines	8	0.3	2 crackers, 2 in. square	35
Cranberry juice, canned	125	4.4	$\frac{1}{2}$ cup or 1 small glass, ascorbic acid added	85
Cranberry sauce, canned	69	2.4	$\frac{1}{4}$ cup, strained and sweetened	85
Cream, coffee (light cream)	15	0.5	1 tbsp	30
Cream, half-and-half	15	0.5	1 tbsp	20
Cream, heavy, whipping	15	0.5	1 tbsp, unwhipped (volume doubled when whipped)	55
Creamer, coffee (imitation cream)	2	—	1 tsp powder	10
Cucumber, raw	50	1.8	6 slices, pared, $\frac{1}{8}$ in. thick	5
Custard, baked	124	4.3	$\frac{1}{2}$ cup	143
Dates, pitted	45	1.6	$\frac{1}{4}$ cup or 8 dates	123
Dessert topping, whipped	11	0.4	2 tbsp (low-calorie, with) nonfat dry milk)	17
Doughnuts, cake-type	32	1.1	1 (enriched flour)	125
Egg, raw, boiled, or poached	50	1.8	1 whole egg	80
Egg white, raw	33	1.2	1 egg white	15
Egg yolk, raw	17	0.6	1 egg yolk	60
Eggs, creamed	113	4.0	$\frac{1}{2}$ cup (1 egg in $\frac{1}{4}$ cup white sauce)	190
Eggs, fried	54	1.9	1 egg, cooked in 1 tsp fat	115
Eggs, scrambled	64	2.2	1 egg, with milk and fat	110
Endive, curly, raw	57	2.0	3 leaves (includes escarole)	10
Farina, cooked	163	5.7	$\frac{2}{3}$ cup (quick, enriched)	70
Fats, cooking, lard	13	0.5	1 tbsp solid fat	115
Fats, cooking, vegetable	13	0.5	1 tbsp solid fat	110
Figs, dried	21	0.7	1 large fig, 1×2 in.	60
Figs, fresh raw	114	4.0	3 small, $1\frac{1}{2}$ in. dia.,	90
Fish (see various kinds of fish)				

PROTEIN G	FAT G	CARBOHYDRATE G	CALCIUM MG	IRON MG	VITAMIN-A ACTIVITY IU	ASCORBIC ACID MG	THIAMIN MG	RIBOFLAVIN MG
1	2	6	2	0.1	64	0	0.02	0.01
3	1	16	2	0.5	310	7	0.09	0.08
3	1	20	5	0.5	345	7	0.04	0.06
2	tr	18	1	0.5	100	0	0.07	0.05
3	4	19	42	0.7	120	tr	0.08	0.09
3	tr	28	5	0.5	0	0	0.15	0.03
11	2	108	8	4.0	610	0	0.61	0.36
15	2	1	38	0.7	—	—	0.07	0.07
1	1	10	6	0.2	0	0	0.01	0.03
1	1	6	2	0.1	0	0	tr	tr
tr	tr	21	7	0.4	tr	20	0.02	0.02
tr	tr	21	4	0.1	13	1	0.01	0.01
1	3	1	15	tr	130	tr	tr	0.02
1	2	1	16	tr	70	tr	tr	0.02
tr	6	1	11	tr	230	tr	tr	0.02
tr	1	1	1	tr	tr	—	—	—
tr	tr	2	8	0.2	tr	6	0.02	0.02
7	7	14	139	0.5	435	1	0.05	0.24
1	tr	33	26	1.3	23	0	0.04	0.04
1	—	3	20	—	1	1	0.01	0.04
1	6	16	13	0.4	30	tr	0.05	0.05
6	6	tr	27	1.1	590	0	0.05	0.15
4	tr	tr	3	tr	0	0	tr	0.09
3	5	tr	24	0.9	580	0	0.04	0.07
9	14	7	103	1.2	928	tr	0.07	0.25
6	10	tr	28	1.1	590	0	0.05	0.15
7	8	1	51	1.1	690	0	0.05	0.18
1	tr	2	46	1.0	1870	6	0.04	0.08
2	tr	14	98	0.5	0	0	0.08	0.05
0	13	0	0	0	0	0	0	0
0	13	0	0	0	—	0	0	0
1	tr	15	26	0.6	20	0	0.02	0.02
1	tr	23	40	0.7	90	2	0.07	0.06

| | WEIGHT | | APPROXIMATE MEASURE | |
FOOD	G	OZ	AND DESCRIPTION	KCAL
Fish, creamed (tuna, salmon, or other, in white sauce)	136	4.8	$\frac{1}{2}$ cup	220
Fish sticks, breaded, cooked	114	4.0	5 sticks, each 3.8 × 1.0 × 0.5 in.	200
Frankfurter, heated	56	2.0	1 frankfurter	170
French toast, fried	79	2.8	1 slice (enriched bread)	180
Fruit balls, raw (dried apricots, dates, nuts)	11	0.4	1 ball, 1 in. dia.	45
Fruit cocktail, canned	128	4.5	$\frac{1}{2}$ cup, with heavy syrup	98
Gelatin, plain, dry	7	0.3	1 tbsp (1 envelope)	25
Gelatin dessert, plain	120	4.2	$\frac{1}{2}$ cup, ready to eat	70
Gingerbread	63	2.2	1 piece (mix), $\frac{1}{9}$ of 8-in.-square cake	175
Grapefruit, white, raw (as purchased)	241	8.4	$\frac{1}{2}$ medium, $3\frac{3}{4}$ in. dia.	45
Grapefruit, white, canned	125	4.4	$\frac{1}{2}$ cup, syrup pack	88
Grapefruit juice, canned	124	4.3	$\frac{1}{2}$ cup, unsweetened	50
Grapefruit juice, dehydrated crystals	124	4.3	$\frac{1}{2}$ cup or 1 small glass, prepared, ready to serve	50
Grapes, raw American-type	153	5.4	1 cup or 1 medium bunch (slip skin, as Concord)	65
Grapes, raw European-type	160	5.6	1 cup or 40 grapes (adherent skin, as Tokay)	95
Grape juice, canned	127	4.4	$\frac{1}{2}$ cup	83
Greens, collards, cooked	95	3.3	$\frac{1}{2}$ cup	28
Greens, dandelion, cooked	90	3.2	$\frac{1}{2}$ cup	30
Greens, kale, cooked	55	1.9	$\frac{1}{2}$ cup, leaves and stems	15
Greens, mustard, cooked	70	2.5	$\frac{1}{2}$ cup	18
Greens, spinach, cooked	90	3.2	$\frac{1}{2}$ cup	20
Greens, turnip, cooked	73	2.6	$\frac{1}{2}$ cup	15
Guavas, raw	82	2.8	1 guava	50
Haddock, fried	85	3.0	1 fillet, 4 × $2\frac{1}{2}$ × $\frac{1}{2}$ in.	140
Ham, boiled	57	2.0	1 slice, $6\frac{1}{4}$ × $3\frac{3}{4}$ × $\frac{1}{8}$ in.	135
Ham, cured, roasted	85	3.0	2 slices, $5\frac{1}{2}$ × $3\frac{3}{4}$ × $\frac{1}{8}$ in.	245
Ham, luncheon, canned	57	2.0	2 tbsp, spiced or unspiced	165
Hamburger (see beef, hamburger)				
Honey, strained	21	0.7	1 tbsp.	65
Hot dog (see frankfurter)				
Ice cream, plain	50	1.8	1 container, 3 fluid oz (factory packed)	95
Ice cream, plain brick	71	2.5	1 slice, $\frac{1}{8}$ of qt brick	145
Ice milk	66	2.3	$\frac{1}{2}$ cup	100

PROTEIN G	FAT G	CARBOHYDRATE G	CALCIUM MG	IRON MG	VITAMIN-A ACTIVITY IU	ASCORBIC ACID MG	THIAMIN MG	RIBOFLAVIN MG
20	13	8	81	0.9	385	tr	0.05	0.18
19	10	8	13	0.5	—	—	0.05	0.08
7	15	1	3	0.8	—	—	0.08	0.11
6	12	14	78	1.0	568	tr	0.09	0.17
1	1	8	10	0.4	285	tr	0.02	0.02
1	tr	25	12	0.5	180	3	0.03	0.02
6	tr	0	—	—	—	—	—	—
2	0	17	—	—	—	—	—	—
2	4	32	57	1.0	tr	tr	0.02	0.06
1	tr	12	19	0.5	10	44	0.05	0.02
I	tr	22	16	0.4	10	38	0.04	0.02
1	tr	12	10	0.5	10	42	0.04	0.02
1	tr	12	11	0.1	10	46	0.05	0.03
1	1	15	15	0.4	100	3	0.05	0.03
1	tr	25	17	0.6	140	6	0.07	0.04
1	tr	21	14	0.4	—	tr	0.05	0.03
3	1	5	145	0.6	5130	44	0.14	0.19
2	1	6	126	1.6	10,530	16	0.12	0.15
2	1	2	74	0.7	4070	34	—	—
2	1	3	97	1.3	4060	34	0.00	0.10
3	I	3	84	2.0	7290	25	0.07	0.13
2	tr	3	126	0.8	4135	34	0.08	0.17
1	tr	12	21	0.5	180	212	0.05	0.03
17	5	5	34	1.0	—	2	0.03	0.06
11	10	0	6	1.6	0	—	0.25	0.09
18	19	0	8	2.2	0	—	0.40	0.16
8	14	1	5	1.2	0	—	0.18	0.12
tr	0	17	1	0.1	0	tr	tr	0.01
2	5	10	73	0.2	220	1	0.02	0.11
3	9	15	87	0.1	370	1	0.03	0.13
3	4	15	102	0.1	140	1	0.04	0.15

FOOD	WEIGHT		APPROXIMATE MEASURE AND DESCRIPTION	KCAL
	G	OZ		
Jams, jellies, preserves	20	0.7	1 tbsp	55
Kale (*see* greens)				
Lamb chop, cooked	137	4.8	1 thick chop with bone	400
Lamb, leg, roasted	85	3.0	2 slices, $3 \times 3\frac{1}{4} \times \frac{1}{8}$ in., lean and fat, no bone	235
Lard (*see* fats, cooking)				
Lemon juice, fresh	15	0.5	1 tbsp	5
Lemonade	248	8.7	1 cup (made from frozen, sweetened concentrate)	110
Lentils, dry, cooked	100	3.5	$\frac{1}{2}$ cup	120
Lettuce, headed, raw	454	16.0	1 head (compact, as iceberg), $4\frac{3}{4}$ in. dia.	60
Lettuce, loose leaf, raw	50	1.8	2 large leaves or 4 small leaves	10
Lime juice, canned	62	2.2	$\frac{1}{4}$ cup	15
Liver, beef, fried	57	2.0	1 slice, $5 \times 2 \times \frac{1}{3}$ in.	130
Liver, calf, fried	74	2.6	1 slice, $5 \times 2 \times \frac{1}{2}$ in.	230
Liver, chicken, fried	85	3.0	3 medium livers	235
Liver, pork, fried	70	2.5	1 slice, $3\frac{3}{4} \times 1\frac{3}{4} \times \frac{1}{2}$ in.	225
Macaroni, cooked	105	3.7	$\frac{3}{4}$ cup (enriched)	115
Macaroni and cheese, baked	150	5.3	$\frac{3}{4}$ cup (enriched macaroni)	325
Mackerel, broiled	85	3.0	1 piece	200
Mangoes, raw	198	7.0	1 medium mango	90
Margarine	14	0.5	1 tbsp or $\frac{1}{8}$ stick (fortified with vitamin A)	100
Marshmallows	9	0.3	1, $1\frac{1}{4}$ in. dia.	25
Meat loaf, beef, baked	77	2.7	1 slice, $3\frac{3}{4} \times 2\frac{1}{4} \times \frac{3}{4}$ in.	240
Milk, dry skim (nonfat)	17	0.6	$\frac{1}{4}$ cup powder, instant	61
Milk, dry whole	26	0.9	$\frac{1}{4}$ cup powder	129
Milk, evaporated, canned	126	4.4	$\frac{1}{2}$ cup, undiluted and unsweetened	173
Milk, fluid, skim or buttermilk	245	8.6	1 cup ($\frac{1}{2}$ pt)	90
Milk, fluid, whole	244	8.5	1 cup ($\frac{1}{2}$ pt), 3.5% fat	160
Milk, malted, plain	353	12.4	1 fountain size glass (about $1\frac{1}{2}$ cup)	368
Milkshake, chocolate	342	12.0	1 fountain size glass	420
Molasses, cane, black-strap	20	0.7	1 tbsp, 3rd extraction	45
Molasses, cane, light	20	0.7	1 tbsp, 1st extraction	50
Muffins, plain	40	1.4	1 muffin, $2\frac{3}{4}$ in. dia. (enriched white flour)	120
Mushrooms, canned	122	4.3	$\frac{1}{2}$ cup, solids and liquid	20
Noodles, egg, cooked	120	4.2	$\frac{3}{4}$ cup (enriched)	150
Nuts, almonds	36	1.3	$\frac{1}{4}$ cup shelled	213
Nuts, cashew, rosted	35	1.2	$\frac{1}{4}$ cup	196
Nuts, peanuts (*see* peanuts, roasted)				
Nuts, pecan halves	27	0.9	$\frac{1}{4}$ cup	185
Nuts, walnut halves	25	0.9	$\frac{1}{4}$ cup, English or Persian	163

PROTEIN G	FAT G	CARBOHYDRATE G	CALCIUM MG	IRON MG	VITAMIN-A ACTIVITY IU	ASCORBIC ACID MG	THIAMIN MG	RIBOFLAVIN MG
tr	tr	14	4	0.2	tr	tr	tr	0.01
25	33	0	10	1.5	—	—	0.14	0.25
22	16	0	9	1.4	—	—	0.13	0.23
tr	tr	1	1	tr	tr	7	tr	tr
tr	tr	28	2	tr	tr	17	tr	0.02
9	tr	22	12	2.5	200	0	0.20	0.09
4	tr	13	91	2.3	1500	29	0.29	0.27
1	tr	2	34	0.7	950	9	0.03	0.04
tr	tr	6	6	0.1	5	13	0.01	0.01
15	6	3	6	5.0	30,280	15	0.15	2.37
15	15	4	5	9.0	19,130	30	0.18	2.65
20	15	5	15	6.4	27,370	17	0.19	2.11
17	15	3	8	15.3	12,070	19	0.34	2.53
4	1	24	6	1.0	0	0	0.15	0.08
13	17	30	272	1.4	645	tr	0.15	0.30
19	13	0	5	1.0	450	—	0.13	0.23
1	—	23	12	0.3	8380	55	0.08	0.07
tr	12	tr	3	0	470	0	—	—
tr	0	8	2	0.2	0	0	0	tr
19	17	3	34	2.9	138	—	0.10	0.21
6	tr	9	220	0.1	5	1	0.06	0.30
7	7	10	234	0.1	290	2	0.08	0.38
9	10	12	318	0.2	405	2	0.05	0.43
9	tr	12	296	0.1	10	2	0.09	0.44
9	9	12	288	0.1	350	2	0.07	0.41
17	15	42	476	1.1	885	3	0.21	0.74
11	18	58	363	0.9	687	4	0.12	0.55
—	—	11	137	3.2	—	—	0.02	0.04
—	—	13	33	0.9	—	—	0.01	0.01
3	4	17	42	0.6	40	tr	0.07	0.09
3	tr	3	8	0.6	tr	2	0.02	0.30
5	2	28	12	1.1	83	0	0.17	0.11
7	19	7	83	1.7	0	tr	0.09	0.33
6	16	10	13	1.3	35	—	0.15	0.09
3	19	4	20	0.7	35	1	0.23	0.04
4	16	4	25	0.8	8	1	0.08	0.03

FOOD	WEIGHT		APPROXIMATE MEASURE AND DESCRIPTION	KCAL
	G	OZ		
Oatmeal or rolled oats, cooked	160	5.6	$\frac{2}{3}$ cup (regular or quick-cooking)	87
Oils, salad or cooking	14	0.5	1 tbsp	125
Okra, cooked	43	1.5	4 pods, 3 × $\frac{5}{8}$ in.	13
Olives, green	16	0.6	4 medium or 3 large	15
Olives, ripe	10	0.4	3 small or 2 large	15
Onions, raw	110	3.9	1 onion, 2$\frac{1}{2}$ in. dia.	40
Onions, cooked	105	3.7	$\frac{1}{2}$ cup or 5 onions, 1$\frac{1}{4}$ in. dia.	30
Onions, young green	50	1.8	6 small, without tops	20
Oranges	180	6.3	1 orange, 2$\frac{5}{8}$ in. dia. (all commercial varieties)	65
Orange juice, fresh	124	4.3	$\frac{1}{2}$ cup or 1 small glass (all varieties)	55
Orange juice, canned unsweetened	125	4.4	$\frac{1}{2}$ cup or 1 small glass	60
Orange juice, frozen concentrate	125	4.4	$\frac{1}{2}$ cup or 1 small glass, diluted, ready to serve	60
Orange juice, dehydrated crystals	124	4.3	$\frac{1}{2}$ cup or 1 small glass, prepared, ready to serve	60
Oysters, raw	120	4.2	$\frac{1}{2}$ cup or 8–10 oysters	80
Oyster stew, milk	230	8.1	1 cup with 3–4 oysters	200
Pancakes, wheat	27	0.9	1 griddle cake, 4 in. dia. (enriched flour)	60
Papayas, raw	91	3.2	$\frac{1}{2}$ cup in $\frac{1}{2}$-in. cubes	35
Parsley, raw	4	0.1	1 tbsp chopped	tr
Parsnips, cooked	77	2.7	$\frac{1}{2}$ cup	50
Peaches, canned halves or slices	129	4.5	$\frac{1}{2}$ cup, solids and liquid, syrup-pack	100
Peaches, canned whole	123	4.3	$\frac{1}{2}$ cup, solids liquid (water pack)	38
Peaches, raw sliced	84	2.9	$\frac{1}{2}$ cup fresh or frozen	33
Peaches, raw whole	114	4.0	1 peach, 2 in. dia.	35
Peanuts, roasted	36	1.3	$\frac{1}{4}$ cup halves, salted	210
Peanut butter	32	1.1	2 tbsp	190
Pears, canned	117	4.1	2 medium halves with 2 tbsp juice (syrup pack)	90
Pears, raw (as purchased)	182	6.3	1 pear, 3 × 2$\frac{1}{2}$ in. dia.	100
Peas, cowpeas, dry, cooked (blackeye peas or frijoles)	124	4.3	$\frac{1}{2}$ cup	95
Peas, green, cooked	80	2.8	$\frac{1}{2}$ cup	58
Peas, pigeon, dry raw (gandules)	99	3.5	6 tbsp	310
Peas, split, dry cooked	125	4.4	$\frac{1}{2}$ cup	145
Peppers, green, stuffed	113	4.0	1 medium pepper, cooked with meat stuffing	200
Peppers, hot red (see chili powder)				
Peppers, pimientos, canned	38	1.3	1 medium pod	10
Peppers, raw sweet green	74	2.6	1 medium pod without stem and seeds, 5 pods per lb	15

PROTEIN G	FAT G	CARBOHYDRATE G	CALCIUM MG	IRON MG	VITAMIN-A ACTIVITY IU	ASCORBIC ACID MG	THIAMIN MG	RIBOFLAVIN MG
3	1	15	15	0.9	0	0	0.13	0.03
0	14	0	0	0	—	0	0	0
1	tr	3	39	0.2	210	9	0.06	0.08
tr	2	tr	8	0.2	40	—	—	—
tr	2	tr	9	0.1	10	—	tr	tr
2	tr	10	30	0.6	40	11	0.04	0.04
2	tr	7	25	0.4	40	7	0.03	0.03
1	tr	5	20	0.3	tr	12	0.02	0.02
1	tr	16	54	0.5	260	66	0.13	0.05
1	1	13	14	0.3	250	62	0.11	0.04
1	tr	14	13	0.5	250	50	0.09	0.03
1	tr	15	13	0.1	275	60	0.11	0.01
1	tr	14	13	0.3	250	55	0.10	0.04
10	2	4	113	6.6	370	—	0.17	0.22
11	12	11	269	3.3	640	—	0.13	0.41
2	2	9	27	0.4	30	tr	0.05	0.06
1	tr	9	18	0.3	1595	51	0.04	0.04
tr	tr	tr	8	0.2	340	7	tr	0.01
1	1	12	35	0.5	25	8	0.06	0.07
1	tr	26	5	0.4	550	4	0.01	0.03
1	tr	10	5	0.4	550	4	0.01	0.03
1	tr	8	8	0.4	1115	6	0.02	0.04
1	tr	10	9	0.5	1320	7	0.02	0.05
9	18	7	27	0.8	—	0	0.12	0.05
8	16	6	18	0.6	—	0	0.04	0.04
tr	tr	23	6	0.2	tr	2	0.01	0.02
1	1	25	13	0.5	30	7	0.04	0.07
7	1	17	21	1.6	10	tr	0.21	0.06
5	1	10	19	1.5	430	17	0.22	0.09
22	2	50	140	4.0	169	0	0.45	0.34
10	1	26	14	2.1	50	—	0.19	0.11
12	14	12	31	1.9	637	64	0.09	0.14
tr	tr	2	3	0.6	870	36	0.01	0.02
1	tr	4	7	0.5	310	94	0.06	0.06

FOOD	WEIGHT		APPROXIMATE MEASURE AND DESCRIPTION	KCAL
	G	OZ		
Peppers, raw sweet red	60	2.1	1 medium pod without stem and seeds	20
Perch, ocean, fried	85	3.0	1 piece, $4 \times 3 \times \frac{1}{2}$ in.	195
Persimmons, raw (Japanese)	125	4.4	1 fruit, $2\frac{1}{2}$ in. dia.	75
Pickle relish	15	0.5	1 tbsp	20
Pickles, cucumber, bread and butter	42	1.5	6 slices, $\frac{1}{4} \times 1\frac{1}{2}$ in. diameter	30
Pickles, cucumber, dill	65	2.3	1 large pickel, $3\frac{3}{4} \times 1\frac{1}{4}$ in.	10
Pickles, cucumber, sweet	15	0.5	1 pickle, $2\frac{1}{2} \times \frac{3}{4}$ in. diameter	20
Pie, apple	135	4.7	4-in. sector or $\frac{1}{7}$ of 9-in.-dia. pie (unenriched flour)	350
Pie, cherry	135	4.7	4-in. sector or $\frac{1}{7}$ of 9-in.-dia. pie (unenriched flour)	350
Pie, custard	130	4.6	4-in. sector or $\frac{1}{7}$ of 9-in.-dia. pie (unenriched flour)	285
Pie, lemon meringue	120	4.2	4-in. sector or $\frac{1}{7}$ of 9-in.-dia. pie (unenriched flour)	305
Pie, mince	135	4.7	4-in. sector or $\frac{1}{7}$ of 9-in.-dia. pie (unenriched flour)	365
Pie, pumpkin	130	4.6	4-in. sector or $\frac{1}{7}$ of 9-in.-dia. pie (unenriched flour)	275
Pineapple, canned crushed	130	4.6	$\frac{1}{2}$ cup (syrup pack)	100
Pineapple, canned slices	122	4.3	1 large or 2 small slices, 2 tbsp juice (syrup pack)	90
Pineapple, raw	70	2.5	$\frac{1}{2}$ cup, diced	38
Pineapple juice, canned	125	4.4	$\frac{1}{2}$ cup or 1 small glass	68
Pizza (cheese)	75	2.6	$5\frac{1}{2}$-in. sector or $\frac{1}{8}$ of 14-in.-dia. pie	185
Plantain, raw, green	100	3.5	1 baking banana, 6 in.	135
Plums, canned	128	4.5	$\frac{1}{2}$ cup or 3 plums with 2 tbsp juice (syrup pack)	100
Plums, raw	60	2.1	1 plum, 2 in. diameter	25
Popcorn, popped	9	0.3	1 cup (oil and salt) added	40
Pork chop, cooked	99	3.5	1 thick chop, trimmed, with bone	260
Pork roast, cooked	85	3.0	2 slices, $5 \times 4 \times \frac{1}{8}$ in.	310
Potato chips	20	0.7	10 medium chips, 2 in. diameter	115
Potatoes, baked	99	3.5	1 medium potato, about 3 per pound raw	90
Potatoes, boiled	122	4.3	1 potato, peeled before boiling	80
Potatoes, French fried	57	2.0	10 pieces, $2 \times \frac{1}{2} \times \frac{1}{2}$ in., cooked in deep fat	155
Potatoes, mashed	98	3.4	$\frac{1}{2}$ cup (milk and butter added)	95
Poultry (chicken or turkey) potpie	227	7.9	1 indiv. pie, $4\frac{1}{4}$ in. diameter	535
Pretzels	3	0.1	5, $3\frac{1}{8}$-in. sticks	10
Prunes, dried, cooked	105	3.7	5 medium prunes with 2 tbsp juice, sweetened	160
Prune juice, canned	128	4.5	$\frac{1}{2}$ cup or 1 small glass	100
Pudding, chocolate blanc mange	130	4.6	$\frac{1}{2}$ cup	190

PROTEIN G	FAT G	CARBOHYDRATE G	CALCIUM MG	IRON MG	VITAMIN-A ACTIVITY IU	ASCORBIC ACID MG	THIAMIN MG	RIBOFLAVIN MG
1	tr	4	8	0.4	2670	122	0.05	0.05
16	11	6	1.1	1.1	—	—	0.08	0.09
1	tr	20	6	0.4	2740	11	0.03	0.02
tr	tr	5	3	0.1	—	—	—	—
tr	tr	7	13	0.8	80	4	0.01	0.02
1	tr	1	17	0.7	70	4	tr	0.01
tr	tr	6	2	0.2	10	1	tr	tr
3	15	51	11	0.4	40	1	0.03	0.03
4	15	52	19	0.4	590	tr	0.03	0.03
8	14	30	125	0.8	300	0	0.07	0.21
4	12	45	17	0.6	200	1	0.04	0.10
3	16	56	38	1.4	tr	1	0.09	0.05
5	15	32	66	0.7	3210	tr	0.04	0.13
1	tr	25	15	0.4	60	9	0.10	0.03
tr	tr	24	13	0.4	50	8	0.09	0.03
1	tr	10	12	0.4	50	12	0.06	0.02
1	tr	17	19	0.4	60	11	0.06	0.02
7	6	27	107	0.7	290	4	0.04	0.12
1	—	32	8	0.8	380	28	0.07	0.04
1	tr	27	11	1.1	1485	2	0.03	0.03
tr	tr	7	7	0.3	140	3	0.02	0.02
1	2	5	1	0.2	—	0	—	0.01
16	21	0	8	2.2	0	—	0.63	0.18
21	24	0	9	2.7	0	—	0.78	0.22
1	8	10	8	0.4	tr	3	0.04	0.01
3	tr	21	9	0.7	tr	20	0.10	0.04
2	tr	18	7	0.6	tr	20	0.11	0.04
2	7	20	9	0.7	tr	12	0.07	0.04
2	4	12	24	0.4	165	9	0.08	0.05
23	31	42	68	3.0	3020	5	0.25	0.26
tr	tr	2	1	tr	0	0	tr	tr
1	tr	42	21	1.5	733	1	0.03	0.06
1	tr	25	18	5.3	—	3	0.02	0.02
6	8	26	158	0.9	211	1	0.06	0.27

FOOD	WEIGHT		APPROXIMATE MEASURE AND DESCRIPTION	KCAL
	G	OZ		
Pudding, cornstarch (plain blanc mange)	124	4.3	½ cup	140
Pudding, rice with raisins (old-fashioned)	136	4.8	½ cup	300
Pudding, tapioca	74	2.6	½ cup	140
Radishes, raw	40	1.4	4 small	5
Raisins, seedless	10	0.4	1 tbsp pressed down	30
Raspberries, raw, red	62	2.2	½ cup	35
Rhubarb, cooked	136	4.8	½ cup (sugar added)	190
Rice, parboiled, cooked	131	4.6	¾ cup (enriched)	140
Rice, puffed	15	0.5	1 cup (nutrients added)	60
Rice flakes	30	1.1	1 cup (nutrients added)	115
Rolls, bagel (egg)	55	1.9	1 roll, 3 in. diameter	165
Rolls, barbecue bun	40	1.3	1 bun, 3½ in. diameter (enriched)	120
Rolls, hard	52	1.8	1 round roll	160
Rolls, plain, white	28	1.0	1 commercial pan roll (enriched flour)	85
Rolls, sweet, pan	43	1.5	1 roll	135
Rutabagas, cooked	77	2.7	½ cup	25
Salad, chicken	125	4.4	½ cup, with mayonnaise	280
Salad, egg	128	4.5	½ cup, with mayonnaise	190
Salad, fresh fruit (orange, apple, banana, grapes)	125	4.4	½ cup, with French dressing	130
Salad, jellied, vegetable	122	4.3	½ cup, no dressing	70
Salad, lettuce	130	4.6	¼ solid head, with French dressing	80
Salad, potato	139	4.9	½ cup, with mayonnaise	185
Salad, tomato aspic	119	4.2	½ cup, no dressing	45
Salad, tuna fish	102	3.6	½ cup, with mayonnaise	250
Salad dressing, blue cheese	15	0.5	1 tbsp	75
Salad dressing, boiled	16	0.6	1 tbsp, home-made	25
Salad dressing, commercial	15	0.5	1 tbsp, mayonnaise-type	65
Salad dressing, French	16	0.6	1 tbsp	65
Salad dressing, low-calorie	26	0.9	2 tbsp (cottage cheese, nonfat dry milk, no oil)	17
Salad dressing, mayonnaise	14	0.5	1 tbsp	100
Salad dressing, Thousand Island	16	0.6	1 tbsp	80
Salmon, boiled or baked	119	4.2	1 steak, 4 × 3 × ½ in.	200
Salmon, pink, canned	85	3.0	½ cup	120
Salmon loaf	113	4.0	½ cup or 1 slice, 4 × 1¼ × 1¼ in.	235
Sardines, canned oil	57	2.0	5 small fish, 3 × 1 × ¼ in.	120
Sauce, chocolate	40	1.4	2 tbsp	75
Sauce, custard	31	1.1	2 tbsp (low calorie, with nonfat dry milk)	45
Sauce, hard	17	0.6	1 tbsp	90

PROTEIN G	FAT G	CARBOHYDRATE G	CALCIUM MG	IRON MG	VITAMIN-A ACTIVITY IU	ASCORBIC ACID MG	THIAMIN MG	RIBOFLAVIN MG
5	5	20	145	0.1	195	1	0.04	0.20
8	8	52	243	0.8	313	3	0.10	0.35
5	5	12	104	0.4	327	1	0.04	0.19
tr	tr	1	12	0.4	tr	10	0.01	0.01
tr	tr	8	7	0.4	2	tr	0.01	0.01
1	1	9	14	0.6	80	16	0.02	0.06
1	tr	50	106	0.8	110	9	0.03	0.08
3	tr	31	25	1.1	0	0	0.14	0.02
1	tr	13	3	0.3	0	0	0.07	0.01
2	tr	26	9	0.5	0	0	0.10	0.02
6	2	28	9	1.2	30	0	0.14	0.10
3	2	21	30	0.8	tr	tr	0.11	0.07
5	2	31	24	0.4	tr	tr	0.03	0.05
2	2	15	21	0.5	tr	tr	0.08	0.05
4	4	21	37	0.3	30	tr	0.03	0.06
1	tr	6	43	0.3	270	18	0.04	0.06
25	19	1	20	1.7	200	1	0.04	0.15
6	18	1	35	1.3	630	1	0.06	0.16
—	6	21	25	0.6	154	22	0.06	0.05
3	—	16	14	0.2	25	20	0.03	0.02
1	6	5	28	0.7	618	9	0.05	0.10
2	12	17	21	0.8	40	17	0.11	0.05
5	0	7	12	0.5	1441	22	0.07	0.05
21	18	1	14	1.2	98	1	0.04	0.09
1	8	1	12	tr	30	tr	tr	0.02
1	2	2	14	0.1	80	tr	0.01	0.03
tr	6	2	2	tr	30	—	tr	tr
tr	6	3	2	0.1	—	—	—	—
2	0	2	31	0	18	1	0.01	0.06
tr	11	tr	3	0.1	40	—	tr	0.01
tr	8	3	2	0.1	50	tr	tr	tr
34	7	tr	—	1.4	—	—	0.12	0.33
17	5	0	167	0.7	60	—	0.03	0.16
29	10	5	43	1.8	332	2	0.08	0.20
13	6	0	248	1.7	127	—	0.01	0.11
1	4	9	32	0.2	87	—	0.01	0.05
2	1	7	56	0.2	89	—	0.02	0.09
—	6	11	1	0	231	0	0	0

	WEIGHT			
FOOD	G	OZ	APPROXIMATE MEASURE AND DESCRIPTION	KCAL
Sauce, hollandaise (mock)	26	0.9	2 tbsp	75
Sauce, lemon	28	1.0	2 tbsp	40
Sauerkraut, canned	118	4.1	$\frac{1}{2}$ cup, solids and liquid	25
Sausage, bologna	57	2.0	2 slices, 4.1 × 0.1 in.	173
Sausage, frankfurters (see frankfurters)				
Sausage, liverwurst	57	2.0	3 slices, $2\frac{1}{2}$ in. diameter $\frac{1}{4}$ in. thick	150
Sausage, pork, cooked	26	0.9	2 small patties or links	125
Sausage, Vienna	16	0.6	1 canned sausage, about 2 in. long	40
Shad, baked	85	3.0	1 piece, 4 × 3 × $\frac{1}{2}$ in.	170
Sherbet, orange	97	3.4	$\frac{1}{2}$ cup	130
Shrimp, canned	85	3.0	$\frac{1}{2}$ cup, meat only	100
Syrup, table blends	21	0.7	1 tbsp, light and dark	60
Soup, bean with pork, canned	250	8.8	1 cup, ready to serve	170
Soup, beef broth, bouillon, consommé, canned	240	8.4	1 cup, ready to serve	30
Soup, chicken noodle, canned	250	8.8	1 cup, ready to serve	65
Soup, clam chowder, canned	255	8.9	1 cup, ready to serve	85
Soup, cream of vegetable (e.g., tomato, mushroom), canned	240	8.4	1 cup, ready to serve	135
Soup, minestrone, canned	245	8.6	1 cup, ready to serve	105
Soup, tomato, canned	245	8.6	1 cup, ready to serve	90
Soup, vegetable, canned	250	8.8	1 cup, ready to serve	80
Spaghetti, cooked	105	3.7	$\frac{3}{4}$ cup (enriched)	115
Spaghetti, in tomato sauce, with cheese	188	6.5	$\frac{3}{4}$ cup	200
Spaghetti, in tomato sauce, with meat balls	186	6.5	$\frac{3}{4}$ cup	250
Spinach (see greens)				
Squash, summer, cooked	105	3.7	$\frac{1}{2}$ cup, diced	15
Squash, winter, baked	103	3.6	$\frac{1}{2}$ cup, mashed	65
Stew, beef and vegetable	176	6.2	$\frac{3}{4}$ cup	160
Strawberries, raw	75	2.6	$\frac{1}{2}$ cup, capped	30
Sugar, brown	14	0.5	1 tbsp firmly packed	50
Sugar, granulated	11	0.4	1 tbsp (beet or cane)	40
Sugar, lump	6	0.2	1 domino, $1\frac{1}{8}$ × $\frac{3}{4}$ × $\frac{3}{8}$ in.	25
Sugar, powdered	8	0.3	1 tbsp	30
Sweet potatoes, baked	110	3.9	1 medium potato, about 6 oz raw	155
Sweet potatoes, candied	175	6.1	1 potato, $3\frac{1}{2}$ × $2\frac{1}{4}$ in.	295
Tangerine	116	4.1	1 medium tangerine, $2\frac{3}{8}$ in. diameter	40

PROTEIN G	FAT G	CARBOHYDRATE G	CALCIUM MG	IRON MG	VITAMIN-A ACTIVITY IU	ASCORBIC ACID MG	THIAMIN MG	RIBOFLAVIN MG
2	7	3	36	0.2	353	1	0.02	0.06
0	1	8	—	—	34	2	—	—
1	tr	5	43	0.6	60	17	0.04	0.05
7	16	1	4	1.0	—	—	0.09	0.12
10	12	1	5	3.1	3260	0	0.10	0.63
5	11	tr	2	0.6	0	—	0.21	0.09
2	3	tr	1	0.3	—	—	0.01	0.02
20	10	0	20	0.5	20	—	0.11	0.22
1	1	30	16	tr	60	2	0.01	0.03
21	1	1	98	2.6	50	—	0.01	0.03
0	0	15	9	0.8	0	0	0	0
8	6	22	63	2.3	650	3	0.13	0.08
5	0	3	tr	0.5	tr	—	tr	0.02
4	2	8	10	0.5	50	tr	0.02	0.02
2	3	13	36	1.0	920	—	0.03	0.03
2	10	10	41	0.5	70	tr	0.02	0.12
5	3	14	37	1.0	2350	—	0.07	0.05
2	3	16	15	0.7	1000	12	0.05	0.05
3	2	14	20	0.8	3250	—	0.05	0.02
4	1	24	8	1.0	0	0	0.15	0.08
7	7	28	60	1.7	810	10	0.18	0.14
15	9	30	93	2.8	1193	17	0.20	0.23
1	tr	4	26	0.4	410	11	0.05	0.08
2	1	16	29	0.8	4305	14	0.05	0.14
11	8	11	21	2.1	1733	11	0.10	0.13
1	1	7	16	0.8	45	44	0.02	0.05
0	0	13	12	0.5	0	0	tr	tr
0	0	11	0	tr	0	0	0	0
0	0	6	0	tr	0	0	0	0
0	0	8	0	tr	0	0	0	0
2	1	36	44	1.0	8910	24	0.10	0.07
2	6	60	65	1.6	11,030	17	0.10	0.08
1	tr	10	34	0.3	360	27	0.05	0.02

FOOD	WEIGHT		APPROXIMATE MEASURE AND DESCRIPTION	KCAL
	G	OZ		
Tartar sauce (*see* salad dressing, mayonnaise)				
Toast, melba	6	0.2	1 slice, $3\frac{3}{4} \times 1\frac{3}{4}$ in.	20
Tomato catsup	15	0.5	1 tbsp	15
Tomato juice, canned	122	4.3	$\frac{1}{2}$ cup or 1 small glass	23
Tomatoes, canned	121	4.2	$\frac{1}{2}$ cup	25
Tomatoes, raw	200	7.0	1 tomato, about 3 in. diameter, $2\frac{1}{8}$ in. high	40
Topping, whipped	4	0.1	1 tbsp, pressurized	10
Tortillas	20	0.7	1 tortilla, 5 in. diameter	50
Tuna fish, canned in oil	85	3.0	$\frac{1}{2}$ cup, drained solids	170
Tuna salad (*see* salad, tuna fish)				
Turnip greens (*see* greens)				
Turnips, cooked	78	2.7	$\frac{1}{2}$ cup, diced	18
Veal cutlet, breaded (wiener schnitzel)	136	4.8	2 slices, $2\frac{1}{2} \times 2\frac{1}{2} \times \frac{3}{4}$ in.	315
Veal cutlet, broiled	85	3.0	1 cutlet, $3\frac{3}{4} \times 3 \times \frac{1}{2}$ in.	185
Veal roast, cooked	85	3.0	2 slices, $3 \times 2\frac{1}{2} \times \frac{1}{4}$ in.	230
Vinegar	15	0.5	1 tbsp	2
Waffles	75	2.6	1 waffle, 7 in. diameter (enriched flour)	210
Watermelon, raw	925	32.4	1 wedge, 4×8 in., with rind	115
Welsh rarebit	125	4.4	$\frac{1}{2}$ cup	330
Wheat flour, white enriched	115	4.0	1 cup, sifted	420
Wheat flour, white unenriched	110	3.9	1 cup, sifted	400
Wheat flour, whole wheat	120	4.2	1 cup, hard wheat	400
Wheat germ	9	0.3	2 tbsp	30
Wheat flakes	30	1.1	1 cup (nutrients added)	105
Wheat, shredded	25	0.9	1 biscuit, $4 \times 2\frac{1}{4}$ in.	90
White sauce (medium)	65	2.3	$\frac{1}{4}$ cup	110
Yeast, brewers, dry	8	0.3	1 tbsp	25
Yeast, compressed	28	1.0	one 1-oz cake	25
Yeast, dry active	28	1.0	four $\frac{1}{4}$-oz packages	80
Yogurt, plain	245	8.6	1 cup (made from partially skimmed milk)	125

PROTEIN G	FAT G	CARBOHYDRATE G	CALCIUM MG	IRON MG	VITAMIN-A ACTIVITY IU	ASCORBIC ACID MG	THIAMIN MG	RIBOFLAVIN MG
1	tr	4	5	0.1	0	0	0.01	0.01
tr	tr	4	3	0.1	210	2	0.01	0.01
1	tr	5	9	1.1	970	20	0.06	0.04
1	1	5	7	0.6	1085	21	0.06	0.04
2	4	9	24	0.9	1640	42	0.11	0.07
tr	1	tr	tr	—	20	—	—	0
1	1	10	22	0.4	40	—	0.04	0.01
24	7	0	7	1.6	70	—	0.04	0.10
1	tr	4	27	0.3	tr	17	0.03	0.04
26	21	5	37	4.2	295	—	0.22	0.41
23	9	—	9	2.7	—	—	0.06	0.21
23	14	0	10	2.9	—	—	0.11	0.26
0	—	1	1	0.1	—	—	—	—
7	7	28	85	1.3	250	tr	0.13	0.19
2	1	27	30	2.1	2510	30	0.13	0.13
19	26	6	534	0.7	1118	—	0.04	0.40
12	1	88	18	3.3	0	0	0.51	0.30
12	1	84	18	0.9	0	0	0.07	0.05
16	2	85	49	4.0	0	0	0.66	0.14
2	1	4	6	0.8	0	0	0.17	0.06
3	tr	24	12	1.3	0	0	0.19	0.04
2	1	20	11	0.9	0	0	0.06	0.03
3	8	6	76	0.1	305	tr	0.03	0.11
3	tr	3	17	1.4	tr	tr	1.25	0.34
3	tr	3	4	1.4	tr	tr	0.20	0.47
12	tr	12	12	4.4	tr	tr	0.69	1.52
8	4	13	294	0.1	170	2	0.10	0.44

Alcoholic Beverages

BEVERAGE	AMOUNT	NUMBER OF CALORIES
Beer	8-oz glass	100
Eggnog, holiday variety, made with whiskey and rum	½ cup	225
Whiskey, gin, rum, vodka		
100 proof	1 jigger (1½ oz)	125
90 proof	1 jigger (1½ oz)	110
86 proof	1 jigger (1½ oz)	105
80 proof	1 jigger (1½ oz)	100
70 proof	1 jigger (1½ oz)	85
Wines		
table wines (such as chablis, claret, Rine wine and sauterne)	1 wine glass (about 3 oz)	75
dessert wines (such as muscatel, port, sherry, or Tokay)	1 wine glass (about 3 oz)	125

Specialty and Fast Food Items (Dashes indicate information not provided by sources.)

	WT (G)	KCAL	PRO-TEIN (G)	FAT (G)	CAR-BOHY-DRATE (G)	CAL-CIUM (MG)	IRON (MG)	VITAMIN A ACTIVITY (IU)	ASCORBIC ACID (MG)	THIA-MIN (MG)	RIBO-FLAVIN (MG)
BURGER CHEF											
Big Shef	186	542	23	34	35	189	3.4	282	2	0.34	0.35
Cheeseburger	104	304	14	17	24	156	2.0	266	1	0.22	0.23
Double Cheeseburger	145	434	24	26	24	246	3.1	430	1	0.25	0.34
French Fries	68	187	3	9	25	10	0.9	tr	14	0.09	0.05
Hamburger, Regular	91	258	11	13	24	69	1.9	114	1	0.22	0.18
Mariner Platter	373	680	32	24	85	137	4.7	448	24	0.37	0.40
Rancher Platter	316	640	30	38	44	57	5.1	367	24	0.30	0.37
Shake	305	326	11	11	47	411	0.2	10	2	0.11	0.57
Skipper's Treat	179	604	21	37	47	201	2.5	303	1	0.29	0.30
Super Shef	252	600	29	37	39	240	4.2	763	9	0.37	0.43
Source: Burger Chef Systems, Inc., Indianapolis, Ind. 1978 (analyses obtained from USDA Handbook No. 8).											
BURGER KING											
Cheeseburger	—	305	17	13	29	141	2.0	195	0.5	0.01	0.02
Hamburger	—	252	14	9	29	45	2.0	21	0.5	0.01	0.01
Whopper	—	606	29	32	51	37	6.0	641	13.0	0.02	0.03
French Fries	—	214	3	10	28	12	1.0	0	16.0	0.01	0.01
Vanilla Shake	—	332	11	11	50	390	0.2	9	tr	0.01	0.05
Whaler	—	486	18	46	64	70	1.0	141	1.3	0.01	0.01
Hot Dog	—	291	11	17	23	40	2.0	0	0	0.04	0.02
Source: Chart House, Inc., Oak Brook, Ill., 1978.											
DAIRY QUEEN											
Big Brazier Deluxe	213	470	28	24	36	111	5.2	—	<2.5	0.34	0.37
Big Brazier Regular	184	184	27	23	37	113	5.2	—	<2.0	0.37	0.39
Big Brazier W/Cheese	213	553	32	30	38	268	5.2	495	<2.3	0.34	0.53
Brazier W/Cheese	121	318	18	14	30	163	3.5	—	<1.2	0.29	0.29
Brazier Cheese Dog	113	330	15	19	24	168	1.6	—	—	—	0.18
Brazier Chili Dog	128	330	13	20	25	86	2.0	—	11.0	0.15	0.23
Brazier Dog	99	273	11	15	23	75	1.5	—	11.0	0.12	0.15
Brazier French Fries, 2.5 oz.	71	200	2	10	25	tr	0.4	tr	3.6	0.06	tr
Brazier French Fries, 4.0 oz.	113	320	3	16	40	tr	0.4	tr	4.8	0.09	0.03
Brazier Onion Rings	85	300	6	17	33	20	0.4	tr	2.4	0.09	tr

	WT (G)	KCAL	PRO-TEIN (G)	FAT (G)	CAR-BOHY-DRATE (G)	CAL-CIUM (MG)	IRON (MG)	VITAMIN A ACTIVITY (IU)	ASCORBIC ACID (MG)	THIA-MIN (MG)	RIBO-FLAVIN (MG)
DAIRY QUEEN (cont.)											
Brazier Regular	106	260	13	9	28	70	3.5	—	<1.0	0.28	0.26
Fish Sandwich	170	400	20	17	41	60	1.1	tr	tr	0.15	0.26
Fish Sandwich W/Cheese	177	440	24	21	39	150	0.4	100	tr	0.15	0.26
Super Brazier	298	783	53	48	35	282	7.3	—	<3.2	0.39	0.69
Super Brazier Dog	182	518	20	30	41	158	4.3	tr	14.0	0.42	0.44
Super Brazier Dog W/Cheese	203	593	26	36	43	297	4.4	—	14.0	0.43	0.48
Super Brazier Chili Dog	210	555	23	33	42	158	4.0	—	18.0	0.42	0.48
Banana Split	383	540	10	15	91	350	1.8	750	18.0	0.60	0.60
Buster Bar	149	390	10	22	37	200	0.7	300	tr	0.09	0.34
DQ Chocolate Dipped Cone, sm.	78	150	3	7	20	100	tr	100	tr	0.03	0.17
DQ Chocolate Dipped Cone, med.	156	300	7	13	40	200	0.4	300	tr	0.09	0.34
DQ Chocolate Dipped Cone, lg.	234	450	10	20	58	300	0.4	400	tr	0.12	0.51
DQ Chocolate Malt, sm.	241	340	10	11	51	300	1.8	400	2.4	0.06	0.34
DQ Chocolate Malt, med.	418	600	15	20	89	500	3.6	750	3.6	0.12	0.60
DQ Chocolate Malt, lg.	588	840	22	28	125	600	5.4	750	6.0	0.15	0.85
DQ Chocolate Sundae, sm.	106	170	4	4	30	100	0.7	100	tr	0.03	0.17
DQ Chocolate Sundae, med.	184	300	6	7	53	200	1.1	300	tr	0.06	0.26
DQ Chocolate Sundae, lg.	248	400	9	9	71	300	1.8	400	tr	0.09	0.43
DQ Cone, sm.	71	110	3	3	18	100	tr	100	tr	0.03	0.14
DQ Cone, med.	142	230	6	7	35	200	tr	300	tr	0.09	0.26
DQ Cone, lg.	213	340	10	10	52	300	tr	400	tr	0.15	0.43
Dairy Queen Parfait	284	460	10	11	81	300	1.8	400	tr	0.12	0.43
Dilly Bar	85	240	4	15	22	100	0.4	100	tr	0.06	0.17
DQ Float	397	330	6	8	59	200	tr	100	tr	0.12	0.17
DQ Freeze	397	520	11	13	89	300	tr	200	tr	0.15	0.34
DQ Sandwich	60	140	3	4	24	60	0.4	100	tr	0.03	0.14
Fiesta Sundae	269	570	9	22	84	200	tr	200	tr	0.23	0.26
Hot Fudge Brownie Delight	266	570	11	22	83	300	1.1	500	tr	0.45	0.43
Mr. Misty Float	404	440	6	8	85	200	tr	120	tr	0.12	0.17
Mr. Misty Freeze	411	500	10	12	87	300	tr	200	tr	0.15	0.34

Source: International Dairy Queen, Inc., Minneapolis, Minn. 1978. Dairy Queen stores in the State of Texas do not conform to Dairy Queen-approved products. Any nutritional information shown does not necessarily pertain to their products.

KENTUCKY FRIED CHICKEN											
Original Recipe Dinner*	425	830	52	46	56	150‡	4.5‡	750‡	27.0‡	0.38‡	0.56‡
Extra Crispy Dinner*	437	950	52	54	63	150‡	3.6‡	750†	27.0‡	0.38‡	0.56‡
Individual Pieces†											
(Original Recipe)											
Drumstick	54	136	14	8	2	20	0.9	30	0.6	0.04	0.12
Keel	96	283	25	13	6	—	0.9	50	1.2	0.07	0.13
Rib	82	241	19	15	8	55	1.0	58	<1.0	0.06	0.14
Thigh	97	276	20	19	12	39	1.4	74	<1.0	0.08	0.24
Wing	45	151	11	10	4	—	0.6	—	<1.0	0.03	0.07
9 Pieces	652	1892	152	116	59	—	8.8	—	—	0.49	1.27

Source: Nutritional Content of Average Serving, Heublein Food Service and Franchising Group, June 1976.
* Dinner comprises mashed potatoes and gravy, cole slaw, roll, and three pieces of chicken, either 1) wing, rib, and thigh; 2) wing, drumstick, and thigh; or 3) wing, drumstick, and keel.
† Edible portion of chicken.
‡ Calculated from percentage of US RDA.

TACO BELL											
Bean Burrito	166	343	11	12	48	98	2.8	1657	15.2	0.37	0.22
Beef Burrito	184	466	30	21	37	83	4.6	1675	15.2	0.30	0.39
Beefy Tostada	184	291	19	15	21	208	3.4	3450	12.7	0.16	0.27
Bellbeefer	123	221	15	7	23	40	2.6	2961	10.0	0.15	0.20
Bellbeefer W/Cheese	137	278	19	12	23	147	2.7	3146	10.0	0.16	0.27
Burrito Supreme	225	457	21	22	43	121	3.8	3462	16.0	0.33	0.35
Combination Burrito	175	404	21	16	43	91	3.7	1666	15.2	0.34	0.31
Enchirito	207	454	25	21	42	259	3.8	1178	9.5	0.31	0.37
Pintos 'N' Cheese	158	168	11	5	21	150	2.3	3123	9.3	0.26	0.16

	WT (G)	KCAL	PRO-TEIN (G)	FAT (G)	CAR-BOHY-DRATE (G)	CAL-CIUM (MG)	IRON (MG)	VITAMIN A ACTIVITY (IU)	ASCORBIC ACID (MG)	THIA-MIN (MG)	RIBO-FLAVIN (MG)
TACO BELL (*cont.*)											
Taco	83	186	15	8	14	120	2.5	120	0.2	0.09	0.16
Tostada	138	179	9	6	25	191	2.3	3152	9.7	0.18	0.15

Sources: Menu Item Portions, July 1976. Taco Bell Co., San Antonio, Tex.
Adams CF: *Nutritive Value of American Foods in Common Units.* USDA Agricultural Research Service, Agricultural Handbook No. 456, November 1975.
Church CF, Church HN: *Food Values of Portions Commonly Used,* ed 12. Philadelphia, J. P. Lippincott Co., 1975.
Valley Baptist Medical Center, Food Service Department: Descriptions of Mexican-American Foods, NASCO, Fort Atkinson, Wisc.

BEVERAGES											
Coffee, 6 oz.	180	2	tr	tr	tr	4	0.2	0	0	0	tr
Tea, 6 oz.	180	2	tr	tr	—	5	0.2	0	1	0	0.04
Orange Juice, 6 oz.	183	82	1	tr	20	17	0.2	366	82.4	0.17	0.02
Chocolate Milk, 8 oz.	250	213	9	9	28	278	0.5	330	3.0	0.08	0.40
Skim Milk, 8 oz.	245	88	9	tr	13	296	0.1	10	2.0	0.09	0.44
Whole Milk, 8 oz.	244	159	9	9	12	188	tr	342	2.4	0.07	0.41
Coca-Cola, 8 oz.	246	96	0	0	24	—	—	—	—	—	—
Fanta Ginger Ale, 8 oz.	244	84	0	0	21	—	—	—	—	—	—
Fanta Grape, 8 oz.	247	114	0	0	29	—	—	—	—	—	—
Fanta Orange, 8 oz.	248	117	0	0	30	—	—	—	—	—	—
Fanta Root Beer, 8 oz.	246	103	0	0	27	—	—	—	—	—	—
Mr. Pibb, 8 oz.	245	93	0	0	25	—	—	—	—	—	—
Mr. Pibb Without Sugar, 8 oz.	237	1	0	0	tr	—	—	—	—	—	—
Sprite, 8 oz.	245	95	0	0	24	—	—	—	—	—	—
Sprite Without Sugar, 8 oz.	237	3	0	0	0	—	—	—	—	—	—
Tab, 8 oz.	237	tr	0	0	tr	—	—	—	—	—	—
Fresca, 8 oz.	237	2	0	0	0	—	—	—	—	—	—

Sources: Adams CF: *Nutritive Value of American Foods in Common Units.* USDA Agricultural Research Service, Agricultural Handbook No. 456, November 1975.
Coca-Cola Company, Atlanta, Ga., January 1977.
American Hospital Formulary Service. Washington, American Society of Hospital Pharmacists, Section 28:20, March 1978.

LONG JOHN SILVER'S											
Breaded Oysters, 6 pc.	—	460	14	19	58	—	—	—	—	—	—
Breaded Clams, 5 oz.	—	465	13	25	46	—	—	—	—	—	—
Chicken Planks, 4 pc.	—	458	27	23	35	—	—	—	—	—	—
Cole Slaw, 4 oz.	—	138	1	8	16	—	—	—	—	—	—
Corn on Cob, 1 pc.	—	174	5	4	29	—	—	—	—	—	—
Fish W/Batter, 2 pc.	—	318	19	19	19	—	—	—	—	—	—
Fish W/Batter, 3 pc.	—	477	28	28	28	—	—	—	—	—	—
Fryes, 3 oz.	—	275	4	15	32	—	—	—	—	—	—
Hush Puppies, 3 pc.	—	158	1	7	20	—	—	—	—	—	—
Ocean Scallops, 6 pc.	—	257	10	12	27	—	—	—	—	—	—
Peg Leg W/Batter, 5 pc.	—	514	25	33	30	—	—	—	—	—	—
Shrimp W/Batter, 6 pc.	—	269	9	13	31	—	—	—	—	—	—
Treasure Chest 2 pc. Fish, 2 Peg Legs	—	467	25	29	27	—	—	—	—	—	—

Source: Long John Silver's Seafood Shoppes, Jan. 8, 1978 (nutritional analysis information furnished in study conducted by the Department of Nutrition and Food Science, University of Kentucky).

McDONALD'S											
Egg McMuffin	132	352	18	20	26	187	3.2	361	1.6	0.36	0.60
English Muffin, Buttered	62	186	6	6	28	87	1.6	106	<0.7	0.22	0.14
Hot Cakes, W/Butter & Syrup	206	472	8	9	89	54	2.4	255	<2.1	0.31	0.43
Sausage (Pork)	48	184	9	17	tr	13	0.9	36	<0.5	0.22	0.13
Scrambled Eggs	77	162	12	12	2	49	2.2	514	<0.8	0.07	0.60
Big Mac	187	541	26	31	39	175	4.3	327	2.4	0.35	0.37
Cheeseburger	114	306	16	13	31	158	2.9	372	1.6	0.24	0.30
Filet O Fish	131	402	15	23	34	105	1.8	152	4.2	0.28	0.28
French Fries	69	211	3	11	26	10	0.5	<52	11.0	0.15	0.03

	WT (G)	KCAL	PRO-TEIN (G)	FAT (G)	CAR-BOHY-DRATE (G)	CAL-CIUM (MG)	IRON (MG)	VITAMIN A ACTIVITY (IU)	ASCORBIC ACID (MG)	THIA-MIN (MG)	RIBO-FLAVIN (MG)
McDONALD'S *(cont.)*											
Hamburger	99	257	13	9	30	63	3.0	231	1.8	0.23	0.23
Quarter Pounder	164	418	26	21	33	79	5.1	164	2.3	0.31	0.41
Quarter Pounder W/Cheese	193	518	31	29	34	251	4.6	683	2.9	0.35	0.59
Apple Pie	91	300	2	19	31	12	0.6	<69	2.7	0.02	0.03
Cherry Pie	92	298	2	18	33	12	0.4	213	1.3	0.02	0.03
McDonaldland Cookies	63	294	4	11	45	10	1.4	<48	1.4	0.28	0.23
Chocolate Shake	289	364	11	9	60	338	1.0	318	<2.9	0.12	0.89
Strawberry Shake	293	345	10	9	57	339	0.2	322	<2.9	0.12	0.66
Vanilla Shake	289	323	10	8	52	346	0.2	346	<2.9	0.12	0.66

Source: "Nutritional analysis of food served at McDonald's restaurants." WARF Institute, Inc., Madison, Wisc., June 1977.

	WT (G)	KCAL	PRO-TEIN (G)	FAT (G)	CAR-BOHY-DRATE (G)	CAL-CIUM (MG)	IRON (MG)	VITAMIN A ACTIVITY (IU)	ASCORBIC ACID (MG)	THIA-MIN (MG)	RIBO-FLAVIN (MG)
PIZZA HUT*											
Thin 'N' Crispy											
Beef†	—	490	29	19	51	350	6.3	750	<1.2	0.30	0.60
Pork†	—	520	27	23	51	350	6.3	1000	<1.2	0.38	0.68
Cheese	—	450	25	15	54	450	4.5	750	<1.2	0.30	0.51
Pepperoni	—	430	23	17	45	300	4.5	1000	<1.2	0.30	0.51
Supreme	—	510	27	21	51	350	7.2	1250	2.4	0.38	0.68
Thick 'N' Chewy											
Beef†	—	620	38	20	73	400	7.2	750	<1.2	0.68	0.60
Pork†	—	640	36	23	71	400	7.2	750	1.2	0.90	0.77
Cheese	—	560	34	14	71	500	5.4	1000	<1.2	0.68	0.68
Pepperoni	—	560	31	18	68	400	5.4	1250	3.6	0.68	0.68
Supreme	—	640	36	22	74	400	7.2	1000	9.0	0.75	0.85

Source: Research 900 and Pizza Hut, Inc., Wichita, Kan.
*Based on a serving size of one half of a 10-inch pizza (3 slices).
†Topping mixture of ingredients

Appendix C

Metabolic Computations in Open-Circuit Spirometry

STANDARDIZING GAS VOLUMES: ENVIRONMENTAL FACTORS

Gas volumes obtained during physiologic measurements are usually expressed in one of three ways: (1) *ATPS*, (2) *STPD*, or (3) *BTPS*.

ATPS refers to the volume of gas at the specific conditions of measurement, which are therefore at *A*mbient *T*emperature (273°K + ambient temperature°C), ambient *P*ressure, and *S*aturated with water vapor. Gas volumes collected during open-circuit spirometry and pulmonary function tests are initially measured at ATPS.

The volume of a gas varies, however, depending on its temperature, pressure, and content of water vapor, even though the absolute number of gas molecules remains constant. These environmental influences are summarized as follows:

Temperature: The volume of a gas varies *directly* with temperature. Increasing the temperature causes the molecules to move more rapidly; the gas mixture expands, and the volume increases proportionately (*Charles' Law*).

Pressure: The volume of a gas varies *inversely* with pressure. Increasing the pressure on a gas forces the molecules closer together, causing the volume to decrease in proportion to the increase in pressure (*Boyle's Law*).

Water vapor: The volume of a gas varies depending on its water vapor content. The volume of a gas is greater when the gas is saturated with water vapor than it is when the same gas is dry (i.e., contains no moisture).

These three factors—temperature, pressure, and the relative degree of saturation of the gas with water vapor—must be considered, especially when gas volumes are to be compared under different environmental conditions and subsequently used in metabolic and physiologic calculations. The standards that provide the frame of reference for expressing a volume of gas are either STPD or BTPS.

STPD refers to the volume of a gas expressed under *S*tandard conditions of *T*emperature (273°K or 0°C), *P*ressure (760 mm Hg), and *D*ry (no water vapor). Expressing a gas volume STPD, for example, makes it possible to evaluate and compare the volumes of expired air measured while running in the rain at high altitude, along a beach in the cold of winter, or in a hot desert environment below sea level. *In all metabolic calculations, gas volumes are always expressed at STPD.*

1. To reduce a gas volume to standard temperature (ST), the following formula is applied:

$$\text{Gas volume ST} = V_{\text{ATPS}} \times \frac{273°\text{K}}{273°\text{K} + \text{T}°\text{C}} \tag{1}$$

where T°C = temperature of the gas in the measuring device and 273°K = absolute temperature Kelvin, which is equivalent to 0°C.

TABLE C-1. *Vapor pressure (P_{H_2O}) of wet gas at temperatures normally encountered in the laboratory*

$T(°C)$	$P_{H_2O(mm\ Hg)}$	$T(°C)$	$P_{H_2O(mm\ Hg)}$
20	17.5	31	33.7
21	18.7	32	35.7
22	19.8	33	37.7
23	21.1	34	39.9
24	22.4	35	42.2
25	23.8	36	44.6
26	25.2	37	47.1
27	26.7	38	49.7
28	28.4	39	52.4
29	30.0	40	55.3
30	31.8		

2. The following equation is used to express a gas volume at standard pressure (SP):

$$\text{Gas volume SP} = V_{ATPS} \times \frac{P_B}{760 \text{ mm Hg}} \tag{2}$$

where P_B = ambient barometric pressure in mm Hg and 760 = standard barometric pressure at sea level, mm Hg.

3. To reduce a gas to standard dry (SD) conditions, the effects of water vapor pressure at the particular environmental temperature must be subtracted from the volume of gas. Because expired air is 100% saturated with water vapor, it is not necessary to determine its percent saturation from measures of relative humidity. The vapor pressure in moist or completely humidified air at a particular ambient temperature can be obtained in Table C-1 and is expressed in mm Hg. This vapor pressure (P_{H_2O}) is then subtracted from the ambient barometric pressure (P_B) to reduce the gas to standard pressure dry (SPD) as follows:

$$\text{Gas volume SPD} = V_{ATPS} \times \frac{P_B - P_{H_2O}}{760} \tag{3}$$

By combining equations (1) and (3), any volume of moist air can be converted to STPD as follows:

$$\text{Gas volume STPD} = V_{ATPS} \left(\frac{273}{273 + T°C}\right)\left(\frac{P_B - P_{H_2O}}{760}\right) \tag{4}$$

Fortunately, these computations need not be carried out, because the appropriate *STPD correction factors* have already been calculated for moist gas in the range of temperatures and pressures ordinarily encountered in most laboratories. These factors are presented in Table C-2. Multiplying any gas volume ATPS by the appropriate correction factor gives the same gas volume STPD that would be obtained if values for the ambient temperature, barometric pressure, and water vapor pressure were substituted in equation (4).

The term *BTPS* refers to a volume of a gas expressed at *Body Temperature* (usually 273°K + 37°C or 310°K), ambient *Pressure* (whatever the barometer reads), and *Saturated* with water vapor with a partial pressure of 47 mm Hg at 37°C. Conventionally, pulmonary physiologists express lung volumes such as vital capacity, inspiratory and expiratory capacity, residual lung volume, and the dynamic measures of lung function such as maximum breathing capacity at body temperature and moist, or BTPS. The following equation converts a gas volume ATPS to BTPS:

$$\text{Gas volume BTPS} = V_{ATPS} \left(\frac{P_B - P_{H_2O}}{P_B - 47 \text{ mm Hg}}\right) \left(\frac{310}{273 + T°C}\right) \tag{5}$$

TABLE C-2. *Factors to reduce moist gas to a dry gas volume at 0°C and 760 mm Hg.*

BARO-METRIC READING	TEMPERATURE, °C																	
	15°	16°	17°	18°	19°	20°	21°	22°	23°	24°	25°	26°	27°	28°	29°	30°	31°	32°
700	0.855	851	847	842	838	834	829	825	821	816	812	807	802	797	793	788	783	778
702	857	853	849	845	840	836	832	827	823	818	814	809	805	800	795	790	785	780
704	860	856	852	847	843	839	834	830	825	821	816	812	807	802	797	792	787	783
706	862	858	854	850	845	841	837	832	828	823	819	814	810	804	800	795	790	785
708	865	861	856	852	848	843	839	834	830	825	821	816	812	807	802	797	792	787
710	867	863	859	855	850	846	842	837	833	828	824	819	814	809	804	799	795	790
712	870	866	861	857	853	848	844	839	836	830	826	821	817	812	807	802	797	792
714	872	868	864	859	855	851	846	842	837	833	828	824	819	814	809	804	799	794
716	875	871	866	862	858	853	849	844	840	835	831	826	822	816	812	807	802	797
718	877	873	869	864	860	856	851	847	842	838	833	828	824	819	814	809	804	799
720	880	876	871	867	863	858	854	849	845	840	836	831	826	821	816	812	807	802
722	882	878	874	869	865	861	856	852	847	843	838	833	829	824	819	814	809	804
724	885	880	876	872	867	863	858	854	849	845	840	835	831	826	821	816	811	806
726	887	883	879	874	870	866	861	856	852	847	843	838	833	829	824	818	813	808
728	890	886	881	877	872	868	863	859	854	850	845	840	836	831	826	821	816	811
730	892	888	884	879	875	871	866	861	857	852	847	843	838	833	828	823	818	813
732	895	890	886	882	877	873	868	864	859	854	850	845	840	836	831	825	820	815
734	897	893	889	884	880	875	871	866	862	857	852	847	843	838	833	828	823	818
736	900	895	891	887	882	878	873	869	864	859	855	850	845	840	835	830	825	820
738	902	898	894	889	885	880	876	871	866	862	857	852	848	843	838	833	828	822
740	905	900	896	892	887	883	878	874	869	864	860	855	850	845	840	835	830	825
742	907	903	898	894	890	885	881	876	871	867	862	857	852	847	842	837	832	827
744	910	906	901	897	892	888	883	878	874	869	864	859	855	850	845	840	834	829
746	912	908	903	899	895	890	886	881	876	872	867	862	857	852	847	842	837	832
748	915	910	906	901	897	892	888	883	879	874	869	864	860	854	850	845	839	834
750	917	913	908	904	900	895	890	886	881	876	872	867	862	857	852	847	842	837
752	920	915	911	906	902	897	893	888	883	879	874	869	864	859	854	849	844	839
754	922	918	913	909	904	900	895	891	886	881	876	872	867	862	857	852	846	841
756	925	920	916	911	907	902	898	893	888	883	879	874	869	864	859	854	849	844
758	927	923	918	914	909	905	900	896	891	886	881	876	872	866	861	856	851	846
760	930	925	921	916	912	907	902	898	893	888	883	879	874	869	864	859	854	848
762	932	928	923	919	914	910	905	900	896	891	886	881	876	871	866	861	856	851
764	936	930	926	921	916	912	907	903	898	893	888	004	079	874	869	864	858	853
766	937	933	928	924	919	915	910	905	900	896	891	886	881	876	871	866	861	855
768	940	935	931	926	922	917	912	908	903	898	893	888	883	878	873	868	863	858
770	942	938	933	928	924	919	915	910	905	901	896	891	886	881	876	871	865	860

As was the case with the correction to STPD, appropriate BTPS *correction factors* are available for converting a moist gas volume at ambient conditions to a volume BTPS. These BTPS factors for a broad range of ambient temperatures are presented in Table C-3. These factors have been computed assuming a barometric pressure of 760 mm Hg, and small deviations ($\pm$ 10 mm Hg) from this pressure introduce only a minimal error.

CALCULATION OF OXYGEN CONSUMPTION

In determining oxygen consumption by open-circuit spirometry, we are interested in knowing how much oxygen has been removed from the *inspired air*. Because the composition of inspired air remains relatively constant (CO_2 = 0.03%, O_2 = 20.93%, N_2 = 79.04%), it is possible to determine how much oxygen has been removed from the inspired air by measuring the amount and composition of the expired air. When this is done, the expired air contains more carbon dioxide (usually 2.5% to 5.0%), less oxygen (usually 15.0% to 18.5%), and more nitrogen (usually 79.04% to 79.60%). It should be noted, however, that nitrogen is inert in terms of metabolism; any change in its concentration in expired air reflects the fact that the number of oxygen molecules removed from the

TABLE C-3. *BTPS* correction factors*

T(°C)	BTPS	T(°C)	BTPS
20	1.102	29	1.051
21	1.096	30	1.045
22	1.091	31	1.039
23	1.085	32	1.032
24	1.080	33	1.026
25	1.075	34	1.020
26	1.068	35	1.014
27	1.063	36	1.007
28	1.057	37	1.000

*Body temperature, ambient pressure, saturated with water vapor.

inspired air is not replaced by the same number of carbon dioxide molecules produced in metabolism. This results in the volume of expired air (V_E, STPD) being unequal to the inspired volume (V_I, STPD). For example, if the respiratory quotient is less than 1.00 (i.e., less CO_2 produced in relation to O_2 consumed), and 3 liters of air are inspired, *less* than 3 liters of air will be expired. In this case, the nitrogen concentration is higher in the expired air than in the inspired air. This is not to say that nitrogen has been produced, only that nitrogen molecules now represent a larger percentage of V_E compared to V_I. In fact, V_E differs from V_I in direct proportion to the change in nitrogen concentration between the inspired and expired volumes. Thus, V_I can be determined from V_E using the relative change in nitrogen in an equation known as the *Haldane transformation*.

$$V_I, \text{STPD} = V_E, \text{STPD} \times \frac{\%N_{2_E}}{\%N_{2_I}} \tag{6}$$

where $\%N_{2_I} = 79.04$ and $\%N_{2_E}$ = percent nitrogen in expired air computed from gas analysis as $[(100 - (\%O_{2_E} + \%CO_{2_E})]$.

The volume of O_2 in the inspired air (Vo_{2_I}) can then be determined as follows:

$$Vo_{2_I} = V_I \times \%O_{2_I} \tag{7}$$

Substituting equation (6) for V_I,

$$Vo_{2_I} = V_E \times \frac{\%N_{2_E}}{79.04\%} \times \%O_{2_I} \tag{8}$$

where $\%O_{2_I} = 20.93\%$

The amount or volume of oxygen in the expired air (Vo_{2_E}) is computed as

$$Vo_{2_E} = V_E \times \%O_{2_E} \tag{9}$$

where $\%O_{2_E}$ is the fractional concentration of oxygen in expired air determined by gas analysis (chemical or electronic methods).

The amount of O_2 removed from the inspired air each minute ($\dot{V}o_2$) can then be computed as follows:

$$\dot{V}o_2 = (\dot{V}_I \times \%O_{2_I}) - (\dot{V}_E \times \%O_{2_E}) \tag{10}$$

By substitution

$$\dot{V}O_2 = \left\{ \left[\left(\dot{V}_E \times \frac{\%N_{2_E}}{79.04\%} \right) \times 20.93\% \right] - \left(\dot{V}_E \times \%O_{2_E} \right) \right\} \tag{11}$$

where $\dot{V}O_2$ = volume of oxygen consumed per minute, expressed in milliliters or liters, and $\dot{V}_E$ = expired air volume per minute expressed in milliliters or liters.
Equation (11) can be simplified to:

$$\dot{V}O_2 = \dot{V}_E \left[\left(\frac{\%N_{2_E}}{79.04\%} \times 20.93\% \right) - \%O_{2_E} \right] \tag{12}$$

The final form of the equation is:

$$\dot{V}O_2 = \dot{V}_E [(\%N_{2_E} \times .265) - \%O_{2_E}] \tag{13}$$

The value obtained within the brackets in equations (12) and (13) is referred to as the *true* O_2; this represents the "oxygen extraction" or, more precisely, the percentage of oxygen consumed for any volume of air *expired*.

Although equation (13) is the equation most widely used to compute oxygen consumption from measures of expired air, it is also possible to calculate $\dot{V}O_2$ from direct measurements of both $\dot{V}_I$ and $\dot{V}_E$. In this case, the Haldane transformation is not used, and oxygen consumption is calculated directly as

$$\dot{V}O_2 = (\dot{V}_I \times 20.93) - (\dot{V}_E \times \%O_{2_E}) \tag{14}$$

In situations where only $\dot{V}_I$ is measured, the $\dot{V}_E$ can be calculated from the Haldane transformation as

$$\dot{V}_E = \dot{V}_I \frac{\%N_{2_I}}{\%N_{2_E}}$$

By substitution in equation (14), the computational equation is:

$$\dot{V}O_2 = \dot{V}_I \left[\%O_{2_I} - \left(\frac{\%N_{2_I}}{\%N_{2_E}} \times \%O_{2_E} \right) \right] \tag{15}$$

CALCULATION OF CARBON DIOXIDE PRODUCTION

The carbon dioxide production per minute ($\dot{V}CO_2$) is calculated as follows:

$$\dot{V}CO_2 = \dot{V}_E (\%CO_{2_E} - \%CO_{2_I}) \tag{16}$$

where $\%CO_{2_E}$ = percent carbon dioxide in expired air determined by gas analysis, and $\%CO_{2_I}$ = percent carbon dioxide in inspired air, which is essentially constant at 0.03%.
The final form of the equation is:

$$\dot{V}CO_2 = \dot{V}_E (\%CO_{2_E} - 0.03\%) \tag{17}$$

CALCULATION OF RESPIRATORY QUOTIENT

The respiratory quotient (R.Q.) is calculated in one of two ways:

1. R.Q. = $\dot{V}CO_2 / \dot{V}O_2$ \hfill (18)

or

2. R.Q. $= \dfrac{(\%CO_{2_E} - 0.03\%)}{\text{``true'' } O_2}$ (19)

SAMPLE METABOLIC CALCULATIONS

The following data were obtained during the last minute of a steady-rate, 10-minute treadmill run performed at 6 miles per hour at a 5% grade.

$\dot{V}_E$: 62.1 liters, ATPS
Barometric pressure: 750 mm Hg
Temperature: 26°C
%O_2 expired: 16.86 (O_2 analyzer)
%CO_2 expired: 3.60 (CO_2 analyzer)
%N_2 expired: [100 − (16.86 + 3.60)] = 79.54

Determine the following:
1. $\dot{V}_E$, STPD
2. $\dot{V}O_2$, STPD
3. $\dot{V}CO_2$, STPD
4. R.Q.
5. kcal · min^{-1}

1. $\dot{V}_E$, STPD (use equation 4 or STPD correction factor in Table C-2).

$$\dot{V}_E, \text{STPD} = \dot{V}_E, \text{ATPS}\left(\frac{273}{273 + T°C}\right)\left(\frac{P_B - P_{H_2O}}{760}\right)$$

$$= 62.1\left(\frac{273}{299}\right)\left(\frac{750 - 25.2}{760}\right)$$

$$= 62.1\,(.913 \times .954)$$

$$= 54.07 \text{ liters} \cdot \text{min}^{-1}$$

2. $\dot{V}O_2$, STPD (use equation 13)
$$\dot{V}O_2, \text{STPD} = \dot{V}_E, \text{STPD}\,[(\%N_{2_E} \times .265) - \%O_{2_E}]$$

$$= 54.07\,[(.7954 \times .265) - .1686]$$

$$= 54.07\,(.0422)$$

$$= 2.281 \text{ liters} \cdot \text{min}^{-1}$$

3. $\dot{V}CO_2$, STPD (use equation 17)
$$\dot{V}CO_2, \text{STPD} = \dot{V}_E, \text{STPD}\,(CO_{2_E} - 0.03\%)$$

$$= 54.07\,(.0360 - .0003)$$

$$= 54.07\,(.0357)$$

$$= 1.930 \text{ liters} \cdot \text{min}^{-1}$$

4. R.Q. (use equation 18 or 19)
$$\text{R.Q.} = \dot{V}CO_2 / \dot{V}O_2$$

$$= \frac{1.930 \text{ liters } CO_2/\text{min}}{2.281 \text{ liters } O_2/\text{min}}$$

$$= 0.846$$

or

$$R.Q. = \frac{(\%CO_{2_E} - 0.03\%)}{\text{"true } O_2\text{"}}$$

$$= \frac{3.60 - .03}{4.22}$$

$$= 0.846$$

Because the exercise was performed in a steady rate of aerobic metabolism, the obtained R.Q. of 0.846 can be applied in Table 8-1 to obtain the appropriate caloric transformation. In this way, the exercise oxygen consumption can be transposed to kcal of energy expended per minute as follows:

5. Energy expenditure (kcal $\cdot$ min^{-1}) = $\dot{V}O_2$ (liters $\cdot$ min^{-1}) $\times$ caloric
        equivalent per liter O_2 at the given steady-rate R.Q.
    Energy expenditure = 2.281 $\times$ 4.862

$$= 11.09 \text{ kcal} \cdot \text{min}^{-1}$$

Assuming that the R.Q. value reflects the nonprotein R.Q., a reasonable estimate of both the percentage and quantity of fat and carbohydrate metabolized during each minute of the run can be obtained from Table 8-1.

Percentage kcal derived from fat = 50.7%
Percentage kcal derived from carbohydrate = 49.3%
Grams of fat utilized = 0.267 g per liter of oxygen or approximately 0.61 g per minute (.267 $\times$ 2.281 l O_2)
Grams of carbohydrate utilized = 0.580 g per liter of oxygen or approximately 1.36 g per minute (.580 $\times$ 2.281 l O_2)

Appendix D*

Energy Expenditure in Household, Recreational, and Sports Activities (in kcal · min⁻¹)

ACTIVITY	kcal·min⁻¹·kg⁻¹	kg lb	50 110	53 117	56 123	59 130	62 137	65 143	68 150
Archery	0.065		3.3	3.4	3.6	3.8	4.0	4.2	4.4
Badminton	0.097		4.9	5.1	5.4	5.7	6.0	6.3	6.6
Bakery, general (F)	0.035		1.8	1.9	2.0	2.1	2.2	2.3	2.4
Basketball	0.138		6.9	7.3	7.7	8.1	8.6	9.0	9.4
Billiards	0.042		2.1	2.2	2.4	2.5	2.6	2.7	2.9
Bookbinding	0.038		1.9	2.0	2.1	2.2	2.4	2.5	2.6
Boxing									
in ring	0.222		6.9	7.3	7.7	8.1	8.6	9.0	9.4
sparring	0.138		11.1	11.8	12.4	13.1	13.8	14.4	15.1
Canoeing									
leisure	0.044		2.2	2.3	2.5	2.6	2.7	2.9	3.0
racing	0.103		5.2	5.5	5.8	6.1	6.4	6.7	7.0
Card playing	0.025		1.3	1.3	1.4	1.5	1.6	1.6	1.7
Carpentry, general	0.052		2.6	2.8	2.9	3.1	3.2	3.4	3.5
Carpet sweeping (F)	0.045		2.3	2.4	2.5	2.7	2.8	2.9	3.1
Carpet sweeping (M)	0.048		2.4	2.5	2.7	2.8	3.0	3.1	3.3
Circuit-training	0.185		9.3	9.8	10.4	10.9	11.5	12.0	12.6
Cleaning (F)	0.062		3.1	3.3	3.5	3.7	3.8	4.0	4.2
Cleaning (M)	0.058		2.9	3.1	3.2	3.4	3.6	3.8	3.9
Climbing hills									
with no load	0.121		6.1	6.4	6.8	7.1	7.5	7.9	8.2
with 5-kg load	0.129		6.5	6.8	7.2	7.6	8.0	8.4	8.8
with 10-kg load	0.140		7.0	7.4	7.8	8.3	8.7	9.1	9.5
with 20-kg load	0.147		7.4	7.8	8.2	8.7	9.1	9.6	10.0
Coal mining									
drilling coal, rock	0.094		4.7	5.0	5.3	5.5	5.8	6.1	6.4
erecting supports	0.088		4.4	4.7	4.9	5.2	5.5	5.7	6.0
shoveling coal	0.108		5.4	5.7	6.0	6.4	6.7	7.0	7.3
Cooking (F)	0.045		2.3	2.4	2.5	2.7	2.8	2.9	3.1
Cooking (M)	0.048		2.4	2.5	2.7	2.8	3.0	3.1	3.3
Cricket									
batting	0.083		4.2	4.4	4.6	4.9	5.1	5.4	5.6
bowling	0.090		4.5	4.8	5.0	5.3	5.6	5.9	6.1

* Data from E. W. Bannister and S. R. Brown, The relative energy requirements of physical activity in H. B. Falls, ed., *Exercise Physiology,* Academic Press, New York, 1968; E. T. Howley and M. E. Glover, The caloric costs of running and walking one mile for men and women, *Medicine and Science in Sports* 6:235, 1974; R. Passmore and J. V. G. A. Durnin, Human energy expenditure, *Physiological Reviews* 35:801, 1955.

Note: Symbols (M) and (F) denote experiments for males and females, respectively. See page 115 for instructions on how to use this appendix.

| 71 | 74 | 77 | 80 | 83 | 86 | 89 | 92 | 95 | 98 |
157	163	170	176	183	190	196	203	209	216
4.6	4.8	5.0	5.2	5.4	5.6	5.8	6.0	6.2	6.4
6.9	7.2	7.5	7.8	8.1	8.3	8.6	8.9	9.2	9.5
2.5	2.6	2.7	2.8	2.9	3.0	3.1	3.2	3.3	3.4
9.8	10.2	10.6	11.0	11.5	11.9	12.3	12.7	13.1	13.5
3.0	3.1	3.2	3.4	3.5	3.6	3.7	3.9	4.0	4.1
2.7	2.8	2.9	3.0	3.2	3.3	3.4	3.5	3.6	3.7
9.8	10.2	10.6	11.0	11.5	11.9	12.3	12.7	13.1	13.5
15.8	16.4	17.1	17.8	18.4	19.1	19.8	20.4	21.1	21.8
3.1	3.3	3.4	3.5	3.7	3.8	3.9	4.0	4.2	4.3
7.3	7.6	7.9	8.2	8.5	8.9	9.2	9.5	9.8	10.1
1.8	1.9	1.9	2.0	2.1	2.2	2.2	2.3	2.4	2.5
3.7	3.8	4.0	4.2	4.3	4.5	4.6	4.8	4.9	5.1
3.2	3.3	3.5	3.6	3.7	3.9	4.0	4.1	4.3	4.4
3.4	3.6	3.7	3.8	4.0	4.1	4.3	4.4	4.6	4.7
13.1	13.7	14.2	14.8	15.4	15.9	16.5	17.0	17.6	18.1
4.4	4.6	4.8	5.0	5.1	5.3	5.5	5.7	5.9	6.1
4.1	4.3	4.5	4.6	4.8	5.0	5.2	5.3	5.5	5.7
8.6	9.0	9.3	9.7	10.0	10.4	10.8	11.1	11.5	11.9
9.2	9.5	9.9	10.3	10.7	11.1	11.5	11.9	12.3	12.6
9.9	10.4	10.8	11.2	11.6	12.0	12.5	12.9	13.3	13.7
10.4	10.9	11.3	11.8	12.2	12.6	13.1	13.5	14.0	14.4
6.7	7.0	7.2	7.5	7.8	8.1	8.4	8.6	8.9	9.2
6.2	6.5	6.8	7.0	7.3	7.6	7.8	8.1	8.4	8.6
7.7	8.0	8.3	8.6	9.0	9.3	9.6	9.9	10.3	10.6
3.2	3.3	3.5	3.6	3.7	3.9	4.0	4.1	4.3	4.4
3.4	3.6	3.7	3.8	4.0	4.1	4.3	4.4	4.6	4.7
5.9	6.1	6.4	6.6	6.9	7.1	7.4	7.6	7.9	8.1
6.4	6.7	6.9	7.2	7.5	7.7	8.0	8.3	8.6	8.8

ACTIVITY	kcal·min⁻¹·kg⁻¹	kg lb	50 110	53 117	56 123	59 130	62 137	65 143	68 150
Croquet	0.059		3.0	3.1	3.3	3.5	3.7	3.8	4.0
Cycling									
leisure, 5.5 mph	0.064		3.2	3.4	3.6	3.8	4.0	4.2	4.4
leisure, 9.4 mph	0.100		5.0	5.3	5.6	5.9	6.2	6.5	6.8
racing	0.169		8.5	9.0	9.5	10.0	10.5	11.0	11.5
Dancing									
ballroom	0.051		2.6	2.7	2.9	3.0	3.2	3.3	3.5
choreographed			8.4	8.9	9.4	9.9	10.4	10.9	11.4
"twist," "wiggle"	0.168		5.2	5.5	5.8	6.1	6.4	6.7	7.0
Digging trenches	0.145		7.3	7.7	8.1	8.6	9.0	9.4	9.9
Drawing (standing)	0.036		1.8	1.9	2.0	2.1	2.2	2.3	2.4
Eating (sitting)	0.023		1.2	1.2	1.3	1.4	1.4	1.5	1.6
Electrical work	0.058		2.9	3.1	3.2	3.4	3.6	3.8	3.9
Farming									
barn cleaning	0.135		6.8	7.2	7.6	8.0	8.4	8.8	9.2
driving harvester	0.040		2.0	2.1	2.2	2.4	2.5	2.6	2.7
driving tractor	0.037		1.9	2.0	2.1	2.2	2.3	2.4	2.5
feeding cattle	0.085		4.3	4.5	4.8	5.0	5.3	5.5	5.8
feeding animals	0.065		3.3	3.4	3.6	3.8	4.0	4.2	4.4
forking straw bales	0.138		6.9	7.3	7.7	8.1	8.6	9.0	9.4
milking by hand	0.054		2.7	2.9	3.0	3.2	3.3	3.5	3.7
milking by machine	0.023		1.2	1.2	1.3	1.4	1.4	1.5	1.6
shoveling grain	0.085		4.3	4.5	4.8	5.0	5.3	5.5	5.8
Field hockey	0.134		6.7	7.1	7.5	7.9	8.3	8.7	9.1
Fishing	0.062		3.1	3.3	3.5	3.7	3.8	4.0	4.2
Food shopping (F)	0.062		3.1	3.3	3.5	3.7	3.8	4.0	4.2
Food shopping (M)	0.058		2.9	3.1	3.2	3.4	3.6	3.8	3.9
Football	0.132		6.6	7.0	7.4	7.8	8.2	8.6	9.0
Forestry									
ax chopping, fast	0.297		14.9	15.7	16.6	17.5	18.4	19.3	20.2
ax chopping, slow	0.085		4.3	4.5	4.8	5.0	5.3	5.5	5.8
barking trees	0.123		6.2	6.5	6.9	7.3	7.6	8.0	8.4
carrying logs	0.186		9.3	9.9	10.4	11.0	11.5	12.1	12.6
felling trees	0.132		6.6	7.0	7.4	7.8	8.2	8.6	9.0
hoeing	0.091		4.6	4.8	5.1	5.4	5.6	5.9	6.2
planting by hand	0.109		5.5	5.8	6.1	6.4	6.8	7.1	7.4
sawing by hand	0.122		6.1	6.5	6.8	7.2	7.6	7.9	8.3
sawing, power	0.075		3.8	4.0	4.2	4.4	4.7	4.9	5.1
stacking firewood	0.088		4.4	4.7	4.9	5.2	5.5	5.7	6.0
trimming trees	0.129		6.5	6.8	7.2	7.6	8.0	8.4	8.8
weeding	0.072		3.6	3.8	4.0	4.2	4.5	4.7	4.9
Furriery	0.083		4.2	4.4	4.6	4.9	5.1	5.4	5.6
Gardening									
digging	0.126		6.3	6.7	7.1	7.4	7.8	8.2	8.6
hedging	0.077		3.9	4.1	4.3	4.5	4.8	5.0	5.2
mowing	0.112		5.6	5.9	6.3	6.6	6.9	7.3	7.6
raking	0.054		2.7	2.9	3.0	3.2	3.3	3.5	3.7
Golf	0.085		4.3	4.5	4.8	5.0	5.3	5.5	5.8
Gymnastics	0.066		3.3	3.5	3.7	3.9	4.1	4.3	4.5
Horse-grooming	0.128		6.4	6.8	7.2	7.6	7.9	8.3	8.7
Horse-racing									
galloping	0.137		6.9	7.3	7.7	8.1	8.5	8.9	9.3

| 71 | 74 | 77 | 80 | 83 | 86 | 89 | 92 | 95 | 98 |
157	163	170	176	183	190	196	203	209	216
4.2	4.4	4.5	4.7	4.9	5.1	5.3	5.4	5.6	5.8
4.5	4.7	4.9	5.1	5.3	5.5	5.7	5.9	6.1	6.3
7.1	7.4	7.7	8.0	8.3	8.6	8.9	9.2	9.5	9.8
12.0	12.5	13.0	13.5	14.0	14.5	15.0	15.5	16.1	16.6
3.6	3.8	3.9	4.1	4.2	4.4	4.5	4.7	4.8	5.0
11.9	12.4	12.9	13.4	13.9	14.4	15.0	15.5	16.0	16.5
7.3	7.6	7.9	8.2	8.5	8.9	9.2	9.5	9.8	10.1
10.3	10.7	11.2	11.6	12.0	12.5	12.9	13.3	13.8	14.2
2.6	2.7	2.8	2.9	3.0	3.1	3.2	3.3	3.4	3.5
1.6	1.7	1.8	1.8	1.9	2.0	2.0	2.1	2.2	2.3
4.1	4.3	4.5	4.6	4.8	5.0	5.2	5.3	5.5	5.7
9.6	10.0	10.4	10.8	11.2	11.6	12.0	12.4	12.8	13.2
2.8	3.0	3.1	3.2	3.3	3.4	3.6	3.7	3.8	3.9
2.6	2.7	2.8	3.0	3.1	3.2	3.3	3.4	3.5	3.6
6.0	6.3	6.5	6.8	7.1	7.3	7.6	7.8	8.1	8.3
4.6	4.8	5.0	5.2	5.4	5.6	5.8	6.0	6.2	6.4
9.8	10.2	10.6	11.0	11.5	11.9	12.3	12.7	13.1	13.5
3.8	4.0	4.2	4.3	4.5	4.6	4.8	5.0	5.1	5.3
1.6	1.7	1.8	1.8	1.9	2.0	2.0	2.1	2.2	2.3
6.0	6.3	6.5	6.8	7.1	7.3	7.6	7.8	8.1	8.3
9.5	9.9	10.3	10.7	11.1	11.5	11.9	12.3	12.7	13.1
4.4	4.6	4.8	5.0	5.1	5.3	5.5	5.7	5.9	6.1
4.4	4.6	4.8	5.0	5.1	5.3	5.5	5.7	5.9	6.1
4.1	4.3	4.5	4.6	4.8	5.0	5.2	5.3	5.5	5.7
9.4	9.8	10.2	10.6	11.0	11.4	11.7	12.1	12.5	12.9
21.1	22.0	22.9	23.8	24.7	25.5	26.4	27.3	28.2	29.1
6.0	6.3	6.5	6.8	7.1	7.3	7.6	7.8	8.1	8.3
8.7	9.1	9.5	9.8	10.2	10.6	10.9	11.3	11.7	12.1
13.2	13.8	14.3	14.9	15.4	16.0	16.6	17.1	17.7	18.2
9.4	9.8	10.2	10.6	11.0	11.4	11.7	12.1	12.5	12.9
6.5	6.7	7.0	7.3	7.6	7.8	8.1	8.4	8.6	8.9
7.7	8.1	8.4	8.7	9.0	9.4	9.7	10.0	10.4	10.7
8.7	9.0	9.4	9.8	10.1	10.5	10.9	11.2	11.6	12.0
5.3	5.6	5.8	6.0	6.2	6.5	6.7	6.9	7.1	7.4
6.2	6.5	6.8	7.0	7.3	7.6	7.8	8.1	8.4	8.6
9.2	9.5	9.9	10.3	10.7	11.1	11.5	11.9	12.3	12.6
5.1	5.3	5.5	5.8	6.0	6.2	6.4	6.6	6.8	7.1
5.9	6.1	6.4	6.6	6.9	7.1	7.4	7.6	7.9	8.1
8.9	9.3	9.7	10.1	10.5	10.8	11.2	11.6	12.0	12.3
5.5	5.7	5.9	6.2	6.4	6.6	6.9	7.1	7.3	7.5
8.0	8.3	8.6	9.0	9.3	9.6	10.0	10.3	10.6	11.0
3.8	4.0	4.2	4.3	4.5	4.6	4.8	5.0	5.1	5.3
6.0	6.3	6.5	6.8	7.1	7.3	7.6	7.8	8.1	8.3
4.7	4.9	5.1	5.3	5.5	5.7	5.9	6.1	6.3	6.5
9.1	9.5	9.9	10.2	10.6	11.0	11.4	11.8	12.2	12.5
9.7	10.1	10.6	11.0	11.4	11.8	12.2	12.6	13.0	13.4

ACTIVITY	kcal·min⁻¹·kg⁻¹	kg lb	50 110	53 117	56 123	59 130	62 137	65 143	68 150
Horse-racing									
trotting	0.110		5.5	5.8	6.2	6.5	6.8	7.2	7.5
walking	0.041		2.1	2.2	2.3	2.4	2.5	2.7	2.8
Ironing (F)	0.033		1.7	1.7	1.8	1.9	2.0	2.1	2.2
Ironing (M)	0.064		3.2	3.4	3.6	3.8	4.0	4.2	4.4
Judo	0.195		9.8	10.3	10.9	11.5	12.1	12.7	13.3
Knitting, sewing (F)	0.022		1.1	1.2	1.2	1.3	1.4	1.4	1.5
Knitting, sewing (M)	0.023		1.2	1.2	1.3	1.4	1.4	1.5	1.6
Locksmith	0.057		2.9	3.0	3.2	3.4	3.5	3.7	3.9
Lying at ease	0.022		1.1	1.2	1.2	1.3	1.4	1.4	1.5
Machine-tooling									
machining	0.048		2.4	2.5	2.7	2.8	3.0	3.1	3.3
operating lathe	0.052		2.6	2.8	2.9	3.1	3.2	3.4	3.5
operating punch press	0.088		4.4	4.7	4.9	5.2	5.5	5.7	6.0
tapping and drilling	0.065		3.3	3.4	3.6	3.8	4.0	4.2	4.4
welding	0.052		2.6	2.8	2.9	3.1	3.2	3.4	3.5
working sheet metal	0.048		2.4	2.5	2.7	2.8	3.0	3.1	3.3
Marching, rapid	0.142		7.1	7.5	8.0	8.4	8.8	9.2	9.7
Mopping floor (F)	0.062		3.1	3.3	3.5	3.7	3.8	4.0	4.2
Mopping floor (M)	0.058		2.9	3.1	3.2	3.4	3.6	3.8	3.9
Music playing									
accordion (sitting)	0.032		1.6	1.7	1.8	1.9	2.0	2.1	2.2
cello (sitting)	0.041		2.1	2.2	2.3	2.4	2.5	2.7	2.8
conducting	0.039		2.0	2.1	2.2	2.3	2.4	2.5	2.7
drums (sitting)	0.066		3.3	3.5	3.7	3.9	4.1	4.3	4.5
flute (sitting)	0.035		1.8	1.9	2.0	2.1	2.2	2.3	2.4
horn (sitting)	0.029		1.5	1.5	1.6	1.7	1.8	1.9	2.0
organ (sitting)	0.053		2.7	2.8	3.0	3.1	3.3	3.4	3.6
piano (sitting)	0.040		2.0	2.1	2.2	2.4	2.5	2.6	2.7
trumpet (standing)	0.031		1.6	1.6	1.7	1.8	1.9	2.0	2.1
violin (sitting)	0.045		2.3	2.4	2.5	2.7	2.8	2.9	3.1
woodwind (sitting)	0.032		1.6	1.7	1.8	1.9	2.0	2.1	2.2
Painting, inside	0.034		1.7	1.8	1.9	2.0	2.1	2.2	2.3
Painting, outside	0.077		3.9	4.1	4.3	4.5	4.8	5.0	5.2
Planting seedlings	0.070		3.5	3.7	3.9	4.1	4.3	4.6	4.8
Plastering	0.078		3.9	4.1	4.4	4.6	4.8	5.1	5.3
Printing	0.035		1.8	1.9	2.0	2.1	2.2	2.3	2.4
Running, cross-country	0.163		8.2	8.6	9.1	9.6	10.1	10.6	11.1
Running, horizontal									
11 min, 30 s per mile	0.135		6.8	7.2	7.6	8.0	8.4	8.8	9.2
9 min per mile	0.193		9.7	10.2	10.8	11.4	12.0	12.5	13.1
8 min per mile	0.208		10.8	11.3	11.9	12.5	13.1	13.6	14.2
7 min per mile	0.228		12.2	12.7	13.3	13.9	14.5	15.0	15.6
6 min per mile	0.252		13.9	14.4	15.0	15.6	16.2	16.7	17.3
5 min, 30 s per mile	0.289		14.5	15.3	16.2	17.1	17.9	18.8	19.7
Scraping paint	0.063		3.2	3.3	3.5	3.7	3.9	4.1	4.3
Scrubbing floors (F)	0.109		5.5	5.8	6.1	6.4	6.8	7.1	7.4
Scrubbing floors (M)	0.108		5.4	5.7	6.0	6.4	6.7	7.0	7.3
Shoe repair, general	0.045		2.3	2.4	2.5	2.7	2.8	2.9	3.1

| 71 | 74 | 77 | 80 | 83 | 86 | 89 | 92 | 95 | 98 |
157	163	170	176	183	190	196	203	209	216
7.8	8.1	8.5	8.8	9.1	9.5	9.8	10.1	10.5	10.8
2.9	3.0	3.2	3.3	3.4	3.5	3.6	3.8	3.9	4.0
2.3	2.4	2.5	2.6	2.7	2.8	2.9	3.0	3.1	3.2
4.5	4.7	4.9	5.1	5.3	5.5	5.7	5.9	6.1	6.3
13.8	14.4	15.0	15.6	16.2	16.8	17.4	17.9	18.5	19.1
1.6	1.6	1.7	1.8	1.8	1.9	2.0	2.0	2.1	2.2
1.6	1.7	1.8	1.8	1.9	2.0	2.0	2.1	2.2	2.3
4.0	4.2	4.4	4.6	4.7	4.9	5.1	5.2	5.4	5.6
1.6	1.6	1.7	1.8	1.8	1.9	2.0	2.0	2.1	2.2
3.4	3.6	3.7	3.8	4.0	4.1	4.3	4.4	4.6	4.7
3.7	3.8	4.0	4.2	4.3	4.5	4.6	4.8	4.9	5.1
6.2	6.5	6.8	7.0	7.3	7.6	7.8	8.1	8.4	8.6
4.6	4.8	5.0	5.2	5.4	5.6	5.8	6.0	6.2	6.4
3.7	3.8	4.0	4.2	4.3	4.5	4.6	4.8	4.9	5.1
3.4	3.6	3.7	3.8	4.0	4.1	4.3	4.4	4.6	4.7
10.1	10.5	10.9	11.4	11.8	12.2	12.6	13.1	13.5	13.9
4.4	4.6	4.8	5.0	5.1	5.3	5.5	5.7	5.9	6.1
4.1	4.3	4.5	4.6	4.8	5.0	5.2	5.	5.5	5.7
2.3	2.4	2.5	2.6	2.7	2.8	2.8	2.9	3.0	3.1
2.9	3.0	3.2	3.3	3.4	3.5	3.6	3.8	3.9	4.0
2.8	2.9	3.0	3.1	3.2	3.4	3.5	3.6	3.7	3.8
4.7	4.9	5.1	5.3	5.5	5.7	5.9	6.1	6.3	6.6
2.5	2.6	2.7	2.8	2.9	3.0	3.1	3.2	3.3	3.4
2.1	2.1	2.2	2.3	2.4	2.5	2.6	2.7	2.8	2.8
3.8	3.9	4.1	4.2	4.4	4.6	4.7	4.9	5.0	5.2
2.8	3.0	3.1	3.2	3.3	3.4	3.6	3.7	3.8	3.9
2.2	2.3	2.4	2.5	2.6	2.7	2.8	2.9	2.9	3.0
3.2	3.3	3.5	3.6	3.7	3.9	4.0	4.1	4.3	4.4
2.3	2.4	2.5	2.6	2.7	2.8	2.8	2.9	3.0	3.1
2.4	2.5	2.6	2.7	2.8	2.9	3.0	3.1	3.2	3.3
5.5	5.7	5.9	6.2	6.4	6.6	6.9	7.1	7.3	7.5
5.0	5.2	5.4	5.6	5.8	6.0	6.2	6.4	6.7	6.9
5.5	5.8	6.0	6.2	6.5	6.7	6.9	7.2	7.4	7.6
2.5	2.6	2.7	2.8	2.9	3.0	3.1	3.2	3.3	3.4
11.6	12.1	12.6	13.0	13.5	14.0	14.5	15.0	15.5	16.0
9.6	10.0	10.5	10.9	11.3	11.7	12.1	12.5	12.9	13.3
13.7	14.3	14.9	15.4	16.0	16.6	17.2	17.8	18.3	18.9
14.8	15.4	16.0	16.5	17.1	17.7	18.3	18.9	19.4	20.0
16.2	16.8	17.4	17.9	18.5	19.1	19.7	20.3	20.8	21.4
17.9	18.5	19.1	19.6	20.2	20.8	21.4	22.0	22.5	23.1
20.5	21.4	22.3	23.1	24.0	24.9	25.7	26.6	27.5	28.3
4.5	4.7	4.9	5.0	5.2	5.4	5.6	5.8	6.0	6.2
7.7	8.1	8.4	8.7	9.0	9.4	9.7	10.0	10.4	10.7
7.7	8.0	8.3	8.6	9.0	9.3	9.6	9.9	10.3	10.6
3.2	3.3	3.5	3.6	3.7	3.9	4.0	4.1	4.3	4.4

ACTIVITY	kcal·min⁻¹·kg⁻¹	kg lb	50 110	53 117	56 123	59 130	62 137	65 143	68 150
Sitting quietly	0.021		1.1	1.1	1.2	1.2	1.3	1.4	1.4
Skiing, hard snow									
level, moderate speed	0.119		6.0	6.3	6.7	7.0	7.4	7.7	8.1
level, walking	0.143		7.2	7.6	8.0	8.4	8.9	9.3	9.7
uphill, maximum speed	0.274		13.7	14.5	15.3	16.2	17.0	17.8	18.6
Skiing, soft snow									
leisure (F)	0.111		4.9	5.2	5.5	5.8	6.1	6.4	6.7
leisure (M)	0.098		5.6	5.9	6.2	6.5	6.9	7.2	7.5
Skindiving, as frogman									
considerable motion	0.276		13.8	14.6	15.5	16.3	17.1	17.9	18.8
moderate motion	0.206		10.3	10.9	11.5	12.2	12.8	13.4	14.0
Snowshoeing, soft snow	0.166		8.3	8.8	9.3	9.8	10.3	10.8	11.3
Squash	0.212		10.6	11.2	11.9	12.5	13.1	13.8	14.4
Standing quietly (F)	0.025		1.3	1.3	1.4	1.5	1.6	1.6	1.7
Standing quietly (M)	0.027		1.4	1.4	1.5	1.6	1.7	1.8	1.8
Steel mill, working in									
fettling	0.089		4.5	4.7	5.0	5.3	5.5	5.8	6.1
forging	0.100		5.0	5.3	5.6	5.9	6.2	6.5	6.8
hand rolling	0.137		6.9	7.3	7.7	8.1	8.5	8.9	9.3
merchant mill rolling	0.145		7.3	7.7	8.1	8.6	9.0	9.4	9.9
removing slag	0.178		8.9	9.4	10.0	10.5	11.0	11.6	12.1
tending furnace	0.126		6.3	6.7	7.1	7.4	7.8	8.2	8.6
tipping molds	0.092		4.6	4.9	5.2	5.4	5.7	6.0	6.3
Stock clerking	0.054		2.7	2.9	3.0	3.2	3.3	3.5	3.7
Swimming									
backstroke	0.169		8.5	9.0	9.5	10.0	10.5	11.0	11.5
breast stroke	0.162		8.1	8.6	9.1	9.6	10.0	10.5	11.0
crawl, fast	0.156		7.8	8.3	8.7	9.2	9.7	10.1	10.6
crawl, slow	0.128		6.4	6.8	7.2	7.6	7.9	8.3	8.7
side stroke	0.122		6.1	6.5	6.8	7.2	7.6	7.9	8.3
treading, fast	0.170		8.5	9.0	9.5	10.0	10.5	11.1	11.6
treading, normal	0.062		3.1	3.3	3.5	3.7	3.8	4.0	4.2
Table tennis	0.068		3.4	3.6	3.8	4.0	4.2	4.4	4.6
Tailoring									
cutting	0.041		2.1	2.2	2.3	2.4	2.5	2.7	2.8
hand-sewing	0.032		1.6	1.7	1.8	1.9	2.0	2.1	2.2
machine-sewing	0.045		2.3	2.4	2.5	2.7	2.8	2.9	3.1
pressing	0.062		3.1	3.3	3.5	3.7	3.8	4.0	4.2
Tennis	0.109		5.5	5.8	6.1	6.4	6.8	7.1	7.4
Typing									
electric	0.027		1.4	1.4	1.5	1.6	1.7	1.8	1.8
manual	0.031		1.6	1.6	1.7	1.8	1.9	2.0	2.1
Volleyball	0.050		2.5	2.7	2.8	3.0	3.1	3.3	3.4
Walking, normal pace									
asphalt road	0.080		4.0	4.2	4.5	4.7	5.0	5.2	5.4
fields and hillsides	0.082		4.1	4.3	4.6	4.8	5.1	5.3	5.6
grass track	0.081		4.1	4.3	4.5	4.8	5.0	5.3	5.5
plowed field	0.077		3.9	4.1	4.3	4.5	4.8	5.0	5.2
Wallpapering	0.048		2.4	2.5	2.7	2.8	3.0	3.1	3.3
Watch repairing	0.025		1.3	1.3	1.4	1.5	1.6	1.6	1.7
Window cleaning (F)	0.059		3.0	3.1	3.3	3.5	3.7	3.8	4.0
Window cleaning (M)	0.058		2.9	3.1	3.2	3.4	3.6	3.8	3.9
Writing (sitting)	0.029		1.5	1.5	1.6	1.7	1.8	1.9	2.0

| 71 | 74 | 77 | 80 | 83 | 86 | 89 | 92 | 95 | 98 |
157	163	170	176	183	190	196	203	209	216
1.5	1.6	1.6	1.7	1.7	1.8	1.9	1.9	2.0	2.1
8.4	8.8	9.2	9.5	9.9	10.2	10.6	10.9	11.3	11.7
10.2	10.6	11.0	11.4	11.9	12.3	12.7	13.2	13.6	14.0
19.5	20.3	21.1	21.9	22.7	23.6	24.4	25.2	26.0	26.9
7.0	7.3	7.5	7.8	8.1	8.4	8.7	9.0	9.3	9.6
7.9	8.2	8.5	8.9	9.2	9.5	9.9	10.2	10.5	10.9
19.6	20.4	21.3	22.1	22.9	23.7	24.6	25.4	26.2	27.0
14.6	15.2	15.9	16.5	17.1	17.7	18.3	19.0	19.6	20.2
11.8	12.3	12.8	13.3	13.8	14.3	14.8	15.3	15.8	16.3
15.1	15.7	16.3	17.0	17.6	18.2	18.9	19.5	20.1	20.8
1.8	1.9	1.9	2.0	2.1	2.2	2.2	2.3	2.4	2.5
1.9	2.0	2.1	2.2	2.2	2.3	2.4	2.5	2.6	2.6
6.3	6.6	6.9	7.1	7.4	7.7	7.9	8.2	8.5	8.7
7.1	7.4	7.7	8.0	8.3	8.6	8.9	9.2	9.5	9.8
9.7	10.1	10.6	11.0	11.4	11.8	12.2	12.6	13.0	13.4
10.3	10.7	11.2	11.6	12.0	12.5	12.9	13.3	13.8	14.2
12.6	13.2	13.7	14.2	14.8	15.3	15.8	16.4	16.9	17.4
8.9	9.3	9.7	10.1	10.5	10.8	11.2	11.6	12.0	12.3
6.5	6.8	7.1	7.4	7.6	7.9	8.2	8.5	8.7	9.0
3.8	4.0	4.2	4.3	4.5	4.6	4.8	5.0	5.1	5.3
12.0	12.5	13.0	13.5	14.0	14.5	15.0	15.5	16.1	16.6
11.5	12.0	12.5	13.0	13.4	13.9	14.4	14.9	15.4	15.9
11.1	11.5	12.0	12.5	12.9	13.4	13.9	14.4	14.8	15.3
9.1	9.5	9.9	10.2	10.6	11.0	11.4	11.8	12.2	12.5
8.7	9.0	9.4	9.8	10.1	10.5	10.9	11.2	11.6	12.0
12.1	12.6	13.1	13.6	14.1	14.6	15.1	15.6	16.2	16.7
4.4	4.6	4.8	5.0	5.1	5.3	5.5	5.7	5.9	6.1
4.8	5.0	5.2	5.4	5.6	5.8	6.1	6.3	6.5	6.7
2.9	3.0	3.2	3.3	3.4	3.5	3.6	3.8	3.9	4.0
2.3	2.4	2.5	2.6	2.7	2.8	2.8	2.9	3.0	3.1
3.2	3.3	3.5	3.6	3.7	3.9	4.0	4.1	4.3	4.4
4.4	4.6	4.8	5.0	5.1	5.3	5.5	5.7	5.9	6.1
7.7	8.1	8.4	8.7	9.0	9.4	9.7	10.0	10.4	10.7
1.9	2.0	2.1	2.2	2.2	2.3	2.4	2.5	2.6	2.6
2.2	2.3	2.4	2.5	2.6	2.7	2.8	2.9	2.9	3.0
3.6	3.7	3.9	4.0	4.2	4.3	4.5	4.6	4.8	4.9
5.7	5.9	6.2	6.4	6.6	6.9	7.1	7.4	7.6	7.8
5.8	6.1	6.3	6.6	6.8	7.1	7.3	7.5	7.8	8.0
5.8	6.0	6.2	6.5	6.7	7.0	7.2	7.5	7.7	7.9
5.5	5.7	5.9	6.2	6.4	6.6	6.9	7.1	7.3	7.5
3.4	3.6	3.7	3.8	4.0	4.1	4.3	4.4	4.6	4.7
1.8	1.9	1.9	2.0	2.1	2.2	2.2	2.3	2.4	2.5
4.2	4.4	4.5	4.7	4.9	5.1	5.3	5.4	5.6	5.8
4.1	4.3	4.5	4.6	4.8	5.0	5.2	5.3	5.5	5.7
2.1	2.1	2.2	2.3	2.4	2.5	2.6	2.7	2.8	2.8

Appendix E

Correction for Water Density at Different Temperatures

TEMPERATURE, C°	DENSITY	TEMPERATURE, C°	DENSITY
4	1.00000	31	0.99537
10	0.99973	32	0.99505
15	0.99913	33	0.99473
20	0.99823	34	0.99440
25	0.99707	35	0.99406
26	0.99681	36	0.99371
27	0.99654	37	0.99336
28	0.99626	38	0.99299
29	0.99595	39	0.99262
30	0.99567	40	0.99224

Index

Page numbers in *italics* refer to figures; page numbers followed by "t" refer to tables.